THE MIND IN SLEEP:
Psychology and Psychophysiology

THE MIND IN SLEEP:
Psychology and Psychophysiology

EDITED BY

ARTHUR M. ARKIN
JOHN S. ANTROBUS
STEVEN J. ELLMAN

*The City College of the
City University of New York*

 LAWRENCE ERLBAUM ASSOCIATES, PUBLISHERS
1978   Hillsdale, New Jersey

DISTRIBUTED BY THE HALSTED PRESS DIVISION OF

JOHN WILEY & SONS
New York   Toronto   London   Sydney

Lawrence Erlbaum Associates, Inc., Publishers
62 Maria Drive
Hillsdale, New Jersey 07642

Distributed solely by Halsted Press Division
John Wiley & Sons, Inc., New York

Library of Congress Cataloging in Publication Data

Main entry under title:

The mind in sleep.

    Bibliography: p.
    Includes indexes.
    1. Dreams—Physiological aspects. 2. Sleep—
Physiological aspects. I. Arkin, Arthur M.
II. Antrobus, John S., 1932- III. Ellman, Steven J.
[DNLM: 1. Sleep. 2. Sleep, Rem. 3. Mental
processes. 4. Psychophysiology. WL108 M663]
QP426.M56   154.6'2   78-6025
ISBN 0-470-26369-5

Printed in the United States of America

Contents

Preface

Our book deals largely with the following four questions:

1. What goes on in the mind during sleep?
2. How do we come by such knowledge?
3. What relationships between physiological and mental events have been brought to light by electrographic and other controlled study of sleep mentation?
4. To what extent are the research findings of the past 25 years valid?

An indispensable component of the data base of scientific dream psychology is the dream report — that sleep experience or mentation sequence which the dreamer recalls as what he dreamt, and to which Freud (1900) referred as the "manifest dream." In 1953, a revolutionary advance in sleep and dream studies was initiated by the employment of new electrographic technology. (Aserinsky and Kleitman 1953, Dement and Kleitman 1957 a&b). Prior to this time dream report data, with rare exceptions, consisted of whatever residual, often skimpy recall of dreams unreliably remained accessible to the subject on awakening the following morning, or after even longer intervals between dream events and recording them. Think what a marvelous technical advantage it is to have a dependable *objective* method capable of indicating to dream investigators when ongoing dreams were in progress! They would then possess the scientific luxury of the closest possible access to the living phenomena they were studying. Surely, reports of dreams in progress only seconds before laboratory awakenings would provide more faithful, comprehensive accounts of dreaming than reports obtained at some relatively remote time. And such a method has been precisely one of the cardinal contributions of modern psychophysiological electrography.

Has the only yield of this new line of work been greater availability of "fresh" dream reports? Surely not. The research accumulated since 1953 has demonstrated varieties of dreams which are associated in differential fashion with diverse physiological events, times of the night, individual subject differences, and so forth. It has also produced a large body of intriguing information in such areas as the effects of a host of experimental variables on dream content, the psychological and physiological effects of attempts to deprive subjects of that type of sleep in which most vivid dreams occur, common sleep abnormalities such as sleep-talking, nightmares and night-terrors. Not unexpectedly, the findings have posed inescapable challenges to prevailing theories of dream psychology, dream interpretation and philosophical thought concerned with mind-brain relationships.

Accordingly, the main goal of our book is to provide a comprehensive history and critical account of sleep mentation research since the introduction of the new electrographic techniques. Progress in this area has been marked throughout by vigorous scientific controversy, the main current outcome of which differs in major significant ways from such earlier formulations as nocturnal dreaming is coterminal with REM sleep, REM deprivation is the equivalent of dream deprivation and is especially harmful to the point that it is likely to result in psychosis. Such ideas have lingered in the minds of readers of the early literature of the 1960s who have lost touch with developments since.

Although other excellent books and reviews have appeared covering similar ground, they are either out of date, do not provide coverage of equal scope, or else have not taken as a specific point of departure the dream or sleep mentation report itself within the operational context of eliciting and evaluating such material. This fundamental focus, this essential data base component has been the source of much critical research. At first glance, one might expect that obtaining sleep mentation reports by experimental awakenings is a perfectly straightforward uncomplicated matter from which useful, unequivocal scientific data could be easily produced. This is not altogether untrue but actually simplistic; methodological problems have plagued the field. Findings from one laboratory to the next have often shown great, even embarrassing disparities. Much of this has been due to differences in methods of evaluation of sleep mentation reports, and inadequate control of variables. Reliable findings and knowledge have been slow in coming.

Our book is organized chiefly in accordance with topic headings covering areas of sleep mentation research which are of common interest. Separate chapters are devoted to methodology, critical reviews of REM deprivation studies, and relationships between sustained and short-lived physiological conditions and sleep mentation, the main findings of phenomenological studies of sleep mentation throughout the night and in various sleep stages, the effects of a host of experimental variables on sleep mentation, clinical phenomena such as sleep talking, nightmares and night-terrors insofar as they reflect sleep mentation processes, and finally a section on implications of the work presented for clinical practice and cognitive psychology.

The main audiences for which the book has been prepared are scientists and scholars working in the field of sleep mentation including dreams, psychophysiologists, cognitive psychologists, graduate and advanced undergraduates in psychology, psychiatrists and neurologists, psychiatric and neurological residents desiring a comprehensive introduction to this new field, and possibly philosophers interested in the mind-brain problem.

We acknowledge and thank the staff of Lawrence Erlbaum Associates for their generous cooperation and patience in helping this book see the light of day.

ARTHUR M. ARKIN
JOHN S. ANTROBUS
STEVEN J. ELLMAN

Acknowledgments

The editors would like to thank Jane Woolman, Phyllis Gross, Agnes Salinger, Gerry Levin, and Bruna Ciceran for their indefatigable industry, patience and good humor in the course of getting this book together — secretaries non pareil!

In addition, we should like to express our deep appreciation to the staff of the New York Academy of Medicine Library for their bibliographical assistance.

Acknowledgments

To the National Institute of Mental Health —
the major source of the work described herein,
and to the APSS.

1

Introduction

Arthur M. Arkin

City University of New York

Until 20 years ago the most influential body of scientific and scholarly thought about dreaming was derived from clinical observations. Freud's (1900/1953c) monumental Traumdeutung dominated the field and continues to be a major force. In addition, Jung, Adler, Stekel, and others had made highly significant contributions. To be sure, there had previously been a slowly growing scientific literature describing attempts to investigate dreaming by laboratory methods but despite many provocative and even valid studies (Ramsey, 1953), it was not a field which commanded the interest of many research scientists.

In 1953, a new era in sleep and dream research began with the publication of Aserinsky and Kleitman's "Regularly Occurring Periods of Eye Motility and Concomitant Phenomena During Sleep." Their work demonstrated that during human sleep, recurrent episodes of distinctive electrographically recordable events were typically associated with dreaming experience as reported by subjects when awakened on such occasions. Actually Aserinsky and Kleitman were attempting to study the behavior of the eye during sleep, and for this purpose employed continuous electrical recording of eye movements (the electro-oculogram, EOG). They were struck by the occurrence of epochs of behavioral sleep featuring bursts of conjugate rapid eye movements, or REMs, in conjunction with low-voltage mixed brain-wave frequencies (LVM), and that following experimental awakenings on such occasions, subjects would regularly report the contents of a vivid dream.[1] By contrast, awakenings from sleep in the absence of the above electrographic patterns were said to result in little or no recall of sleep mentation. This finding was confirmed and extended in a series of studies conducted by Dement et al. (Dement & Kleitman, 1957a, b; Dement & Wolpert,

[1] Such epochs are referred to as Stage REM sleep, whereas all other sleep is called non-REM or simply NREM.

1958b) and it was only a matter of a few years until scientists from all over the world, like enthusiastic treasure hunters, were absorbed in research on the psychophysiology of sleep and dreaming.

For the first time in history, a reliable, objective, quantifiable index of the occurrence of dreams seemed to be available. So enthusiastic was the dedication of the researchers that in 1960, the Association for the Psychophysiological Study of Sleep (APSS) was founded. The unflagging labors of its membership have produced an enormous scientific literature on varied aspects of sleep and dreaming. Because research in this field is complex, expensive, and most arduous (even exhausting), preliminary findings were based on a relatively small number of selected subjects. As time passed, with the accumulation of new observations on larger and diversified subject populations, early conclusions underwent revision, sometimes to a drastic degree. We feel, therefore, that the time has come to prepare a definitive review of the current state of the art in that part of the field which is of central interest to psychologists: mental processes and their manifestations as they occur in sleep, that is, sleep mentation.

The presentation of any scientific field appropriately starts with its observational base. Accordingly, in the creation of his psychoanalytic work on dreaming, Freud utilized the following set of items:

1. the content of the dreaming experience as recalled and reported by his patient-subjects (including himself) usually on the morning following the dream. Freud referred to such reports as the *manifest* content of the dream; in laboratory research, the equivalent term is the *sleep-mentation report.*

2. the psychological context within which the dream occurred. This included the mosaic of the day's events previous to the dream as well as a multidimensional conception of the total life history and the specific psychological difficulties and personality of the dreamer. It was usually possible to discern some intelligible relationship between these psychological context materials and aspects of the manifest dream.

3. the psychological associations of the dreamer to the various components of the manifest content.

A psychoanalyst listening to an array of such information is often able to formulate interpretations of various aspects of the dream. Such interpretation might include making explicit the components of the dream which had previously been unintelligible or inaccessible to wakeful conscious understanding; or it might include articulating the complex psychological pathways traversed by unconscious elements in the course of acquiring final representation in the dream experience of sleep, what Freud called the *manifest* dream. The psychological totality of such unconscious elements — the "underlying" thoughts, urges, images, memories, fantasies, emotions, and so on — Freud defined as the *latent* content of the dream. The complicated intervening process through which the latent content became transformed into the manifest dream, he referred to as the *dreamwork*. (The details of dreamwork mechanisms such as condensation, displacement, influence of intrapsychic censorship, and so on are outside the scope of this discussion.)

Although other contributors to dream theory (Jung, Adler, Maeder, and others) differed with Freud in many respects, it is to be emphasized that they all used, along with Freud, the "manifest" dream report as their point of departure, as did Joseph, Daniel, Aesculapius and Artemidorus.

In summary, modern ideas about dreaming have arisen from two main sources: clinical and laboratory investigation. In both cases, the fundamental observational base is the sleep-mentation report as it is produced in relation to multidimensional contexts. In the laboratory approach, the context includes the data derived from electrographic and behavioral methods as well as the laboratory situation itself. In the clinical approach, the context derives from the specific clinical theory, the method and personality of the investigator, as well as the particular clinical situation itself.

The sleep mentation report occupies, therefore, a key position in any basic and applied science of dreaming, and a valid general science of dreaming must derive from the most complete investigation possible of the dream report within related standard contexts. In view of this consideration, it is essential to note that the samples of dreams available to us when we awaken in the morning, or which are remembered for a psychotherapeutic session, are always incomplete versions of a larger, more elaborate sleep experience. That is, an imponderable amount of forgetting of dream content occurs as well as subsequent distortion and editing in the ensuing wakefulness. By contrast, dream reports elicited in the laboratory are as "hot off the griddle" as we can get and even though they do not contain a "complete" record of sleep consciousness, they do provide us with the most direct possible access to dream content with minimal loss of information.

Laboratory studies have made clear that much more than dreaming goes on in the mind during sleep; rather, dreaming occupies an imprecisely defined area within a larger continuum of sleep experience. Thus, sleep mentation includes all sleep-associated cognitive processes: dreaming, thinking, unelaborated imagery, emotions, and so on. Inasmuch as laboratory method has unique advantages over other approaches to the problem, the principal focus of this book will be on sleep mentation as observed by laboratory method. All scientific scholarly and clinical approaches to dreaming must ultimately be consistent or capable of articulation with valid laboratory findings on reported sleep mentation.

As we present in detail in subsequent chapters, a fascinating finding obtained in the course of psychophysiological sleep research pertains to sequellae of deprivation of Stage REM sleep. It should be noted, by way of introduction, that under baseline conditions, healthy subjects experience more or less stable proportions of the various sleep stages (including Stage REM) during a night's sleep. For example, Stage REM comprises 20-25% of the total nightly sleep of young adults. This observation, in conjunction with the demonstrated association between recall of vivid dreams and Stage REM led Dement (1960) to wonder what would happen if humans were prevented from experiencing REM sleep. Would this deprive them of all dreaming experience as well? Would the effects be deleterious? Accordingly, a laborious experiment was carried out requiring subjects to sleep a series of consecutive nights in the laboratory, during which their sleep was electrographically monitored.

First, a set of undisturbed nights were employed to establish baseline levels of Stage REM. Then, on following nights, subjects were deprived of REM by awakening them each time they entered this stage. With succeeding nights, a striking phenomenon was observed: the number of awakenings required to deprive the subject of Stage REM increased progressively, for example, on the first experimental night, a particular subject might be effectively Stage REM-deprived by 7 awakenings, but by the fifth night, over 30 such awakenings would be necessary to bring about REM suppression. It seemed as though with increased amounts of deprivation, subjects made correspondingly increased "attempts" to obtain the Stage REM being denied to them. Furthermore, when the subjects were allowed to sleep undisturbed once more during the next few consecutive nights, the proportion of Stage REM was initially far in excess over that of baseline levels.

Could they be trying to make up their lost Stage REM? Neither of the above results were obtained when an equal number of control awakenings from NREM sleep was made. Thus, the findings could not be attributed to mere deprivation of sleep per se but rather stemmed specifically from Stage REM deprivation. Subsequently, additional studies revealed that when subjects were Stage REM deprived, they tended to enter their first REM period of the night sooner than on baseline nights; and, also the frequency of REMs themselves (REM density) increased under conditions of REM deficit. These findings suggested that when subjects are REM deprived, a potential tendency to produce Stage REM is established somewhat in proportion to the degree of deprivation. Furthermore, Dement (1960) noted that as REM deprivation progressed, subjects experienced distressing behavioral changes and mental symptoms in their daily *wakeful* behavior. For example, intense anxiety, hunger, irritability, apathy, difficulties in concentration, undue suspiciousness, and hallucinatory tendencies were observable. It was concluded that humans have a biological "need" for a certain amount of REM sleep each night and that if this is suppressed, a REM "pressure" will arise, producing a rebound or compensatory increase of Stage REM on subsequent undisturbed (or recovery) nights. Similar results have been obtained in a large number of studies on a variety of infrahuman mammals.

This demonstration of a biological "need" for Stage REM in combination with associated psychological and behavioral disturbance suggested to Fisher and Dement (1963) that there might be some validity to earlier speculations (Volkan, 1962) linking clinical psychosis to dreaming. For example, one often cited formulation defined psychosis as dreaming while awake (Jung, 1944). Thus, if REM deprivation results in increased REM "pressure," and if Stage REM is that phase of sleep in which vivid dreams occur, might the behavioral disturbances associated with Stage REM deprivation represent tendencies of dreaming experience to "spill over" into wakeful consciousness? And could Stage REM deprivation, if continued long enough, result in clinical psychosis?

An ancillary question also arose: Besides a biological need for Stage REM might there be a separate but related psychological need for nocturnal dream experience per se?

A further contribution on the significance of REMs was the demonstration of a high positive correlation between REM density (number of REMs per unit time) and the degree to which an awakened subject reports active involvement in or watching dramatic dream events containing much movement as opposed to reports of passively observing more or less static scenes (the latter being positively correlated with the absence of REMs; Berger & Oswald, 1962).[2]

These three early conclusions: the close association between vivid dream recall and Stage REM; the establishment of a biological need (and possibly psychological need as well) for this sleep stage; and the positive correlation between REM density and the subjects active involvement in dramatic dreams have provided stimuli for a vast amount of research, the critical review and discussion of which forms most of the substance of this volume. The relevant material lends itself for organization around the following topics:

METHODOLOGY

A striking and disquieting feature of reported results in sleep-mentation investigations has been the marked variability from one laboratory to the next. Much of these discrepancies are due to interlaboratory differences in the techniques of measurement of sleep mentation and the related difficult methodological problems. Accordingly, Antrobus and co-workers, in Chapter 2, deal extensively with

---

[2]This conclusion has been brought into doubt in recent years. Three studies have indicated that the original finding reflected a time of night effect. Dreams occurring later at night are more likely to possess high visual activity. It was the sparseness of REMs in the first REM period that was responsible for the correlation; and when data from the first REM period are excluded, the relationship initially reported between REM activity and visually active dreams vanishes (Firth & Oswald, 1975; Hauri & Van de Castle, 1973b; Keenan & Krippner, 1970). On the other hand, Ellman et al. (1974), comparing mentation reports from the same approximate time of the night, and keeping elapsed time of REMPs constant (2-4 min after REMP onset), found a weak but statistically significant positive relationship between the immediately prior presence of REM bursts and "dream-like" mentation reports; and with the prior absence of REMs, reports from equivalent durations of elapsed REMPs were less dreamlike (see Ellman's foreword to Chapter 7, and also Chapter 6, this volume.)

the nature of these problems and describe the cautions and criteria necessary for adequate measurement, evaluation and comparison of sleep mentation reports.

An epitomizing example of such interlaboratory disparate results is provided by the variability of findings on NREM recall. Herman and co-workers, in Chapter 3, explore this puzzle in depth. The question of whether NREM mentation actually exists, or should be taken seriously, has occasioned zestful partisanship in the field. And since several studies have proven that biases and expectancies of the investigator may critically influence the nature of the raw data obtained, it is good to have the information provided by well-designed work on the effects of experimenter bias on sleep mentation reports. Thus, Herman and co-workers present their ingenious study in the second part of Chapter 3.

REVIEWS OF SLEEP-MENTATION STUDIES

First in order of the night's sequence, mentation associated with the transition from wakefulness to sleep seems an appropriate point of embarkation. Actually, much dream-like experience occurs during this interval. Vogel has been a leading investigator in this field and his work must be taken into account by all theorists interested in formulating models of sleep mentation. Vogel, in Chapter 4, provides a comprehensive review of the phenomenology of sleep onset, a conceptual scaffolding and a discussion of the implications of the hypnogogic state.

In Chapter 5, we are given a detailed review of the topic of dream recall — an immensely complicated area. Factors affecting the amount and nature of what we remember of our dreams have long concerned clinicians, theoreticians, and philosophers. According to Freud and Bertram Lewin, variables related to intrapsychic "censorship" and repression are of cardinal importance. Do laboratory findings support this claim? If not, what are the most influential factors involved? Goodenough deals with these matters in a profound and gracious manner and relates them to more general concerns.

Chapter 6 is more difficult to introduce. Actually, we are not satisfied with its title; yet, we could think of none better. There is a heterogeneous assortment of topics which deserve review, or at least mention, in a book such as this. Methodological considerations not covered earlier, the content of children's dreams, dreams in relation to the menstrual cycle, dreams of the blind, work in the area of psychophysiological parallelism not extensively covered in other chapters, dreams in relation to psychopathological syndromes, and theories of relationships between wakeful life and sleep mentation are all touched on in varying degree. There is some overlap with material in other chapters, yet the emphasis is different. All, in some way, relate to phenomenology and qualitative aspects of sleep mentation. We could have included more — it was difficult to know when to stop.

PSYCHOPHYSIOLOGICAL MODELS OF SLEEP MENTATION

The earlier scientific work on sleep psychophysiology employed as an organizing principle the dichotomy between REM and NREM sleep. So distinctive and remarkable were the characteristics of REM sleep that it was referred to as a "third organismic state" of mammalian life, different from both wakefulness and ordinary sleep. The high positive association between dream-like experience and REM sleep was an integral feature of this concept. As will be described by Pivik in Chapter 7, Moruzzi proposed a useful scheme in which both REM and NREM sleep stages were viewed as possessing sustained, state-like properties during which sporadic, short lived events occurred. The former were categorized as *tonic states* and the latter, *phasic events*. With the progress of investigation, reports appeared claiming that dream-like mentation tended to be more closely associated with phasic event components of REM sleep rather than the tonic state aspects per se. For example, an influential study claimed that intervals of REM sleep devoid of eye movements were associated with thought-like rather than dream-like mentation, whereas the opposite was true when mentation reports were obtained in the presence of REM bursts. The question then arose as to whether the more useful organizing principle was the tonic state-phasic event dichotomy regardless of sleep stage, rather than the older REM-NREM sleep stage distinction. Was REM-phasic event sleep the "true dreaming sleep" and should REM nonphasic event and NREM sleep be lumped together as the relatively undream-like sleep? Pivik conducts the reader through the relevant scientific territory in a masterful manner.

EFFECTS OF EXPERIMENTAL VARIABLES
ON SLEEP MENTATION

The reader may well imagine that the new availability of detectable physiological events as likely indicators of dreaming provoked a frenzy of experimentation testing the effects of independent variables on sleep mentation. In Chapter 8, Cartwright considers in comprehensive fashion the effects of the laboratory situation and the person of the experimenter on sleep mentation. Taken up are such questions as whether dreaming is different at home as compared to the laboratory, and whether personal attributes of the experimenter are influential factors. In addition, she presents intriguing data from her own work.

Chapter 9 deals with a painstaking investigation, still in progress, of the effects of sustained alteration of sensory experience on dream content. Specifically, if a person were to wear colored spectacles during the entire wakeful day, would this affect the sensory qualities of dreams in some systematic manner? If red goggles were so worn, would dreams be dominated by reddish colors, or would complementary greens suffuse visual dream life as if to compensate for the daily overdose of red? And would effects appear throughout the night's dreams, mostly the earlier or mostly the later ones? If effects are detectable, do they become manifest with the first night of dreaming after a red-goggle day, or is there a time lag? And, is there an analogous lag on termination of goggle wearing? That is, even after the subjects cease wearing goggles, do related color effects linger on for several nights afterward? All of these questions and many more are explored in depth by Roffwarg and his colleagues in their chapter.

In contrast to the previous two focused chapters of Cartwright and Roffwarg and co-workers, Chapter 10 attempts a panoramic review of the effects of external stimuli applied prior to or during sleep on ongoing mentation. Do we dream about scary or sexually exciting movies viewed prior to sleep? Do words uttered below waking threshold find their way into ongoing dreams? If so, do they appear unchanged or in "disguise" (that is, indirectly)? Is it possible to control dream content by posthypnotic suggestion? Does serious wakeful stress influence dream content? These are but a few of the questions taken up in this part of the book.

Finally, Chapter 11 is devoted to presenting what is known or claimed regarding the effects of various drugs on dream content. As we see, the assessment of such effects is difficult and the work done thus far, on the whole, leaves much unanswered.

EFFECTS OF REMP DEPRIVATION

As mentioned above, assessing the effects of REMP deprivation on a host of variables has understandably received much attention in the field. Accordingly Chapters 12, 13, and 14 are occupied by a comprehensive exploration of this realm. First, REMP deprivation research in humans and animals is generally reviewed by Ellman and co-workers. Methodological considerations and outcomes of studies are covered in detail. Next, we, the editors, present our own research on the effects of REMP deprivation on sleep mentation. If subjects are prevented from experiencing REMP sleep, does NREM mentation become more dream-like? Does REM mentation acquire increased dream-like intensity under conditions of REM deficiency? Is it psychologically important to have sufficient quantities of dream experience? This latter question is discussed further by Hoyt and Singer where the research dealing with wakeful effects of REMP deprivation is reviewed. For example, if we are deprived of REM sleep, do we experience intrusions of dream experience into wakefulness? If, as is claimed by some, psychosis is a form of dreaming in wakefulness, does REM deprivation seem capable of producing incipient psychotic states? How does REMP deprivation affect wakeful cognition generally? Hoyt and Singer also give additional discussion of the extent to which experimental results are consistent with theoretical formulations regarding the functions of sleep.

CLINICAL PHENOMENA IN RELATION TO
SLEEP MENTATION

In both common sleeptalking and the less common night terrors, subjects verbalize in close proximity to sleep. What might such verbalizations tell us about the content of sleep mentation? Does sleeptalking reflect ongoing dreaming? Does sleep speech betray personal secrets? Is a night terror an unusually intense bad dream? What physiological changes occur in the course of a night terror? Such questions are representative of those taken up in Chapters 15 by Arkin and 16 by Kahn, Fisher and Edwards.

IMPLICATIONS AND FUTURE DIRECTIONS

Chapter 17 considers the bearing of the new sleep-research findings on the ways in which dreams are utilized clinically. Are such findings inconsistent with attempts to interpret dreams? To what extent are changes in prevalent clinical theories of dream interpretation necessitated by experimental results?

In Chapter 18, Antrobus presents his ideas on relationships between sleep mentation and the general field of cognitive psychology. Is the latter enriched by experimental work on sleep mentation? And how might work in the cognitive psychology of wakefulness lead to better understanding of sleep mentation processes?

In concluding this section, we repeat that our chief concern has been the thorough presentation of the current state of sleep-mentation study as derived mainly from laboratory investigation. The field has not stood still. It has not progressed smoothly, building on a solid, well-established body of knowledge undisturbed by dissonant new findings and difficulties in replication of older ones. Much has happened to stimulate discussion, ferment, controversy, and revision; hence it is time to step back and critically review the field.

We end our introduction with a plea for the readers' indulgence. As we have indicated, the early reports of Aserinsky, Kleitman, and Dement were filled with germinal, provocative, exciting data and conclusions regarding specific relationships of sleep mentation to sleep stages, biopsychological needs for REM sleep, and the like. This body of information comprising the early history of our subject is like the hub of a wheel from which the various chapter topics radiate in spoke-like fashion. As editors, we considered the possibility of reducing redundancy to a minimum by confining such historical material to one preliminary section and thereby eliminating as much repetition as possible from the introductory paragraphs of each chapter. When we attempted it, however, we had the feeling that an important element of unity was lost — the authors had taken their departure from the hub and used a review of it as an overture and frame for the succeeding material, each in their own way, to best achieve their overall goals. We, therefore, decided to retain this background material in each chapter, redundant though much of it may be.

A NOTE ON THE USAGE OF TERMS IN THIS BOOK

In accordance with the recommendations of Rechtschaffen and Kales (1968), we have employed the terms Stage REM or REM sleep. The recurrent intervals occupied by such sleep are called REM periods and are often abbreviated as REMPs. Correspondingly, NREM or NREMP are also used. Finally, in an effort to avoid the hydraulic implications of "REM pressure," we use instead the term REM deficit or deprivation.

ORIENTING REMARKS ON ELECTROGRAPHIC FEATURES OF THE SLEEP CYCLE

For the sake of completeness, we include a concise description of features of the sleep cycle. It has become standard laboratory procedure in sleep research to continually measure at least three electrographic parameters: the EEG, EOG, and chin EMG (Rechtschaffen & Kales, 1968).

The EEG is usually recorded from sites C3 or C4 as defined by the Ten Twenty Electrode System of the International Federation for Electroencephalography and Clinical Neurophysiology. The EOG is usually recorded from both eyes with electrodes applied to a site slightly lateral to and above the outer canthi. In both EEG and EOG, reference electrodes are attached to the contralateral and homolateral earlobe (or mastoid process) respectively. The EMG is recorded bilaterally from the muscle areas on and beneath the chin and it is often termed the mental or submental EMG.

We will now continue with the essential features and changes registered by these electrographic indicators during the course of a night's sleep of "normal" young adults (see figures at end of section).

When the usual subject is lying quietly in a darkened bedroom immediately after receiving permission to go to sleep, the EEG is likely to show prolonged intervals of more or less sustained alpha rhythm (8-13 Hz; 25-100μv in amplitude), often with varying admixtures of low-voltage mixed frequencies (LVM); the EOG may contain REMs and eyelid blinks, and the tonic chin EMG is relatively high. This condition is termed Stage W.

Presently, as the subject becomes progressively drowsy, there is gradual fragmentation of the sustained epochs of alpha frequencies giving way to shorter intervals of alpha, interspersed with LVM, and finally more or less complete disappearance of alpha and replacement by LVM with 2-7 Hz activity prominent. Vertex sharp waves may appear. REMs and blinks disappear from the EOG and are replaced by slow rolling eye movements (SEMs) or minimal or no eye-movement activity. The tonic EMG is generally below that of the preceding Stage W. This condition is termed Stage 1 NREM or Sleep Onset Stage 1.

After 5-10 min of Stage 1 NREM elapse, sleep spindles and K complexes appear. The former consist of recurrent groups of sinusoidal waves 12-14 Hz in frequency and at least .5 sec in duration The latter are biphasic EEG forms exceeding 0.5 sec with initial negative sharp wave and succeeding positive components. EOG activity is minimal or absent and the EMG continues at a level lower than relaxed Stage W. Such an electrographic picture defines Stage 2.

After a varying interval, high-voltage, slow waves occur. These occupy a range in excess of 75 up to $200\mu v$ and are 2 Hz or less in frequency. At first they appear sporadically but gradually increases and come to dominate the EEG.

When such slow waves comprise 20-50% of the EEG, the sleep stage is termed Stage 3; and when in excess of 50%, it is termed Stage 4. The EOG and EMG continue more or less as before in both stages (sometimes called slow-wave sleep, or SWS, collectively). Stages 1 through 4 are also grouped as NREM or non rapid eye-movement sleep.

Finally, sometime during the second hour of sleep, polygraphic changes occur which indicate the presence of REM sleep. The EEG consists of relatively low-voltage mixed frequencies with occasional bursts of lower than waking-frequency alpha and "saw-toothed" waves (averaging about 3 Hz). This configuration is correlated with intense CNS activation. The EOG by striking contrast to NREM sleep contains repeated clusters of one or more conjugate rapid eye movements. Finally, the EMG is at its lowest tonic level of the night. The latter corresponds to massive inhibition of muscular activity. Occasionally, brief episodes of increased EMG activity are interspersed with this general background.

These intervals of REM sleep are termed REM periods or REMP(s). The first REMP of the night is usually the shortest, tends to contain the smallest number of REMs, is occasionally omitted entirely, and compared to the subsequent REMPs of the night, likely to be associated with less mentation and less dream-like mentation. REMPs may last from a few minutes to times well in excess of a half hour. REMPs reappear on the average of 90 min throughout the night. With the passage of time they tend to become longer and the intervals between them shorter. Healthy young adults have 3-5 REMPs per night (7-8 hrs of sleep).

Following the termination of the REMP, Stage 1 NREM typically reappears briefly, and is followed by Stage 2. In the first half of the night, Stages 3 and 4 succeed Stage 2 as before; but in the second half, slow-wave sleep is usually insignificant in amount.

The events from Sleep-Onset Stage 1 NREM to the end of the first REMP comprise the first sleep cycle; and subsequent components of the sleep cycle are bounded by events from the end of one REMP to the end of the next, regardless of whether in the last half of the night slow-wave sleep occurs in between. Thus, the typical night of a healthy young adult is characterized by recurrent sleep cycles as described.

In summary, the chief typical electrographic features of the sleep-cycle stages are as follows:

Stage W or wakefulness (see Figs. 1.1, 1.2)
>EEG: More or less sustained alpha activity, and/or LVM
>EOG: Various amounts of REMs and blinks
>EMG: relatively high tonic level.

Stages NREM
>Stage 1 (Fig. 1.2)
>>EEG: LVM, vertex sharp waves
>>EOG: SEMs or no EM activity
>>EMG: lower than Stage W
>Stage 2 (Fig. 1.3)
>>EEG: sleep spindles and K-complexes with a background of LVM
>>EOG: absence of significant EM activity
>>EMG: lower than Stage W
>Stage 3 (Fig. 1.4)
>>EEG: moderate accounts of high amplitude, slow wave activity comprising 20-50% of the epoch.
>>EOG: as in Stage 2
>>EMG: as in Stage 2
>Stage 4 (Fig. 1.5)
>>EEG: large amounts of high amplitude slow wave activity comprising more than 50% of the epoch
>>EOG: as in Stage 2
>>EMG: as in Stage 2
>Stage REM (Figs. 1.6, 1.7)
>>EEG: LVM, saw-toothed waves, alpha bursts at slightly lower than Stage W frequency.
>>EOG: recurrent episodes of the conjugate REMs
>>EMG: lowest tonic EMG of the night.

ORIENTATION TO FIGURES IN INTRODUCTION CHAPTER

The following series of tracings are all from the same night with a 25 year old normal male college student as subject. The specimens were recorded on a Grass Model IV-C electroencephalograph. The paper speed was 15mm./sec. The time constant for the EEG & EOG was 0.3 sec and the calibration was 1cm=50 microvolts. The time constant for the EMG was 0.03 sec and the calibration was 1 cm=10 microvolts.

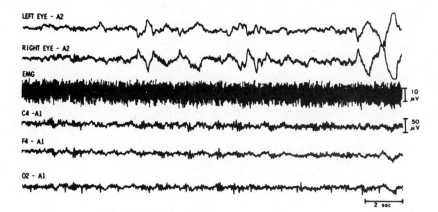

FIG. 1.1. A tracing illustrating unambiguous stage W (from Rechtschaffen & Kales, 1968). Note high EMG, sustained Alpha and REMs.

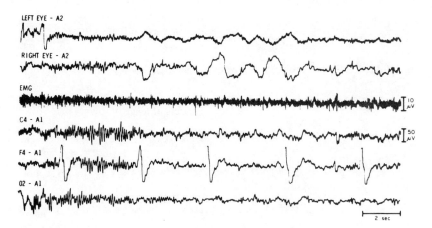

FIG. 1.2. A tracing illustrating the transition between Stage W and Stage 1 NREM. Note low voltage activity replacing alpha, high EMG and slow eye movements. (From Rechtschaffen & Kales, 1968).

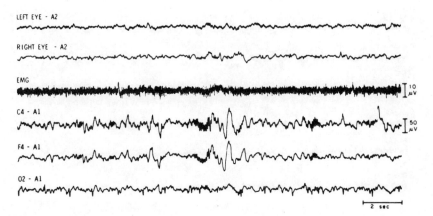

FIG. 1.3. A tracing of unambiguous Stage 2. Note spindles and K-complexes (From Rechtschaffen & Kales, 1968).

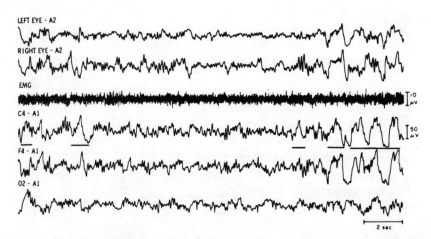

FIG. 1.4. A tracing of Stage 3. Note approximately 28% high amplitude slow wave activity. (From Rechtschaffen & Kales, 1968).

14

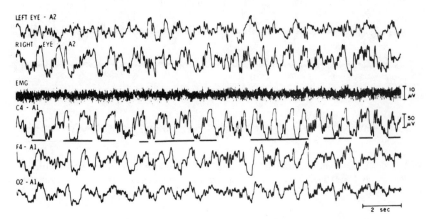

FIG. 1.5.   A tracing of unambiguous Stage 4. Note predominance of high amplitude slow wave activity. (From Rechtschaffen & Kales, 1968).

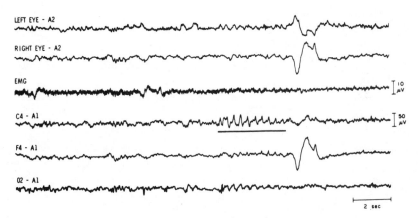

FIG. 1.6.   A tracing illustrating transition from Stage 2 to Stage REM. Note REMs relatively low voltage mixed frequencies, saw-toothed waves in C4-A1 derivation (underlined) and decreased tonic EMG. (From Rechtschaffen & Kales, 1968).

15

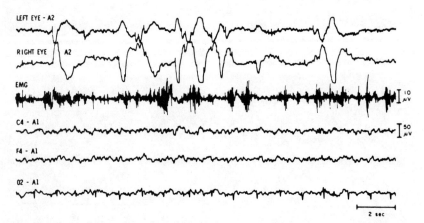

FIG. 1.7. Unambiguous stage REM. Note REMs, low voltage tonic EMG with phasic twitching, and relatively low voltage mixed EEG frequencies. (From Rechtschaffen & Kales, 1968).

Part I

METHODOLOGY AND
SLEEP MENTATION STUDIES

2

Measurement and Design in Research on Sleep Reports

John S. Antrobus
George Fein
Larry Jordan
Steven J. Ellman
Arthur M. Arkin

The City College of The City University of New York

In the broad sense of the term, the "measurement" of the characteristics of sleep reports ranges from the clinical "interpretation of dreams" to formal psychometric scaling procedures. The notion that the interpretation of dreams constitutes a form of judgment or multidimensional measurement of the characteristics of the sleeper and the sleeper's cognitive processes has not been developed in the research literature and for that reason is not discussed futher in this chapter.

In this chapter we will consider certain issues regarding the subject's report of the sleep experience, particularly the method of eliciting the sleeper's report, the optimum number of reports to obtain, order effects in the sleep report, memory and attention during sleep, and postawakening biases in the report. We then consider methods for improving judgments based upon sleep reports. Finally, we compare the merits of several research designs together with their statistical models for determining the association of sleep-report variables (judgments) and physiological events and states.

For our purposes, the measurement of the characteristics of sleep reports includes any systematic procedure whereby judgments about certain qualities are made by an individual, upon awakening, about an experience, a private event, which in the individual's judgment occurred while asleep. A subsequent judgment may often be made by a second person or judge, based upon the verbal report, or occasionally on a drawing, produced by the awakened sleeper.

For the purpose of analyzing the measurement issue in this area, it is useful to classify the judgments or measures on two factors: (1) according to whether the judgments are made only by the sleeper or jointly in a sleeper-second-judge sequence; and (2) whether or not the judgments are to be compared with an independent criterion such as Stage REM versus NREM sleep.

THE SLEEPER AS DREAMER AND JUDGE

Let us begin with a look at the subject awakened from sleep and asked to report on whatever was going through the subject's mind before being awakened. *We propose here that the "verbal report" itself be regarded as a set of judgments, albeit unsystematic judgments, about the subject's private experience prior to awakening.* The subject judges the names of the persons, objects, and events "seen" and "heard;" and he judges the color and brightness of the images, kinesthetic sensations, and intentions of the dream characters. Second, the subject judges how many of these judgments-statements are required for a report that will satisfy the experimenter. Thus, remembering a very long dream sequence, the subject may summarize the visual detail in order to report the plot within a reasonable interval of time. Recalling almost nothing, the sleeper may stretch one or two vague images into several sentences. This tendency will attenuate the distinction between REM and NREM reports. It may be counteracted by asking the subject for as much detail as possible.

Finally, we present evidence which suggests that, at least in REM sleep, the subject may make judgments while asleep about the relevance of the sleep experience to the experiment (or psychotherapy), and thus make the experience more available for subsequent recall.

As scientists, who also dream, we would like to take the subject's report at face value as an accurate description of the sleeper's prior state. Yet there are clear limits to our gullibility. Interestingly, in the two cases in which discrepancies exist between the sleeper's report and independent evidence concerning the validity of the report, we rule the report in error. There is the child who believes that there was a bad man in the room and we know there really wasn't. Then there is the subject who claims being awake and thinking despite the fact that posture and EEG indicate sound sleep. We reject the subject's judgment about wakefulness. After reading Goodenough's (1967) account of a subject who said he was *thinking* and who gave a vivid account of going to the rear of the classroom, operating a pinball machine which spilled out all its contents, and then observed an oil well under the machine, we are also disinclined to accept the subject's judgment, that he was thinking rather than dreaming. But in the absence of an independent measure of the sleeper's thought and imagery we too easily tend to take the report uncritically.

Experimenter Bias

One plausible, potential factor affecting subjects' report-judgments is experimenter bias. Inasmuch as this issue is dealt with more fully in Chapter 3, we make only a passing comment here. Since the beginning of sleep-mentation research we have been concerned about the possibility that the experimenters might unintentionally communicate to the subject something about the experimenter's knowledge of the EEG waking criterion. Thus, the experimenter might inadvertently alter the inflection or loudness of voice, or be more likely to repeat a question if aware that the subject was awakened from Stage REM rather than from NREM sleep. Fortunately, this problem can be managed by tape recording the awakening stimulus (usually the subject's name) and all subsequent questions.

Dependence of Judges on Subjects' Judgments

In most sleep mentation studies, the standard requests utilized are: (1) "Tell me everything that was going through your mind;" and, when the subject finishes, (2) "Was there anything else?" Since the questions are open ended, the subject is quite free to decide how much information to provide. For example, if the subject is struck by an odd or bizarre combination of elements in the dream, little information may be provided about the hallucinatory quality of the experience. Now let us suppose that we wish to have an independent set of persons judge or rate the strength of such different qualities of the sleep experience as: (1) vividness of the visual imagery; (2) bizarreness; and (3) hallucinatory quality. This second set of judges must base their judgments upon the judgment-reports of the subject. Like the subjects' judgments, those of the independent set of judges are about the private experience of the sleeper, but the qualities judged are generally more abstract. If the subject has made a number of judgment-reports or simple statements about the bizarreness of the experience, the judges will have a reasonable basis for making a more abstract rating of this quality. If there is no specific statement about the vividness of the visual imagery, then a judgment about this quality may be inferred from the number, or perhaps, relative frequency of concrete nouns, action verbs, and so on in the original report. If no specific mention is made about the hallucinatory quality of the experience, then the judges may have little choice other than to infer its absence. In other words, the validity of the judges's judgments is totally at the mercy of how much information is contained in the judgment-reports of the subject.

Open-ended Versus Specific Questions

Foulkes (1966) and other investigators have attempted to rectify this matter by asking the subject to make judgments in the form of simple descriptive statements about several specific qualities of interest to the investigator. Following the first two questions mentioned above, the subject may be asked, "How vivid was the visual imagery?" "How much emotion . . ." and "How real . . ." As the procedure is repeated the subject eventually learns to report on each of these dimensions when responding to the first question, that is, without a reminder from the specific questions. In a recent study, we also asked the subject to make a numerical rating of the magnitude of these qualities. Although the results have not yet been formally analyzed, the numerical response appears promising.

How Many Questions?

In the course of replicating the Molinari and Foulkes' (1969) phasic-tonic study, Foulkes and Pope (1972) did produce some evidence suggesting that judgments and ratings are more valid when based only upon the response to the first two questions. When judges in the Foulkes and Pope study were given subjects' responses to one open-ended question plus five specific questions regarding the sensory quality of the sleep experience, there was no distinction between the phasic and tonic sleep reports. When, however, they used only the responses to the initial open-ended questions, they obtained a statistically significant difference between the two. Foulkes and Pope ask whether the significance is spurious or whether subjects' responses tend to be more similar from condition to condition when they are question cued about specific qualities of their sleep experience. Obviously, further examination of the matter is appropriate.

We decided to study the discriminability of Stage REM and Stage 2 reports among the 20 subjects in the Arkin, Antrobus, and Ellman study reported in Chapter 13. We compared responses to only two open-ended questions versus all 5 questions, the last 3 of which were: "How vivid and clear was the sleep experience you just described?," "What feelings were you aware of in the course of the sleep experience?," and "To what extent did the experience seem like it was really happening?" Each subject contributed one Stage REM and one Stage 2 report from each of the first 2 baseline nights. Each report was rated on the basis of the response to the first 2 baseline nights. Each report was rated on the basis of the response to the first 2 questions and on the response to all 5. The entire pool of 160 reports from 80 awakenings were rated for magnitude of dreaming (see Appendix 2.1) on an 8-point forced-normal distribution. Eight judges were arranged so that each judge rated 80 reports, 40 2-question reports, and 40 5-question reports, from 80 awakenings. That is, no judge rated a 2-question and a 5-question item from the same awakening.

Judges rated the five-question responses higher on dreaming than the two-question reports (5.1 and 4.7 respectively; $F = 13.6$; $p \leq .01$) on an eight-point scale, collapsing sleep stages. The difference between Stage REM and Stage 2 reports was 0.87, identical for the two-and five-question responses ($F = 27.7$; $p \leq .01$). In short, the main effects for sleep stage, number of questions, and order of session were statistically significant, but no interaction existed between number of questions and sleep stage. That is, the discriminability of sleep stage was independent of the number of questions asked.

Order Effects

Whenever possible, sleep studies are designed so that all subjects go through all experimental conditions. The data is analyzed by means of a randomized block analysis-of-variance solution which is a powerful statistical procedure, but one which is quite sensitive to violations of the statistical assumptions upon which it is based. Violations of compound symmetry of the variance-covariance matrix (Winer, 1971) are commonly caused by a host of order effects which properly should be checked before proceeding with the analysis of variance. Failure to satisfy the assumptions results in significance levels that purport to be better than they really are, and the bias increases as the sample size decreases.

Antrobus, Arkin, and Toth (1972) found that word count of subjects' reports decreases as a function of number of baseline nights in the lab (see Figure 2.1). Employing a partial sleep-deprivation procedure bounded by a pair of pre- and a pair of postdeprivation baseline nights, we found that word count decreased from the first to the last baseline night; the drop being larger for Stage REM awakenings than for Stage 2. Since we decided to modify the procedures after running only 10 subjects, the decrements, while sizable, were not statistically significant. Changes in fatigue or motivation seemed likely reasons for the

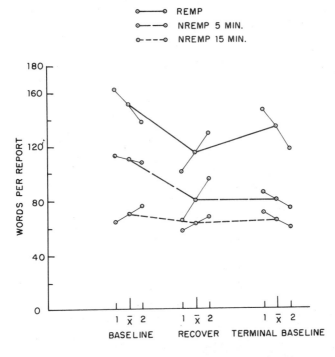

FIG. 2.1.   Word count per report from REMP, NREMP 5 min. after REMP and NREMP, 15 min. after REMP, before, during, and after recovery from REM deprivation.

decrement in word count. Fatigue was ruled out, however, because the last two nights were preceded by normal home sleep so that the decrement could not be attributed to sleep loss or similar short-term experimental effects.

First-night-report effect. The final version of this experiment (see Chapter 13, this volume) was designed to give more careful attention to order effects, particularly inasmuch as each of 20 subjects went through both Stage 1 REM, and 2 deprivation. Night 1 was preceded by 3 adaptation nights in which no awakenings for sleep reports were made. Night 3 was preceded by at least 3 nights of normal home sleep, but Night 5 was preceded by a laboratory recovery night, which in turn was preceded by 3 nights of either Stage 1 REM, or 2 deprivation. Postadaptation laboratory nights 1 and 2, 3, and 4, and 5 and 6 were established as first, middle, and terminal baseline nights. The reports were rated on an 8-point scale for dream-like quality (see Dreaming in Appendix 2.1). (For a complete description of the procedures and results, see Chapter 11, this volume). The mean ratings by night, early and late half of the night, and sleep stage are presented in Figure 2.2.

Some of the order effects in Figure 2.2 are among the strongest effects of any kind reported in the sleep-mentation literature. They have important implications for the interpretation of the Stage 1 REM-NREM effect and for the design of sleep-mentation studies. First, we see that within each of the three pairs of nights, dreaming is always lower in the second member of the pair (mean of Stages 1, REM, and 2 awakenings). Since normal home sleep did not precede Night 5, a statistical test on the difference between first and second members of a pair was carried out only on Nights 1, 2, 3 and 4 ($F_{1, 19}$ = 18.38; $p \leq .01$). By far the largest within-pair drop occurs within Stage 1 REM from Night 1 to 2.

The within-night, within-sleep stage effects are not particularly consistent. In general, dreaming is higher during the second half of the night. The order is reversed within the first night, Stage 1 REM, so that the largest contrast in dreaming between Stage 1 REM and Stage 2 occurs during the first half of the first night (see Figure 2.2). Within Stage REM only, there is a strong negative linear trend across the three night pairs, but the linear trend for pairs of nights averaged across sleep stages is not significant ($F_{1,19}$ = 1.48; p = .24).

Looking at the whole-night differences between Stages 1 REM and 2 dreaming scores, we find the largest contrast occurring during the first night. Figure 2.2 shows how the significance levels vary if we were to carry out tests on different baseline nights. F drops from 49 on Night 1 to F = 4.6, barely significant at the .05 level, on Night 2; and just under the .10 level of significance on Night 6.

Throughout this chapter we insist that statistical tests of significance are only gross estimators of the size of experimental effects. We want to know the *magnitude* of the differences between Stages 1 REM and 2, not simply that the differences are significantly different from zero. If we collapse the design to a

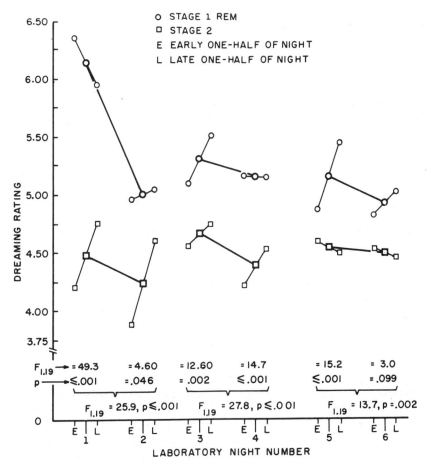

FIG. 2.2.   Dreaming ratings for 20 subjects by number of nights in the laboratory, and early versus late halves of the night.

simple sleep stage x subjects randomized blocks design and compute omega, the size of effect variable proposed by Hays (1973), omega drops from .68 on Night 1 to .10 on Night 6. That is, the REM/NREM effect accounts for 68% of the Night 1 variance, or variability among scores, but only 10% of the Night 6 variance.

The strongest effect in the data appears to be a "novelty" effect associated with verbal report-response. This novely effect appears strongest within Stage REM; it appears largely dissipated by the second night in which reports are elicited. Being absent from the laboratory appears to revive the novelty motivation (Night 3); but sleeping in the laboratory without being asked to report "What was going through your mind. . .?" (Night 1 versus 3) may further enhance the effect. The decrement in dreaming may be caused by an effort or cost of attending to one's REM mentation such that the negative cost effect accumulates over time in REM sleep.

Interaction of Order Effect with Sleep Stage

We may now return to the original issue of distinguishing what goes on within the sleeper's experience from possible biases in the verbal report-description of the experience. By bias, we refer to variation in the attention, selectivity, motivation, alertness, and memory for the original sleep experience. The problem may be limited somewhat by looking only at the difference in the responses to two states or stages of sleep. Biases that are common to both states may thereby be cancelled out. Since, however, we do not have an independent measure of the sleeper's internal experience, we cannot easily determine whether the response biases are equal in the two states. In the case of the first night effect and first half-night effect in Figure 2.2, such simple motivational response sets as the subject wanting to perform well and please the experimenter by giving a thorough detailed report cannot by itself account for an effect that occurs in only Stage REM. Perhaps Williams, Hammack, Daly, Dement, & Lubin's (1964) finding is pertinent that, compared to NREM sleep, subjects in REM sleep show a large drop in response threshold to a "significant stimulus" (response avoids loud noise) relative to a stimulus that was not paired with the noxious noise. The significance or consequences of responding to the stimulus were "interpreted" by the sleeper during Stage REM sleep whereas the physical qualities of the stimulus were the sole determiners of probability of response within NREM sleep. To interpret the relevance of the perceptual and cognitive elements of one's sleeping experience in terms of a potential future request for a verbal report-response is an operation similar to that required of Williams et al's. (1964) sleepers — an operation which might well be characteristic of Stage REM sleep.

The quality of Stage REM sleep may differ on Night 1 in some way that distinguishes it both from preceding nights in which no reports were elicited and from subsequent nights when dreaming scores were lower. One might expect more signs of phasic events, for example, during Night 1 (Chapter 7, this volume). But just as the physiological description of Stage REM sleep has not advanced our understanding of the cognitive processes by which the dream is constructed, so too, the identification of physiological characteristics unique to the first night effect might neither add nor detract from a cognitive explanation of the process. The most promising way to test the preawakening explanations of the first-night effect is to manipulate, by means of instructions, the subject's expectation of the night that sleep will be disrupted.

Memory and Dream Modification

If the first-night-report effect operates within sleep, it will be essential to determine whether the effect is simply to improve attention to and recall of the stimulus events of the sleep experience or whether the elementary events of the sleep experience, like dreams, are themselves altered in some way. We may think of the sleeper as carrying through time an open-ended box of continuously decaying memory where the rate of decay or loss at one end of the box is approximately equal to the rate of entry of new items. Let us suppose that the first-night-report-effect operates by increasing the length of the box, that is, the number of events in memory or available for report. If the sequence of events generated in the dream is determined in part by the presence of the preceding dream events in the box, then the dream should become more consistent from one moment to the next as the size of the memory box increases. In this case, not only recall of the sleep experience, but the nature of the experience itself would be affected by the first-night report effect.

On the other hand, the elements of the sleeper's experience available to the sleeper immediately before the awakening stimulus may be the same on all nights; Night 1 may differ only with respect to what happens *after* the awakening stimulus. For example, on Night 1 the subject may awaken faster and reach a higher level of arousal before giving the report. Such a possibility could be tested by showing subjects a 5-sec visual or audio-visual movie sequence immediately upon awakening and determine whether their description-reports of the sequence showed the same night-to-night order effect as the Stage REM report trend.

Long-Term Order Effects

The long-term order effects are somewhat puzzling because of the tendency of Stage 2 dreaming to move in the opposite direction from Stage REM dreaming (see Figure 2.2). Perhaps the small positive slope within Stage 2 should await replication before interpretation. The net result of the respective positive and negative slopes is a sizable linear decrease in the difference between Stage REM and Stage 2 as the subjects move through the three baseline night pairs (1 and 2; 3 and 4; and 5 and 6). As the trend continues, the Stage REM-NREM effect disappears below statistical significance.

Pre- and Postawakening Biases: Summary.

We have argued that order effects possibly involving a sense of novelty or other motivational factors may be associated with postawakening processes such as the retrieval of the sleep experience (visual and auditory images) as well as the manner in which these images are judged and reported by the subject. We have stated that the motivational factor may also operate within sleep, at least Stage REM sleep, to improve the amount of imagery events stored and possibly even the manner in which the images are generated. We have suggested some research routes to determine whether the first-night-report effect is a pre- or postawakening effect or both.

The Real Effect Versus Bias

In general, it seems reasonable to assert that postawakening effects would constitute "response bias" whereas preawakening experimental effects, unless they
are specific to the experimental procedure, belong to a larger class of factors
which affect the sleeper's perceptual-cognitive sleep experience. Let us look at
the implications of these alternatives. If the first-night-report effect operates
only as a postawakening one and is restricted to Stage REM, and if the effect of
order on Stage 2 awakenings is trivial, then the first night and other order biases
can be removed by comparing the two stages only after the bias asymptotes,
for example, after several nights of laboratory awakenings. Even then we cannot
be assured that the bias is equal in both sleep stages, but we can be assured that
we have removed a very large source of differential bias. We would, thereby,
sacrifice considerable detail in the Stage REM report in order to make a less
biased estimate of the magnitude of the true difference in dreaming, or any
other scale, between Stages REM and 2. If all of the order effect is response bias,
then the asymptote in Figure 2.2 implies that there is no real difference in REM
and NREM mentation.

If the first-night-report effect operates only during the preawakening interval,
we would assume that the instructional stimuli which elicit the motivation are
part of a larger class of stimuli which could be described experimentally. If the
class can be abstracted and defined operationally as a variable, then we might
conclude that the effect of Stage REM on dreaming or visual imagery is contingent upon the state of that motivational variable; or, that dreaming is a joint
function, possibly both linear and interactive of sleep stage and motivation. In
other words, the REM/NREM effect on dreaming may not stand alone, or, if
it does, only rather weakly.

If the first-night-report effect operates only during the postawakening interval, we could conclude nothing about the size of the REM/NREM effect on
dreaming or other variables unless we found a way to measure and match across
the two stages the magnitude of the motivation effect or remove its influence by
by means of some covariance procedure.

Consequences for Research Design

If a particular effect does actually exist among a population of subjects, we
want our experiment which uses only a sample of subjects to pick up, or be sensitive to, this effect. The probability that the experiment will do so is called the
power of the experiment. Statistical power is a function of one's significance
level, the size of the real effect in the population and, in general, one's sample
size. With respect to the difference between Stages REM and 2, it is clear that
the largest difference occurs within the first night, and in particular, the first
half of the first night. We have, therefore, optimum statistical power or sensitivity, if we make awakenings only from one night, or for the matter, only from

the first half of the first night. Not only is the statistical power lower on all other nights, but it decreases as we combine data from the first night with that of any other night (see Figure 2.2). Of course, the interpretation of all data so gathered must be qualified by the issues raised in the preceding section.

Individual Differences

Individual differences are the brick and mortar of personality theory. Attempts have been made to demonstrate a link between individual differences in sleeping fantasy and daytime fantasy, schizophrenia, and adjustment (Cartwright, 1972; Fisher & Dement, 1963; Foulkes, 1966; Singer & Schonbar, 1961). For those investigators interested in effects that hold across subjects in general, such individual differences constitute a random, nuisance variable. Because misconceptions exist respecting the size and consequences of the nuisance, we would like to devote some space to its consideration.

The statistical model underlying the typical sleep-mentation study is

$$X_{ij} = \mu + \tau_j + \pi_i + \tau\pi_{ij} + \epsilon_{ij},$$

in which:

X_{ij} = the imagery score of the ith subject under the jth sleep stage;

μ = the mean score of all possible subjects under all j conditions, a constant;

τ_j = the mean of all possible subjects in the jth condition, not just the subjects in the particular sample;

π_i = the mean of the ith subject;

$\tau\pi_{ij}$ = the interaction of the ith subject in the jth sleep stage;

ϵ_{ij} = all residual unidentified variability, essentially differences between different awakenings under the same condition (j), of a specific subject (i). Where subjects are observed only once in each treatment condition or sleep stage, no separate estimate of ϵ_{ij} is available (see Hays, 1973; Winer, 1971).

In personality research (see Singer & Schonbar, 1961) in which the interest is in individual differences in imagery regardless of sleep stage (that is, averaged across sleep stages), the component of interest is π_i. In testing personality models, however, some investigators explicitly refer to individual difference within a specific treatment condition, such as Stage REM or REM deprivation. Such individual differences are the sum of $\pi_i + \tau\pi_{ij} + \epsilon_{ij}$. That reports from a specific condition be reliably different from reports averaged across all conditions assumes that the treatment-by-subject term, $\tau\pi_{ij}$, is appreciably $\neq 0$. For example, are individual differences in REM imagery reliably different from individual differences in imagery averaged over all states? With the exception of Foulke's and Vogel's (1965) comparison of REM and sleep onset imagery, to our knowledge, no one studying individual differences has ever tested this assumption in sleep mentation.

We examined individual differences in the effect of Stage REM versus Stage 2 (REM/2) on dreaming during the first two control nights of our recent study and found that r ranged from .92 to −.44 for the 20 subjects, with 4 subjects lying between .1 and −.44.

Do all subjects do their own thing? If so, what does the test of the main effect (across subjects) of sleep stage on dreaming mean? The main effect is essentially the effect of the hypothetical "average subject." Under conditions of substantial $\tau\pi$ effects, some investigators have given up testing the main τ effect and proceeded to test a main effect separately on each subject ($\tau + \tau\pi$). This approach is reasonable only if some method of combining the results of several subjects is available, or, of independently distinguishing subjects who respond differently to the treatment conditions. It seems to us that the randomized block analysis of variance (ANOVA) combined with estimates of both ω_τ^2 and $\omega_{\tau\pi}^2$ (Fleiss, 1969) remains the best solution. Thus, individual differents in the sleep stage effect may account for 30% of the dreaming variance ($\hat{\omega}_{\tau\pi}^2$ May = .3), but it is still worthwhile to know whether the main sleep stage or "average subject" effect ($\hat{\omega}_\tau^2$) = 0 or .5. Conversely, if $\hat{\omega}_\tau^2$ = .5 and $\hat{\omega}_{\tau\pi}^2$ = .1, the "average subject" tells nearly the whole story! (See Arkin, Antrobus, & Ellman, Chapter 13, this volume.)

Before estimating the size of ω_τ^2 and $\omega_{\tau\pi}^2$, however, it is appropriate to test the null hypothesis for each. It is possible, as we shall see, for there to be large "individual differences" in scores which are simply due to ϵ_{ij}, while true individual differences, π and $\tau\pi$ remain essentially = 0.

Since we were not interested in π in the study described in Chapter 11, we eliminated the term and held response scale magnitude constant for all subjects by judging each subject's reports independently on a forced-normal distribution with subject mean and variance = constant. $\tau\pi_{ij}$, however, was free to vary. In designs in which there are no replications in the design, $\tau\pi_{ij}$ = 0 may be tested by Tukey's nonadditivity test (see Winer, 1971). Where replicated observations exist, as in our recent study with 6 control nights, $\tau\pi_{ij}$ can be tested directly by the randomized blocks ANOVA or by examining the night-to-night stability of individual differences in dreaming during Stage REM versus Stage 2. Taking the latter route, we first computed the signed difference in dreaming between Stage REM and 2 separately on each of 6 control nights and then correlated the differences between all pairs of nights. The mean of the 15 correlations was .03! Apparently, the interaction of REM/2 and dreaming, $\tau_j\pi_i$, is reasonably close to 0. Since visual imagery, hallucinatory quality, and so on correlate strongly with dreaming, it is a reasonably safe hunch that $\tau\pi$ = 0 for these variables also.

Because this finding is at variance with the working assumptions of many investigators, it should be replicated and the limits within which it holds should be identified. Note that this result carries absolutely no implication about the significance of the π_i component. This analysis suggests that more attention should be given to our working assumptions about the magnitude of the components of the individual differences in sleep mentation. In the meantime, the main implication of the zero treatment-by-subject interaction is that *the "average subject" model fits nearly all subjects*. There is, therefore, no need or advantage of making separate tests of the REM/NREM effect for each subject. From a statistical point of view, if $\tau_j \pi_i = 0$, then a simpler statistical model may be employed for the randomized blocks design: $X_{ij} = \mu + \pi_i + \tau_j + \epsilon_{ij}$ (see Winer, 1971). In this model, $MS_{\text{Treatment x Subject}}$ or MS_{Residual} is an estimator simply of σ_ϵ^2. To the extent that the treatment-by-subject interaction = 0 for other treatment effects, such as REM deprivation versus control night, the various subject interactions may be pooled to give a single pooled MS_{Residual} which is a stable estimate of σ_ϵ^2. Further, the computations of the error terms for factorial models are greatly simplified if all MS_{Residual}s estimate the same σ_ϵ^2.

Subjects versus Nights

This is perhaps a good point to draw attention to an important procedural issue in sleep mentation research: whether to put one's money into subjects or nights. The traditional sleep experiment tends to run a few subjects over and over again. Is this preference for nights over subjects the "best" experimental strategy? Is it the most powerful in the sense of being most likely to identify relationships that do, in fact, exist in the population of subjects at large — within the constraints of an investigator's time and resources. The strategy with the greatest power or sensitivity is the one with the smallest error term. Since most sleep studies run each subject through all or most conditions, variation from subject to subject, the π_i effects, are eliminated from the error term which is then associated only with $\tau\pi_{ij}$, the treatment-by-subject interactions and ϵ_{ij}, residual unidentified errors of measurement and variation from occasion to occasion within a subject, order effects, variations in experimental procedures, and so on. We have just presented evidence that the $\tau\pi_{ij}$ effects are negligible, at least for dreaming and sleep stage, thereby assigning all unidentified variation to the ϵ_{ij}. If multiple awakenings are made on each subject, then the expression on page 29 changes so that X_{ij} becomes $\overline{X}_{ij}$ = the mean dreaming score of the ith subject in the jth sleep stage, and ϵ_{ij} similarly becomes $\overline{\epsilon}_{ij}$ which is generally smaller than ϵ_{ij}. Using the familiar

$$\sigma_{\overline{\epsilon}}^2 = \frac{\sigma_\epsilon^2}{N},$$

the estimate of the error term, $\hat{\sigma}_{\overline{\epsilon}}^2$, can be reduced by half by doubling the number of observations. If $\sigma_{\tau\pi_{ij}}^2$ is close to 0, then $\hat{\sigma}_\sigma^2$ should be reduced equally well either by increasing subjects or awakenings within the same subject(s). That is, 40 nights on one subject is as good as 40 subjects, one night each.

As a check on this conclusion, we examined 19 studies of the dreaming-sleep stage relationship in order to see how subject sample size and number of observations per subject was associated with power. Sample size ranged from 3 to 25. Number of awakenings per subject was essentially independent of sample size. We were able to construct a 2 x 2, dreaming/not dreaming-by-Stage 1 REM/ NREM table for each study, and for each study computed a phi coefficient. We then plotted one against the other (see Figure 2.3). The range of phi with the small sample sizes runs from .22 (Foulkes, Larson, Swanson & Rardin, 1969) to .84 (Wolpert & Trosman, 1958) with sample sizes of 5 and 10 respsectively. As the sample size increases to 25, the largest sample size we could locate (Orlinsky, 1962), the range of phi narrows sharply. The entire plot appears to point toward a best estimate for phi of approximately .45.

Figure 2.4, which plots phi coefficients against number of awakenings per subject, shows little consistent effect of number of awakenings upon the stability of phi from one study to another. The modest negative slope of the plot

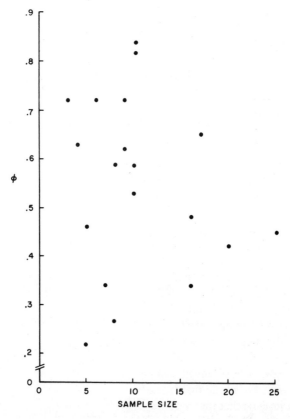

FIG. 2.3.   PHI coefficients of association between dreaming and stage. REM versus NREM sleep plotted against sample size for 19 studies.

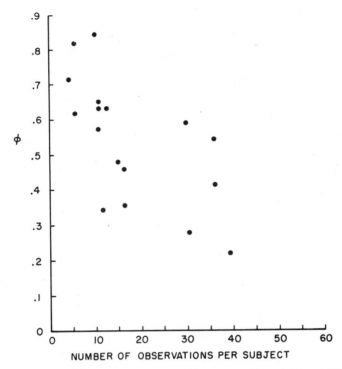

FIG. 2.4.   PHI coefficients of associations between dreaming and Stage 1 REM versus NREM sleep plotted against number observations per subject.

($r = -.19$) is completely consistent with the first-night-report effect in which the maximum degree of association between dreaming and sleep stage was on the first half of the first night. Unlike the previous distribution, there is no tendency for the variability among studies to decrease as more awakenings are made per subject.

The chief conclusion to be drawn from this analysis is that increasing the number of observations-reports by increasing the number of observations per subject does not increase the statistical power of the design, but increasing the number of observations by increasing sample size does. Furthermore, sample sizes less than 20 are completely useless for the purpose of estimating the strength of the relationship between sleep-stage and sleep-report variables. Inasmuch as the indices of association between sleep stage and dreaming most commonly quoted are the highest estimates and are based upon studies of only 5 subjects, this analysis calls for a large downward shift in our estimates — unless, perhaps we restrict our estimates to the first laboratory night.

Our analysis suggests that the preferred design observes each of 20-40 subjects on only 1 night each. We cannot make this suggestion a firm recommendation, however, until some of the assumptions about the first-night-report effect are tested. In the meantime it is clearly advisable to analyze reports separately by laboratory-night order and perhaps by early versus late half of the night. It is entirely plausible that some of the discrepancies among different studies come from the fact that some used only 1 or 2 nights, thereby obtaining high estimates of degree of association and others used many nights, thereby obtaining low estimates. We should like to note parenthetically that there is a tendency ($r = -.25$) for phi to decrease with sample size (see Figure 2.3). We interpret this as an inclination of experimenters to stop running subjects if their initial results are strong.

JUDGMENTS BASED UPON SLEEP REPORTS

The purpose of judging, measuring or scaling different qualities of sleep reports is to directly or indirectly obtain a description of the sleep report or experience. When a judge, other than the subject who made the sleep report, makes a judgment based upon that report, the judge generally makes an implicit or explicit judgment about the private experience of the sleeping subject prior to the subject's awakening. Notable exceptions are simple counts of the total number of words and other syntactic classifications. Nevertheless, when a judge counts the total number of humans or architectural objects in the report, the judge is, in our opinion, assuming that these events occurred in the original sleep experience. For the most part, therefore, judgments based upon sleep reports are judgments about characteristics of sleep experience or, what we have come to call, sleep mentation. The discussion of the first-night-report effect in the previous portion of this chapter suggests some ways to test the presumed invariance between the mentation and report.

Global Ratings Versus Counts of Simple Events

Judgments about qualities of sleep reports vary from global judgments of complex, loosely defined classes such as dreaming to a count of the total number of concrete (visualizable) nouns in the report. In general, the greater the detail with which a scale is defined, the less latitude there is for the judges to impose their own personal set of assumptions and response biases. For example, should a report of a "red car" receive the same visual-imagery rating if it is the only visual object in a one-hundred-word report as it would if it made up the entire report? Some judges may tend toward a proportional rating whereas others may judge the absolute number of visual items. To what extent should reports of color and movement be weighted against the number of different objects or number of words in the report? Despite the prominent role of visual imagery in discriminating between Stage REM and NREM sleep reports, the private "rules" by which judges weight these various properties have never been investigated.

Perhaps the time has come for us to combine some of the techniques of psycholinguistics for the analysis of sentence structure with the methods developed by Paivio (1971) for scaling visual imagery.

Although high interjudge reliabilities tend to be associated with precise definitions, global judgments about dreaming, visual imagery, and related scales have generally yielded high interjudge agreement even when the judgment class is defined in no more than a single sentence.

The single major limitation of the global rating is that the meaning of the quality judged lies unarticulated in the head of the judge. The very fact that the experimenter cannot describe the rules of definition to the judge suggests that even the experimenter may be unable to define explicitly the quality under study. It is our position that the psychophysiological model of sleep mentation will not be complete until we are able to define precisely the nature of judgment operation performed on the sleep report.

The difficulty with the precise, countable qualities, on the other hand, is that standing alone they tend to be of only trivial interest. The variables of greatest interest to many investigators are multidimensional in nature. Accordingly, rules, arbitrary or empirical, must be devised for combining elementary classes into the larger judgment classes of interest to the investigator. Even a simple quality such as visual imagery may consist of some weighted combination of a count of several elementary judgment classes: concrete nouns, visual modifiers of the nouns, action verbs, and spatial prepositions. *A Psycholinguistic Scoring Manual for Mentation Reports* (Antrobus, Schnee, Offer, Lynn, & Silverman, 1976), currently being tested in our laboratories shows that a count of the number of words in any of these four classes is highly correlated with a global rating of Visual Imagery and is also a good discriminator of REM/NREM sleep stages.

It seems impossible, however, to define complex constructs such as dreaming, bizarreness, or regressive thought in terms of a count of words standing in isolation. Rather than instructing judges to make a direct judgment concerning the presence of a complex, abstract class, it seems better to define several less abstract classes of events which constitute regressive thought. Thus Vogel, Foulkes, and Trosman (1966) defined regressive thought as a report which had one or more of six qualities such as: single isolated images, incomplete or fragmentary scenes, inappropriate or distorted imagery, magical or omnipotent thought.

Scoring Unit

The Gottschalk-Gleser (1969) content analysis scales are, to our knowledge, the most elaborate scoring system to be applied to the analysis of sleep reports. The system provides for the scoring of several affects: anxiety, hostility directed outward, and inward and ambivalent hostility, as well as a social alienation-personal disorganization (schizophrenic) scale. The Gottschalk-Gleser scales were developed for the analysis of verbal behavior in a psychiatric-clinical psychology setting where the basic operating assumptions are psychoanalytic. But regardless of his affiliation with the psychoanalytic model, the reader will find the author's detailed description of their procedures and explicit consideration of their assumptions and the testing of some of these assumptions most instructive. Instead of using the entire sleep report to obtain a global judgment, Gottschalk, Winget and Gleser (1969) divide the report into a sequence of clauses which are then used as a basis for all subsequent judgments. Although the authors describe several procedural rules for defining the clauses, they do not indicate the realibility of this operation. Although the clause may be the best unit for judging complex qualities such as anxiety and hostility, we have found that the individual word is a satisfactory scoring unit for visual imagery. The variable bizarreness, on the other hand, which has figured prominently as a characteristic of dreaming, would seem to require the entire sleep report as the scoring unit. Objects and events in a dream often assume their bizarre quality because they are improbable in the larger context in which they appear. A suitable scoring unit must therefore preserve an adequately large context. Certainly, the analysis of sleep reports could benefit from a comparison of different sizes of coding units.

Word Count

Consideration of the size of the scoring unit inevitably raises the issue of the effect of the length of the total sleep report on judgments made from the reports. In our own data, word count shares a significant portion of the variance of most of our scales. In our most recent study (see Chapter 13, this volume) we estimated the correlation of dreaming with word count from the pooled regression coefficient in an analysis of covariance design: $r = .35$; $r^2 = .12$. That is, when treatment conditions were held constant, word count shared 12% of the between-treatments term, holding subject and time of night constant, word count shared .41-.48 of the variance of dreaming. The proportion was invariant for Nights 1 and 2 of our recent study despite the fact that the mean word count dropped by one-third from Night 1 to 2. Word count shared .35 to .60 of the variance of 7 out of 10 of the global ratings we employed. Nevertheless, there is a sizable portion of predictive variance that a simple word count does not share. If we use the scales to discriminate the 2 stages of sleep from which the reports were gathered, dreaming accounts for .48 of the REM/NREM variance whereas word count manages only .32. If we first partial out the word count variance, dreaming adds .173 to word count. To put it another way, the correlation of dreaming with Stage 1 REM/NREM, corrected for word count, drops to $\sqrt{.173} = .42$ from .69, using a set of 115 Stage 1 REM/NREM report pairs.

Whether one corrects a variable for word count depends entirely upon the quality or purpose of the construct under study. In general, if one wishes to isolate particular components of a complex variable, it is entirely appropriate to clean up a variable by partialling out other unwanted variance. Let us suppose, however, that sleep reports consisted almost entirely of descriptions of visual imagery, that is, the correlation between visual imagery and word count was .90. To partial out word count would simply wipe out almost all the visual-imagery variance! Obviously, a word count correction should be used cautiously.

The chief consideration, in our opinion, is whether the variation in word count is attributable only to the amount of material available in memory immediately prior to awakening. In this case one assumes that memory and speech functions at the time of making the report are the same for all subjects under all conditions. If, on the other hand, subjects are more articulate and fluent upon awakening from REM sleep, one could measure this articulacy by instructing subjects to describe a briefly presented, postawakening, audiovisual event. Such an independent word count could be used to statistically correct for variation in waking report fluency. Yet if such waking fluency were an integral part of the preawakening cognitive processes, the statistical correction would be inappropriate. At best one might parcel variance into a fluency-memory component and a visual-imagery component.

A major consideration with respect to whether one should or shouldn't partial out word count is whether one regards the variable in question, say visual-imagery, as an intensity or total-magnitude variable. If we are concerned with the cognitive processes involved in generating, storing, and retrieving visual or auditory images, we may want a total-magnitude judgment and would, therefore, not partial out word count. On the other hand, if we want to find out whether people are more anxious in REM than NREM sleep or whether one set of subjects is more anxious than another, then we might prefer an intensity variable. Thus, Gottschalk, Winget and Gleser (1969) argue that anxiety and similar variables should be independent of word count. Although the Gottschalk et al. (1969) scoring procedure has been applied to the analysis of sleep reports, it was originally developed for the analysis of psychotherapy protocols. The fluency factors which determine total word output in the waking state differ considerably from the consolidation and retrieval factors which presumably account for differences in the word count of reports from sleep states. We are asking simply that the assumption of independence of word count, which Gottschalk, Winget and Gleser (1969) make for the analysis of waking protocols, not be applied uncritically to the analysis of sleep reports. The assumption of independence does seem plausible for anxiety and hostility where we are looking at an average quality of an experience, but a total count of recalled items seems more appropriate as a measure of visual imagery. The soundness of these options is open to empirical test. For example, if anxiety has higher predictive validity when corrected for word count, the independence assumption is supported.

Gottschalk, Winget and Gleser (1969) point out that the reliability of their scales begins to decrease rapidly as the word count falls below 100. They recommend that their scales not be applied on samples of fewer than 70 words. The scales would be unsuitable, therefore, for sleep reports particularly from NREM sleep or from any sleep stage after multiple nights in the laboratory. In our recent

REM-deprivation study, we found that word count decreased from a mean of 84 words/report on Night 1 to 67 on Night 2. Gottschalk and Gleser's reliability problem would appear to stem from their use of the word-count correction. When a variable, such as dreaming, is correlated with word count, decreasing the range of word count by using samples of more than 75 words will decrease rather than increase all measures of reliability. We must conclude, therefore, that correction for word count may lower predictive validity simply because of decreased reliability.

Explicit Assumptions

One of the most refreshing things about the construction of the Gottschalk-Gleser scales is their attempt to make explicit assumptions by which they infer an affect such as anxiety or hostility from speech. Although the assumptions are based upon the psychoanalytic model, some nonpsychoanalytic investigators may find the assumptions quite acceptable while, conversely, some psychoanalysts may disagree with certain features. The great virtue of the Gottschalk *et al.* (1969) effort is that we know what the authors think it is measuring and we have an informed basis for accepting or rejecting their scales. Let us illustrate this point by once again referring to their anxiety scale. One of their key assumptions is that:

> the more anxiety a person is experiencing, the more likely he will speak of incidents in which he reports being directly threatened. . . . When the anxiety is somewhat less potent, the subject is more likely to express it indirectly by externalization or displacement and, hence, more likely to refer to others as being hurt or in a dangerous situation, and even more remotely, in terms of inanimate objects being injured or destroyed [Gottschalk, *et al.*, 1969].

The authors then assign interval weights of 3, 2, and 1, respectively, to the three ordinal classes of self, animate others, and inanimate others. Thus "Boredom and finances, that's what's killing me," and "He was so mad he might have killed me," receive a weight of 3 under death anxiety. "He took his own life," and "They caught a beauty of a trout," are weighted 2, and, "The baby pulled the doll apart," and "The whole motorcycle was demolished," are each weighted 1. An additional arbitrary weight of 1 is added to an item which is amplified by a modifier. Thus, "I am terribly afraid of being hurt," receives an additional point for the presence of "terribly." This weighting system is repeated across the six subtypes of scaled anxiety. Although the authors state that each subtype receives equal weight because the scores of each subtype are summed to create a total score, the subtypes are, in fact, weighted by the proportion of variance they contribute to the variance of the total score and this proportion, in turn, is determined empirically by the frequency of clauses scored in each subclass. This latter particular procedure is, therefore, neither arbitrary nor objectionable. The assumption that anxiety is a decreasing negative function (weights 3, 2, and 1) plus 1/0 for an amplifying modifier is, however, very much in need of empirical justification. Fortunately, the assumptions are sufficiently explicit so that they can be independently tested. Gottschalk and his colleagues have vigorously sought out empirical support for their scales, but, alas, most of their studies test the predictive validity only of the total-scale scores. In a general sense, all of the scales seem to be doing what they are supposed to but only independent tests of the various assumptions will make it possible to improve the weights of the component parts of the scales. In our opinion, the advantage of a weighted over an unweighted system must be reliably demonstrated. If weighted scores are to be used, the weights must be determined by a discriminant function analysis or multiple regression. Finally, the relative advantage of alternative scaling models must be estimated from the proportions of predicted variance accounted for, $\hat{\omega}$, rather than from simple significance tests.

We recommend that investigators studying imagery and thought during sleep follow the example of Gottschalk, Winget and Gleser (1969) in making explicit all of the assumptions underlying their judgment and scaling processes. Only by so doing can measurements based upon sleep reports have a public meaning shared by all investigators and their readers. Otherwise the meaning of a scale remains the private subjective property of the judges who scored the reports, whose assumptions are hoped to be somewhat similar to the general public's.

Validity

For the purpose of considering the validity of sleep-mentation judgments, we find it useful to divide the judgments into two classes. The first are concerned primarily with whether the persons making the sleep, particularly REM, reports have certain personality characteristics such as hostility or anxiety. Such judgments may be validated in the same manner as any other measure of individual differences as described in every textbook in psychometrics. The second attempts to compare the cognitive and affective qualities of certain physiological states such as Stage REM/NREM. The validity issue is somewhat simplified by the opportunity to use the physiological states, discrete or continuous, as criteria variables. Research strategies and statistical models appropriate to this second effort are the subject of the remainder of this chapter.

MULTIDIMENSIONALITY OF VARIABLES: RESEARCH STRATEGIES

Research on sleep mentation has, from the outset, involved multidimensional variables both on the physiological and cognitive side of the fence. Not only were the sleep stages defined jointly by EEG and eye movements and subsequently EMG, but the EEG variable involves a combination of frequency, pulse duration, and amplitude. Dreaming, the most commonly used cognitive variable in sleep research, remains an obscure multidimensional conglomerate of an hallucinatory belief in the actual occurrence of an imagined experience which, in turn, tends to be an extended visual, sometimes bizarre, drama. The first question asked of that rapid-eye-movement interval of sleep called Stage REM was of its association with dreams (Aserinsky & Kleitman, 1953; Ladd, 1892). The high degree of association repeatedly observed in the initial studies of the late 1950s promoted the compelling assumption that there was a one-to-one association between the two. As subsequent research forced the abandonment of the one-to-one model, it became necessary to broaden the search. Several variations on both the cognitive and physiological side of the fence needed consideration.

Thus the research problem became essentially a multivariate one. Yet investigators have continued to employ univariate models, at least in their data analyses. In an effort to clarify some of the issues involved, we would like to propose four research strategies relevant to the multivariate, psychophysiological study of sleep mentation:

1. one physiological variable, one cognitive variable, repeated measures on each subject; for example, phasic-tonic sleep, bizarreness;

2. multiple physiological variables, one cognitive variable, multiple measures on each subject; for example, sleep stage and phasic tonic sleep, dreaming;

3. one physiological variable, multiple cognitive variables, repeated measures on each subject;

4. multiple physiological variables, multiple cognitive variables, multiple measures per subject.

In general, most investigators think in terms of Strategy 4, but research with Strategy 1! Strategy 1 encourages the endless collection of countless psychophysiological relations but allows no way to distinguish unique associations from redundant ones. In his excellent review of "Mental Activity During Sleep," Rechtschaffen (1973) concludes that those few variables which are reliably associated with dreaming and related cognitive variables appear simply to be sharing variance that has previously been identified in what are regarded as more fundamental associations. He cites the association of dreaming within Stage REM to low-rectal temperature, pointing out that both variables are associated with REM activity, and the association of dreaming with REMs within the sleep stage is stronger than the association with rectal temperature. Rechtschaffen rightly recommends that future studies in this area must examine several variables jointly and use some kind of statistical technique to correct for the overlap among the physiological-predictor variables. Specifically, he suggests the use of partial correlation. For example, the correlation of rectal temperature with dreaming should be statistically corrected for the correlation of both with rapid eye movements.

Because of the multiple-measures-per-subject feature there is no single existing statistical data-analysis method suitable for Strategy 4. Canonical correlation comes closest since it identifies the relationship between two sets of multivariables — physiological and cognitive. Since a canonical correlation analysis generally requires a minimum of 40 independent observations per variable, working with only 5 variables in each set, we would require either one set of scores from each of 400 subjects or 400 observations on each subject. In the latter case, several subjects would be required for replications.

To avoid the blind piecemeal approach of Strategy 1 and the statistical problems as well as the high cost of Strategy 4, then, we recommend the middle ground of Strategies 2 and 3 — together with a strong background in neurophysiology! Before proceeding to examine these strategies in detail, let us say in passing that factor analysis is not appropriate as a formal analysis of data that crosses such diverse domains as cognition and physiology. If such a statistical procedure were attempted, it would tend to produce separate cognitive and physiological factors. Factor analysis is useful for reducing a large number of correlated variables to a small number of orthogonal vectors, but provides no unique shortcut to "truth." Thus, if one constructs separate scales for the measurement of purple, violet, and yellow dreams, one will obtain a "purple versus yellow dreams factor," and in grape country it might embrace a Bacchus scale! Since one can, in effect, create a factor simply by intensively building or sampling variables in the area of one's interest rather than systematically sampling within the domain of inquiry, one's factor analysis may simply mirror one's prior personal conception of the domain under study.

Having so said, we would nevertheless encourage investigators to make free use of factor analysis and canonical correlation as an intermediate step in data analysis, simply to identify patterns of organization among variables in the two domains. Appreciation of such patterns can make the subsequent steps in formal data analysis more efficient and intelligently focused.

Criterion Variable

In Strategies 2 and 3, the weights given to the multivariables in one domain are determined by, or anchored to, a single empirical point, the "criterion" variable, and thereby relatively immune to the response variable sampling problems of factor analysis. These strategies, therefore, require the judicious choice of a criterion. Should a better criterion turn up, the research must be done all over again. As the multivariate experiment increases in sample size, more and more cost and effort hang on the adequacy of criterion variables derived from the sleep reports. If the choice of a cognitive variable (Strategy 2) is a poor one, there is always some consolation in knowing one can obtain judgments or ratings on an indefinite set of variables once the sleep reports have been obtained. This is not true when the criterion is a physiological variable, in which the measurement of each variable requires a unique electromechanical system and the total number of such systems is limited to the number of channels on one's polygraph.

Despite the greater potential freedom of choice, there must be sufficient consensus among sleep researchers as to the significance of a given criterion so that it will be employed by several investigators.

When a single-criterion variable is employed it should, if possible, derive its significance from some more fundamental or larger system of variables. REMs and PIPs (phasic integrated potentials) derive their importance from their presumed relation to the PGO (parietal-geniculate-occipital) neural system. Visual imagery derives its significance from the fact that vision is one of the fundamental sensory modalities. The virtue of recall of any content as a dichotomous all-or-nothing variable is that it avoids the arbitrary selection of any dimensions within the recall universe. It is thus a crude first approximation to any variable which might be derived from "content." The significance of dreaming comes from its universal use in the vernacular of all cultures since the beginning of recorded history. More precise psychophysiological models, however, might well employ more specific cognitive criteria, for example, primary visual experience (Molinari & Foulkes, 1969) might be an appropriate criterion for a psychophysiological model of right hemispheric dominance in sleep (multiple-EEG predictors); bizarreness might be more appropriate for measures of phasic activity, including PIPs and REMs (Rechtschaffen, 1973).

Strategy 2. Multiple Physiological Variables, One Cognitive-Criterion Variable, Multiple Measures per Subject

Statistical models: Cognitive variable, continuous; physiological variables, discrete or continuous.   Again, because of the multiple-measures-per-subject feature, if a large number (20-100) of awakenings are obtained from each of, for example, 5-40 subjects, no single statistical model is available to handle the analysis. The simplest alternative is to carry out separate multiple-linear-regression (MLR) solutions for each subject, entering the physiological "predictor" variables in the same order for all subjects, carrying out incremental F tests on each added variable using a liberal alpha level because of the small N per subject. The order should be determined by a psychophysiological model rather than by an empirical criterion as in the case of stepwise MLR. The significance of the combined F tests from all subjects may be estimated by the chi-square test for combined tests (Winer, 1971, p. 49-51). Fisher z transformations can be used to estimate the average incremental contribution, R^2, of a particular variable.

Because this model handles correlated physiological variables, it permits the investigator, by means of the incremental F test, to look at the correlation between, say, dreaming and penile erection, with sleep stage partialled out.

Cognitive variable: Continuous; physiological variables: discrete and orthogonal.   This method of analysis was employed by Pivik (1971) when he examined the joint effects of sleep stage and phasic-tonic sleep on several cognitive variables. Pivik treated four sleep stages x phasic-tonic sleep as orthogonal independent variables in a randomized blocks ANOVA design. Thus, the main effect of phasic-tonic sleep is independent of sleep stage and, therefore, analogous to the effect of phasic-tonic sleep with sleep stage partialled out. This orthogonal design is a powerful technique as a test of significance, but since the two "independent" variables are, in fact, strongly dependent or correlated in normal sleep, the analysis does not present as accurate a picture of their joint action as does MLR in the statistical models discussed above.

Strategy 3

Question 3 asks the psychophysiological question from the other end: *not,* "What are the physiological correlates of a particular cognitive variable, such as dreaming?" but, "What are the cognitive correlates of a particular physiological criterion variable, such as Stage REM versus NREM sleep?" We remind the reader that the two questions are identical so long as we confine ourselves to simple bivariate relationships, such as correlations and differences between means. The purpose of our discussion, however, has been to assess the improved power of multivariate models and to compare the relative merits of three different classes of multivariate psychophysiological models: where the physiological, cognitive, or both domains involve two or more variables considered jointly, as in partial, multiple, or canonical correlation.

The selection of a single physiological-criterion variable against which to describe the joint association of several cognitive variables is just as critical as the choice of the cognitive criterion for Question 2. Two dichotomous variables, Stage REM/NREM and tonic-phasic sleep, have been acknowledged for several years as fundamental physiological classifications of sleep. They are possibly the strongest candidates for criterion variables associated with characteristics of sleep mentation. Although details in the measurement of these states are under constant revision, there are sufficient occasions during sleep which can be unequivocally classified that Stage REM/NREM sleep is quite suitable as a criterion variable. Within Stage REM, REMs themselves are acquiring longevity as a measure of phasic-tonic sleep. Other physiological criteria should probably be evaluated under Strategy 2 before being used to supercede REM/NREM sleep as a physiological criterion.

Statistical Models

Dichotomous physiological criterion; multiple, continuous cognitive variables, correlated pairs.   Each subject contributes data from both, say, Stages REM and 2 awakenings. If there are a large number of awakenings per subject, and multiple-cognitive scores derived from each awakening, a complete multiple-regression solution may be obtained for each subject, similar to the solution of page 42 of this volume. Not only is the 50-100 observations/subject impractical, however, but the order effects of motivation (p 23-7, this volume) may wash out real effects that exist. If each subject is run one or two nights, the scores from each sleep state should be averaged over all awakenings so that each subject contributes a Stages REM and 2 score for each cognitive measure. The difficulty encountered in handling this data is that not only are the cognitive variables correlated, but the two members of the pairs are correlated (Stages REM with 2).

It is instructive to examine briefly the available statistical models that don't quite do the job. If half of the subjects were observed only in one physiological state, such as Stage REM, and the remaining subjects in Stage 2, the multiple-linear-regression (MLR) model would provide an ideal solution. The physiological state would constitute a dichotomous criterion variable and the multiple-cognitive measures, the "predictors," one set of predictor scores for each subject. But if every subject provides two sets of predictor scores, that is, paired scores, the assumption of independence of the N observations is violated so that MLR analysis cannot be used, at least in its usual form.

Although Hotelling's T^2 (Timm, 1975) and discriminant function as well as multivariate analysis of variance (MANOVA) were not designed to handle the repeated measures or treatments-within-subjects design with multiple-dependent variables, special cases of each can be used to analyze this data. Hotelling's one-sample T^2 may be used to test whether the Stage REM minus Stage 2 difference scores for a set of cognitive variables simultaneously equals zero (Timm, 1975, pp. 226-229; Tatsuoka, 1971, pp. 76-81). Unfortunately, the overall significance test for the set of multiple-cognitive variables provided by the one-sample Hotelling's T^2 is not adequate for this data-analysis problem inasmuch as we are attempting to add cognitive variables to the basic REM-dreaming association which is already statistically significant. Fortunately, Rao (1973, sections 8c.4 and 8d.1) has developed a multivariate significance test, which provides a significance test for the increment in "prediction" afforded by the addition of successive cognitive measures to the model. Rao's solution is a "repeated measures" analog of the incremental F test in MLR. Unfortunately, these statistical tests were published after the analyses reported on the following pages was completed. Furthermore, we have not yet been able to derive a size of effect index from the Hotelling's T^2. Accordingly, a "repeated measures" variation of MLR developed by Antrobus (Appendix 2.2) continues to be the best statistical model for this particular type of data.

"Repeated measures" MLR

This analysis is described for the experiment in which each subject is observed in only two treatment conditions, REM and NREM. The method could, of course, be extended to multiple-treatment conditions by means of orthogonal contrasts. The basic transformation changes all raw scores to deviation scores about each subject's mean — for each subject on each of J variables. If multiple awakenings are obtained in REM and NREM sleep, the scores on each variable in a given sleep stage are averaged before obtaining a single deviation score for each stage, thereby creating a $2 \times J$, sleep stage $\times$ cognitive scale, matrix for each subject. The scores for N subjects are combined to produce a $2N \times J$ matrix, that is, each subject contributes two observation sets, one for each sleep stage. Sleep stage or any other dichotomous state (coded 1, −1, or 2, 1; see Cohen & Cohen, 1975) constitutes the criterion variable which may be regressed onto any combination of the J cognitive variables.

Version A. One may then proceed with a MLR analysis with one modification. Because of the redundancy of the paired deviation scores, the *df* for the denominator are $N - J$ = number of rows/2 − J, rather than the usual: number of rows − 1 − J.

Version B. For the price of one *df*, one may cut the card punching in half and enjoy the advantage of the standard MLR F tests in which N = number of subjects = number of observation sets. Divide the sample into two equal halves (odd, even numbered subjects), creating the dummy variable (odd/even) which costs one *df*. Let the odd subjects represent one sleep state, for example REM, and the even represent the other, Stage 2. Let the two states be the criterion variable as before (coded 2 and 1). For the odd-REM subjects, let the J cognitive predictors equal REM deviation scores

$(d_{REM_{ij}})$, where

$$d_{REM_{ij}} = \overline{X}_{REM_{ij}} - (\overline{X}_{REM_{ij}} + \overline{X}_{2_{ij}})/2$$

where $\overline{X}_{REM_{ij}}$ is the mean REM score for the ith REM subject on the jth cognitive variable, averaged over all REM reports and over all judges of those reports. For the Stage 2 subjects, the predictors are calculated as

$$d_{2_{ij}} = \overline{X}_{2_{ij}} - \frac{(\overline{X}_{REM_{ij}} + \overline{X}_{2_{ij}})}{2}.$$

This transformation of the one-sample (mixed-model) univariate problem to a two-sample (fixed-effects-model) univariate problem is described in some detail in Appendix 2.2. The extension to a multivariate problem entails no special features (Cohen & Cohen, 1975).

Statistical Models

Continuous physiological criterion; multiple, discrete and continuous cognitive variables. The analysis of this type of data must follow the approach demonstrated for the first variation of Strategy 2.

Results Using the First Variation of Strategy 3

In conclusion, we describe what we have learned to date using the first variation of Strategy 3. We have examined three data sets. Set 1, 115 REM/NREM report pairs comes from, unfortunately only, 34 subjects (see Table 2.1). Reports were obtained from different laboratories under similar baseline conditions. Sets 2 (see Table 2.2) and 3 (see Table 2.3) come from the 20 subjects described in Chapter 13 of this volume and consist of 37 REM/NREM pairs on Night 1 and 39 pairs on Night 2. Data Set 1 was rated by 6 judges; Set 2, by 4 judges. Intercorrelations generated by the 3 data sets and 2 judge sets are compared in Table 2.4. Judges were undergraduate seniors and graduate students with A standing in psychology or English. Considering the comparison of 19 studies in Figure 2.3, we are of the opinion that the size of the correlations with REM/NREM for Data Set 1 are higher than exist in the population at large though they appear to be similar to first-night results of Table 2.2. In general, Judge Set 1 seems to be better than Set 2. The relative improvement of detail and clarity of report over dreaming as a discriminator of REM/NREM sleep may represent a slight improvement in the written instructions of detail and clarity for the second set of judges.

The major limitation of the 3 data sets is that their small subject size permits the evaluation only of gross-multivariate models. We are currently assembling a data set of 90 subjects to carry out such tests. Contributions of additional data from our colleague-readers will be gratefully accepted. Our target of 200 subjects will permit us to generate statistical solutions on half of the set and replicate them on the remaining 100.

Paired-Comparison Judgments

All three data sets were scored by presenting reports in REM/NREM pairs, in which members of each pair were matched for subject and time of night. Each judge decided which member of a pair had the most of a particular quality, like, dreaming. If four judges in Set 1 judged the REM member of the pair to be most dreamlike, the score would be 4, that is, the sum of six independent, binary judgments of 1 or 0. With six judges, scores ranged from 0 to 6. Interjudge reliabilities ran above .9, as high as .99 for some variables.

With several variables, each sharing a major portion of the cognitive variance of REM/NREM sleep, there are a variety of multivariate models which can be constructed to maximize the amount of REM/NREM variance shared with the cognitive variables. Two different criteria may be employed for developing these models:

1. Empirical: Find the combination of variables that accounts for the largest portion of REM/NREM variance. The size of this proportion tells us, in effect, the magnitude of the psychophysiological bridge within sleep, although it does not illuminate us greatly about its structure. The two statistical routes for the

TABLE 2.1

Intercorrelations Among 12 Ratings and Stages REM versus 2 Criterion
(Data Set 1: 115 REM-2 Pairs, 6 Judges)

Variables.

	1	2	3	4	5	6	7	8	9	10	11	12	13
1. Stage REM-2	—	.84	.80	.78	.78	.67	.80	.34	.62	.49	-.07	-.25	.71
2. Dreaming	—	—	.92	.85	.87	.75	.88	.48	.76	.53	.00	-.16	.83
3. Visual imagery	—	—	—	.87	.85	.71	.82	.43	.73	.53	-.08	-.24	.78
4. Movement	—	—	—	—	.83	.76	.81	.34	.67	.45	-.04	-.23	.74
5. Bizarreness	—	—	—	—	—	.66	.76	.43	.65	.47	.01	-.19	.76
6. Hallucinatory	—	—	—	—	—	—	.86	.43	.75	.44	.05	-.08	.73
7. Detail and clarity	—	—	—	—	—	—	—	.50	.86	.54	.10	-.11	.82
8. Speech and verbal thinking	—	—	—	—	—	—	—	—	.52	.44	.27	.27	.53
9. Number of words	—	—	—	—	—	—	—	—	—	.42	.20	.04	.78
10. Number of "ahs" and "uhms"	—	—	—	—	—	—	—	—	—	—	.09	.02	.49
11. Reference to lab	—	—	—	—	—	—	—	—	—	—	—	.60	.06
12. Recent events	—	—	—	—	—	—	—	—	—	—	—	—	-.06
13. Emotions	—	—	—	—	—	—	—	—	—	—	—	—	—

TABLE 2.2

Intercorrelations Among 12 Ratings and Stage 1 REM versus 2 Criterion
(Data Set 2: 37 REM-2 Pairs, 4 Judges, Night 1)

	Variables												
	1	2	3	4	5	6	7	8	9	10	11	12	13
1. Stage 1 REM-2	—	.73	.60	.47	.68	.63	.79	-.24	.56	.52	-.05	.72	.37
2. Dreaming		—	.76	.68	.77	.52	.81	-.27	.66	.44	-.13	.75	.33
3. Visual imagery			—	.86	.72	.61	.87	-.27	.82	.54	.07	.61	.34
4. Movement				—	.65	.55	.74	-.34	.71	.46	.20	.54	.24
5. Bizarreness					—	.52	.71	-.19	.76	.43	-.12	.76	.28
6. Hallucinatory						—	.69	.02	.42	.42	.10	.62	.34
7. Detail and clarity							—	-.29	.78	.61	.09	.77	.28
8. Speech and verbal thinking								—	-.25	-.25	.35	-.04	-.34
9. Number of words									—	.51	.04	.62	.20
10. Number of "ahs" and "uhms"										—	.12	.36	.31
11. Recent events											—	-.07	-.36
12. Emotions												—	.20
13. Depth													—

48

TABLE 2.3

Intercorrelations Among 12 Ratings and Stage 1 REM versus 2 Criterion
(Data Set 3: 39 REM-2 Pairs, 4 Judges, Night 2)

	Variables												
	1	2	3	4	5	6	7	8	9	10	11	12	13
1. Stage 1 REM-2	—	.25	.29	.30	.14	.44	.40	-.15	.30	.16	-.13	.32	.31
2. Dreaming	—	—	.80	.74	.62	.72	.73	-.05	.53	.64	.36	.62	.23
3. Visual imagery	—	—	—	.88	.64	.81	.90	-.12	.64	.68	.24	.73	.43
4. Movement	—	—	—	—	.58	.72	.90	-.05	.63	.67	.35	.77	.22
5. Bizarreness	—	—	—	—	—	.33	.56	-.17	.55	.37	.08	.37	.21
6. Hallucinatory	—	—	—	—	—	—	.79	.06	.53	.60	.39	.69	.31
7. Detail and clarity	—	—	—	—	—	—	—	.04	.64	.71	.30	.77	.31
8. Speech and verbal thinking	—	—	—	—	—	—	—	—	.02	-.04	.61	.01	-.32
9. Number of words	—	—	—	—	—	—	—	—	—	.54	.19	.48	.10
10. Number of "ahs" and "uhms"	—	—	—	—	—	—	—	—	—	—	.26	.75	.13
11. Recent events	—	—	—	—	—	—	—	—	—	—	—	.33	-.29
12. Emotions	—	—	—	—	—	—	—	—	—	—	—	—	.31
13. Depth	—	—	—	—	—	—	—	—	—	—	—	—	—

TABLE 2.4

Correlation of Rating Scales with Stage 1 REM versus 2 Criterion
Across Samples, Nights, and Judges

| Scales | Judge Set 1 (6 Judges) | Judge Set 2 (4 Judges) | | |
| | Data Set 1 35 Subjects 115 Pairs | Data Set 1 35 Subjects 115 Pairs | Data Set 2 20 Subjects | |
			Night 1: 37 Pairs	Night 2: 39 Pairs
1. Dreaming	.84	.69	.73	.25
2. Visual Imagery	.80	.71	.60	.29
3. Movement	.78	.68	.47	.30
4. Bizarreness	.78	.70	.68	.14
5. Hallucinatory	.67	.65	.63	.44
6. Detail & Clarity	.80	.77	.79	.40
7. Speech & Verbal Thinking	.34	−.15	−.24	−.15
8. No. of Words	.62	.57	.56	.30
9. No. of "Ahs" "Uhms"	.49	.36	.52	.16
10. Ref. to Lab	−.07	−	−	−
11. Recent Events	−.25	.20	−.05	−.13
12. Emotions	.71	.66	.72	.32
13. Depth of Sleep	−	.14	.37	.31

empirical approach, employing MLR, are: (a) all possible predictors; and (b) stepwise MLR (see Kerlinger & Pedhazur, 1973). The stepwise method eliminates unnecessary redundancy in the predictor equation, so that the number of predictors is reduced to the smallest number possible.

2. Theoretical: In the interests of understanding the nature of the cognitive qualities which distinguish REM from NREM sleep, one may enter variables into the MLR equation in an order prescribed by a theoretical model of interest to the investigator. Thus, one investigator might start with regressive thought and emotionality variables. The investigator might then examine the size and significance of the semipartial correlation coefficients of the variables not yet entered before deciding on a third or subsequent variable to add.

Our own preference is to start with the conceptually simplest variables first and add variables identifying higher-order cognitive processes last. Thus, we would prefer to start with visual imagery. If the semipartial r for auditory imagery or speech is significant, we would add that next. As we move on to the higher-order cognitive qualities and processes, there is no obvious order in which significant semipartial rs should be added. Other criteria, such as the relative size of the semipartial rs and the simplicity and nature of the assumptions involved in defining the scales, should be considered. Thus, bizarreness is preferred over dreaming because bizarreness can be defined simply in terms of improbable combinations of objects and events in time and space; the definition of dreaming is much more complex.

If several variables which correlate highly with REM/NREM are also highly intercorrelated with each other, the choice of a particular subset of variables to define the cognitive-affective characteristics of REM/NREM may be somewhat arbitrary. Our best estimate from existing data sets is that cognitive variables share between .65 and .71 of the REM/NREM variance (Antrobus, Pass, Luck, Sanders, Ellman, & Arkin, 1974; Antrobus, Rich, Pass, Nelson, & Sanders, 1973). There are several combinations of variables which will sum to this value.

As soon as we can assemble a data set of 200 REM/NREM report pairs, we hope to determine reliable estimates of the weights and proportion of contributed variance of each cognitive variable to REM/NREM sleep. Having done this, we will turn to other classifications of sleep to determine at what point the strongest psychophysiological bridge may be erected.

We also intend to use waking-state reports as a reference-state point for all sleep-state multidimensional models. As Foulkes and Fleisher (1975) have shown, our presumptions about the relation of mentation from various sleep stages to waking mentation have been off mark. If we are to develop a systematic model of the cognitive operations underlying the sleep report, we must have a better understanding of the dimensions which best describe the characteristics of waking mentation. It is, after all, only the contrast to waking thought that makes the study of sleeping mentation interesting.

APPENDIX 2.1: INSTRUCTIONS TO JUDGES: DREAMING SORT

You will be given a complete set of reports obtained from a subject awakened from sleep. There will be about ____ reports in each set.

The nature of this task is to sort the reports into eight piles on a continuum of dreaming. The piles should be arranged in ascending order: Pile 1, least like a dream; Pile 8, most like a dream.

Keep in mind that the major characteristics of a dream are the presence of visual imagery, a succession of scenes often somewhat bizarre, and a strong sense that the fantasy is real.

You are asked to read each report carefully and place it in one of the eight piles according to how dreamlike you think it is. After this first sorting, count the number of reports you have in each file. The number allowed in each pile is recorded under the pile number (for example, Pile 1, N = 4 or 5). If your number does not correspond to the number allowed, re-sort them until they match the given number.

When you have finished sorting, enter the random number (located on the top left hand corner of each report) for each report in each of your piles in the appropriate column on the data sheet supplied to you.

Note: There are a number of reports in which the subject states inability to remember anything from the sleep experience. *These constitute the least dreamlike reports.* If you can make any distinctions between these reports do so. Place the least dreamlike in Pile 1. If there are more of these reports than Pile 1 can accommodate, place them in Pile 2. If Pile 2 overflows, place them in Pile 3, and so on.

APPENDIX 2.2: TRANSFORMATION OF REPEATED MEASURES DATA (TWO CONDITIONS) INTO BETWEEN GROUPS FORMAT FOR MULTIPLE CORRELATION ANALYSIS

The preliminary data array consists of one REM (R) and one NREM (NR) score for each subject $(1 \ldots i \ldots N)$ on each variable. Each score may be a single rating or word count, or the mean of several such scores averaged over several mentation reports from the same sleep stage or awakening condition. These scores $(X_{i,R}$ and $X_{i,NR})$ yield a 2 x N matrix for each variable. This appendix describes a transformation which is carried out on each of such 2 x N matrices. It then shows how these transformed matrices may be analyzed by means of a conventional one-way analysis of variance (ANOVA) with 1 and N-2 degrees of freedom. The entire set may be analyzed by means of multiple correlation/regression, with REM versus NREM as the criterion variable (see Cohen & Cohen, 1975).

The first step is to produce a matrix of deviation scores (d_i) where

$$d_{i,R} = X_{i,R} - \frac{(X_{i,R} + X_{i,NR})}{2} = \frac{X_{iR} - X_{i,NR}}{2}$$

$$d_{i,NR} = X_{i,NR} - \frac{(X_{i,R} + X_{i,NR})}{2} = \frac{X_{i,NR} - X_{i,R}}{2}$$

The subjects are then divided into 2 "dummy" samples by any random procedure such as odd (O) and even (E) numbered subjects:

Dummy Variable		Criterion State	
	Subject	REM	NREM
Odd (O)	1	$d_{1,O,R}$	$d_{1,O,NR}$
	3	$d_{3,O,R}$	$d_{3,O,NR}$
	⋮	⋮	⋮
	$N-1$	$d_{N-1,O\,R}$	$d_{N-1,O,NR}$
		$\overline{d}_{.O,R}$	$\overline{d}_{.O,NR}$
Even (E)	2	$d_{2,E,R}$	$d_{2,E,NR}$
	4	$d_{4,E,R}$	$d_{4,E,NR}$
	⋮	⋮	⋮
	N	$d_{N,E,R}$	$d_{N,E,NR}$
		$\overline{d}_{.E,R}$	$\overline{d}_{.E,NR}$
		$\overline{d}_{..R}$	$\overline{d}_{..NR}$

We now proceed to compare the Odd group in REM ($\overline{d}_{.O,R}$) with the Even group in NREM ($\overline{d}_{.E,NR}$). We will show that the F test on 1 and $N-2$ df between these means is equivalent to the more familiar correlated means test between $\overline{d}_{..R}$ and $\overline{d}_{..NR}$. It is proven in section A that $\overline{d}_{.E,R} - \overline{d}_{.O,NR} = \overline{d}_{..R} - \overline{d}_{..NR}$, providing $n_O = n_E$, and therefore, that $\overline{d}_{.E,R} - \overline{d}_{.O,NR}$ provides an unbiased estimate of $\mu_R - \mu_{NR}$. Further it may be shown that the pooled MS$_\text{Within Groups}$ provides an unbiased estimate of and any Treatment x Subject interactions which may exist (see Section B). The usual mixed model, randomized block ANOVA F test with 1 and $N-1$ df is thus converted into a fixed effects ANOVA F test with 1 and $N-2$ df. The loss of 1 df tends to be offset by slightly larger F values, so that no loss in significance level is incurred.

A. Proof that

$$\overline{d}_{.O,R} - \overline{d}_{.E,NR} = \overline{d}_{..R} - \overline{d}_{..NR} \qquad (1)$$

Since

$$\overline{d}_{.O,R}$$

and

$$\overline{d}_{.E,R}$$

are based on independent samples, they will not necessarily $= \overline{d}_{..R}$.

Let

$$\overline{d}_{.O,R} + a = \overline{d}_{..R}. \tag{2}$$

For the sake of simplicity, consider the case where $n_1 = n_2$, and therefore,

$$\overline{d}_{..R} = \frac{\overline{d}_{.O,R} + \overline{d}_{.E,R}}{2} \tag{3}$$

Substituting, 2 into 3,

$$\overline{d}_{.E,R} - a = \overline{d}_{..R}. \tag{4}$$

Since

$$\overline{d}_{i,O,R} = -\overline{d}_{i,O,NR} \tag{5}$$

then

$$\overline{d}_{.O,R} = -\overline{d}_{.O,NR}, \tag{6}$$

and

$$\overline{d}_{..R} = -\overline{d}_{..NR} \tag{7}$$

Substituting into equation 3,

$$\overline{d}_{.O,NR} = -\overline{d}_{..R} + a = \overline{d}_{..NR} + a$$

and,

$$\overline{d}_{.O,NR} - a = \overline{d}_{..NR}. \tag{8}$$

Similarly,

$$\overline{d}_{.E,NR} + a = \overline{d}_{..NR}. \tag{9}$$

Substituting in equations 2 and 9,

$$\overline{d}_{.O,R} - \overline{d}_{.E,NR} = (\overline{d}_{..R} - a) - (\overline{d}_{..NR} - a) = \overline{d}_{..R} - \overline{d}_{..NR}.$$

B. Statistical Models

Each score may be partitioned as follows:

$$\overline{d}_{ij-k} = \overline{d}_{...} + (\overline{d}_{.j.} - \overline{d}_{...}) + (\overline{d}_{.j-k} - \overline{d}_{.j.}) + (\overline{d}_{ijk} - \overline{d}_{.j-k})$$

where i is subject within group, j is one of two criterion (R or NR) conditions, k is Odd or Even sample, $j - k$ indicates the intersection of a particular level of j with a particular level of k, for example, Odd-REM, and $\overline{d}_{...} = 0$.

If we subtract $\overline{d}_{...}$ from each side of the equation, square each side, and sum over all subjects in the two condition combinations, Odd-REM and Even-NREM (see Section A), the three cross-product terms cancel out and we are left with

$$\sum_{j-k} \sum_i (\bar{d}_{i,\,j-k} - \bar{d}_{...})^2 \;=\; \sum_{j-k} n_{j-k}(\bar{d}_{.j.} - \bar{d}_{...})^2 + \sum_{j-k} n_{j-k}(\bar{d}_{j-k} - \bar{d}_j)^2$$
$$+ \sum_{j-k} \sum_i (\bar{d}_{i,\,j-k} - \bar{d}_{j-k})^2.$$

$$\sum_{j-k} \sum_i (\bar{d}_{i,\,j-k} - \bar{d}_{...})^2 \;=\; SS_{total},$$

which is partitioned into

$$\sum_{j-k} n_{j-k}(\bar{d}_{.j.} - \bar{d}_{...})^2 \;=\; SS_{between_{j-k}}$$
$$=\; SS_{between\ treatments\ (REM\ vs.\ NREM)},$$

$$\sum_{j-k} n_{j-k}(\bar{d}_{j-k} - \bar{d}_j)^2 \;=\; SS_{jxk\ treatment\ by\ group\ interaction},$$

and

$$\sum_{j-k} \sum_i (\bar{d}_{i,\,j-k} - \bar{d}_{j-k})^2 \;=\; SS_{within\ treatments}.$$

The sums of squares of (SS) of this model have the following relationships to the sums of squares of the more familiar $2 \times N$ randomized blocks ANOVA*:

$$SS_{between\ treatments} \quad\quad = \; \tfrac{1}{2}SS^*_{between\ treatments}$$

$$SS_{treatment\ by\ group\ interaction} = \; \tfrac{1}{2}SS^*_{treatment\ \times\ subject\ interaction}$$

$$SS_{within\ groups,\ treatments} \quad = \; \tfrac{1}{2}SS^*_{within\ groups} \quad\quad (since\ subject\ effect\ has\ been\ removed)$$

$$MS_{between\ treatments} \quad\quad = \; \frac{SS_{between}}{1}.$$

Following Hays (1973), Chapter 12),

$$E(MS_{between\ treatments}) \quad = \; \sigma_e^2 + \frac{\overline{\sum_{j-k} n_{j-k}\sigma_{j-k}^2}}{1}.$$

The $SS_{treatment\ by\ group\ interaction}$ constitutes a nuisance factor on 1 df, and is discarded. The remaining $SS_{within\ groups,\ treatments}$ are associated with $J(N - 1)$ or $N - J\ df$. Following Hays (1973, Chapter 12), $E(MS_{within\ groups,\ treatments})$ = σ_e^2, and therefore constitutes the appropriate denominator for the F test of the group treatment effect.

In summary, the between treatment effect has been converted from a within subject to a between group difference; the error term, converted from a treatment-by-subject interaction to a within-subject effect. The loss of 1 df in the error term tends to be offset by a smaller $SS_{within\ groups}$.

EDITORS' INTRODUCTION TO CHAPTER 3

This chapter presents a deeply thoughtful review and analysis of the problem of NREM mentation and describes an unique experiment dealing with important issues at the heart of sleep research. Its central approach to the subject involves a study of the effects of experimenter bias on the content of both REM and NREM mentation reports. It is probable that an experiment of this kind cannot be done often. Attempts to replicate it would very likely be hampered by the technical staff being "wised-up" to the various conditions entailed by the design features because the true aims of the principal investigator could not remain in concealment; that is, similar work would have been carried out in so many laboratories that alert, scientifically informed technicians would have suspicions about the hypotheses being tested such that an authentic double blind design would be difficult of implementation. We are, therefore, fortunate to have this beautifully executed piece of work to provide us with clear-cut results before experiments of this sort become popular in the field.

3

The Problem of NREM
Dream Recall Re-examined

John H. Herman

*Department of Psychiatry, Southwestern Medical School,
University of Texas Health Science Center, Dallas, Texas*

Steven J. Ellman
Department of Psychology, The City University of New York.

Howard P. Roffwarg
*Department of Psychiatry, Southwestern Medical School,
University of Texas Health Science Center, Dallas, Texas*

INTRODUCTION

The study of when dreaming occurs in sleep has produced the most confusing literature of any in the sleep field. Though the controversies are complex, the dialogue essentially boils down to whether or not (and to what extent) dreaming occurs in NREM sleep. Making sense of whether dreaming is found in more than one sleep stage on the basis of the reports in the literature is difficult, though it appears that careful examination and comparison of various studies permit the formation of some reasonable inferences. It is our contention that, even with attempts at neutralization of differences among studies, an irreducible and inexplicable discrepancy remains between the data from two main camps of investigators.

The student of this field is confronted with one group of papers that virtually writes off NREM dreaming and another that claims high rates (over 50%) for this phenomenon (see Table 3.3, column 4). Certainly, in view of these massive differences in the data from several of the major laboratories in sleep research, presumably working on the same problem, a suspicion is raised as to whether, indeed, the same experimental question was really being researched. In this review we examine several key variables that were not treated in the same way by investigators and show how the differing methods appear to have influenced reported rates of REM and NREM recall.

Because dissimilarities in the design and execution of studies of dream recall do not completely reconcile the conflicting data in this area, there exists the possibility that experimenter bias played some role. We speak of experimenter bias in the sense of a heightening of data expectancies owing to theoretical convictions as well as failures to control for the influence of these expectancies on the putative findings. Experimenter expectancy can blind an investigator to the importance, or even the existence, of certain material in the field of view by affecting definitional loadings and choice of design. The investigator may, as a result, unwittingly predetermine the outcome of the experiment or possibly promulgate results in fashions and in contexts that skew their implications.

In this chapter we selectively review certain prototypical groups of studies. Matters of definition, criterion, method, and interpretation are explored in terms of the effects that, in our view, they may have had on the reported findings. Additionally, we examine a possible cause of sharply divided experimenter expectancies that is rooted in the models of certain experimenters vis-à-vis physiological differences between the sleep stages and their implications for dreaming. Such a review is particularly timely since the most recent development, the phasic-tonic model (Grosser & Siegel, 1971; Moruzzi, 1963), is currently accepted by many as the best means available of explaining the physiological concomitants of dreaming (Molinari & Foulkes, 1969).

Finally, we present an experiment that actually attempted to study whether varying experimenter expectancies which were built into several of the conditions of a study examining dream recall affected the reported incidence of dream recall. By appraising the several sources of variation and the "bias" experiment presented in Part 2, we hope to assess to what extent, if any, experimenter and subject expectancy may have affected the results in earlier work on dream recall. Though it is impossible to prove that bias was or was not operative in any given study, we hypothesize that in some instances it was a concealed factor in setting the different directions taken by the data. However, such matters are not easy to unravel and will, of course, remain largely in the realm of speculative reconstruction.

PART 1: AN EXAMINATION OF THE METHODOLOGICAL
APPROACHES AND DIVERGENT DATA

Dreaming and the Psychology of Sleep

The first proposed physiological correlate of dreaming was the presence of eye movements. In both the Aserinsky and Kleitman (1953) paper and a follow-up by Dement (1955, p. 273), experimental awakenings were performed when eye movements were present, and control awakenings were performed at a time during sleep when eye movements were absent but the electroencephalogram was similar to that of the experimental awakenings. The concept of stage of sleep, or state, had not yet been developed. These two studies reported 74 to 92% vivid dream recall respectively when eye movements were present in sleep and 7 and 0% recall respectively when they were absent. These studies appeared to demonstrate that vivid dreams occurred in conjunction with eye movements, and that they occurred infrequently, if at all, in their absence. Dement (1955), noting this psychophysiological correlation, stated that "the appearance of eye movements themselves suggested that they were a direct result of visual experience. . . [p. 268]." Thus, dreaming was considered a correlate of ocular activation. The control awakenings were done when no eye movements were recorded and the EEG was similar to that when eye movement awakenings were done. Presumably, the control awakenings were done from light NREM sleep and not from ocular quiescent moments within the REM periods, but this is not at all certain. In any event, the key link to the dream imagery seemed to be eye activity, and the REM awakenings were apparently done at the moment of REM bursts, but this was not explicit. Several later studies (Dement & Kleitman, 1957a; Kales et al., 1967; Wolpert & Trosman, 1958) emphasized that dreaming was most likely to occur during the periods of REM sleep, not in the intervening periods lacking eye movements when a synchronized EEG was present (non-REM or NREM sleep).

Dement and Kleitman's (1957a) paper, "An Objective Method for the Study of Dreaming," reported 79% dream recall from REM awakenings and only 7% recall of dreams following NREM awakenings. After finding 85% detailed recall from REM awakenings and 0% following NREM awakenings, Wolpert and Trosman (1958) concluded that the "dream investigations have culminated in the demonstration that the physiological correlate of visual dreaming consists of low voltage, nonspindling brain wave patterns associated with the presence of rapid eye movements [p. 603]." Believing that they had identified stage REM as the indicator of dreaming mentation, Dement and Kleitman (1957) suggested that "the few instances of dream recall during NREM periods are best accounted for by assuming that the memory of the preceding dream persisted for an unusually long time [p. 341]."

Studies that demonstrated the high correlation between REM and dreaming were not confined to the 1950s. In 1967, Kales, Hoedemaker, and Jacobson found 81% REM recall and 7% recall from NREM. This group, in another paper, summed up their findings by observing, ". . . it appears that except for sleep onset. dreaming is infrequent during subsequent NREM sleep throughout the night [Kales et al., 1966, p. 136]."

The discovery of rapid eye movements during sleep and their association with dreaming was quickly followed by the uncovering of a large number of physiological variables that behave differently within the REM sleep envelope than without. Consequently, a shift in emphasis took place so that dreaming began to be considered the mental homologue of the *state* of REM sleep, and not simply of eye movements. REM-NREM rapidly began to assume a differing role; that is, observable registrations of particular parameters available at the time were taken to be only the most superficial markers of a massive and basic organismic dichotomization. Investigators treated REM and NREM as differing states that superceded the few known differences in CNS and autonomic patterns. REM sleep was even termed "a third state of human existence [Snyder, 1965]," and Kramer (1969) stated that during REM sleep "the organism is neither asleep nor awake."

The distinction between REM sleep and dreaming was often overlooked. REM (or "activated" or "paradoxical") became synonymous with dreaming — a derivative of a host of shifts in mentation quality from that in NREM sleep. Dement spoke of "dream depriving" cats as though the purported correlations between Stage REM and dreaming in humans were absolute and universal in all mammalian species. Cats and dogs can also be said to look as if they are dreaming when twitching, pedalling their paws and breathing irregularly. Wolpert and Trosman (1958), in a study of the frequency of dream recall stated, as was typical for the time, that awakenings were done at the "beginning, middle," and "after dreams were over," having in actuality performed early-, middle-, and late-REM awakenings.

In addition to the above studies, which demonstrated that dream recall occurs most frequently following REM awakenings, various experiments were performed with the express purpose of uncovering the psychophysiological links in the chain relating REM sleep to dreaming. Indications of a quantitative relationship between the state and the amount of dream material were reported by Wolpert and Trosman (1958), who found that the length of a dream narrative was positively correlated with the length of a given REM period. Although Dement (1955, p. 268) had reported no correlation between REM-period length and the length of dream report in earlier work, later, more systematic study of this relationship supported the Wolpert-Trosman findings, (Dement & Wolpert, 1958b).

Other findings also came to light from the early studies and seemed to lend weight to the model that REM sleep and dreaming are integral to each other. A correlation was found between the amount of time a subject *thought* was spent dreaming and the span of REM time (Dement & Wolpert, 1958b); Wolpert and Trosman already had reported in 1958 that a body movement in the course of a REMP seems to end a dream episode or scene and signals the start of a new one. A further assertion was that REM periods that contained two or more dream scenes were found to be punctuated by gross body movements whereas continuous scenes came from relatively body movement-free REM period sequences. Stimulation of subjects in REM with light flashes, water spray, and so on frequently found its way as clear incorporations into concurrent REM (Dement (1965a).

Research examining the possibility of a quantitative relationship between ocular activity during REM and reported visual activity grew out of the certainty that REM sleep was dreaming sleep. Dement and Wolpert (1958a) as well as Berger and Oswald (1962) had noted that REM periods with many eye movements yielded mentation reports with more physical activity than did REM sleep awakenings associated with ocular quiescence. This was the first line of evidence suggesting that not only was dreaming related to REM sleep but that the quantity of REMs had a correlate in the nature of the mentation. Recently, however, both Krippner, Calvallo, & Keenan (1972), and Hauri and Van de Castle (1973b) have not been able to confirm the relationship between ocular and dreamed physical activity.

In 1965a, Dement stated that "the most conclusive evidence that dreaming takes place during the REM period . . . is the demonstrable correspondence between the specific directional patterns of REMs and the spatial orientation of events in the dream [p. 173]." Roffwarg et al. (1962) made the focus of a discrete investigation the possibility of a specific point-for-point relationship between the direction of polygraphically registered eye movement and hallucinated shift of gaze reported by the dreamer. This group attempted to assess the goodness of fit between the number and direction of the actual eye movements immediately prior to the awakening and a prediction by an interrogator of those parameters. The latter was based on a careful assessment of the subject's visual narrative. A "good" concordance between eye movements and imagery was reported in a sizeable proportion of all electrooculogram/dream narrative pairs. It is not necessary to demonstrate an intimate relationship between eye-movement incidence and imagery alteration (let alone a directional uniformity) to prove simply that dreaming and REM sleep are related. But, if true, there would be specific, predictable, and quantitative equivalences of components of the presumed physiological substratum with variations in the visual dream. Later studies by Moskowitz and Berger (1969) and Jacobs, Feldman, and Bender (1971) have not been able to confirm this relationship. Roffwarg (1975) has since acknowledged a methodological fault in his 1962 data analysis. Nevertheless, researchers still have difficulty questioning that the eye movements of REM are not simply the physical counterpart of hallucinated gaze shifts in the dream. (For a full and elegant discussion of the REM-imagery experiments, see Rechtschaffen, 1973).

The purported isomorphism between REM sleep and dreaming was based upon the high dream-recall rates in that state as well as upon assertions of specific associations between physiological REM components and appropriate dream actions. Such correspondences between dreaming and specific physiologic components of the REM state have continued to be uncovered. Watson (1972) recently offered evidence that phasic bursts of extraorbitally recorded electrophysiological activity were associated with the appearance of swift change, ("bizarreness") in the dream content. Roffwarg, Herman and Lamstein (1975) found correspondences between middle-ear muscle activity in REM sleep and auditory components of the dream. Gardner et al. (1975) were able to demonstrate a statistically significant correlation between limb action in the dream and the appropriate actual limb action. Such findings have given support to the presumed tie of the REM state to dreaming.

The "Intrusion" of NREM Dreaming

Given the widespread acceptance of the marriage of dreaming and the REM state, and the corollary that dreams recalled in NREM sleep are residues left over from previous REM experience, the emphatic claim of Foulkes (1962) that dreaming was also a property of NREM sleep caused a theoretical upheaval and a scrambling for new positions.

Foulkes (1962) reported that far more mentation occurs during NREM sleep than had previously been reported (see Table 3.3, column 4). Additional studies which reported higher recall following NREM awakenings soon followed (Orlinksy in 1962 reported 43% NREM recall; Kamiya in 1961, 46%; Goodenough et al. in 1959, 35%; Foulkes in 1962, 74%; Foulkes and Rechtschaffen in 1964, 62%; and Pivik and Foulkes in 1968, 64%). Not only did these experimenters find more mentation in NREM than did the early studies, but Foulkes (1966) observed that subjects more frequently than not thought they had been awakened from a "dream" following NREM arousals. In this study, visual recall was present in 62%, at least one character other than the dreamer in 50%, and two or more scenes in 38% of NREM awakenings. As a matter of fact, because subjects frequently described NREM mentation as dreamlike, visual, and as containing more than one episode, no criterion or set of criteria was found (or has yet been developed) that qualitatively differentiates REM content from NREM content. Foulkes (1967b) alleged that "the modal NREM experience is not described by subjects as a thought but as a dream . . . perhaps different more in degree than in kind from the REM experience [p. 35]."

Nevertheless, experimenters who observed frequent and dream-like NREM mentation lacked a physiological underpinning that would lend validity to their assertions. At the time, there was little evidence of singular neurophysiologic activity and motor outflow in NREM sleep. Therefore, NREM "dream" proponents were faced with the burden of proving that their results were not artifactual. Controls not thought to be necessary for studies of REM recall were performed by this group in order to demonstrate that what was being reported was indeed mentation from NREM sleep. Foulkes and Rechtschaffen (1964) controlled for the possibility that NREM reports might have been the memory of previous REM sleep, and found that NREM recall rates were not affected if the subject was interrogated following the previous REM period. (No one has ever checked to see if REM reports are the memory of a prior NREM experience.) Goodenough et al. (1965), as well as Foulkes (1967b), found that the abrupt, quickly gathered NREM report is no more likely to produce dream recall than is a report gathered following a gradual awakening. Since subjects who on a suggestibility scale were found not to be compliant or amenable to suggestions have the same rate of NREM as those who are, Foulkes (1967b) argued that NREM recall is not a product of confabulation or an attempt to please the NREM-interested experimenter.

In the cross discussion concerning the nature of NREM mentation, several developments emerged:

1. Virtually all observers came to agree that at least some mental content occured during NREM. No longer could it simply be entertained that the mind lay dormant, in NREM, only to spring alive with phantasms in REM.

2. Studies of REM versus NREM mentation showed that it was a difficult but possible task for blind judges to distinguish reliably between the two (Monroe, 1965); and the conclusion, which has gained wide currency in the field, was drawn that, in general but not always, NREM mentation is "more poorly recalled, more like thinking and less like dreaming, less vivid, less visual, more conceptual (Rechtschaffen, Verdone & Wheaton, 1963 [p. 411]).

3. Dement (1965a) saw real "dreams" as "experiences that include primarily perceptual activity in both a physiological and psychological sense." However, Dement incorporated later observations that small quantities of phasic activity are found in NREM into a neurophysiological argument for the existence of NREM mentation. From Dement's own laboratory came information that the K complexes of Stage 2 sleep were frequently associated with phasic EMG suppression. The imagery of NREM was expected to be lower in grade than in REM because there is vastly more central phasic discharge in the latter (Dement, 1975a).

In recent years, both the REM and NREM dream camps have found the phasic-tonic physiological model an effective supplanter of the REM-NREM state model in terms of dreaming. It allowed both Dement to persist in a perceptual/phasic model of dreaming, and Foulkes to claim anew that REM-NREM dream differences are, in effect, only a matter of degree.

An Attempt to Understand the Divergent Claims of REM/NREM Discriminability

With the foregoing discussion as a backdrop, we are now in a position to examine the early recall experiments with respect to their content yield from NREM sleep. The reported rates of "dream" recall from NREM sleep were so contradictory that it is necessary to clarify the process by which a number of serious investigators, purporting to research the same problem, arrived at such widely divergent results.

We will first evaluate definitional and methodological differences.

Subject Selection and Population

Most dream-recall studies have suffered from a small subject population. That this is not a new problem can be seen in Table 3.1, column 1. Of the 11 studies,

TABLE 3.1

Comparative Methodologies of NREM
Recall studies: some quantitative parameters

Studies	No. of Subjects	Subject population	Number of Nights	Number of awakenings		When in REM awakened	When in NREM awakened	How awakenings distributed through night
				REM	NREM			
Aserinsky and Kleitman (1953)	10	"Normal adults"	14	27	19 (?)	Eye-movement burst	Probably Stage 2, 30 min after REM	Not described
Dement (1955)	13	Medical students who dreamt once or twice a month at most, 22-32 years old	?	50(EM)	19(NoEM)	During eye movements, 5-50 min	EEG pattern similar to REM EEG	?
Dement and Kleitman (1957a)	9	Medical students	61, of which 40 were from 3 subjects	191	160	Eye-movement burst	Stages 2, 3, and 4	Approximately ¼ every 2 hrs
Wolpert and Trosman (1958)	10	"Men"	51, 32 of which from 2 subjects	54	26	"Middle" of the "dream"	At least 10 min after EMs ceased	Not described
Kales, Hoedmaker, and Jacobson (1967)	3	The 3 authors	40	134	108	2-10 min after REMP onset	15 min at least, after previous REMP from any NREM sleep stage	6 awakenings divided equally by halves of night
Goodenough, Shapiro, Holden, and Steinschriber (1959)	16	8 college students who reported dreaming every night and 8 who dreamt less than once per month	48	91	99	EM burst 5-15 min into REMP	At least 10 min after REMP	2 REM, 2 NREM per night

Study								
Kamiya (1961)	25	?	250	—	400	None	?	?
Foulkes (1962)	8	Age 17-27	56	108	136	Balanced long, medium, and short time into REM	Stages 1, 2, 3, and 4	Counterbalanced schedule
Hobson, Goldfrank, and Snyder (1965)	10	"Selected on the basis of their interest and ability to express themselves	4-6 nights each	195	102	Stage REM half with and half without EMs	Stages 2, 3, and 4	Not described
Pivik and Foulkes (1968)	20	College students	40	—	158	—	30 min after prior REMP	Stages 2, 3, or 30 min into NREMP, balanced evenly throughout the night
Molinari and Foulkes (1969)	10	Persons likely to be adept at introspective discrimination	40	40	40	½ REM eye movement burst, ½ REM ocular quiescence	Stage 2	Done in counter-balanced order
Foulkes and Pope (1973)	14	College students with high "openness to experience" score	3 per subject	186	—	78 REM burst, 54 sawtooth, no REM. 54 quiescent for REM and sawtoothing		Random order of awakening categories

7 listed have 10 or fewer subjects. The small subject populations could well be a factor in what may have been an excessive REM/NREM differentiation. For instance, Rechtschaffen (1973) wondered whether "a very fortuitous selection of subjects [pp. 5-6]" might have contributed to the high REM-low NREM recall figures. But why a small number of subjects should lead to *this* type of error and not the reverse is not easily apparent. Furthermore, Dement in 1955, used 13 medical students and, in another experiment (Dement and Kleitman, 1957b, see Table 3.1) used 9. However, in the 1957 study, 40 of the 61 nights were from 3 of the 9 subjects and it is possible that these 3 had recall patterns more congenial to the hypothesized model.

Perhaps the early studies employed subjects who were naturally "good" recallers, thus yielding the high REM-recall percentages. However, Dement (1955) states that, of 13 subjects, "none admitted dreaming more frequently than once or twice a month [p. 264] ... " And he also remarks that some of them "stated that they dreamt only once or twice a year [Dement, 1955, p. 268] ... " This population seems similar to Goodenough et al.'s (1959) "nondreamers," yet Dement's figures of 90% REM recall and 0% NREM recall are far different from Goodenough's findings of 46% REM recall and 17% NREM recall. Another study that showed very high-REM and very low NREM recall was that of Kales, Hoedemaker, and Jacobson (1967). In this study, the three authors constituted the subject population themselves and can be said to be "aware" or knowledgeable as to the criteria of dream content evaluation as well as of the hypothesized REM/NREM-recall differences.

In fact, it appears that most of the studies that showed high REM and practically no NREM recall, shared the feature of a knowledgeable subject population. Perhaps the awareness by the subject of the key differentiators was a variable of some import in producing the high REM-low NREM-recall figures.

In terms of differentiating REM from NREM, little can be done with the awakening that produces no content or the vaguest of memories. Surely, the subjects who serve in the laboratory have to produce dreams for analysis. For that purpose the frequency and type of home dream recall has been increasingly utilized as a screening parameter. But probably more critical factors than the incidence of previous home recall are the analytic and resolving abilities of the subject: sophistication about the quality of the information imparted, capacity to be precise and deal in detail, the orientation the subject has (or is given) to the individual's importance in the study and, of course, motivation to perform honestly and objectively in a demanding situation without feedback.

Perhaps much of the deficiency in distinguishing REM from NREM sleep is related to using a subject population that is ill-equipped to describe accurately the exact qualities of the mentation preceeding arousal. In truth, few individuals are truly "excellent recallers." Only by carefully selecting those rare individuals who are able to give rich and detailed reports from most awakenings is it possible to assess the extent to which mentation from the two sleep states overlap. For example, Foulkes and Pope (1973) report 50% auditory recall from phasic and tonic REM awakenings while 2 of the authors of this chapter (Roffwarg, Herman & Lamstein, 1975) observed more than 90% audition from awakenings in a subject population that was demandingly screened (less than 1 subject accepted of every 50 applicants) for excellent dream recall. A fair chance exists that the better the recall ability of the subject population, the more the experiment would be able to demonstrate any subtle nuances of recall quality that differentiate REM from NREM mentation.

We speculate that the subjects in the early Dement (see Table 3.1) studies were "knowledgeable," being comprised of fellow students and friends with whom the experimenter shared concepts about "real" dreams appearing at only certain times in sleep and not others. The highly polarized REM/NREM recall rates in these studies, we believe, represent not only the subject's memory of the actual mentation, but the unwitting superimposition of a decision grid as well. The subject, to some degree, judges the mentation himself and engages in an out-of-awareness decision as to whether it will be accepted as dream-like by the experimenter. Imagery above a certain threshold of vividness is sensed and presented as a "dream." Imagery at any level below that threshold does not pass muster as a "dream," and is, therefore, not reported. This amplifying and reducing process, we feel, effected a bimodal sharpening of the differences in imagery in the 2 states, a sharpening into a too dichotomized misrepresentation of the actual states of mentation. Accordingly, the data from the early studies, in which we infer that the "apex" REM experience was the de facto criterion of dreaming, operated not so much to demonstrate the incidence of imagery in each state as they purported to, but to demonstrate that under certain conditions the mental content in REM and NREM could be successfully differentiated in 2 groupings as it is known judges can do fairly well (Monroe et al., 1965). Antrobus and Fisher (1965) have shown also that subjects can distinguish between REM and NREM awakening. In the "dreaming or not" type of design the subject could conceivably "learn" that only a certain quality of mentation or "state" was sufficient and the materials that did not meet the criteria of this "state" could be disregarded. This could well have the effect of training the subject to exclude certain types of reports and emphasize the more vivid ones.

The Influence of How Dreaming Was Defined on Rates of NREM Recall

A prime factor leading to very dissimilar NREM "dream" recall rates was the patent lack of agreement as to what defined a dream. Dement (see Table 3.2) applied terms in his definition of dreaming such as "quite vividly," "fairly detailed," and "coherent" whereas Foulkes (see Table 3.2) in his definitions, used the terms "occurrences," "recall," or "mentation." Such striking differences make it clear that Foulkes and Dement had designed experiments to examine different hypotheses. Therefore, the reported recall figures obtained from their experiments are not comparable.

TABLE 3.2

Comparative Methodologies of NREM recall studies: Interrogational procedures.

Studies	What was the initial question asked	Definition of dreaming used by experimenter
Aserinsky and Kleitman (1953)	?	"Detailed dreams"
Dement (1955)	?	"Remembered dreaming and were able to recall the content quite vividly."
Dement and Kleitman (1957) (*b*)	Asked to state whether or not they had been dreaming.	"A coherent, fairly detailed description of dream content."
Wolpert and Trosman (1958)	Subject "asked to report his dream, if any . . ."	"Detailed" or "fragmentary" dreams.
Kales, Hoedmaker, and Jacobson (1967)	Subject pretrained, not questioned when awakened.	The presence of any sensory imagery with development and progression of mental activity.
Goodenough, Shapiro, Holden, and Steinschriber (1959)	Subject pretrained, not questioned when awakened.	"A dream was recalled in some detail."
Kamiya (1961)	Subject questioned for all able to remember.	At least a "short but coherent dream, the parts of which seem related to each other."
Foulkes (1962)	Asked subject "if he were dreaming" and if not, "what was going through his mind."	"Any occurrences with visual, auditory, or kinesthetic imagery."
Hobson, Goldfrank, and Snyder (1965)	Subject pretrained to "recount what was going on in your mind for the last 30 seconds."	"Complex visual imagery which had undergone some development."
Pivik and Foulkes (1968)	Subject asked, "What was going through his mind."	The presence of "some mentation."
Molinari and Foulkes (1969)	Subject pretrained, not questioned when awakened.	Some visual experience.
Foulkes and Pope (1973)	"What was the very last thing going through your mind just before I called you?"	Total recall: any mentation recalled "very well" determined by subject.

Not only are the definitions of dreaming quite vague in most of the studies, but behind each of them was the experimenter's concept of what was a "true" dream and where in sleep it resided. The early idea of what is a dream was an unquestioned concept, something the investigators believed would be intuitively understood. However, the stated definitions contained in their published reports were at best only (to their group) internally meaningful descriptions of what is commonly meant by "dreaming" (see Table 3.2, coulmn 2). The greater the difference between certain unstated parameters in the definition employed in their analysis of the data and the public definition contained in their report, the more misunderstanding and nonreplicability could and did result.

These experimenters, in a sense, thought they "knew" what a dream was. Dreams were surely vivid, sensory, coherent, sequential, and strong in the temporal dimension (some of these criteria were not explicitly stated in the definition at the time; Dement, 1965a). Presuming to know what a dream was, the investigators took it as their task to find when in sleep it could be found. The REM dream (actually the "apex" or most vivid REM dream) came to define all dreaming. A high threshold was unwittingly set for imagery to be defined as dreaming. In effect, the more vivid and striking REM dream was accepted as the definition for the standard dream, and so it was the "apex" REM dream that was searched out in all stages. This might have predetermined where it would be found — in REM sleep almost exclusively. Experimenters and subjects (from whom there was no apparent reason to shield the defining characteristics of dreaming) together erected a filter that screened out vague and fragmentary imagery. It is perhaps possible that "apex" REM dreaming, as against more standard REM dreaming (both in contrast with mentation), occupies only 0-7% of NREM recall.

The fascination of the early experimenters with the active and floridly discharging REM state, we feel, provided a seductive framework for acceptance of only sharp and interwoven perceptual-like imagery as dreaming. Such a state, it was felt, must have a unique subjective component, and that component must be the pure-vein REM dream. In other words, given dilution by the vagaries of dream memory and narration, the sense was that but for those filters, the "apex" dream must be the standard dream experience in REM sleep.

When Foulkes (1962) was attempting to demonstrate that a subject could report mentation from any stage of sleep, he deserted the term "dreaming" in his definition and set off on his own to observe what forms and types of recall were reported subsequent to NREM arousals. His opening question to his subjects was to ask if they "were dreaming." The dream-like fantasy (DF) scale was the first to be subjected to rigid reliability checks (the inter-rater reliability was found to vary between .85 and .99, Foulkes, Spear, & Symonds, 1966; Larson & Foulkes, 1969; Pivik and Foulkes, 1968). However, this scale was acknowledged by Foulkes to be superior for the categorization of NREM recall than for REM recall. It is a poor tool for assessing REM-NREM mentation differences because the scale reaches its "ceiling" with the scoring of relatively brief and static images that, to many investigators, do *not* constitute sufficient material for a "dream." The percentage-recall figures that Foulkes (1962) reported from both REM and NREM sleep can be confusing since he has never provided a definitional point on his scale that minimally corresponds to what is ordinarily considered dreaming. Foulkes, in effect, sidestepped the issue of when, and to what extent, dreaming occurs. From the definitional (really conceptual) point of view, it is clear that at first he felt unwilling to classify a "dream" as any particular sort of mental activity. His methods accorded with his theoretical suppositions; namely, that imagery and mentation can take many forms and it is arbitrary to categorize one type as dreaming and another as not. His investigative role and his technique aimed at bringing all sleep mentation into scientific view.

The Influence of the Initial Question Asked and How the Subject Was Interrogated on Reported Recall

Enormous variations in types of dream content may be obtained in the laboratory depending on how the subject is questioned (see Table 3.2). For example, asking only for the last 10 sec of the dream content, in contradistinction to the whole dream, may make it much more apparent whether clarity of detail exists. Also, in studies in which specifics of imagery (features on a face, precise description of how the gaze shifted from one point to another, and so on) are probed for, the differentiation of a clear perceptual experience from similar but less perceptual content becomes possible. However, this is done more in psychophysiological correlation studies than in dream-recall studies.

Asking whether or not the subject has been dreaming can have a vastly different impact than asking the subject to report all that can be recalled. If the subject was asked whether or not a dream had occurred, the subject might well recall mentation but, as has been pointed out above, might prejudge it and consider it too fragmentary or thought-like to label a dream. The subject would then fail to report material that the experimenter might consider dream-like. On the other hand, if the subject is asked to report anything that can be recalled, this will elicit all mentation and allow the experimenter to evaluate whether or not the content is dream-like on the basis of the experimenter's criteria.

Dement and Kleitman asked their subjects "to state whether or not they had been dreaming." Quite differently, Foulkes asked the subjects to say what had been going through their minds if at first they did not recall a dream (see Table 3.2, column 1); Pivik and Foulkes asked the subject "What was going through your mind,"akin to the question of Hobson, Goldfrank, and Snyder, who asked their subjects to "recount what was going on in your mind for the last 30 seconds" (see Table 3.2, column 1).

One possible danger in the technique of requesting any and all contents of mental activity from the awakened subject is the possibility that the "set" will be to feel always responsible to produce something, anything. (Similarly, the subject who is asked if he was dreaming might feel pushed towards reporting dream material.)

This attitude conceivably may cause the subject to blur the distinction some-what between the preawakening and during-the-awakening (hypnogogic) processes, providing any wisp of sensation from either to a content-sensitive scale. In any event, the experimenter, using the "total recall" method, is at least in a position to make assessments of the nature of the content. The experimenter who uses the "all-or-none" interrogation can never evaluate what has not been told.

Different methods of interrogating the subject may also lead to differing results. At one extreme is the method of pretraining the subject and requiring spontaneous reporting of recall. Kales, Hoedemaker, & Jacobson (1967), as well as Goodenough et al. (1959), pretrained their subjects to recount all they recalled spontaneously; the subjects were not interrogated following awakenings. At the other extremes are the preconstructed interview format (Foulkes, 1966) and the technique of allowing the interrogator free reign to question the subject as desired.

Each method has advantages and disadvantages. Obviously, not having to question subjects at all or having the questions on tape are the only ways to eliminate the possibly biasing effects of the voice of the experimenter. However, this method does not allow the experimenter to ask questions that the subjects might have neglected to answer, or to make sure sleepy subjects are fully alert and have reported all they can recall. The open interview format does not safeguard the experimenters from interjecting their own bias and influencing subjects. On the other hand, the preconstructed interview does not generally allow the experimenter the option to pursue a new line of questioning or to adapt the questioning techniques to what might best be utilized in a specific awakening. For instance, if a subject were to describe a visual scene in response to the standard queries, additional questioning might reveal that this scene is actually either fragmentary or rich in perceptual detail.

Was Recall Rated by a Scale or on an All-or-None Basis?
Were Reports Evaluated by Blind Judges?

Many of the studies of dream recall scored the subjects' report as either positive or negative, dream or no dream, and so on based on a given set of criteria. Other experiments (Kamiya, 1961; Pivik & Foulkes, 1968) used a predefined scale for recall and placed the recall at the best-fitting level (see Table 3.3, column 3). As noted above, with this method all recall is given a rating and may later be appraised.

The all-or-none type of design has the effect of creating a dichotomy (dreaming or not) when, in actuality, the material would be more accurately graded according to a continuum. This polarization of findings is reinforced by the ease of

TABLE 3.3

Comparative Methodologies of NREM recall studies: procedures for rating recall.

Studies	Was recall rated relatively objectively?	Were recall reports evaluated blindly?	Was recall scored by a scale or on an all or none basis?	REM-NREM rates of recall
Aserinsky and Kleitman (1953)	No	No	All or none	74% (eye movement) EM dreaming 11% NEM dreaming 22% NEM total recall
Dement (1955)	No	No	All or none	92% eye movement dream recall 0% ocular quiescence dream recall
Dement and Kleitman (1957b)	No	No	All or none	80% REM dreaming 7% NREM dreaming
Wolpert and Trosman (1958)	No	No	All or none	85% REM detailed 6% REM fragmentary 4% NREM fragmentary 96% NREM "none"
Kales, Hoedemaker, and Jacobson (1967)	No	No	All or none	81% REM dreaming 2% thinking 7% NREM dreaming 28% thinking
Goodenough, Shapiro, Holden, and Steinschriber (1959)	Yes	Yes	All or none	93% REM for "dreamers" 53% NREM for "dreamers" 46% REM for "nondreamers" 17% NREM for "nondreamers"

Study				
Kamiya (1961)	Yes	No	Scale	27% NREM dreaming 46% NREM total recall
Foulkes (1962)	Yes	Yes	All or none	82% REM dreaming 54% NREM dreaming 74% NREM total recall
Hobson, Goldfrank, and Snyder (1965)	Yes	Yes	All or none	76% REM dreaming 14% NREM dreaming 37% NREM total content
Pivik and Foulkes (1968)	Yes	Yes	Scale	72% Stage 2 recall 64% Stage 3 recall 46% Stage 4 recall
Molinari and Foulkes (1969)	Yes	Yes	All or none	100% REM "phasic" 58% REM "tonic" 75% NREM
Foulkes and Pope (1973)	Yes	Yes	Scale(s)	Total recall: 95% REM burst 87% sawtooth 87% no REM or sawtooth Recalled "very well": 45% REM burst 50% sawtooth 50% no REM or sawtooth

reducing a study to a single recall figure following REM and another following NREM awakenings, thus lending a superficial clarity to the results.

The frequency of dreaming in a particular stage is commonly reported by a single-percentage-recall figure. This type of data may derive from either an all-or-none questioning technique ("were you dreaming?") or from a scale in which, at some point, an arbitrary cutoff is created, above which the report is considered a dream and below which it is not. That a large proportion of the awakenings might have yielded material that was barely more or less dreamlike than required is never elucidated in the single-percentage method of reporting results. Most of the studies utilizing scaled responses make the frequency of response at each scale point available in the reports.

What is apparent is that many of the early all-or-none studies might well have given higher ratings to NREM content if all impressions were drawn from the subjects and scaled. Wolpert and Trosman (1958) would have found 28 rather than 0% recall had they included their "fragment-only" category as content that was scaled positively.

In terms of a separate issue, potential dangers existed in the early studies with regard to the objectivity of information gathered from the subjects. Foulkes' DF scale rated recall along four dimensions that were clearly specified and relatively objective. In contrast, most earlier studies had definitional clauses for dreaming but no relative priorities of importance or specified scoring methods. Foulkes' scale is designed for use in conjunction with a particular format in which the interrogator is pretrained and interrater reliability tests are performed (Pivik & Foulkes, 1968; NREM, $r = .97$). Similarly, Goodenough et al. (1965) taped their interviews and had them rated by a judge who had no knowledge of the awakening condition. In the experiment described subsequently in this chapter the definitions of dreaming are also objectified.

In contrast to these studies stand others in which more fluid classificatory techniques were employed. In many (Dement; Dement & Kleitman; Kales, Hoedemaker, & Jacobson), it is not specified that the interrogators and perhaps even the judgement makers were fully aware of the awakening condition. Not blind to the awakening condition, they gathered the information and may have made on-the-spot decision as to whether or not the report was a dream. Since the definitions employed were circular, or at least private (that is, a dream was often *defined* as " a dream" or "dream-like," see Table 3.2, column 2), there existed a relative paucity of objective criteria according to which the report could be evaluated. A similar problem is presented in a recent study (Molinari & Foulkes, 1969) in which classificatory categories were created and clearly specified but only after the experimenters listened to and evaluated the recall reports. The authors acknowledged the use of these post hoc definitions to distinguish what was to be termed phasic from what was labeled tonic recall. They believed their effort would have heuristic value. But the pitfalls of compromised study procedures and data analysis are demonstrated by the fact that later studies of this duality of mentation by Foulkes and colleagues (Foulkes and Pope, 1973) have not been clearly confirmatory of the original suggestions.

The Possible Influence of the Schedule of Awakenings on Recall Rates

There is indication from some research that "time of night" may prove to be as significant a variable as stage of sleep in explaining recall variance. Pivik and Foulkes (1968) reported that Stage 2 recall increased from 14% in the beginning of the night to 75% by the second half of the night. It has also been noted by many, but recently commented on by Krippner et al. (1972) that REM recall is poorer and less active during the first REM period. Thus, controlling for time of night is especially important in any study of differences in recall purportedly attributable to stage of sleep. When not controlled, and the awakening distribution not made clear, as was frequent in most early studies, time of night may greatly enhance REM/NREM dream-recall differences.

REM periods are of briefer duration in the first half of the night. While approximately 18-25% of all sleep is scored as REM, approximately half of the last two hours of a normal night consists of REM sleep. Unless carefully controlled, it would be easy to conduct a study of REM-NREM recall in which a majority of the REM awakenings occurred later in the night. This leads to a frequently unanalyzed interaction of time-of-night factors with stage of sleep. Most studies have not described how their awakenings were distributed throughout the night, and of those that have, very few matched the REM and NREM reports by time of night.

Another temporal consideration of some importance is the moment within the REM and NREM periods when awakenings are performed. Again, most early studies set, at best, loose limits for how long into a period an awakening could be executed. Apparently, NREM recall is very poor immediately after the termination of the prior REM period and then improves during the subsequent interval of NREM sleep. Baldridge, Whitman, and Kramer (1962) found that recall was 16% from 7 to 15 min after the cessation of eye movements, and 70% 31 to 63 min after eye movements ceased. For example, it is possible that Kales, Hoedemaker, and Jacobson, who found only 7% NREM recall, might have produced this low figure as a result of having done all their NREM awakenings 15 min after the end of a REM period rather than later in NREM sleep (see Table 3.1, column 6). Similarly, Wolpert and Trosman (1958), who failed to observe any detailed NREM recall, only stated that they waited "at least ten minutes after eye movements ceased." Pivik and Foulkes (1968), at the other extreme waited until at least 30 min of NREM sleep had occurred and noted 72% Stage 2 recall.

PART 2 – A STUDY OF THE EFFECT OF EXPERIMENTER
EXPECTANCY ON NON-REM RECALL

It is reasonable to suppose that early investigators were highly expectant of vast state differences in dream recall between REM and NREM sleep. They were ready to assume a connection in REM between the prolonged sequences of phenomenal activity and concomitant, perceptual-like mentation. On the other hand, it would appear that those who were first to find substantial NREM imagery had been scientifically offended by either or both the theory and the adequacy of the early data that dreaming occurred exclusively in REM sleep.

With hindsight, it now appears that an array of definitional, procedural, and data-treatment variables had a part to play in the divergence of the evidence from the two groups. Many of the differences now seem amenable to some degree of reconciliation. However, on analysis, it does not appear that accounting for the study differences simply in terms of design and execution can account for the totality of the almost astonishing discrepancies. At root is the question: Since mentation is now widely accepted as observable in NREM, how was it the early studies failed to report it?. One is pushed to look for additional explanations.

As pointed out earlier, the several experimenters had different theoretical expectations of how the mind functions in the NREM phases of sleep. Their findings seemed to confirm these expectations. Is it possible that their opposite dispositions may have selectively affected the directions of the recall data? To illustrate, if an examination is made of the findings, holding, for example, the definition of dreaming fairly constant, how much would the data differences be reduced? Kamiya (1961) stated that the criteria he employed to accept sleeping mentation as dreaming ("the subject remembers a short but coherent dream, the parts of which seem related to each other") is approximately as restrictive as that used by Dement and Kleitman (1957), who had defined dreaming as a "... coherent, fairly detailed description of dream content." Notwithstanding, though the explicit definitions are reasonably alike, Kamiya found four times as much NREM recall as did Dement and Kleitman (27% versus 7%). Goodenough et al. (1959), requiring that the dream be recalled "in some detail", observed 35% NREM recall, whereas Dement (1955) found 0% NREM recall when he asked the subjects "to recall the content quite vividly."

These observations force certain conclusions:

1. Differences in rates of recall that were reported by different studies cannot be entirely reconciled by standartizing definitions of dreaming.

2. The high degree of discriminability between REM and NREM recall reported in several studies (Aserinsky & Kleitman, 1953; Dement, 1955; Dement & Kleitman, 1957a; Kales, Hoedemaker, & Jacobson, Kales, Paulson, Wilson,

1967; Wolpert & Trosman, 1958) did not result only from differences in their published definitions of dreaming.

3. Factors other than the definition of dreaming must have influenced how much mentation a subject reported from REM and NREM awakenings in many of these studies.

It is difficult, of course, to be sure even when studies are equilibrated along lines of the definitional parameter, that they were not at the same time dissimilar on methodological or data-treatment grounds. It is likely that the design of no two studies that yielded different data can be brought completely into apposition. Accordingly, the idea that extraprocedural factors played a role as well will probably remain inconclusive even at the end of this exploration.

Inevitably, the subject of bias has to be approached, and its examination may yield some useful leads about interrogation studies in general and dream-recall studies in particular. In approaching it, we make the assumption that no worker in the dream-recall field knowingly skewed data just to make it come out to subjective liking. Rather, our point of view is that investigators may, at times, have been unaware victims of their scientific passions. Further, they may have been blinded to interactions of their biases with study procedures. For example, in the early studies, there were few barriers to the experimenter's communicating a host of cues to the subject, including when recall was or was not expected. The pairing of this experimenter expectancy with an interview situation in which the subject was asked to report simply whether or not "dreaming" had occurred left more than ample room for the possible incursion of bias. These uncontrolled factors, we believe, may have led to sizable differences in outcome between early work and later research that employed rank and scaling questionnaires for all mentation. We believe that the former methods had a vastly different impact on subject narratives than the later methods that examined all that the subject could recall.

Beyond the published accounts of initial question and interrogational procedures in mentation studies, it is imperative to examine the demand characteristics that are exerted upon the subject in the experimental situation. The gathering and judging of narratives by the experimenter is susceptible to influence, if, and whenever, the experimenter is aware of hypothesis and condition. Likewise, the responses of a subject are affected whenever performance is evaluated by a hypothesis-persuaded (biased) experimenter. The demand characteristics of a study are defined as *the effect of all the interpersonal expectations that the subject perceives that are not intended investigational variables.*

In the experiment on dream recall carried out in this laboratory, we explored whether or not bias may influence subject responses. We did so in the hope of shedding some light on the question of why subjects' dream recall seemed to discriminate differentially between REM and NREM sleep far more acutely in some studies than in others. In other words, beyond differences in methods of awakening, leadoff questions to subjects, and definitions of dreaming, could the subjects' responses have been influenced also by experimenter expectancy?

We explore this issue further by reviewing some landmark studies that threw light on the subtle but powerful effect that the attitude of the experimenter can induce. They have been conducted to demonstrate the conditions necessary for an experimenter biasing effect to occur and the extent to which bias may influence results. Perhaps the best-studied area has been that of person perception. Fifty-seven experiments have been reported that evaluated the bias effects and were reviewed by Rosenthal and Rosnow (1969).

In an illustrative experiment (Rosenthal & Fode, 1963), 10 advanced undergraduate and graduate students in psychology were utilized as "experimenters," all of whom had experience in conducting research experimentation. The "experimenter" showed 10 photographs of faces to each of 10 subjects individually. The subject's task was to evaluate the degree to which the faces suggested the success or failure of the individuals. A scale of +10 to −10 was was provided (+10 indicating extreme success, and −10 indicative of utter failure). The photographs had been preselected to be as neutral as possible on this dimension; that is, to produce a mean of 0. All 10 experimenters were given identical instructions to read to their subjects. Half the experimenters were led to believe that a "well-established" result from such ratings, was a mean of +5; the other half were given a mean of −5 as "well-established." The result was that all experimenters expecting higher ratings obtained higher ratings than those expecting lower ratings.

Adair and Epstein (1967), found that a tape recording of a biased experimenter's instructions to subjects is sufficient to significantly influence the subject's responses in the direction of the expectancy, whereas other research has shown that certain conditions fail to produce a significant biasing effect. Some examples include equal status of experimenter and subject (Barber et al., 1969) or when the experimenter remains mute (Moffat, 1966).

Experiments have been conducted repeatedly to demonstrate this biasing potential in areas as diverse as learning (Kennedy et al., 1968), intelligence testing, (Getter, Mulry, Holland, & Walker, 1967), psychophysical judgment (Weiss, (1967), reaction time (Wessler, 1968), projective tests (Masling, 1965), and animal learning (Rosenthal & Fode, 1963). Even when an intermediary (that is, a technician) is hired to work with subjects, protection against the bias of the experimenter is not conferred. Research has demonstrated that a principal investigator's expectations were more closely related to the subject's responses than the latter was to the expectations of the hired research assistant who had direct contact with the subject (Rosenthal, 1966). This finding may have special relevance to sleep-dream research because of the common utilization of research assistants.

Furthermore, it has been shown by Rosenthal, Friedman, and Kurland (1966) that the manner in which an experimenter reads standardized questions to a subject will influence the nature of the subject's responses. The influence, or bias, always turns out to be in the direction of the experimenter's investigational hypothesis. Similarly, Raffetto (1968) found that the experimenter's expectancy influenced the frequency with which subjects reported hallucinatory experiences while in a 1-hr sensory restriction experience. This occurred even though the data gathering interview consisted of well-structured questions to be answered mostly by "yes" or "no."

From these studies, we may speculate that whenever a sleep-dream investigator is aware of the experimental hypothesis and the condition of the awakening, he is in a position to influence the nature and extent of reported mentation. The explicit wording of the experimenter's questions may not reveal the emphasis of the experimenter and the actual demands placed upon the subject.

As we have already observed in regard to the dream recall studies, we feel there is reason to believe that the initial question asked by the experimenter, the manner in which the subject was questioned, and the demand characteristics of the experiment had particular effects on the results of a considerable number of the dream-recall studies, though the extent to which they were affected still remains a matter of conjecture. None of them was performed under totally double-blind conditions. The experiment we carried out was designed to assess the extent to which bias could influence results of an otherwise rigidly controlled-sleep laboratory dream experiment.

We realize that it is never possible to demonstrate retrospectively that bias was, in fact, operative and that it did indeed influence the results of previously performed work. However, we feel it would be instructive to learn what lapses in method can produce recall-rate differences. It is also reasonable to examine what precautionary measures dream-recall studies could undertake in order to insure that the theoretical attitudes of the authors did not influence the experimental results. Our review of several studies suggests to us that most were ripe for the possible incursion of experimenter bias. We are led, consequently, to ask to what extent may experimental bias influence rates of REM and NREM recall?

We performed an experiment that replicated the techniques utilized by other laboratories in the collection and analysis of dream reports. However, in addition, we manipulated the bias of the experimenter and subjects in an otherwise carefully controlled experiment. REM and NREM recall were gathered from four experimental groups that were identical except for procedures intended to affect expectancy.

The expectancy, or bias, of the experimenters assigned the tasks of collecting the subjects' dream reports was manipulated by leading them to believe that they were studying the effect of nortriptyline (Aventyl) on dream recall. The experimenters were told that this drug previously had been found to increase recall dramatically from all stages of sleep. (In fact, only a placebo would be administered). The differences in rates of dream recall between the various groups in this study would be attributable to the anticipation of an increase in recall supposedly caused by the drug.

A second variable examined was the effect on recall of instructions given to the subjects. Half the subjects who were supposedly administered the drug were instructed to expect recall on every awakening. The "experimenters" gave the other half of the subject group instructions intended to minimize the expectancy. As a result, the subject population was divided equally into drug and nondrug halves, which subdivided into high-recall and low-recall expectancy. This design allowed manipulation of the bias of both the "experimenters" and subjects either together or independently of each other. Accordingly, the effect of experimenter bias, subject bias, and the cumulative effect of the two could be studied against a fourth group in which neither experimenter nor subject was intentionally biased.

Since the experimental manipulation was the introduction of a bias intended to increase recall, it was expected that the most demonstrable changes in mentation rates would be from NREM sleep inasmuch as the rates from REM might already be at a "ceiling" level. Although this study was of both REM and NREM recall, and bias was equally imposed upon both states, we presumed that a bias towards REM state recall already existed in the mind of the "experimenters." We reasoned that the main effect would be in NREM in which a similar expectancy was being introduced. This would work to neutralize the normal differential in recall rate between the two states.

Methods of Inducing and Measuring Bias

Though we wanted our "experimenters" to be disposed to a high-recall expectancy, we were equally concerned that this experiment should be comparable to others in the field. This necessitated: (1) a bias that was not overwhelming; and (2) a natural way of communicating the bias to the "experimenters." Every effort was made to introduce and carry out the "Aventyl experiment" in a manner similar to the way experiments normally proceed in our laboratory, not only as far as the "experimenters" were concerned, but in our dealing with all other laboratory staff, none of whom knew the double nature of the experiment (everyone in the laboratory believed that half the subjects were receiving Aventyl and half placebo, whereas they were all receiving placebo).

The high-recall Aventyl expectancy was induced as follows:

1. The director of this laboratory, in the middle of a laboratory meeting, remarked with interest to investigators and technicians that the tricyclic antidepressant, nortriptyline (Aventyl), which had strong CNS norephinephrine activity, had been found to increase dream recall in a pilot study, and that this laboratory was considering a larger scale and better controlled replication study.

2. A fraudulent three-page mimeographed abstract of the pilot work, under the authorship of a noted sleep investigator, was circulated. It described, in some

detail, how the drug was found to increase NREM recall greatly (from 20 to 92%) as well as REM recall (from 86 to 99%).

3. Experimenters were chosen according to the procedure described below. They were given copies of the Aventyl abstract. The rationale of the experiment was explained to them, and they participated in meetings in which final procedures were determined.

4. Experimenters were given so-called Aventyl capsules in original, "sealed" containers (all of them had already been refilled with placebo). From these, they were instructed to make their own placebo capsules by filling half the Aventyl capsules with lactose.

5. Three Aventyl pilot nights were run by each experimenter in which experienced sleep researchers and confederate colleagues of the principal investigators, serving as pilot subjects (not uncommon in this lab), reported prerehearsed dreams every time they were awakened.

Design

The experiment consisted of a four-cell, matched-groups design. Subjects were assigned to one of the four conditions, on the basis of home dream recall and demographic factors. Two "experimenters" duplicated the complete four-cell design in terms of their independent study populations. The four cells were constituted as follows:

Cell 1: In this group, the experimenter told the subjects that they were receiving Aventyl, a drug that enhanced recall to the point that dreams were usually recalled following every awakening. The experimenters believed they were administering a CNS norepinephrine-increasing medication that, as they were told by the investigators, had been found to increase recall dramatically from both REM and NREM sleep. Thus, both experimenter and subject were biased towards a high dream-recall in this cell.

Cell 2: The subjects in this group received "no-effect" instructions. They characterized the experiment as one in which voice changes were to be studied during different stages of sleep. The experimenter informed the subjects that awakenings were for the purpose of recording voice fluctuations, and the questioning about dreams provided a suitable format, considering the time and circumstances, to have a standardized verbal interchange. The experimenter told the subjects in this cell and in Cell 4 that the pill they were receiving was a salt tablet that reduced skin resistance to better facilitate EEG recordings. Since the experimenters believed they were administering Aventyl to the subjects in this cell the effect of experimenter bias alone could be studied in this group (that is, high recall expected by experimenter only).

Cell 3: Subjects in this group were given the same high-recall instructions as those in Cell 1, but the experimenter believed a placebo was administered. In this cell high dream-recall expectancy was induced in the subject only.

Cell 4: Subjects in this group received the "no-effect" instructions described for Cell 3. Experimenters believed they were administering a placebo (that is, "no-effect" expectations for experimenter and subject).

Each subject spent two nights in only one of the above four conditions. Each of the experimenters recruited their own subject pools and executed the complete four cell design. Five factors were studied:

1. whether both, either, or neither of the experimenters' subject pools were affected by the Aventyl bias;
2. the differential effects of the Aventyl and placebo conditions on recall;
3. the difference in recall rates between the high-recall and no-effect instructions;
4. the effect of the experimental conditions on the subject's first versus second laboratory night, and
5. whether the experimental effects influenced both REM and NREM sleep or only one.

"Experimenters"

Two male undergraduate students administered all phases of the experiment. They were selected by a sleep investigator from another institution who was unaware of the actual purpose of this experiment. This procedure was undertaken in order to rule out the possibility that *we* might choose experimenters who seemed easily malleable to our own biases (cf. Rosenthal & Fode, 1963).

Subjects

Twenty male undergraduates were recruited by each experimenter. Those given high-recall instructions were from different campuses than those given low-recall instructions. This was done to minimize the possibility of contact between subjects in the same experiment, who were given different expectations about the study. Subjects were recruited by means of a public notice that the experimenters placed on the campus advertising for males with "normal sleep patterns." Our departmental secretary received all inquiries and placed names alternately on the list of potential subjects for each of the two experimenters.

Procedure

EEG, EOG, and EMG were simultaneously recorded from each of two subjects in private bedrooms adjoining a master control room. The subjects were awakened by calling their names via a two-way intercom system. All awakenings were taped. A signal marker indicated the moment the subject was called.

The experimenters followed a schedule that required three paired REM and NREM (Stage 2) awakenings on each night according to a sequence that controlled for time of night, order of awakenings (counterbalancing REM-NREM sequence), time in stage, and period number. Following the awakenings, the experimenter questioned the subject according to the Foulkes' DF-scale interrogation format (Foulkes, 1966), and then asked whatever additional questions were necessary to rank the subject's recall on the Orlinsky scale (Kamiya, 1961). Also noted were the EEG stage of awakening, time of night, period number, and elapsed time in stage, as well as elapsed time from the moment the subject was called to: (1) the moment awakened; (2) the moment of first verbal response; and (3) the moment coherent response began.

After subjects were called, they were asked "What was going through your mind just before I called you?" A subject reporting no recall would be asked to "think for a moment or so and see if anything comes back to you."

Rating Scales

As mentioned above, subjects were first questioned according to a flow sheet developed by Foulkes (1962), which enabled the ranking of their recall on a 0 to 7 scale. The Orlinsky scale is identical for scores of 0-1, but requires increasing complexity, multiplicity of scenes, and development of plot in its 2-7 ratings. For instance, a 7 on the Orlinsky scale requires "an extremely long and detailed dream sequence of five or more stages. . . [Kamiya, 1961]" in contrast to a 7 on the Foulkes (1966) scale which requires only a single perceptual, hallucinatory, and bizarre recollection.

The Foulkes DF scale makes fine distinctions between varying types of recall in terms of whether it is conceptual or perceptual, mundane or bizarre. In contrast, the Orlinsky scale is fairly gross at its lower levels, but is the superior instrument of the two scales for differentially assessing long, multiple-scened, narrative dreams. It was expected that the Foulkes DF scale would be a better instrument for measuring the effect of the experimenter and subject bias following NREM awakenings, and that the Orlinsky scale would prove better at measuring bias following REM awakenings.

Results

This study demonstrated that the bias affected both "experimenter" and subject in the predicted direction following NREM awakenings, but not following REM awakenings. The REM rate of recall stayed fairly consistent between conditions. Both the experimenter-expectancy and subject-expectancy manipulations affected NREM recall. We found a cumulative effect when both subject and experimenter were biased. The magnitude of the bias effect was 0.55 standard units when the high experimenter- and subject-expectancy cell (1) is compared to the low-experimenter- and subject-expectancy cell (4), using the Foulkes DF scale (see Figure 3.1). To put 0.55 standard units into perspective, one standard unit on the Foulkes scale was the difference between total REM and NREM rates of recall across all cells in the study. In other words, 0.55 units represents a sizeable

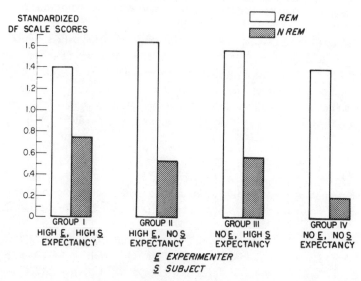

STANDARD SCORES (+1.01) *FOR DF SCALE:*
EFFECTS OF E AND S EXPECTANCY ON REM AND NREM RECALL

FIG. 3.1.   The height of each bar represents the standard score conversions of Foulkes' DF rankings in a specific cell. Standard scores yield a single number that represents recall for REM or NREM in each cell. All the NREM values are below the grand mean.

effect size. Second, the magnitude of the bias remains consistent across all levels of NREM recall for both the Foulkes and Orlinsky scales, contrary to expectations (see Figures 3.1-3.3).

Also of interest are the size of the differences between REM and NREM recall seen in all experimental conditions. In the high experimenter- and subject-expectancy cell (1), REM recall is 0.65 standard units higher than NREM on the Foulkes scale. The REM-NREM scale differences were somewhat larger in the other three cells, reaching more than one standard unit in Cell 4. *The effect of the bias in Cell 1 is as large in magnitude as the stage-of-sleep effect (REM-NREM), indicating that the bias influencing NREM recall is potent and can substantially affect experimental results.*

An analysis of variance of the NREM-recall figures, as assessed by the Foulkes DF scale, showed a nonsignificant, overall F ratio in the comparison of the four conditions. Planned orthogonal comparisons performed on this analysis of variance revealed that the two extreme cells (1 and 4) are significantly different ($t = 1.80; p = .05$), and that the high experimenter-expectancy (Cells 1 and 2) conditions are significantly different from the low experimenter-expectancy (Cells 3 and 4) conditions ($t = 1.76; p = .05$). However, the high subject-expectancy instruction conditions (Cells 1 and 3) did not differ significantly from the "no – effect" instruction conditions (Cells 2 and 4), though they varied in the

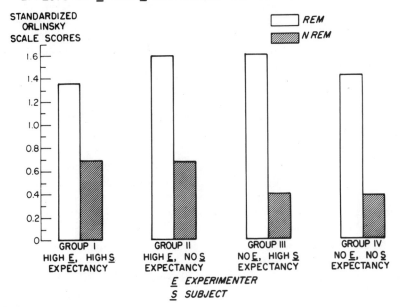

FIG. 3.2. Standardized score for the Orlinsky scale. The levels of recall of REM and NREM were quite similar to the Foulkes scale.

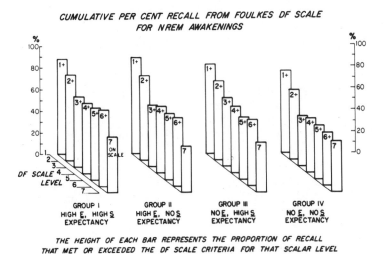

FIG. 3.3. Cumulative percent recall. REM recall in the high experimenter–, high subject expectancy condition is usually greater for any level on the DF scale than is the comparable level in the other three cells.

predicted direction. Further data analysis showed that both experimenters were contributing equally to the between-groups experimental variance, and that the bias effect was present on both of the subject's nights in the laboratory.

Since Rosenthal (1966) reported that later subjects run by an experimenter show more of a bias effect than subjects who are run earlier, we performed a subject-order analysis in our study. It was found that, in general, recall from both REM and NREM increased across *all* experimental conditions as the experiment progressed. This increase did not seem to be typical of the bias effect insofar as Cell 1 showed the smallest change.

An analysis of recall by time of night showed, first, that NREM recall (as measured by Foulkes' DF scale) rises but never reaches REM recall levels in any interval of the sleep period. NREM recall, though consistently lower in ratings than the REM awakenings, towards the end of the night approaches a level that is similar to REM recall at the beginning of the night. Second, with respect to the bias effect, it is more operable towards the early morning hours, though the individual means suffer from too great intragroup variance (the number of observations they represent is extremely small). Also, the differences between recall rates from the first REM-period awakenings and from later REM periods are far smaller than usually reported.

As noted, we found smaller differences between REM and NREM recall than reported in the literature. We believe that, this can be accounted for, to some extent, by the generally poor recall exhibited by most subjects in the course of this study. Because we made an effort to accept the very first 40 subjects who called and who met the widely-ranging criteria for home recall, we accepted some subjects who probably would be exempted from most laboratory studies of dream recall.

Both experimenters' subjects took an average of 2 sec to arouse except for the low experimenter- and subject-expectancy cell (4) in which the latency to arousal was twice as long (perhaps a bias effect, see Figure 3.4). REM awakenings generally showed a slightly greater latency to arousal than did NREM awakenings (see Figure 3.3). Further analysis showed that subjects usually uttered some verbal response within the next .5 sec. The latency to a coherent verbal report is consistently greater in the high-experimenter- and subject-expectancy condition despite this group's shorter latency to arousal. In effect, then, subjects in biased conditions spent more time awake before beginning their reports of recall than did control subjects. In fact, Experimenter 2 waited roughly twice as long to interrogate subjects after NREM awakenings from the highest bias condition than from the other three conditions.

In order to see if the results in this experiment were created mainly by the subject's recall and not by biased ratings by the experimenters of the subjects' recall (independent of actual differences in their mentation), a sample of 28 tape-recorded awakenings, 7 from each of the 4 cells, was sent to 3 independent judges. All 3 of the judges were senior investigators of national repute, who were

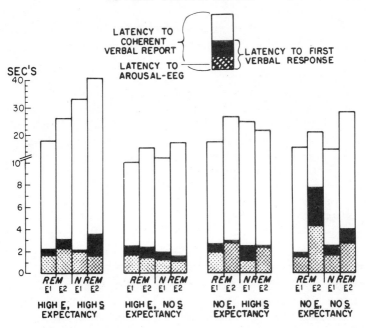

FIG. 3.4.   Latency in seconds to arousal (cross hatch), to the first verbal response (black portion), and to a coherent verbal report (clear portion), for both REM and NREM from each of the two experimenters.

familiar with the use of dream-evaluation scales and had conducted recall experiments of their own. The judges were blind to stage of sleep and condition of awakening. Comparisons were made between their ratings and those from our laboratory. These can be summarized as follows:

1. In all but the low experimenter- and subject-expectancy cell (4), our experimenters rated recall slightly higher than the independent judges. However, this difference was greatest in the low experimenter- and high subject-expectancy group (Cell 4). It did not follow a pattern consistent with the experimental results in which the high experimenter- and high subject-expectancy cell contained the greatest bias effect.

2. Somewhat inexplicably, the tendency for our experimenters to rate recall at a higher scaler level than the judges occurred almost completely for REM awakenings. As a consequence of this tendency, the slightly higher recall rating by our experimenters, compared to the judges, in no way contributed to the main NREM experimental effect. The differences in ratings might well be due to

differences between our "experimenters" and the judges' use of the high end of the rating scales (the portion of the scale most used in REM) rather than as a product of experimenter bias.

3. Each of the three judges was able to ascertain correctly whether an awakening followed REM or NREM sleep approximately 70% of the time (chance = 50%).

4. All three judges reported that they were unable from the taped interrogations to detect any signs of bias on the part of the experimenters towards maximizing or minimizing recall in *any* of the awakenings. However, the judges noted that, at times, one of the experimenters, in the interrogations did not follow the prescribed format and would make not infrequent rambling and humorous side comments. However, these irregularities, when analyzed by condition did not appear to follow a systematic variation.

Discussion and Conclusions

This experiment demonstrates that the expectancies of both the experimenter and subject can have subtle but pervasive effects upon the outcome of sleep-mentation studies. They must be exactingly controlled. One way of interpreting our results is that we were able only to bias NREM recall inasmuch as no appreciable effect upon rates of REM reporting was found. However, we think there is an advantage in viewing the outcome of this experiment as evidence that the degree of *discriminability* of REM and NREM mentation may be clearly altered by experimenter expectancy. In other words, in the highest-expectancy cell (1), the difference between REM and NREM rates of recall is 0.65 standard units as opposed to Cell 4, in which no bias was induced, in which the difference in recall from the two states is 1.19 standard units, almost a twofold increase. Another way of looking at that result is that the discriminability of REM from NREM recall on the DF scale was halved by our bias intervention. In reporting 90% REM and 0% NREM dreaming, Dement (1955) had, in effect, claimed virtually complete discriminability between the two states of sleep. Goodenough and his coworkers' data (92% REM and 53% NREM dreaming; see Table 3.3), differed from Dement's in asserting that far more NREM dreaming exists, but they essentially pointed to a far lower order of discriminability as well.

Our results are in line with those investigators who found substantial amounts of NREM mentation and a relatively small REM-NREM discriminability. Though some NREM recall can be traced to expectancy even in our no bias group (Cell 4), substantial NREM recall was observed.

Notwithstanding this NREM finding, this study also demonstrates the robustness of the by now venerable state theory of sleep. For throughout our four-group design, experimental variance is related chiefly to state of sleep. Bias had a proportionately minor effect. REM recall remains far higher than NREM recall rates despite a number of obstacles. First was the bias that increased NREM recall. Second, though we made an attempt to balance it with excellent and poor recallers, our study population demonstrated poor recall, and Monroe et al. (1965) have shown that a dream is difficult to place correctly into its REM or NREM origins in line with the mediocrity of its recall. Third, the questioning procedure, as employed by our experimenters, was found to be at times incomplete and far from precise. Under such circumstances, the fact that even in our data REM recall was consistently more bizarre, perceptual, and experienced as really happening (the three Foulkes DF-scale dimensions) than NREM recall in all conditions (in all REM periods) speaks well for the belief that vivid mentation is more a phenomenon of REM neurophysiology.

The review of dream-recall research that began this chapter documented that NREM recall rates varied astonishingly and somewhat inexplicably from study to study, whereas REM dreaming rates were consistently high. It could be argued that our investigation sheds some light on this enigma. We have found that reports following REM awakenings are relatively immune to the expectancy of the investigator. Reports subsequent to NREM arousals are significantly influenced by the set of the subject and especially the expectancy of the experimenter. From these findings we may hypothesize that *a possible major source of variance in NREM recall studies is the predisposition of the investigator.* This is supported to some extent by comparing the presumed theoretical underpinnings of an investigator to the rate of NREM recall observed. There appears to be a high degree of concordance between what was expected and what was found. However, as we have shown earlier, this variance, unlike the variance in our study, may have been manifested largely through definitional and methodological (scaled versus all-or-none) factors.

The reader may wonder why we used a recall-*raising* expectancy when a recall-*lowering* expectancy might have enabled us to duplicate the early very small NREM recall frequencies, thereby showing that expectancy alone can explain the disparities in the field. In fact, with the right definition of dreaming, the right bias, and the right questioning mode, we might well have been able to replicate the early work that showed almost no NREM recall. The reason we chose to use a recall-raising expectancy in this investigation was that we were attempting to test a larger hypothesis: that no difference in mentation actually exists between REM and NREM sleep, and that dreaming is as frequent and vivid in both states. Our results thoroughly refute this hypothesis.

This study and review, when taken together, suggest to us that the conclusions about mentation reached by early sleep investigators were overzealously drawn and premature. No matter if definitions of dreaming are equilibrated, it is not possible to manipulate their data to produce the *combination* of 90% REM recall and no NREM recall in any study or group of studies. This has long been quietly understood in the field and is no longer news. The hope that one stage of sleep, or a given physiologic marker, will serve as the sole magic key for vivid dream mentation has all but faded from view (see Chapter 8 in this volume).

For some investigators who long suspected that bias may have influenced the low NREM recall rates reported in some studies and the high rates reported in others, this report can be taken as supportive evidence but not as conclusive confirmation. Though we believe that the definitions reported by some studies should not have been able to differentiate REM from NREM mentation as well as the authors of those investigations claimed, this study has shown again the force of the state-related mentation differences.

ACKNOWLEDGMENTS

This investigation was supported in part by Grants 5 RO 1 MH 26066 (J.H.), Interdepartmental Research Training Grant 2 to 1 MH 06418 to Albert Einstein College of Medicine (J.H.), and 2 RO 1 MH 13269, 5 KO 5 MH 18739 (H.P.R.).

We would like to express our sincerest appreciation to Robert Rosenthal for his extensive help in the formulation and the analysis of this project and to Steven Casolero and Thomas D'Aquinni for serving as the "experimenters" in this study.

Part II

REVIEWS OF
SLEEP-MENTATION
STUDIES

Inasmuch as Stage 1 REM does not include the interval of sleep onset (SO), the discovery by Foulkes and Vogel (1965) that SO dreaming was almost indistinguishable from REM dreaming stood out as the first major exception to the original REM/NREM-dreaming association. Most of the sleep-onset mentation research was carried out by dividing the sleep-onset interval into a sequence of four stages or classes. The stages, however, lack the discrete differences that divide stages REM from NREM sleep. For this reason, Dr. Vogel suggests (page 00 of this chapter) that the discrete events which distinguish phasic from tonic sleep may lead to a better understanding of the physiological substrate of sleep-onset mentation. We have carried out some research along this line which we report in the commentary at the end of the chapter.

The reader who is interested in personality and psychopathology will be pleased with the way Vogel relates differences in mentation between physiological states to individual differences in mentation, including psychotic persons. The reader should be alert to the implicit assumptions about the separation of body and mind that underlie Vogel's psychological model of SO mentation.

John S. Antrobus

4

Sleep-Onset Mentation

Gerald W. Vogel
Georgia Mental Health Institute
and
Emory University School of Medicine

More than a decade elapsed after the initiation of modern laboratory studies of sleep and dreaming (Aserinsky & Kleitman, 1955; Dement & Kleitman, 1957) before the systematic investigation of the psychophysiology of sleep onset (SO) was undertaken. (Foulkes, Spear, & Symonds, 1966; Foulkes & Vogel, 1965; Pope, 1972; Vogel, Barrowclough, & Giesler, 1972; Vogel, Foulkes, & Trosman, 1966.) The findings of these studies were important not only in their own right but because they required alteration of the early generalizations to the effect that REM sleep accompanies dreaming and NREM sleep accompanies either no mental activity, or, as was later reported, more thought-like mentation (Foulkes, 1962; Monroe, Rechtschaffen, Foulkes, & Jensen, 1965). In this chapter I review these findings and some of their implications.

DESCRIPTION OF MENTAL ACTIVITY AT SLEEP ONSET (SO)

Reports of SO mentation were retrieved by "awakening" subjects from one of four consecutive electroencephalographic/electrooculographic stages which cover the transition from wakefulness to sleep. (Foulkes & Vogel, 1965). Usually several SO awakenings of each subject were made each night, each awakening from a randomly selected EEG/EOG SO stage as the subject returned to sleep from a previous awakening. The four SO EEG/EOG stages, in order from wakefulness to sleep, were: (1) alpha EEG, usually continuous, with one or more rapid eye movements a few seconds prior to the "awakenings" (alpha REM); (2) alpha EEG, often continuous, with pronounced slow eye movements (alpha SEM); (3) descending Stage 1 EEG; and (4) descending Stage 2 EEG or .5–2.5-min duration. Subjectively these four successive EEG/EOG stages were usually rated as ranging in succession from awake and alert, or awake but drowsy, through drifting off to sleep, to light sleep. There were individual differences in the match between these subjective states of consciousness and EEG/EOG stage but all subjects did report a steady progression toward sleep with successive SO EEG/EOG stages. Moreover, with each successive EEG/EOG stage there was a steady decline in control over the course of mental activity and an awareness of the immediate environment and a steady rise in the frequency of hallucinatory experience, though again with large individual differences in the EEG/EOG stage at which these changes typically occur.

Recall of at least one item of mental content at SO was very frequent in all four EEG/EOG stages, more so than during REM sleep (83.3%; Dement, 1965a) and during NREM sleep (23-74%, depending on the study; Foulkes, 1967b). Pooled recall percentages of awakenings with content by SO stages were as follows: alpha REM, 96.2%; alpha SEM, 98.1%; S-1, 97.9%; S-2, 89.7% (Foulkes & Vogel, 1965). The length of SO reports (word count of alpha SEM and Stage 1 reports) was not significantly different from the length of REM reports from the same subjects (Foulkes et al., 1966). Thus these data indicated that an awakening from SO is at least as likely to produce as long a report of recalled mentation as an awakening from REM sleep.

The mentation recalled from SO was not simply flashing lights or primarily auditory imagery, or affectively intense and unpleasant as had been indicated by folklore or by earlier anecdotal reports of SO mentation, some of which were obtained by morning questionnaires rather than from on-the-spot awakenings at SO (Critchley, 1955; McKellar, 1957). Like REM mentation, most SO mentation collected "on-the-spot" consisted of meaningful sensory imagery, and again like REM mentation, the imagery was visual (Foulkes & Vogel, 1965). In fact, visual imagery was present in 78-89% of reports depending on the EEG/EOG stage of the awakening. Though auditory imagery occurred occasionally (range of 14 to 37% of reports from each stage), as did undistorted bodily sensations like touch and movement (range of 22 to 32% of reports from each stage), gustatory imagery was never reported and olfactory imagery was very rare (2 to 4%). The systematic data collected on the spot also revealed that affect was usually not intense nor unpleasant, usually peaked during alpha SEM, and thereafter decreased. If anything then, the SO period can be called a period of relatively flat affect. (Of course, that makes some kind of adaptive or teleological sense since it is hard to imagine that SO could proceed successfully to deep sleep with intense affect.)

Since dreaming has previously been assigned exclusively to REM sleep, the most unexpected finding in the initial laboratory study of SO (Foulkes & Vogel, 1965) later replicated in three other studies (Foulkes et al., 1966; Pope, 1973; Vogel et al., 1972), was the presence of substantial dreaming during SO. Dreams, defined as hallucinated, dramatic episodes (not as single scenes or flashing lights or nonhallucinated images) occurred in the following percentages of awakenings from EEG/EOG stages; alpha REM, 31%; alpha SEM, 43%; Stage 1, 76%; Stage

2, 71%. Again, though all subjects dreamed, there were large individual differences in dream frequency and in the EEG/EOG stages at which dreaming became abundant.

> That these [reports classified as dreams] were something other than engrossing waking fantasies was indicated by the following facts: (a) by definition, these experiences had to partake of an hallucinatory quality which is lacking in even the most engrossing of waking fantasies; (b) subjects generally described such experiences as more like night-dreams than any form of waking fantasy; (c) subjects described their state prior to awakenings producing such content as "drowsy," "drifting off to sleep," or "light sleep;" and (d) such content showed distortions and symbolic transformations of a type generally assumed to be absent in voluntary daytime fantasy. To illustrate these four points, let us consider . . . an alpha SEM dream (Foulkes & Vogel, 1965, p. 237).

> "I was looking at sort of a low lazy-Susan type of thing which was on the floor under a typewriter stand. I was in a very peculiar vantage point. I was looking down between the legs there, and never got above this. It was made out of crystal, and it was a platter type of arrangement. In the middle there was a stem and a little ball on the top, and I first saw there was blood in the little glass thing. In the middle it was full of blood; and then as it developed, the blood turned into what looked like sort of cocktail sauce that's served with shrimp; and then as it developed more, little shrimp started appearing around the little glass where the sauce was; and then as it developed more, more shrimp appeared on the platter below; and just as you called, a dog was walking over there and was just about ready to help himself to a few of the shrimp. This was mostly in vague symbols because there was nothing realistic about this at all. The dog was strange too, because his head, you know where his snout comes down to his nose, this part was all, like it was sawed off. In other words, his face was completely squared off and he didn't have any nose, I remember when I saw the dog coming out, I looked at him, made me feel uneasy [Foulkes & Vogel, 1965, p. 237-238]. . . ."

The occurrence of dreams like this one — long, vivid, visual, hallucinated, bizarre — suggested that SO reports might be very similar to REM reports. Three later studies showed this to be the case (Foulkes et al., 1966; Pope, 1973; Vogel et al., 1972). One study compared REM reports with alpha SEM and Stage 1 SO reports and found there were no significant REM-SO report differences in length of report, and in reliably rated sexual content, aggressive content, hedonic tone, and dream-like fantasy (DF) (the last was measured on an eight-point scale by which the formal properties of reported content were rated in terms of increasing dreamlike properties, ranging from no content to conceptual, everydayish content; to conceptual, bizarre content; to perceptual, nonhallucinatory everydayish; to perceptual, hallucinating everydayish; to perceptual, hallucinating, bizarre content; Foulkes et al., 1966). The finding of similar REM-SO DF scores has also been twice replicated. (Pope, 1973; Vogel et al., 1972).

In another study (Vogel et al., 1972), using a different approach, trained judges attempted to discriminate unlabeled REM from unlabeled Stage 1 SO reports on the basis that REM content would be more "dream-like" or regressive than Stage 1 content, that is, compared with Stage 1 SO reports, REM reports would have some combination of being "more visual, more perceptual, more affective, less thoughtlike, less hedonically neutral, less concerned with contemporary life and more concerned with past life; more bizarre, implausible or novel; more "lived in;" under less volitional control; accompanied by less awareness of the environment; and/or more often hallucinatory [p. 450]." Results showed that although the nine judges were able to discriminate Stage 1 SO from REM reports with an overall 70% correct hit ($p < .001$), there was considerable overlap. Approximately 25% of SO reports were called REM reports and approximately 50% of REM reports were called SO. Looked at in terms of regressive or dreamlike mentation, these results confirmed studies indicating that REM reports are often less implausible and more banal than originally thought (Dorus, & Rechtschaffen, 1971; Snyder et al., 1968); more to the point of this review, they again confirmed that SO mentation was often as regressive as the most regressive REM mentation — a fact now shown in four separate studies, two of which indicate that the most dream-like, regressive mentation is retrieved from SO about half as often as from REM sleep (Foulkes et al., 1966; Vogel et al., 1972).

PSYCHIATRIC IMPLICATIONS OF SO MENTATION

Because of the similarities between dreams and psychoses (Freud, 1900, 1955a), psychiatrists have for a long time hypothesized that the physiological correlates of dreaming might be similar to, or clues to, the physiological correlates of psychoses (Jac'son, cited in Jones, 1961). With the initial discovery that REM sleep was a reliable correlate of dreaming and the subsequent early generalization that it was the only correlate of dreaming, this hypothesis took the form that some unique property of REM sleep might be a correlate of psychosis (Fisher & Dement, 1963). Oversimplified, the notion was that psychosis might be a psychological expression of an intrusion of the REM state into wakefulness. Several different experimental approaches to this hypothesis have failed to find support for it (Vogel, 1968) and, although some controversy still exists about this question (Wyatt, Termini & Davis, 1971), the bulk of the evidence is still against it (Vogel, 1972). However, the finding that dreaming frequently occurred during SO in the absence of REM sleep suggests that the failure to find a link between REM sleep and psychosis may not be a complete refutation of the dream-psychosis hypothesis. In other words, if there is some physiological foundation to the psychological similarity of dreaming and psychosis, it may lie in a physiological correlate of SO dreaming or in a common physiological correlate of SO and REM dreaming rather than in a unique property of REM sleep.

In this regard it should be repeated that Stage 1 EEG which is so similar to a Stage REM EEG, is not a strong, or at least a unique, physiological correlate of dreaming because: (1) dreams (hallucinated dramatic episodes) were reported from high percentages of SO awakenings from EEG stages other than Stage 1

(31% of alpha REM; 43% of alpha SEM; and 71% of Stage 2); Foulkes & Vogel, 1965); and (2) dreams were also reported, though infrequently, from NREM sleep (Vogel et al., 1972). Nor is regressive content (i.e., bizarre, implausible content), regardless of whether or not it is hallucinated (dreamed), limited to the Stage 1 EEG pattern, of SO or REM sleep. Although regressive content reports occurred in a significantly greater percentage of reports during SO Stage 1 than during the other SO stages ($p < .002$), (51.2% of Stage 1 reports had regressive content in comparison with 19.2% of alpha REM reports, 27.8% of alpha SEM reports, and 26.9% of Stage 2 reports), only 37.1% of all regressive content reports from SO occurred during Stage 1 (Vogel et al., 1966). Furthermore, regressive content, independent of hallucinations, was reported from only 50% of Stage REM awakenings (Vogel et al., 1972). In short, neither REM sleep nor a Stage 1 EEG is a relatively unique physiological correlate of regressive content or of dreaming.

PSYCHOPHYSIOLOGICAL IMPLICATIONS OF SO FINDINGS

Although the search for other physiological correlates of dreaming and regressive mentation occurred about the same time as the discovery of dreaming at SO, it was independently initiated from an entirely different area of sleep research. What follows is a brief review of this new direction to the search for the physiological correlates of dreaming and of regressive mentation during sleep, and its relation to SO studies.

The new approach was initiated by Moruzzi's (1963; 1965) physiological distinction between tonic and phasic physiological events during REM sleep. Tonic events are continuous ones, for example, the relatively low-voltage, mixed-frequency EEG or the persistent loss of muscle tone. Phasic events are brief and intermittent, like the rapid eye movements, the PGO spikes, changes in autonomic discharge, spike discharges at the extraoccular muscles or the middle ear muscles. Moruzzi's tonic-phasic distinction was soon supported by Pompeiano's (1970) evidence that the vestibular nucleus controls phasic but not tonic events. From the psychological side Aserinsky (1967) suggested that the tonic-phasic distinction might be parallelled by psychologically different kinds of dreams, a suggestion taken up by Molinari and Foulkes (1969) who reasoned that since phasic events occurred not only during REM sleep but also in NREM and SO, they might provide a stronger and temporally more precise parallel to regressive mentation than REM sleep (Moruzzi & Foulkes, 1969). Thus, the phasic-tonic distinction came to supercede the old REM-NREM dichotomy as a hypothetical parallel for regressive-nonregressive content. In very recent investigations not yet replicated, several different phasic events have been reported to be correlates of regressive mentation. These included the following:

1. In visually hallucinated content retrieved from REM sleep, thinking was less likely to occur during REM bursts than during REM quiescence (Molinari &

Foulkes, 1969); the absence of thought or cognitive elaboration was even more strongly related to EEG sawtooth waves, which are unique to REM sleep and often occur during REM bursts (Foulkes & Pope, 1974); and very recently, Pope (1973) generalized and extended this finding to SO by observing that SO theta bursts, which are in the same frequency range as sawtooth waves, were associated with discontinuity in the content reported.

2. Another indicator of phasic activity is the phasic integrated potential (PIP) of the periorbital EMG which is believed to be a correlate of the ponto-geniculate-occipital spike, the presumed generator of many phasic events (Rechtschaffen et al., 1970). These workers found that both REM and NREM content reported from PIP awakenings was more bizarre than that reported from non-PIP awakenings in the same sleep stages (Watson, 1972; Rechtschaffen et al., 1971), although the REM finding was not confirmed (Foulkes & Pope, 1973).

3. Pivik and Dement (1970) found that in the human momentary suppressions of the EMG occur during SO Stage 1 and during NREM which were coincident with phasic H-reflex inhibition. Finally, Pivik's (1971) study of the relationship between the phasic EMG suppressions and NREM mentation found that the EMG suppressions were related to increased aggression and auditory imagery.

In summary, if replicated, several lines in the current investigation of the phasic-tonic dichotomy may provide stronger, and temporally more precise physiological parallels to regressive-nonregressive mentation than the old REM-NREM dichotomy, to which the finding of SO dreaming originally stood as an isolated exception.

PSYCHOLOGICAL ORGANIZATION OF SO

The finding that SO dreams and REM mentation were not correlated with a particular EEG stage — in effect that SO dreams and regressive mentation were not simply EEG stage epiphenomena — not only stimulated the search for other physiological correlates of dreaming and regressive mentation, but it also initiated a search for psychological variables which might be related to SO dreaming and REM mentation.

An early unsuccessful candidate for a correlate of SO regressive content was hallucinatory activity. A priori, it made sense that subjects should have had regressive content when they hallucinated. But the fact was that they often did not. Only 42% of all hallucinated SO reports had regressive content and only 49% of all regressive content reports occurred in the presence of hallucinatory activity (Vogel et al., 1966).

More success was obtained with the relation between regressive content and loss-of-waking control over mentation and reality orientation (Vogel et al., 1966). In this regard, I repeat the findings. During SO subjects first lost their control over the course of mentation; either slightly later or simultaneously they

lost awareness of the environment (did not know they were in bed in the laboratory) and only after these two losses, did they begin to hallucinate (believe that
mental events were really happening in the external world). In psychoanalytic
terms, one might say that over the course of SO there was a progressive withdrawal of interest in (decathexis of) the psychological functions which maintained
waking contact with reality: first, a decathexis of the volitional control over
mentation; then a decathexis of perception; and finally, with hallucination, a
decathexis of reality testing.

Empirically, there was a positive relation between the degree of decathexis
(withdrawal) and the pooled frequency of regressive content reports. Regressive
content occurred in 6% of reports with no decathexis of these functions; in 12%
of reports with only loss of control over mentation; in 31.3% with loss of control over mentation and loss of awareness of environment; and in 50.7% with
complete decathexis, that is, with loss of control over mentation, loss of awareness of environment, and loss of reality testing (hallucinations). Altogether, 94%
of regressive-content reports were accompanied by some degree of decathexis of
contact with reality and only 6% of regressive-content reports were not accompanied by some decathexis (Spearman $r = 0.44$; $p < .001$). This figure was high
enough so that it was concluded that during SO some decathexis of waking contact with reality was a necessary condition for regressive content, and the 6%
exceptions to this rule were interpreted as the result of a decathexis too subtle
for the gross instrument (question with four-point scale) to detect.

And yet this conclusion stood in puzzling contrast to the fact that reports
with the greatest loss of control (hallucination) often had nonregressive content
(for example, 58% of all Stage 2 reports were hallucinated, nonregressive-content
reports). Thus, if some loss of contact were necessary for regressive content, why
should reports with the greatest loss of contact often have had nonregressive
content?

The suggested resolution of this paradox involved the considerations about
the following modal (typical) relation in each EEG stage between kind of content (regressive or nonregressive) and the degree of decathexis of waking controls.
In each alpha stage the modal report had nonregressive content with either no
decathexis of waking control or only a partial one, a combination called a relatively intact ego (I). The percent of I reports in each alpha stage was significantly higher than the percent of I in all reports ($p < .001$), and progressively decreased
during successive EEG/EOG stages (75% of reports in alpha REM; 63% in alpha
SEM; 20% in Stage 1; 15.4% in Stage 2).

In Stage 1 the modal report had regressive content and a partial or complete
decathexis of waking controls, a combination called a destructuralized ego (D).
The percentage of D reports in Stage 1 was significantly higher than the percent
of D in all reports ($p < .002$), and it increased with successive stages to a maximum in Stage 1 after which it decreased (19.2% of reports in alpha REM; 27.8%
in alpha SEM; 51.2% in Stage 1; 26.9% in Stage 2).

In Stage 2 the modal report had a complete decathexis of waking control and paradoxically a return to nonregressive content, a combination called a restructuralized ego (R). The percentage of R reports in Stage 2 was significantly higher than the percentage of R in all reports ($p < .001$) and progressively increased with successive EEG/EOG stages (5.8% of reports in alpha REM; 9.2% in alpha SEM; 28.8% in Stage 1; and 57.7% in Stage 2). Thus the modal SO report was I during alpha EEG; D during Stage 1; and R during Stage 2. An example of the I-D-R sequence follows:

Alpha SEM: intact ego (I):

"I was thinking of sending a clipping to a Russian pianist and I saw an envelope with 15 cents postage." (The subject was a concert pianist. The content was not regressive. The subject reported that during the SO experience he had lost volitional control over content, was unaware of his surroundings, but knew that the image was in his mind and not in the external world.)

Stage 1: destructuralized ego (D):

"I was observing the inside of a pleural cavity. There were small people in it, like in a room. The people were hairy, like monkeys. The walls of the pleural cavity are made of ice and slippery. In the midpart there is an ivory bench with people sitting on it. Some people are throwing balls of cheese against the inner side of the chest wall." (The report contains bizarre, implausibly associated elements, distortions, and so on. The subject reported that during the SO experience there was a complete loss of contact with external reality — including hallucination — during the reported experience.)

Stage 2: restructuralized ego (R):

"I was driving a car, telling other people you shouldn't go over a certain speed limit." (In this report the content is again plausible and realistic. There was a complete loss of contact with external reality (including hallucination) during the reported experience.)

Though the above sequence was the modal psychophysiological parallel during SO, that is, I during alpha EEG, D during Stage 1, and R during Stage 2, there were, among all the reports, numerous departures from this modal psychophysiological parallel. However, the departures seemed to fit in a pattern which suggested that the psychophysiology of SO could be understood as follows: at each SO each subject progresses through the I-D-R psychological sequence and also progresses through the four EEG/EOG sleep stages. Usually the members of the two sequences match in the modal manner, but in some instances they do not, though each sequence still progresses through its individual stages in the typical order. Two kinds of data supported this interpretation. First, in some subjects D usually occurred earlier (during alpha EEG) while in others D usually occurred later (during Stage 2). Among the 9 studied subjects there were 2 subjects in which most of the D reports were in alpha and a higher than expected frequency of R in Stage 1. On the other side, one subject's highest frequency of D was in Stage 2 and a lower than expected frequency of R was in Stage 2. Second, if the ego states I, D, and R were assigned numbers 1, 2, and 3, and each subject's mean ego state was calculated for each EEG stage, all subjects showed a monotonically increasing curve of mean ego state across the four EEG/EOG stages. Of the 27 comparisons of consecutive EEG stages (9 subjects, 3 comparisons between 4 successive EEG stages), 23 were in the expected direction ($p < .001$). The 4 exceptions were in 3 subjects and 3 of these exceptions concern minimal differences between alpha REM and alpha SEM.

In summary, the psychophysiological data about SO can be interpreted as follows: viewed psychologically SO is a sequence of three ego states (I, D and R), and viewed physiologically it is a sequence of four EEG/EOG states. The elements of the two sequences have a typical match with I during alpha EEG, D during Stage 1, and R during Stage 2. But each sequence can and does occur independently of the other, thus accounting for departures from the ideal psychophysiological parallel.

The finding of a sequence of ego states — or psychological changes — that were relatively independent of EEG stages suggested that the individual differences in the frequency of SO dreaming and in the (EEG) interval from wakefulness to dreaming might be more readily explainable in psychodynamic terms than in terms of a psychophysiological parallelism. Thus, the finding that withdrawal from contact with reality preceded regressive mentation suggested that the withdrawal helped induce the regressive content for two reasons. First, SO withdrawal from sensory input (represented by loss of awareness of environment), indicated sensory deprivation and that encouraged the emergence of regressive content. Second, SO "withdrawal" from the usual directed thought of wakefulness (represented by a loss of control over course of mentation), indicated a reduction of the usual waking inhibition of regressive content or of regressive thought connections. Thus, both these aspects of the withdrawal during SO allowed or encouraged the emergence of regressive content (D state). Accordingly, the regressive mentation during SO is not necessary for SO, nor is it the result of endogenous activation of archaic modes of thought. Rather, it is simply an unavoidable side effect of the reduction in focused thought and sensory input which is essential for SO.

> Furthermore, because the D state is so quickly and regularly followed by a restitution (R) (to nonregressive content), it appears that the tendency toward regression which is represented by D, threatens the ego and produces the need for defense. Thus, at this point in the SO period, the ego, in order to sleep, needs a defense which will allow it to continue to withdraw and yet overcome the threatened chaos (D) induced by the withdrawal. The finding that the loss of reality testing is necessary for the return to nonregressive content (at the end of SO) suggests that the inactivation of reality testing is a part of the needed defense which will resolve the conflict and allow the restitution represented by R [Vogel et al., 1966 p. 246-247].

In other words, potentially threatened by the emergence of regressive content, but needing to continue the withdrawal (which only adventitiously fostered the emergence of the regressive content) in order to sleep, the ego gains some control by constructing its own reality in a primitive manner, reminiscent of the defensive renunciation of reality testing used in psychosis.

This psychodynamic view of SO provided an explanation of an empirically significant characteristic of hypnagogic dreaming, namely, the individual variations in the length, frequency, and EEG stage of SO dreams (Vogel et al., 1972). The suggested explanation was

> ... that during SO individuals differ in their tolerance of the potential threat of regression induced by the withdrawal and that these differences are responsible for the variations in the length, frequency, and EEG stage of hypnagogic dreams. This notion is consistent with our clinical impression that the subjects who are free to experience and enjoy their own fantasies had earlier and richer hypnagogic dreams than more anxious and rigid subjects. It appears likely that the more rigid subjects were more threatened by an impending regression and so held on to external reality longer or withdrew in some special way so as to minimize the regression. This is also compatible with the clinical phenomena of hypnagogic dreamlike experiences which abruptly awaken anxious patients who are particularly prone to insomnia [Vogel et al., 1966, p. 247].

PERSONALITY CORRELATES OF SO MENTATION

Some empirical support for the above psychodynamic view of SO has been obtained by the study of personality correlates of individual differences in SO dreaming (Foulkes et al., 1966). In this study subjects contributed both SO (alpha SEM and descending Stage 1) and REM reports, which were reliably rated for their word count (length), manifest aggression, sexuality, hedonic tone, and dream-like fantasy. Personality variables were measured by the California Personality Index (CPI) and by reliable ratings of thematic apperception test (TAT) responses, in terms of aggression, sex, hedonic tone, and imaginativeness.

SO and REM reports did not differ significantly in mean length, dream-like fantasy (DF), aggression, sexuality, and hedonic tone, thus confirming the essential similarity of REM and SO reports. There were, however, some differences in distribution of kinds of reports which were not revealed by the group averages. The frequency of REM bizarre, hallucinatory reports was twice that of the SO frequency. Indeed, REM reports tended to be at either extreme of the dreamlike fantasy scale, having either no content or bizarre hallucinatory content, whereas SO reports were evenly distributed at all points on the DF scale with substantial individual differences in the frequency of hallucinated, bizarre reports. There was no significant intrasubject REM and SO correlation in DF, sex, aggression, and hedonic ratings. It seems then that different psychological mechanisms must determine the mental qualities of SO and REM reports.

This was borne out by the finding that several indicators of waking fantasy were related to SO fantasy (DF rating) and not related to REM fantasy (DF rating). SO fantasy correlated positively and significantly with TAT word count, sex, imagination, and not with REM fantasy. REM fantasy and SO fantasy did, however, both correlate with TAT, aggression, and hedonic tone. By inference, the psychological mechanisms responsible for SO fantasy are strongly related to the mechanisms responsible for waking fantasy and independent of the mechanisms responsible for REM fantasy. Investigation of these mechanisms was begun by a study of the personality differences between SO dreamers and nondreamers (Foulkes et al., 1966). In support of the above psychodynamic view of SO, it was found that SO dreamers were less rigidly defensive than SO nondreamers. On the CPI administered to college students, SO dreamers were more self-accepting, less rigidly conforming to social standards, and more socially poised than SO nondreamers, who, in contrast, scored high on items characteristic of the authoritarian personality (rigid, intolerant, conformist). And none of the personality variables which correlated with SO waking fantasy was related to REM fantasy, which was found in a separate study to be bizarre and vivid in subjects with psychopathology (Foulkes & Rechtschaffen, 1964).

Thus, SO and REM fantasy are independent of each other and independently related to different personality variables. SO fantasy is positively related to a flexible, nonrigid, nondefensive ego which is free to engage in waking fantasy, while REM fantasy is more related to psychopathology. One might reasonably conclude from this that SO fantasy is positively related to ego strength, while REM fantasy is positively related to ego weakness. However, that must be a mistaken oversimplification because SO and REM fantasy are not negatively correlated. They are unrelated.

An explanation for this paradox may be as follows. SO fantasy is related to waking fantasy and both of these are inhibited by rigid defensiveness, while REM fantasy is related to psychopathology. But defensiveness and psychopathology are not correlated, that is, some rigidly defensive subjects have severe psychopathology (like the "frozen" paranoid); some do not (like the inhibited, but well functioning obsessive-compulsive); and some undefensive subjects may have severe psychopathology (like the disorganized schizophrenic), and some do not (like the poised, self-acceptant adult). In a sample of functioning college students, such as the one used in the Foulkes (1966) study, subjects with little defensiveness would more likely be poised and self-acceptant rather than disorganized and disturbed. Hence, such a sample would suggest that high SO fantasy would relate equally well to ego strength and to lack of defensiveness. But it is my hunch that a broader range of subjects including those with undefended disturbances would show that SO fantasy is related to waking fantasy and that both are related to lack of defensiveness independent of ego strength.

Whether or not this explanation (of the paradoxical lack of a negative correlation between REM and SO fantasy) is correct, the central empirical findings whose implications I want to pursue are: (1) that SO and REM fantasy are independent of each other; and (2) that each is related to different waking personality variables.

If each subject's REM and SO fantasy were correlated, then one could easily imagine a common mechanism or control determining each subject's SO and REM fantasy. But the lack of a relation between a subject's REM DF score and

SO DF score implies that SO and REM fantasy must be under separate controls. Thus the evidence implies that there are two independent systems for the production of fantasy including regressive mentation. Let us consider some psychoanalytic implications of this conclusion.

In psychoanalytic terms there are several reasons for classifying SO fantasy — and particularly its regressive mentation — as initiated by ego regression and for classifying the REM fantasy (and its regressive mentation) as initiated by unconscious wishes and needs of the id. (Of course, in psychoanalytic terms both ego and id participate in both SO and REM fantasy. The question here concerns the initiator.) SO fantasy can be classified as initiated by ego regression because it is initiated volitionally; is related to waking fantasy under volitional control; becomes more regressive as the ego's "nutriment," sensory information is reduced. REM fantasy, on the other hand, can be classified as initiated by unconscious wishes and needs because it is never volitionally initiated; is not related to waking mentation under volitional control — on the contrary it is related to nonvolitional waking mentation, namely, psychopathology; is almost invariably associated with the physical signs of sexual arousal (Karacan et al., 1972); and arises with increased endogenous activation (Berger, 1969). Thus, the laboratory evidence that there are two independent, different systems for fantasy production supports psychoanalytic theory, derived from clinical observations, that regressive mentation can result from two such independent, different systems. Further, within my limited knowledge of the psychoanalytic literature, the SO-REM dichotomy is the first systematic, laboratory, empirical evidence supporting the proposition that psychopathology is more related to the system producing nocturnal dreams than to the system which controls waking fantasy. Perhaps, modern psychoanalytic ego psychologists to the contrary, Freud's (1900/1955a) original topographic model is more consistent with these findings than later elaborations of the structural model. Certainly contemporary structural views that psychopathology and the nocturnal dream can better be explained as a result of ego regression than of unconscious "activation" are not supported by this laboratory evidence (Arlow & Brenner, 1964).

The chief argument for Vogel's construction of a psychoanalytic-psychological model of SO mentation is that this mentation is: (1) independent of the concurrently measured psychological states; and (2) in terms of individual differences, independent of REM mentation. In my judgment, the first assumption is invalid, but not essential to Vogel's argument in any event. The finding of some exceptions to a strong relationship (page 00 of this chapter) in no way detracts from the fact that an association is demonstrated by the data. Vogel could argue that the psycho-physiological correlation is spurious, both processes simply being associated with time from "lights out." Furthermore, the independence of a psychological process from one particular class of physiological events, does not mean the psychological processes are independent of *all* physiological events. Those available for measurement on the surface of the scalp are but a tiny portion of the neurophysiological events which might conceivably be causally associated with sleep mentation. Even the id and ego must have physical structure in the broadest sense of that concept. Consequently, if Vogel were to acknowledge the physiological association in his data or were to find an even stronger physiological association, his psychoanalytic model still need not be relinquished.

Statistical independence is a requisite for the postulation of independent cognitive processes, in this case SO fantasy and REM fantasy systems. The absence of a statistically significant association, however, does not constitute evidence of independence. First, since Vogel speaks of a bimodal distribution of DF scores within REM (page 00 of this chapter) the possibility of a nonlinear association between SO and REM DF scores should be examined. The Pearson r estimates only the linear component of an association; and conversely, the absence of a significant linear correlation says nothing about the absence of nonlinear associations.

Second, it is never possible to assure that the true correlation in the population, p, is exactly 0. The sample r, upon which Foulkes, Spear, & Symonds (1966) assert the independence of SO and REM DF = .20. With $N = 32$; $-.16 \leqslant p \leqslant +.51$ and $(-).02 \leqslant p^2 \leqslant .26$. Thus fantasy from the two states could share at least a quarter of their variance.

Third, DF is a multidimensional scale (see Chapter 2 of this volume). It is possible, therefore, for SO and REM fantasy to be independent with respect to some components such as bizarreness but associated with respect to others. Inasmuch as Vogel's psychoanalytic model requires independence only of the bizarre component, the use of the more complex DF scale may have tended to obscure the relationships examined. Given the multivariate character of DF it is similarly important to rule out the possibility that the correlations between SO DF and waking TAT measures are not due simply to correlations with the large visual imagery component of DF. That is the correlations may have nothing to do with bizarreness or regression.

Despite these minor technical comments, I heartily approve of the thorough manner in which Vogel, Foulkes, and their colleagues have pursued this issue of independence. It may be an unfortunate characteristic of the human cognitive apparatus that even scientists tend to conceive of completely unrelated variables as somehow belonging to a single construct. One suspects that further research on waking and sleeping fantasy may uncover yet more independent components.

I also endorse Vogel's recommendation that future studies attempt to locate the changes in alertness and fantasy more precisely in time. Using again the 20 subjects described in Chapter 13 of this volume we obtained 1 SO report on each of 8 nights which had been preceded by uninterrupted sleep. The awakenings averaged 15 min from hour lights out. The awakenings were sampled according to a distribution of eye-movement criteria, ranging from intervals of saccades and blinking, eyes closed, through 3 min of SEMs (Hilddoff, U., Antrobus, J.S., Farber, J., Ellman, S., & Arkin, A., 1974). SEMs, EEG alpha, saccadic EMs, and blinks were scored according to the proportion of the 3-min intervals preceding the awakening which was occupied by these events. The proportion of SEMS ($r^2 = .14$), alpha ($-r^2 = .12$) and saccades ($r^2 = .10$) were associated with alertness, rated from the subjects' response to: "Were you awake or asleep when I called you?" and the remainder of the sleep report. Alertness, in turn was associated with rated continuity of thought ($r^2 = .10$) and a combination of continuity and recent events ($R^2 = .19$). None of the physiological variables correlated directly, however, with any of the sleep-mentation scales, continuity, recent events, detail and clarity, visual imagery, or dreaming. Whatever the physiological variables said about alertness was not the same component of alertness that was associated with continuity and recent events. When we used subjects' latency of response to the experimenter's call, as a second measure of alertness, no correlations were obtained. Even measures of alertness may be independent of one another!

In the process of carrying out this small study we were dismayed at the poor association between formal criteria of sleep onset, on the one hand, and both subjective and behavioral measures of sleep onset, on the other. We urge further research on the combined problem of sleep onset and sleep onset mentation. Vogel and Foulkes have uncovered major trends in sleep onset mentation. More detailed work in the identification of arousal, sleep mentation and physiological covariates is needed.

John S. Antrobus

EDITORS' FOREWORD TO CHAPTER 5

It is truly a pleasure to read this contribution. Goodenough walks through the history of thinking and research on dream recall as though he were conducting a tour through his laboratory. He considers each and every position in turn listing its merits, weaknesses, and the research evidence on either hand. His ability to consider an issue from the point of view of psychoanalysis, psychometrics, experimental psychology, and a host of personality models has always been unusual. His even-handed treatment of widely different points of view in this chapter is exemplary.

John S. Antrobus

5

Dream Recall: History and Current Status of the Field [1]

Donald R. Goodenough

Educational Testing Service

It has long been a matter of common knowledge that we dream far more than we are able to remember the morning after. In the words of Freud (1900/ 1955a):

> ... we are so familiar with the fact of dreams being liable to be forgotten, that we see no absurdity in the possibility of someone having had a dream in the night and of his not being aware in the morning either of what he has dreamt or even of the fact that he has dreamt at all [p. 43].

The widespread belief that dream recall is difficult derives from the everyday observation that many once-recalled dreams are impossible to recover even a few moments after they are vividly in our recollection. During the last two decades it has become increasingly evident how much of our nightly dream life is lost to recall by morning. Since the discovery by Aserinsky and Kleitman (1953) of REM sleep, many studies have been done on the frequency of dream reporting following awakenings from different types of sleep. Snyder (1967) has summarized this work in his excellent review. The consensus of these studies is that dreams can be recalled from about 80% of REM-period awakenings and from a somewhat smaller, although still substantial percentage of NREM awakenings. Since approximately two hours of a normal night are spent in REM sleep, it is clearly possible to collect a large number of dream reports from awakenings during the night. In contrast, ordinary morning recall of a dream occurs in the typical person at the rate of about once every two days (Webb & Kersey, 1967).

One way to account for this huge discrepancy is to suppose that dreams are produced by the awakenings themselves and therefore the more frequent the awakenings, the greater the number of dreams recalled. Such a view has had its historical proponents (e.g., Goblot, cited in Giora, 1973). While arousal (hypnopompic) experiences may occur under certain conditions (Goodenough, Lewis,

[1]This work was supported in part by grant MH 21989.

Shapiro, Jaret, & Sleser, 1965a), the view that all or even many dreams are produced in this way is not taken seriously by current authors for a variety of reasons (Rechtschaffen, 1967; Stoyva & Kamiya, 1968).

An alternative explanation is that most dreams are simply not remembered by morning. In fact, the evidence consistently supports the view that dreams are difficult if not impossible to recall unless the sleeper awakens during or shortly after the dream experience itself. While dream reports may be collected in 80% of awakenings from REM periods, percentage recall drops dramatically if the awakening is delayed for even a few minutes after the end of REM sleep (Goodenough et al., 1965a; Wolpert & Trosman, 1958). Even a slight delay in the process of awakening, produced experimentally by the use of a gradual (as contrasted with an abrupt) awakening procedure, is enough to decrease the frequency of dream reporting substantially, particularly among people who rarely recall dreaming in the morning under everyday conditions (Goodenough, et al., 1965a; Shapiro, Goodenough, & Gryler, 1963; Shapiro, Goodenough, Lewis, & Sleser, 1965). Given all the evidence, the common conclusion that the vast majority of dream experiences are forgotten seems inescapable.

The key question remains as to why dreams are so much more difficult to recall than waking experiences. The answer to this question could be very useful in the attempt to understand memory processes more generally, or so it has seemed, at least, to those involved in the area. It is not surprising, therefore, to find a substantial body of literature on dream recall and a wide variety of proposed answers. Very little research has been directed at this question directly, however. Most studies of dream recall have been concerned with the conditions under which dreams are initially reported, with the conditions under which the rerecall of once reported dreams occurs, or with individual differences in frequency of dream reporting. While these issues may be important in their own right, they are of primary interest in this review to the extent that they bear on our key question.

My purpose in this chapter is to review the most prominent of the theories offered to account for differences in ease of recall between dreams and waking experiences, to summarize the evidence relevant to these theories, and to suggest an arousal-retrieval model as an alternative explanation for some of the generalizations that are emerging from the evidence.

THE DEFINITION OF DREAM-RECALL FAILURES

The fact that dream recall has attracted a fair amount of research attention over the years certainly is not due to a ready access to empirical information in the area. All research approaches attempted so far are beset with difficulties. The major problem involves the definition of recall failures. Defining dream recall failures depends directly on our ability to identify when a dream experience occurs. If we can tell.when dreams occur, then there is no problem in defining recall failures. If we cannot tell, then we cannot easily define recall failures. We may "see no absurdity" in supposing that a dream occurred without the dreamer's recall of it as Freud suggested, but we cannot be certain whether we are dealing with a recall failure or whether the claim that no dream has occurred is in fact correct.

The problem of determining when a dream occurs has been dealt with in a variety of ways. At one extreme, it has been argued that dreams go on continuously during sleep. In this view, failures to report a dream are obviously always failures of dream recall (ignoring for the moment the possibility that subjects may lie about their dream experiences). At the other extreme, some theorists have insisted that the concept of a dream experience is meaningless (e.g., Malcolm, 1959). This view renders the problem of dream-recall failure meaningless as well. One simply equates dreaming with the dream report as does Erickson (1954): "A dream is a verbal report of a series of remembered images, mostly visual, which are usually endowed with affect [p. 17]." Neither one of these extreme positions has many adherents among contemporary sleep researchers.

The proposal by Dement and Kleitman (1957b) that REM sleep be used as an objective, operational definition of the dream state had a dramatic and well-known impact on theories of dreaming. Initially the REM criteria of dreaming seemed to solve the problem of defining dream-recall failures. If REM sleep is the dream state, then one simply awakens the subject from a REM period (or some time thereafter) and counts a failure to report as a failure to recall. Unfortunately this simple solution does not look as appealing today as it once did. A variety of evidence has accumulated since the discovery of REM sleep to indicate that the REM definition of dreaming is inadequate. It seems clear that dreams may occur in NREM sleep, and that REM sleep may occur under conditions which make it unlikely that dreaming can occur (that is, decorticate individuals or neonates). The evidence on these points has been reviewed in detail by a number of authors (e.g., Foulkes, 1966; Rechtschaffen, 1967; Stoyva & Kamiya, 1968). We are left, then, with a reasonable doubt that REM sleep coincides completely with dreaming sleep.

While the uncertainty that exists in defining the dream state represents a substantial problem, it has not paralyzed research efforts. Many current theorists view the concept of the dream experience as a construct which can be approached through sets of converging operations, including physiological ones as well as verbal reports (e.g., Rechtschaffen, 1967; Stoyva & Kamiya, 1968). Similarly, the concept of dream-recall failure may be viewed as a construct. Hypothetical properties may be assigned to the construct, and deductions made on the basis of these properties may be examined empirically. A construct of dream-recall failure of this sort serves a useful function. It has a clear role in generating research hypotheses. In addition, a recognition of its status as a construct may inhibit the uncritical use of data on dream reporting to draw inferences about dream recall failures.

The problems involved in drawing inferences about recall failures from data on dream reporting may be illustrated in the literature on individual differences. In most such studies people either are asked how often they typically dream or are required to keep a diary of the dreams recalled each morning over some representative period at home. Home dream reporters and nonreporters are then selected from the extremes of the resulting distribution of people, and compared on some variable of interest.

The problem of defining dream-recall failures certainly arises in these studies. There are several possible ways to account for differences between home dream reporters and nonreporters without assuming that recall is involved. For example, it has been suggested that some people typically fail to report dreaming merely because their alarm clock is usually set to go off in the morning during NREM rather than during REM sleep (Webb & Kersey, 1967). Since the probability of reporting a dream is lower during NREM sleep, this view raises the question as to whether individual differences in home dream reporting may be due to recall at all. There is a considerable amount of evidence on this point. It is clear that home nonreporters have about the same number of REM periods as home dream reporters (Antrobus, Dement, & Fisher, 1964; Goodenough, Shapiro, Holden & Steinschriber, 1959; Lewis, Goodenough, Shapiro, & Sleser, 1966). The evidence indicates, however, that the total amount of time spent in REM sleep is slightly, but significantly related to the frequency of home reporting (Antrobus, et al., 1964; Baekeland, 1970). This relationship suggests that the probability of the alarm clock going off in the morning during REM sleep may be somewhat greater for home dream reporters than for nonreporters. This issue has been examined directly. Neither Antrobus, et al. (1964) nor Cohen & MacNeilage (1973) found any consistent difference between home dream reporters and nonreporters in the tendency to awaken in the morning from REM sleep in the laboratory. At this point, the evidence is not very persuasive that substantial individual differences exist in the likelihood of awakening from REM sleep in the morning, but the issue is not completely settled.

There are additional grounds for suspecting that individual differences in home dream reporting do not necessarily reflect differences in dream recall. In one laboratory study of subjects identified as home nonreporters (Lewis, et al., 1966), some nonreporters claimed that they were awake and thinking rather than asleep and dreaming each time their REM periods were interrupted by an experimental awakening. They were able to recount the content of their thoughts. These thoughts were bizarre and dreamlike in many ways, raising the possibility that something about the process of labeling their experiences as dreams, rather than recall of their experiences, is responsible for their claim to be "nondreamers." Other subjects among the home-nonreporter group were able to report only an occasional vague fragment of sleep mentation even when awakened from REM periods. In the absence of a definitive method of determining when dreams occur, it is not clear for these latter subjects whether they may be correct in their claim that they rarely dream, even though they have REM periods.

The point should be emphasized that many home nonreporters did recall dreams with no apparent difficulty under relatively ideal conditions in the laboratory (that is, following abrupt awakenings from REM sleep). Even a slight departure from these conditions was enough to significantly decrease dream reporting, however, as would be expected on the assumption that recall difficulties are involved for these people. The evidence from other studies indicates that people who claim that they rarely dream at home are likely to find it particularly difficult to rerecall dreams that they have once reported (Baekeland, 1970; Barber, 1969). It is clear, therefore, that many nonreporters are nonrecallers of dreams.

It is obvious that there are problems involved in attempts to apply the construct of dream-recall failure to the study of individual differences. Since recall factors may not be the sole determinants of home dream reporting, the correlates of individual differences in frequency of home dream reports may be hard to identify. It should not be surprising, therefore, to find only low relationships among variables in this area, and many failures to replicate findings from one study to the next. Just such a picture emerges from the literature. In spite of the problems, the studies of individual differences in dream reporting have produced some interesting results. Moreover, some of these results are relevant to questions about why dreams are more difficult to recall than waking experiences. It seems reasonable to conclude that the construct of dream-recall failure can usefully be applied, even in a research area as problem ridden as is the study of individual differences.

TWO TYPES OF THEORY ABOUT WHY DREAMS ARE HARD TO RECALL

All attempts to explain why dreams are so difficult to recall begin by emphasizing either some characteristic of dream experiences, or of sleep more generally, that is distinctively different from waking life. It is possible to distinguish two classes of explanation in terms of the characteristic so emphasized. One class may be called content centered. This class of explanation focuses on some feature of the content of dream experiences which may make them more difficult to recall than the usual waking experience. A second class focuses on some property of sleep which impairs memory for experiences without regard to content. The ability to recall any experience during sleep, whether endogenously or exogenously produced, is said to be impaired. Something in the memory process is thought to be deficient during sleep.

The distinction between content-centered and memory-process theories of dream forgetting is a very useful one. It serves as a convenient framework for the discussion of alternative explanations of dream forgetting. However, its use is not confined to this didactic function. It is possible to gather evidence which bears on one or the other of these two formal classes of theory without consideration of the specific class members in terms of their substance. In the organization of the discussion to follow, this distinction is therefore given a major role.

Content-Centered Explanations of Dream-Recall Failure

Before examining the literature which bears on specific content-centered theories of dream recall, the evidence on this general class of theory will be considered. The evidence that would be most directly relevant to content-centered theories of dream recall would certainly involve a comparison between dream experiences that are recalled and dream experiences that are not recalled. Unfortunately the content of a dream experience that the subject never recalls is no more available to us than it is to the subject. The only data we have are in the form of the subject's best recollections of some of the dreams. We can compare initial reports of dreams which are subsequently rerecalled or not rerecalled. We can also collect dream reports from subjects who typically fail to report dreams, and compare these with reports from subjects who typically do report dreaming. Both of these techniques involve certain difficulties, but the data are of interest to content-centered theorists.

One study of home dream reporters and nonreporters is particularly relevant to the content-centered class of theories (Barber, 1969). In this study it was possible to collect five dreams from most subjects by waking them at home with a telephone call, although more calls were naturally required for the nonreporters than for the reporters. As might be expected, subsequent rerecall of these initially reported dreams was more likely for the home reporters than for the home nonreporters, but the study did not stop at this point. The novel feature involved teaching the dream reports to subjects other than the ones who produced the dreams. These new subjects were then tested for recall of the dream reports they had learned. Dreams produced by home nonreporters turned out to be more difficult to recall than dreams produced by reporters, not only by the subjects who originally produced the dreams, but by other people as well. These results suggest that at least insofar as once-reported dreams are concerned, there is something about the content of nonreporters' productions that makes them less recallable.

While Barber's (1969) results are interesting, they do not require a content-centered theory of dream recall. As Barber recognized, some forgetting of the dream experience no doubt went on before the subjects reported their dreams initially. This fact leads to a rather simple interpretation of Barber's results. One may begin with the plausible assumption that the subjects who often totally fail to remember dreams (nonreporters) also tend to remember only vaguely the dreams that they do report. There is no reason to believe that the recall of dreams is an all-or-nothing affair. For people who find it easy to recall, more dreams should be reported and the dreams they are able to recall should be more vividly told. In the dreams collected from each nonreporter we may have, then, a set of narratives that are somewhat vaguer and less easily rerecallable than is true for the set of dream narratives collected from the reporters.

In view of the possibility that a very simple explanation of the results may suffice, it seems imprudent, in the opinion of this reviewer, to draw any far-reaching conclusion from these data concerning the content-centered class of theories. More studies of the content of dream reports in relation to rerecall are needed. It is important to recognize, however, that certain kinds of content differences may be expected and may be of trivial consequence.

We turn now to a consideration of the most prominent specific theories within the content-centered class.

The Role of Dream Salience in Recall

The relationship between item salience and recall is well known in classical memory theory. The greater the novelty, bizarreness, affectfulness, or intensity of an experience, the more salient it appears to be, and, other things being equal, the more likely it is to be recalled.

The salience concept appeared very early in the literature on dream recall. For example, according to Strümpell (cited in Freud 1900/1955a):

> When we are awake we regularly forget countless sensations and perceptions at once, because they were too weak or because the mental excitation attaching to them was too slight. The same holds good of many dream images: they are forgotten because they are too weak while stronger images adjacent to them are remembered [p. 43].[2]

Calkins (1893) early discussed the role of dream intensity in recall, while Radestock (cited in Freud, 1900/1955a) believed that the most peculiar dreams are best remembered. Among recent theorists, Cohen (1974) and Goodenough, Witkin, Lewis, Koulack, and Cohen (1974) have also emphasized the role of salience in dream recall.

The evidence leaves no doubt that salience is an important factor in the rerecall of once-reported dreams. Long dream reports are much more easily recalled than short ones (Baekeland & Lasky, 1968; Meier, Ruef, Ziegler, & Hall, 1968; Strauch, 1969; Trinder & Kramer, 1971), and dream reports with great dramatic intensity are better recalled than bland reports (Strauch, 1969; Trinder & Kramer, 1971). Emotional intensity has also been related to morning recall in the data of Meier, et al. (1968) and Goodenough, et al. (1974), but not in the study by Baekeland and Lasky (1968).

There are other hypotheses that may be generated on the assumption that salience of the dream experience is related to morning rerecall of dreams reported immediately after experimental awakenings during the night. One set of hypotheses rests on the known relationship between certain physiological variables during REM sleep and the salience of the dream report obtained at REM-period

---

[2]The extensive review by Freud (1900/1955a) of the early work on dream recall has been used as the source of material for the early non-English literature in this summary.

awakenings. Dement and Wolpert (1958b) provided the earliest demonstration that salience in dream reports can be predicted from REM characteristics. These authors found that frequency of eye movements during REM sleep is related to activity in dreams reported from REM-period awakenings. This finding has often been replicated (e.g., Berger & Oswald, 1962; Goodenough, Lewis, Shapiro, & Sleser, 1965). Eye-movement activity during REM sleep has also been related to dream bizarreness (Goodenough, et al., 1965b), and to intensity and emotionality (Hobson, Goldfrank, & Snyder, 1965; Karacan, Goodenough, Shapiro, & Starker, 1966; Molinari & Foulkes, 1969; Takeo, 1970; Verdone, 1963, 1965). Moreover REM-period respiration rate and irregularity have been related to dream intensity and affect, at least under some conditions (Fisher, Byrne, Edwards, & Kahn, 1970; Goodenough, Witkin, Koulack, & Cohen, 1975; Hauri & Van de Castle, 1970b; Hobson, et al., 1965; Knopf, 1962).

Given these data and the fact that the most salient dream reports of the night are most easily rerecalled, it would not be surprising to find that, among the dream reports given during the night, the ones remembered next morning tend to come from REM periods with frequent eye movements and with the most rapid and irregular breathing. In line with this expectation Baekeland and Lasky (1968) found that eye-movement activity is significantly related to morning re-recall. This finding has since been replicated (Goodenough, et al., 1974). In the latter study, evidence was also found that morning rerecall was better for dream reports collected during the night when the report came from a REM period with relatively irregular respiration. It is interesting to note that in this study the relationship between REM-period respiratory irregularity and morning rerecall was significant only among those subjects who responded to stress when awake by increased breathing irregularity. No such relationship was found among subjects who did not respond in the respiratory channel when awake. Such a finding suggests that this respiratory correlate of emotion is congruent in waking and dreaming states and adds credence to the idea that the relationship between REM-period breathing irregularity and morning recall can be understood in terms of emotional salience.

Since salience plays such a well-documented role in the rerecall of once-remembered dreams, the question should be raised as to whether this principle might be used in interpreting findings from various studies on the initial recall of dreams. In fact, a variety of initial-recall data can be understood in terms of salience theory.

In view of the relationships between REM-period eye-movement activity, breathing rate, breathing irregularity and salience of dreams that are reported, it seems plausible to assume that these REM-period characteristics are related to salience of the dream experience itself, whether or not the dream is ever recalled. If this assumption is correct, and if salience is an important factor in the initial recall of dreams, then failures to remember dreams immediately after REM-period awakenings ought to occur more frequently for REM periods with little eye-movement activity, low respiration rates, and relatively regular breathing. The evidence tends to support these expectations.

Snyder (1960) was one of the first to explore the relationship between REM-period characteristics and dream recall. He showed that respiratory irregularity was related to immediate dream recall, a finding which was replicated by Shapiro, Goodenough, Biederman, and Sleser (1964) and by Goodenough, et al. (1974), although not by Hobson, et al. (1965). Significant relationships between respiratory rate and REM-period dream reporting have been found by Hobson, et al. (1965) and Goodenough, et al. (1974), although not by Shapiro, et al. (1964). In the case of eye-movement activity, significant relationships with dream reporting have been found by Goodenough, et al. (1965b), Hobson, et al. (1965) and Verdone (1965), but not by Goodenough, et al. (1974). Takeo (1970) found no relationship between eye-movement activity and frequency of dream reporting, but dream reports obtained from REM periods with great activity tended to be more complicated and distinct. The data from these studies can be understood by assuming that during REM sleep the most salient dream experiences are the best recalled on awakening.

There is a fair amount of data on the relationship between measures of autonomic functioning during NREM sleep and dream reporting. These data have been summarized repeatedly in the recent literature (e.g., Cohen, 1974; Rechtschaffen, 1973) and, therefore, are not reviewed here. There is some evidence that transient autonomic changes in NREM sleep are related to dream reporting. It is possible to explain these relationships in terms of salience theory (Cohen, 1974). Often, however, these relationships are interpreted in terms of frequency of NREM dreaming rather than in terms of frequency of dream recall. This shift in interpretation as we move from REM to NREM sleep merely underlines the fact that we are dealing with *constructs* of the dream experience and of dream recall failure. In either REM or NREM sleep, the relationship of autonomic activity with frequency of dream reporting may either reflect an underlying relationship with the occurrence of dream experiences or with the frequency of dream recall, and we cannot tell for certain which of these interpretations is correct.

Studies of individual differences in the frequency of dream reporting are also interesting to examine within the framework of salience theory. The suggestion has been made that nonreporters may have less salient dream experiences and have difficulty in dream recall for this reason (Cohen, 1974). Several studies have been done on eye-movement activity during REM sleep in dream reporters and nonreporters, with results that are inconclusive. Baekeland (1970) found that home dream reporters had greater eye-movement activity during REM sleep than home nonreporters, as might be expected if salience is involved. However, Lewis et al. (1966) found no significant relationship between eye-movement activity and frequency of home dream reporting; and Antrobus, et al. (1964) actually found greater eye-movement activity in nonreporters than in reporters.

The weight of this evidence does not favor the salience explanation of individual differences.

Studies which have compared home reporters with nonreporters in the content of reported dreams in the laboratory are also relevant here. These studies have been summarized by Cohen (1974) and are not reviewed in detail here. As Cohen suggests, there is some evidence from these studies to indicate that dream narratives of nonreporters are less salient in some respects than the dream narratives of reporters. As suggested in the preceding section, however, most of these data may mean simply that the nonreporter not only recalls fewer dreams, but when remembering one, memory of the details is less vivid.

In summary, it seems safe to conclude that salience is an important factor determining which dreams will be recalled by a given person. Salience may play some role in individual differences as well. The theory of dream salience has been offered as an alternative to repression theory in the explanation of dream-recall failures (Cohen, 1974; Meier, et al., 1968). Since salience theory suggests that the most ordinary, mundane experiences are the ones most likely to be forgotten, the contrast with the types of dreams that might be considered good candidates for repression is inviting. It should be noted, however, that repression theory does address itself to the question of why dreams are more difficult to recall than waking experiences as well as to the question of why some dreams may be more difficult to recall than others. Salience theory seems to help only in our attempt to answer the second of these questions.

Dream Disorganization

Strümpell (cited in Freud, 1900/1955a) listed disorganization of dream experience as one of the factors considered important in accounting for dream-recall difficulty. There is no doubt that dreams can be chaotic and disorganized experiences. If chaos results in forgetting, then we can easily account for the fact that many dreams are difficult to recall. In fact, however, there is no evidence that dream organization plays a major role in recall. The organization factor has been studied extensively by Barber (1969). She did not find a significant relationship between ratings of organization in initial dream reports and subsequent recall of the reports. Nor were there significant differences between home reporters and nonreporters in degree of dream organization. To further study this issue Barber gave her subjects two types of dream reports to learn: ordinary dream reports and reports for which degree of organization was experimentally increased by changes in the structure of the narratives. No significant difference was found between these two types of dream materials in their recallability. The evidence from these several approaches consistently suggests that organization does not play a substantial role in dream recall.

The Role of Dream Kinesthesia in Recall Failure

Rorschach (1942) is responsible for one little-known but interesting content-centered theory of dream-recall failure. He focused on the fact that the sleeper perceives his own movements in the dream but these movements are not usually overt. Like kinesthetic imagery in the waking state, dream recollection is inhibited by actual body movements, in Rorschach's view. If the dreamer does not move his body or open his eyes, dreams may be retained on awakening, but a movement at arousal is often sufficient to blot out the kinesthetic recollection. Rorschach's view has recently been reemphasized by Lerner (1967).

There is no doubt about the effect on dream recall of distraction. It is a common experience that even momentary distractions at the time of awakening may blot out the recollection of a dream experience. For example, Calkins (1893) early noted the importance of attentional factors:

> To recall a dream requires usually extreme and immediate attention to the content of the dream. Sometimes the slight movement of reaching for paper and pencil or of lighting one's candle seems to dissipate the dream-memory, and one is left with the tantalizing consciousness of having lived through an interesting dream-experience of which one has not the faintest memory [p. 312].

The effect of distractors has been shown very clearly in experiments by Cohen and Wolfe (1973). They collected dreams from home diaries under two conditions. In the distracting condition the subjects were required to telephone the local weather information number at awakening and to record the predicted temperature range at the top of their diary sheet before writing their dream descriptions. Control subjects were asked to lie quietly in bed for a similar period of time before recording their dreams. The distracting telephone call dramatically decreased the number of dreams whose content the subjects were able to report.

That small distractions at awakening do have large effects on dream recall is interesting. It seems doubtful, for example, that telephone calls of the sort used in the study by Cohen and Wolfe (1973) would have such profound effects on waking experiences as they appear to have on dreams. The dramatic effect of distraction is one of the phenomena which must be taken into account by any comprehensive theory of dream recall. There are a number of alternative explanations that are possible, however. For example, according to Whitman (1963), the forgetting of dreams is partly an ego problem at the moment of awakening, "involving the turning of cathexis outward to the sensory or motor demands on the dreamer, thereby depriving the ego of sufficient searching energy to focalize on the dream [p. 65]."

It is possible to view distraction as one of the energy-depriving demands. In addition, Cohen (1974) has suggested that the large effect of distraction on dream recall may be a consequence of state-dependent learning of the dream experience. How this process may work is not entirely clear, however. Still another explanation of the effect of distraction is attempted subsequently in the framework of the proposed consolidation theory of dream recall failures.

In summary, while it is clear that distraction at awakening does impair dream recall, as suggested by Rorschach, the kinesthetic theory is only one among several ways of accounting for this phenomenon. The theory suffers from the fact that no other deductions have been suggested in the area of dream recall. As a consequence, Rorschach's views have not generated much interest among workers in the area.

Disinterest in Dream Content

Another factor suggested by Strümpell to account for dream-recall failures was lack of interest in the content of dream experiences. In stronger terms, Schachtel (1959) has emphasized the lack of importance assigned to dream content in modern western civilization. According to Schachtel, there is a rejection of the useless, irrational dream thoughts when the dreamer enters the logical, reasonable, efficiency-oriented waking state.

Frequency of dream reporting is clearly related to how interested we are in our dream life and how strongly we are motivated to work at the recall process. Psychoanalysts have often commented that patients who rarely recall dreams before entering therapy can do so when motivation increases after entering analysis (e.g., Stekel, 1943). Cohen and Wolfe (1973) have manipulated motivation by varying the instructional set given to their subjects. They were able to collect more dreams by the home diary method from subjects for whom the importance of dreams was emphasized than from control subjects. In another study Reed (1973) was able to collect more dreams from his students when they were highly motivated to report than when interest in the project was not so high.

Evidence which is consistent with the hypothesis that motivational variables play a role in dream recall has also been found in studies of individual differences in dream reporting. According to Strauch (1969), and Cohen and Wolfe (1973) home dream reporters tend to feel that their dreams are meaningful and important, whereas nonreporters more often express disinterest in their dream life.

It seems clear that how much a person wants to remember his dreams may influence how many dreams he can actually report. The importance of motivation may be based on the fact that dream recall requires so much attention at the moment of awakening. In the opinion of this reviewer, however, motivational factors can only account for a limited range of phenomena in the area. Anyone who has struggled to remember a dream or who has observed others do so, would probably reject the idea that dream recall is difficult merely because dreams are uninteresting experiences.

Repression

The Freudian view that repression plays a major role in dream recall failures is also, of course, a content-centered theory, and it has been by far the most influential of all explanations. Lewin (1953) and Kanzer (1959) are among the strongest modern advocates of a repression model. Lewin has expressed the view that *all* dream recall failures are due to repression, a position upon which even Freud appears not to have insisted. For Kanzer, repression of dreams so clearly follows from the nature of dream content that his attention is directed at the question of why dreams are ever recalled, rather than to the problem of recall difficulty. In the recent literature Whitman (1963), Wolpert (1972), and Goodenough (1967) have discussed repression as one of a multiplicity of factors that may be responsible for dream recall failures.

The evidence for the repression explanation of dream-recall failures came initially and still comes primarily from clinical sources which suggest that dreams are often recalled at the moment when resistance to the dream content is lifted during the course of analysis. One interesting study by Whitman, Kramer, and Baldridge (1963) has combined the clinical and laboratory approaches by using subjects who were concurrently visiting a therapist and participating in laboratory dream collection procedures. In some instances, a dream was reported either to the laboratory experimenter or to the therapist, but not to both. Failure to report the dream to one or the other of the two listeners seemed to be a function of the way in which the dream content bore on the developing relationship between the subject and the person to whom the dream was not told. These recall failures were attributed to repression by Whitman et al. (1963).

A number of recent authors have shared Whitman's interest in the communication of dreams to different persons (Kanzer, 1959; Winick & Holt, 1962). In the opinion of this reviewer, Whitman's approach to the study of motivated, content-centered recall of dreams is one of the most promising to appear in the literature. Unfortunately, however, we have only a few instances of selective reporting from Whitman's work, and while these cases are dramatic, they are hardly more than anecdotal in nature.

A number of studies on individual differences in dream reporting have appeared which are based on repression theory. These studies begin by postulating a dimension of individual differences in the organization of defenses against ego-threatening information. At one extreme of this dimension, people are said to be characteristic users of repression, and at the other extreme, users of sensitization or intellectualization as preferred defenses. In this view, nonreporters should be repressors if repression plays a major role in the production of dream recall failures. Three lines of work may be distinguished which take this general approach. One line involves the use of personality questionnaires to identify repressors. Another makes use of projective techniques. Still another involves the use of cognitive style dimensions which are thought to be related to repression as a defensive style. Field dependence, leveling versus sharpening, and convergent versus divergent thinking are among the cognitive dimensions that have been examined.

Field dependence was the first of the cognitive styles to be related to dream recall. The first studies in this area were conducted before the discovery of REM sleep. It had been suggested that field-dependent persons are likely to use repression as a predominant defense (Witkin, Dyk, Faterson, Goodenough, & Karp, 1962/74), and it seemed reasonable, therefore, to expect that field-dependent subjects might have particular difficulty in dream recall (Witkin, 1970). To explore this possibility, Linton and Eagle (cited in Witkin et al., 1962/1974) examined the relationship between frequency of home dream reporting and field dependence. In these studies field-dependent subjects tended to be home nonreporters. Schonbar (1965) was subsequently able to replicate this finding. However, no significant relationship has been found between field dependence and frequency of home reporting in a number of other studies (Baekeland, 1969; Bone, Thomas, & Kinsolving, 1972; Montgomery & Bone, 1970; Starker, 1973).

In view of the fact that people apparently may be nonreporters for a variety of distinctly different reasons, it is not too surprising to find that attempts to replicate the relationship between field dependence and home dream reporting are not very consistent. Fortunately, more detailed laboratory studies are available that clarify the situation. An unpublished finding from an early study of 46 home dream reporters and nonreporters conducted in our laboratory is relevant here (Lewis, et al., 1966). Comparison of the 8 most field-dependent and the 8 most field-independent subjects in the sample showed that 7 of the 8 dependent subjects were nonreporters, in contrast to only 3 of the 8 independent subjects. This difference was only marginally significant ($p < .05$; one-tailed test). It is important to note, however, that the field-dependent nonreporters all came from one subgroup who were able to recall their dreams immediately after abrupt REM-period awakenings. The field-dependent home nonreporters, like the field-independent home reporters recalled some dream content for approximately 80% of their REM-period awakenings. However, with a gradual awakening method, produced by slowly increasing the intensity of a bell until the subject awakened, the percentage of awakenings from which dream content could be collected dropped to about 60% for the field-dependent subjects. In contrast, the method of awakening had no significant effect among field-independent subjects. The results of this study suggest that among the several types of home nonreporters that may be distinguished by analysis of laboratory awakening, only one type is field dependent. In addition, the results suggest that field-dependent people have no difficulty in recalling their dreams under relatively ideal conditions (that is, abrupt awakenings from REM periods), but dream reporting is dramatically reduced by departures from this ideal (for example, gradual awakenings, ordinary morning recall at home).

The results of several other studies are consistent with this view. In one study subsequently described in more detail, frequency of dream reporting from REM-period awakenings was significantly reduced by stress among field-dependent subjects, but no stress effect was found among field-independent subjects (Goodenough, et al., 1974). In another study, Baekeland and Lasky (1968) found no relationship between field dependence and initial reporting of dreams following REM-period awakenings, but subsequent morning recall of these once-reported dreams was significantly less frequent among field-dependent than among field-independent subjects. These laboratory studies support the conclusion that dream recall is disrupted by a variety of conditions among field-dependent people.

While it seems reasonable to conclude that field independence is related to dream recall, the question remains as to whether repression has anything to do with this relationship. We have had an opportunity to examine dreams collected from field-dependent and independent subjects at abrupt REM awakenings. We have not been impressed by any dramatic content differences that might account for the greater difficulty to recall among field-dependent people. It is possible, of course, that the critical content features are subtle ones. Clearly, however, the factor responsible for the poor dream recall among field-dependent people has not yet been persuasively demonstrated.

Turning now to similar research with other cognitive style dimensions, one investigation of leveling-sharpening in relation to individual differences in home dream reporting has been done on the premise that levelers tend to use a repressive defensive style (Lachmann, Lapkin, & Handelman, 1962). The study produced positive, but somewhat equivocal results. Convergent and divergent cognitive styles have been studied extensively by Hudson (1966), who noted that some people (divergers) do better on open-ended intelligence tests than on conventional objective tests, while other people (convergers) are superior on conventional tests. As is the case for field-dependent persons and for levelers, it has been proposed that convergers typically resort to repression as a defense (Hudson, 1966) and it has therefore been hypothesized that convergers will tend to be nonreporters. Austin (1971) did find that convergers reported dreaming less often than divergers immediately after REM awakenings in the laboratory. Holmes (1973), however, failed to find an overall relationship between frequency of dream reporting and convergence-divergence. As in the case of leveling-sharpening, the results available to date with the converger-diverger dimension appear suggestive but inconclusive.

Turning now to more traditional personality-test measures of repression, Levine and Spivak (1964) have examined their Rorschach index of repressive style in relation to frequency of home dream reporting. In women, the hypothesized relationship was found: repressors tended to report fewer dreams. In men, however, just the opposite result obtained: repressors tended to report more dreams.

Equivocal results have also emerged from questionnaire measures of repression. Expected correlations between home report frequency and an interrelated cluster of repression-relevant questionnaire scales (repression-sensitization, anxiety, neuroticism, and ego strength) have occasionally been found, following the work of Schonbar (1959), but these findings have not been confirmed in other studies (Bone, 1968; Bone & Corlett, 1968; Bone, Nelson, & McAllister, 1970;

Cohen, 1969; Domhoff & Gerson, 1967; Foulkes & Rechtschaffen, 1964; Foulkes, Spear, & Symonds, 1966; Larson, 1971; Pivik & Foulkes, 1968; Puryear, 1963; Singer & Schonbar, 1961; Tart, 1962).

In summarizing the findings from these personality tests, it seems prudent to say that the role of repression as an explanation of individual difference in frequency of dream reporting has not been clearly established. Even if it can be shown that one or more of these measures is related to dream reporting, it may be that the relationship is due to differences among the subjects in the importance which they attach to inner-life experiences, a factor which is known to be related to individual differences in dream reporting, as discussed previously, and which may underlie questionnaire and projective-test responses leading to repressor-sensitizer scorings.

Laboratory studies which have examined the effects of presleep stress on dream reporting may also have some bearing on the repression issue. These studies are based on the assumption that more dreams will occur which are good candidates for repression under conditions of stress than under neutral conditions (Goodenough, 1967; Witkin, 1969a; Witkin & Lewis, 1965, 1967). Cartwright, Bernick, Borowitz, and Kling (1969) found less dream reporting at REM awakenings following the viewing of a sexually exciting film. They attributed these effects to the influence of repression. Foulkes, Pivik, Steadman, Spear, and Symonds (1967) also found reduced dream reporting following presleep stress-film viewing, but Foulkes and Rechtschaffen (1964) did not. Karacan, et al. (1966) also failed to find the expected stress-film effects, but this study was complicated by the fact that a penis gauge was used in all sleep sessions. There was reason to believe that the gauge in itself may have been stressful, overwhelming any possible film effects.

Two recent studies have examined individual differences in the effects of stress on frequency of dream reporting. These studies have compared subjects with an hypothesized repressive style, for whom the stress effect should be pronounced, with control subjects. In one of these studies, briefly referred to previously, presleep stress films significantly decreased the frequency of dream reporting from laboratory REM awakenings in field-dependent subjects, but had no effect among field-independent subjects (Goodenough, et al., 1974). Since field-dependent subjects are presumed to be repressors, the fact that the stress films were particularly effective for them is noteworthy. However, no evidence could be found that the stress-produced dream-report failures came from REM periods characterized by physiological arousal as might have been expected (Goodenough, 1967; Koulack, 1970).

In another study, Cohen (1972) examined the effect of stress on home dream reporting in home reporters and nonreporters. In the stress condition used by Cohen, subjects watched a "fake" experiment in which an accomplice, ostensibly in the subject role, apparently received painful treatment. The subjects were led to believe that they themselves would participate in this experiment a few days later. Dream reports were collected from home diaries kept on the morning following this experience and following control (nonstressful) conditions. Cohen found that dream reporting was less frequent under stress conditions for home nonreporters and better under these same conditions for home reporters relative to the control condition. As Cohen pointed out, his results are also consistent with repression theory.

While the studies of stress effects on dream reporting have produced results that are consistent with repression theory, a rather simple alternative explanation seems possible. Both Goodenough, et al. (1974) and Cohen (1974) have emphasized the possibility that anxiety-produced distractions at awakening may have been responsible for the lower frequency of dream reports on stress nights. This interpretation is in line with the known importance of distraction in producing dream-recall failures.

In summary, while repression may be responsible for some instances of dream-recall failure, the role of repression has not been persuasively demonstrated in solving the problem of why so many dreams are so difficult to recall.

Memory-Process Explanations of Dream Recall Failure

To this point, the discussion of dream-recall theories has focused on content-centered explanations of dream-recall failures. We now consider the second major class of theories about dream recall, the "memory-process" class. As suggested earlier, this class of theories is content-free — that is, the ability to recall any experience during sleep is said to be impaired, whether the experience is an endogenous dream or one produced by an exogenous stimulus. In considering content-centered theories it was appropriate to limit the review to studies concerned with the frequency of dream reporting under various conditions. In considering memory-process theories, however, the literature concerning the effects of sleep on memory for events other than dreams is also of interest.

In fact, the acquisition of information is very generally impaired during sleep. This conclusion is so much a part of common experience that it must have been evident early in the history of thought on dream recall. Incidental observations to this effect are repeatedly found in the psychological literature. For example, in their study of retention over periods of sleep, Jenkins and Dallenbach (1924) found that in the morning their subjects sometimes could not remember that tests were given to them during brief nighttime awakenings. During his studies of respiration in sleep, Magnussen (1944) also observed that his subjects frequently failed to recall the fact that they had awakened during the night and had spoken a few words or had performed simple tasks during these awakenings.

These casual observations have been amply supported by more systematic studies of sleep learning conducted during the last 20 years. Since the classical studies by Simon and Emmons (1956) and by Emmons and Simon (1956), it has commonly been concluded that learning does not occur during sleep. In more recent years, however, there has been some revival of interest in the possibility of sleep learning, due primarily, perhaps, to persistent claims of success by Russian workers (e.g., Rubin, 1968). It is important to note that Simon and Emmons did find some learning during EEG stages of sleep which were defined as light or transitional at the time, but which we now know would include REM sleep. While the literature suggests that some sleep learning may be possible during REM, or even during NREM periods, it is clear that learning is at least substantially impaired during all stages.[3]

At one time it was popular to regard sleep as a state of deafferentation. Difficulties in sleep learning were thus understood as failures of stimulus registration. Recent research suggests, however, that auditory stimuli can be discriminated and are effective in evoking responses which have been learned when awake (e.g., Minard, Loiselle, Ingledue, & Dautlich, 1968; Oswald, Taylor, & Treisman, 1960; Williams, Morlock, & Morlock, 1966). It also seems clear that rewards and punishments are effective in motivating performance during sleep (Williams, Morlock, & Morlock, 1966; Wilson & Zung, 1966). These findings suggest that impaired learning during sleep is due to some defect in memory. If we accept this conclusion, then some kind of memory-process theory must be entertained. If sleep impairs recall of all experiences, including dreams, then a theory explaining the more general phenomenon is required. At best, content-centered theories could account for only a limited set of data.

The literature on individual differences in dream reporting also contains some evidence which is relevant to memory-process theory. Home dream reporters and nonreporters have been compared on standard tests of memory in the waking state in a number of studies (e.g., Barber, 1969; Cohen, 1971; Puryear, 1963). Intelligence has been examined in many other studies (e.g., Antrobus, et al., 1964; Ramsey, 1953; Schonbar, 1959; Singer & Schonbar, 1971). There is no persuasive evidence from these studies that nonreporters are less intelligent or are lower in specific waking memory abilities. Of course, these findings do not rule out the possibility that some sleep-memory-ability factor may be found that distinguishes dream reporters from nonreporters. However, they do suggest that whatever the memory dimension may be during sleep, it is not the same dimension tapped by waking memory tests.

Specific theories about the nature of the memory process impaired during sleep are considered in the sections below.

Some Classical Memory Phenomena in the Recall of Dreams

It is not surprising to find that the classical laws of memory apply to the recall of dreams as they do to memory for other types of material. It is important, however, to examine the available data on dream reporting in order to see how much can be understood from this perspective. Attention was drawn in a very dramatic way to the role of these factors in the study of dream reporting by Meier, et al. (1968). These authors studied morning rerecall of dreams that were

---

[3]For an excellent review of learning during sleep, see Aarons, L. (1976).

initially reported during the night. As might be expected, the duration of the interval between the initial report and the morning rerecall was an important factor in determining which dreams were lost. Many more of the dreams reported later in the night were recalled by morning, in contrast to dreams reported earlier in the night. In addition, the number of dreams reported during the night was significantly related to the percentage recalled the next morning. For nights when few dreams were reported, these dreams were much easier to recall the next morning than was the case for nights when many dreams were reported.

The results of Meier, et al. (1968) have been confirmed and extended in several studies. The relationship between number of dreams reported and morning recall has also been found by Trinder and Kramer (1971), Strauch (1969), and by Goodenough, et al. (1974). The recency effect has been noted by Trinder and Kramer (1971), Strauch (1969), and by Baekeland and Lasky (1968) for home nonreporters (but not for subjects who claim that they recall dreams at home almost every morning). Strauch as well as Trinder and Kramer not only found that the last dream of the night is favored, but also found that the first dream report of the night is more easily recalled than reports in the middle positions of the nightly set of dreams.

In this connection, it is interesting to note the results of a different kind of study done in our laboratory (Goodenough, Sapan, Cohen, Portnoff, & Shapiro, 1971). In this study subjects were awakened briefly several times each night, and at each awakening a different word was shown. Next morning the subjects were asked to recall the words. We found that for words, the effects of list length, primacy, and recency appear to be comparable to the effects that have been found for dreams. We did not anticipate these results, perhaps because we did not have a "set" to think of the words shown to the subject at widely separate times during the night as a serial list. However, it is clear that either the dreams of the night or the words of the night may be viewed as a serially occurring list of items with effects on memory that are well known to classical learning theorists.

In summary, serial effects may play an important role in determining which dreams of the night are recalled. However, they do not help us in the attempt to understand why dreams and other types of sleep experiences are more difficult to recall than waking events.

State-Dependent Learning

Another type of memory-process explanation considers dream-recall failures as special cases of state-dependent learning. In this view, any information acquired in the sleeping state is difficult to retrieve from memory storage in the waking state (but theoretically it might be retrieved at a later time during the sleeping state). The concept of state-dependent learning has been used primarily to account for the fact that responses acquired while under the influence of certain drugs can be elicited at a later time when the individual returns to the drugged state, but cannot be elicited under nondrug conditions (e.g., Overton, 1966). If the sleep state is also characterized by state-dependent learning, then it may be possible to account for difficulties of dream recall.

Theories of this general type were popular in the early literature. For example, Strumpell (cited in Freud, 1900/1955a) called attention to the fact that dreams often involve details of waking life which are torn out of the contexts in which they are usually remembered when awake. Given this characteristic of dream content, he believed that recall difficulty was a natural consequence. Similar ideas have been expressed by many theorists since Strumpell. For example, Bonatelli (cited in Freud, 1900/1955a) believed that "the alternation in coenesthesia between the sleeping and waking states is unfavorable to reciprocal reproduction between them [p. 45]." Similarly Prince (1911) proposed that the forgetting of dreams may be a special case of amnesia for experiences in dissociated mental states. Jung (1939) also suggested that the fantastic arrangement of ideas in dreams makes them difficult to connect with waking consciousness. More recently Blum (1961) has suggested that specific contextual circuits are inaccessible during dreaming. Schachtel (1959) has offered a similar argument that, "it seems obvious that the experience and memory schemata developed and formed by man's life in his society are much less suitable to preserve the fantastic world of the dream than to recall conventional waking experience [p. 307]." This tradition is represented in the current literature by Evans and his colleagues (Evans, Gustafson, O'Connell, Orne, & Shor, 1966, 1969, 1970) and by Cohen (1974).

As far as this reviewer is aware, only one series of studies has been directed specifically at this issue (Evans, 1972; Evans, et al., 1966, 1969, 1970). In these studies, subjects were given verbal suggestions during REM sleep of the sort, "Whenever I say the word 'itch,' your nose will feel itchy until you scratch it." Some subjects carried out the suggestion in response to the cue word during REM sleep. That is, they scratched their noses when the experimenter said, "itch," without waking up. The subjects typically had no waking recall of the suggestion the next day, nor did they respond appropriately to the cue word when awake. The most interesting aspect of this work is that the subjects did respond on subsequent nights to the cue words, indicating that the appropriate response was learned, but could only be elicited in the REM state in which the learning had occurred. These experiments did not work in NREM sleep. For REM sleep, at least, Evans, et al. (1969) offer the possibility that "acquisition of new experiences must occur within a particular context of other ongoing experience, aspects of which are necessary at a later time to act as a 'triggering mechanism' for the subsequent recall of the acquired behavior [p. 667]."

It is interesting to note that these findings are related to hypnotic phenomena in several ways. First, the results could be obtained only for good hypnotic subjects (poor hypnotic subjects were apparently awakened by the suggestions). Second, for one subject at least, a posthypnotic suggestion to recall when awake was effective. The complex nature of the relationship between hypnosis, REM

sleep and the ability of the subjects to remember the response contingency is discussed in detail by Evans (1972). While this line of work is intriguing, it is uncertain whether a state-dependent learning model of sleep is necessary to account
for the results, as Evans has pointed out.

It seems likely that state-dependent theories would gain more wide-spread acceptance if it could be shown that habituation readily occurs during sleep. Habituation to a repetitive stimulus should not be difficult during continuous sleep if
the only problem in sleep learning is a state dependency. However, the data on
habituation do not appear to support a state-dependent theory very strongly.

In discussing the literature on habituation, it is important to distinguish between habituation of the awakening response itself, and habituation of other responses like the K complex, orienting responses, and the like, which may occur
without awakenings. This distinction is important because it is only in the latter
case that learning may be said to occur entirely during sleep.

Many studies have been done on habituation of awakening responses. It is evident that a stimulus which may awaken a person when novel, tends to lose its
effectiveness on repeated presentation. Data on this point are reviewed by Oswald
(1962). Habituation, during sleep, of responses that are not accompanied by
awakening appears to be relatively ineffective, however. Unfortunately, the data
on this point are not absolutely clear. By the very nature of the habituation
phenomenon, many stimulus presentations are necessary, and some of these are
likely to produce awakenings even if the response being studied is not a necessary arousal accompaniment. In fact, several studies have reported some evidence
of habituation for K complexes, for galvanic skin responses, and for heart-rate
responses during sleep (e.g., Firth, 1973; Oswald, et al., 1960). However, no evidence of habituation has been found in other studies (e.g., Johnson & Lubin,
1967; Roth, Shaw, & Green, 1956; Tizard, 1968). In still another study, habituation of the orienting response was found to be impaired in a drowsy state as
compared with an alert state (McDonald, Johnson, & Hord, 1964). It is probably
a conservative conclusion to say of these data that if habituation occurs during
sleep, it is much slower and more difficult to demonstrate than is habituation
during the waking state.

In summary, while a state-dependent learning theory of dream-recall failure is
attractive, the evidence for an explanation of this sort is not very compelling at
this time.

Impairment in Memory-Trace Consolidation

Another type of memory-process explanation involves the assumption that
consolidation of memory traces is impaired during sleep. The concept of mem-
ory-trace consolidation has had a long history among learning theorists (Muller &
Pilzecker, 1900). In the most general terms, the consolidation concept implies a
multistage memory trace. For some period of time after an experience occurs,
the trace of that experience is carried in a temporary, short-term form. The more-
or-less permanent traces in long-term memory take time (and perhaps a favorable

state) to become effectively established. As information is transferred from the short-term to the long-term form, trace consolidation is said to occur.

During the history of thought concerning consolidation, a number of variants of the concept have been proposed, and several very different forms have been applied to sleep-related phenomena. It is essential to distinguish among these forms in order to avoid confusion in any discussion of consolidation mechanisms during sleep.

The traditional conception of consolidation was developed in the attempt to account for retrograde amnesias produced by a variety of agents, including electroconvulsive shocks, blows to the head, and certain drugs. In this view the long-term trace may take an hour or more to become fully established. During the process of consolidation, a disrupting agent may destroy the trace or a facilitating agent may enhance trace establishment, but susceptibility to these agents diminishes with time. Several applications of this concept have been applied to sleep phenomena.

Some theorists, attempting to understand the adaptive function of REM sleep, have proposed that the transfer of daytime experiences to long-term memories and/or integration of the temporary memories of these experiences into long-term storage occurs during dreaming (e.g., Dewan, 1968; Fishbein, 1969; Greenberg, 1970; Greenberg & Leiderman, 1966; Shapiro, 1967; Stokes, 1973). In this view, memories are held in short-term storage for hours before the REM periods of the night produce their consolidation. The extensive experimental literature on the possible consolidation function of dreaming are not reviewed here because a mechanism of this sort is irrelevant to an understanding of dream-recall failure.

Another application of traditional consolidation theory has grown out of sleep research on the interference theory of memory. The study of forgetting over periods of sleep attracted early learning theorists because it seemed reasonable to suppose that cognitive activity ought to be minimal during sleeping states. If such activity interferes with memory, then one might expect forgetting to be slight if sleep intervenes between learning and tests of retention. In fact, the early research on this issue suggested that memory tends to be better over periods of sleep than over comparable periods of waking activity (Jenkins & Dallenbach, 1924; Newman, 1939; Van Ormer, 1932, 1933). More recent studies have largely reemphasized this conclusion, particularly for NREM sleep (Barrett & Ekstrand, 1972; Ekstrand, 1967; Fowler, Sullivan, & Ekstrand, 1973; Hockey, Davies, & Gray, 1972; Lovatt & Warr, 1968; Yaroush, Sullivan , & Ekstrand, 1971). It has been suggested by some authors that the less rapid decay of memory during sleep may be due to a facilitation of consolidation during NREM periods rather than to a reduction in interference (Fowler, et al., 1973; Graves, 1936; Grieser, Greenberg, & Harrison, 1972; Heine, 1914; Richardson & Gough, 1963). In this view, consolidation must continue for a considerable period, since subjects typically do not go to sleep until many minutes have elapsed after the end of learning trials. As is the case for the consolidation concept as a REM-period function, difficulties in dream recall cannot be understood in terms of this application of consolidation theory.

The traditional view of the consolidation concept has also been applied in just the opposite way by some authors who have suggested that consolidation may be impaired by NREM sleep. This view is implicit in the work of several authors. It has been suggested, for example, that the transfer of information from short- to long-term memory storage is less effective as arousal level decreases (e.g., Klein-smith & Kaplan, 1963; Walker & Tarte, 1963). It is not easy to characterize REM sleep in terms of its location on a hypothetical arousal continuum. However, during NREM sleep, at least, these theories imply a reduction in effectiveness for the process of long-term memory storage. Hebb (1949) also suggested a consolidation explanation in his discussion of sleep learning problems. In Hebb's theory, memory is a two-stage process: a short-term memory store in the form of reverberating circuits; and a long-term store involving the more permanent growth of "neural knobs." The structural changes involved in the growth of these knobs is believed to be difficult, at least during the synchronized EEG stages of sleep more or less characteristic of many NREM periods. The idea that dream-recall difficulty may be due to consolidation difficulties is explicit in the writing of a number of researchers in the field (e.g., Goodenough, 1967; Goodenough, et al., 1971; Portnoff, Baekeland, Goodenough, Karacan, & Shapiro, 1966; Rechtschaffen, 1964; Williams, 1973; Wolpert, 1972).

The idea that dream-recall difficulty might be due to ineffective consolidation was first suggested by observations indicating a rapid decay in the probability of eliciting the report of a dream after the end of REM periods in the absence of an awakening. It was found that many fewer dream reports are obtainable from NREM awakenings a few minutes after REM periods end than from REM period awakenings (Dement & Kleitman, 1957b; Goodenough, et al., 1965a; Wolpert & Trosman, 1958). It was also found that more dreams can be collected from NREM awakenings shortly after REM periods end than can be obtained after longer delays. These data were originally interpreted to mean that memory for the dream may persist after some minutes of NREM sleep. However, the decline in dream reporting after REM ends may not be part of a forgetting curve. It may reflect, instead, a decrease in NREM dream frequency. The evidence for this conclusion is summarized elsewhere (Goodenough, 1968). In brief, there is good reason to suspect that dreams are never recalled unless the dream experience is interrupted by an awakening.

Given the evidence on rapid loss of dreams, it was easy to imagine that consolidation is impaired during sleep. According to Rechtschaffen (1964), for example:

> Dreams are remembered if there is an awakening following the dream, because consolidation can take place during this wakefulness. However, if the dream is followed by NREM sleep, it is forgotten because of the lack of opportunity for consolidation [p. 165].

There are other sorts of data that can be understood in terms of traditional consolidation theory. Length of time awake at REM awakenings has been related to the rerecall of the dream experience. The longer the subject remains awake after initially reporting a dream, the more likely is dream-recall the next morning (Baekeland & Lasky, 1968; Strauch, 1969). The authors of both studies have interpreted the time spent awake as "consolidation time," under the assumption that more effective consolidation of the long-term traces will occur as a function of more time awake after the dream experiences.

The relationship between length of time awake after an experience and subsequent memory of the experience is not unique to dreams. The same relationship holds for word stimuli (Goodenough, et al., 1971; Portnoff, et al., 1966). In these studies, subjects were awakened several times each night, and immediately after each awakening a word was shown by means of a bedroom slide projector under incidental learning conditions. These studies clearly demonstrate that when the subjects spontaneously remain awake for a relatively long period of time after the words are shown, they are more likely to remember the word the next morning than when they return to sleep more quickly.

This series of studies also produced data that appear to contradict an interpretation in terms of traditional consolidation theory. The studies were designed to determine whether the critical variable that affects memory for the words might be the level of arousal during the minutes that followed the word presentation. For this purpose, on half the trials the subjects were kept awake for about 15 min after the words were shown by requiring them to work on a motor task. Next morning, memory for the words shown under this enforced waking condition was compared with memory for the words shown on trials when the subjects were permitted to return to sleep immediately. Over the range of times examined, longer periods of waking "consolidation time" did not affect retention as was expected. These findings suggest that the relationship between spontaneous time awake and retention must be due to level of arousal at, and/or very shortly after, the word presentation. If the subject is highly aroused at this point in time, then sleep onset is likely to be delayed for some minutes, but delay in sleep onset beyond a few minutes is not in itself sufficient to improve retention. In fact, some evidence was found that instructions to the subjects designed to vary level of arousal within a period of seconds *after* the word presentation did have an effect on subsequent retention. High-arousal instructions tended to favor retention (Goodenough, et al., 1971). Thus, while evidence of an arousal-retention relationship was found, the time during which arousal is effective may be on the order of seconds after the stimulus rather than many minutes after it, as assumed in traditional consolidation theory.

Another problem in the attempt to understand dream recall difficulty in terms of traditional consolidation theory was pointed out by Foulkes (1966), who emphasized the retrieval problem:

There must be something still unknown about the way in which these traces are "filed" that renders them generally inaccessible to consciousness unless wakefulness intervenes very soon after the original impressions are experienced [p.55].

As this statement indicates, Foulkes has emphasized the possibility that recall difficulties may be due to retrieval of the trace from long-term storage at the time of recall, rather than to an impairment in consolidation. From everyday experience we may share with Foulkes (and with Freud, 1900/1955a) the impression that dream recall failures are typically retrieval failures. In many cases, we cannot recall a dream for the moment, but can vividly recall the dream at some later time. Kanzer (1959) has discussed this phenomenon at length. Such cases are troublesome for traditional consolidation theory.

An Arousal-Retrieval Model

The results of these studies suggest still another application of multistage memory theory that involves what might be called a "rapid" consolidation concept (Koulack & Goodenough, 1976). As before, it is assumed that the effectiveness of information transfer from short- to long-term storage is impaired at low levels of arousal and particularly during sleep. However, the duration of the short-term memory is assumed to be on the order of seconds rather than many minutes or hours.

While the existence of a short- as distinct from a long-term memory system is not universally accepted, it seems fair to say that the evidence for a short-term memory form which lasts for a period of seconds is more persuasive than is the evidence for a short-term memory form which lasts for much longer periods. Much of the material for consolidation theory has come from studies on the effects of electroconvulsive shock on memory. In the view of some authors, however, the evidence for a short-term store would support a process lasting less than a minute (Spevack & Suboski, 1969). A short-term memory form of this duration is consistent with a variety of other data, as well. The work of Peterson and Peterson (1959) provided a dramatic impetus to research on theories of short-term memory. In much of the recent work in this area, buffer memory stores have been proposed with very limited capacities in terms of chunks of information and/or time span (e.g., Atkinson & Shiffrin, 1968; Waugh & Norman, 1965).

In many of the recent multistage memory theories, it is assumed that cognitive processing of information in the short-term store facilitates the transfer of information to long-term memory storage. These processes include repetition or recycling of information through the short-term store as well as more complex activities such as recoding, reorganization of the information for insertion into long-term storage and the like. Within this framework it is easy to imagine that sleep impairs or even prevents such processing.

The fact that dream-recall failures are often retrieval failures is easily handled in this view. One may suppose that the information processing steps impaired by sleep are critically involved in the "filing," coding, or addressing of new information for ready retrieval from long-term storage. Thus information may be transferred to long-term storage during sleep, but in a form that is difficult to access.

In this view, dream-recall failures should occur unless the sleeper awakens within a matter of seconds after the dream experience occurs. If arousal takes place during the life of the short-term trace, then the content of the dream experience which immediately preceded the awakening may be retrievable from the short-term store directly. Given this retrieval cue as an entry into the long-term store, the dreamer may then be able to recall some of the preceding content of that dream experience. If the awakening is delayed until the short-term trace has expired, then retrieval may no longer be possible, or it may be much more difficult. Ralph Waldo Emerson (1884) has expressed this state of affairs at awakening in much clearer terms:

> Dreams are jealous of being remembered; they dissipate instantly and angrily if you try to hold them. When newly awakened from lively dreams, we are so near them, still agitated by them, still in their sphere – give us one syllable, one feature, one hint, and we should repossess the whole; hours of this strange entertainment would come trooping back to us; but we cannot get our hand on the first link or fibre, and the whole is lost. There is a strange wistfulness in the speed with which it disperses and baffles our grasp [p. 10].

That distractions at awakening have such a devastating effect on dream recall can also be understood in terms of an arousal-retrieval model. It is easy to suppose that incoming events may compete with the dream experience for attention in the limited-capacity processing system during the critical period after the awakening when effective transfer to long-term memory storage must take place if the dream is to be subsequently recalled.

An arousal-retrieval model also appears to be useful in accounting for a variety of data on sleep learning. There seems to be little doubt that sleep learning is facilitated if the stimuli to be learned are followed within a few seconds by even a transient arousal. This conclusion has been emphasized in a series of studies by Koukkou and Lehmann (e.g., Lehmann & Koukkou, 1973). They found that their subjects could remember sentences read to them during sleep. However, the amount retained was a function of the duration of transient waking alpha induced by the stimuli. Koukkou & Lehmann (1968) suggest that ". . . the duration of the EEG wakefulness pattern after the presentation of the test sentences reflects the time available for long-term storage of the memory material in retrievable form [p. 461]." In other studies (Jus & Jus, 1972; Jus, Kiljan, Kubacki, Losieczko, Wilczak, & Jus, 1969), words and tones were presented during sleep, and recall of these stimuli was also found to be significantly related to the duration of arousal produced. A consolidation explanation of the phenomenon was proposed. In still another study by Evans and Orchard (1969), subjects were presented during sleep with learning materials in the form of "A for apple," "B for ball," and so on, and were subsequently asked to recall the word associated with the letter. In cases of successful recall, alpha responses were found to occur within 30 sec of the stimulus presentations.

SUMMARY AND CONCLUSIONS

Many of the theories which have been advanced to account for difficulty in dream recall can be traced back at least to the beginnings of psychology as a discipline. Despite the fact that dream-recall failures were sufficiently interesting to invite extensive speculation, it was not until the discovery of REM sleep that systematic research in the area became common. During the last 20 years, evidence has accumulated which now makes it possible to evaluate many of these theories.

It is evident that serial position and dream salience are important factors in determining which dreams of the night will be recalled. These factors appear to play the same role in dream recall as they do in the recall of waking experiences. However, they are not very helpful in the attempt to understand why dreams are harder to recall than waking experiences.

In the attempt to understand dream-recall difficulty, several generalizations require central consideration. First among these is the fact that recall difficulties are encountered for any experience during sleep, whether a dream or an experience produced by exogenous stimulation. This generalization is a central one because it limits the type of theory that can account for the effect of sleep on recall. Theories which explain dream-recall difficulty in terms of some factor in dream content are not necessarily incorrect, but they are obviously insufficient to account for the effects of sleep on recall of other experiences. At the least, it is necessary to postulate some effect of sleep on memory processes more generally.

Two additional key generalizations concern the conditions under which sleep experiences can be recalled. One is that dreams or any other type of sleep experience seem to be recalled with ease only if the sleeper is awake within a matter of seconds after the experience occurs. Another is that distractions at the moment of awakening impair dream recall. Conversely, recall is improved if attention is focused on the dream for a period of some seconds after awakening.

We can account for a variety of facts in terms of the need for attention to the dream at awakening. For example, it has been found that interest in dream life is related to dream recall. It seems reasonable to suppose that the effect of interest may be mediated by attentional processes. The fact that salient dreams are most easily recalled may also be due to their attention-demanding quality. Moreover, the fact that stress impairs dream recall may be understood in terms of an anxiety-based distracting effect which interferes with attentional processes at awakening.

An arousal-retrieval model (Koulack & Goodenough, 1976) has been employed in the attempt to understand why sleep experiences seem so difficult to recall unless waking attention is focused on the experience during the period immediately after the experience occurs. It is assumed that cognitive information processing is required to effectively transfer information from short- to long-term memory storage in retrievable form. It is further assumed that sleep or distraction will impair this type of processing. Because of this impairment, transfer to long-term storage of retrievable information about sleep experiences cannot occur effectively unless a distraction-free waking state occurs during the life of the short-term memory trace.

An arousal-retrieval theory of this sort may be capable of accounting for the striking effects of sleep on memory.

Evidence for the key roles of attention, consolidation, and arousal in dream recall is convincing. The first night effect described in Chapter 2 may be taken as additional support for the role of attention. But what is the nature of this attention? Is the attention to REM dreaming the same as to Stage 2 dreaming (see Chapter 7, this volume) and the same as attention to daydreaming (see Singer, 1975)? Or is the attention really unselective? That is, does the person who attends to dreaming also attend to peas under the mattress? How does attention to dreaming actually work? Are there feature detectors for dreams (see Lindsay & Norman, 1972)? Must the individual be first aroused before the attentional processes can operate or is arousal a consequence of attending to a dream? What reinforces or maintains the attention to dreaming? Are the factors which account for individual differences in attention to dreaming the same as those that account for variation from night to night or from one interval to the next with a given REM period? The clinical use of dreams and the clinical interpretation of dream-recall failure provided the major impetus for the study of dream recall. It seems to me that the intelligent clinical interpretation of dream-recall failure must wait for the answers to some of these questions.

John S. Antrobus

6

Qualitative Aspects of
Sleep Mentation

David G. Schwartz
Lissa N. Weinstein
Arthur M. Arkin

City University of New York

In this chapter we emphasize the qualitative aspects of sleep mentation in relation to a heterogeneous assortment of variables. The material presented here is important but is not covered in sufficient depth, or else not at all, elsewhere in this volume. Actually, there is some overlapping in topics dealt with in other chapters but in such instances, the treatment here is usually in greater depth. Thus, important methodological papers, sleep-stage correlates; sleep mentation in association with psychopathologic syndromes, sensory and physical impairments, various age epochs (childhood, adult life and old age), and the menstrual cycle are reviewed; as well as material on dream sequences and psychological meaning and organization of dreams; general theories of dream formation; and personality tests in relation to dreaming; material on psychophysiological parallelism; laboratory studies of dreams of patients in psychotherapy; dreaming in relation to the nondominant cerebral hemisphere; the Pötzl phenomenon; and ESP studies utilizing dreams.

METHODOLOGICAL ISSUES

Since the demise of introspectionist psychology some 50 years ago with the publication of Watson's (1924) behaviorist manifesto, the study of private experience has labored under the double burden of a bad reputation (deserved or not), and real methodological problems. Three papers (Hauri 1975; Rechtschaffen 1967; Stoyva & Kamiya 1968) have surveyed some of these problems and proposed solutions by way of explicating the logic of the scientific investigation of private events.

The central problem of the methodology of dream research is that the dream is not an empirical (publicly observable) event. We rely primarily on verbal report as a best indicator of an already past experience. Rechtschaffen (1967, p. 5)

143

points out that the correspondence between such reports and actual dreams can be diminished by two processes: recall, and what he refers to as "translation" which consists of "the processes which intervene between the recalled dream and the . . . dream report," such as choosing words to describe the dream and actually speaking them. To minimize the distortions of the dream experience introduced by the processes of recall and translation, dream researchers take various appropriate precautions, such as excluding subjects with gross memory defects and structuring the experimental situation so that subjects are encouraged to report freely. Nevertheless, such precautions do not provide us with empirical certainty; and so Rechtschaffen (1967) suggests some guides which he feels are implicit in our assumptions of what constitutes reasonableness in choosing procedures to evaluate dreaming. Briefly, these are as follows:

1. *Parsimony* (or a "preference for the fewest assumptions"): when there is no report it is more parsimonious to assume that there was no dream experience than to assume that there was one which was forgotten.

2. *Prevalence:* we assume those phenomena to be occurring which are most frequent in other contexts, for example, when a subject gives a verbal report, we do *not* assume that gross memory defect influenced it because such conditions are uncommon.

3. *Plausibility:* we assume the occurrence of those unobserved phenomena that are consistent with the situation's characteristics and are frequently observed in similar (analogous) contexts. For example, we assume that subjects tell the truth in experimental situations. (This is mostly an extension of the prevalence principle.)

4. *Private experience:* we assume the existence of phenomena which we believe we have experienced directly.

Rechtschaffen (1967) argues that these principles help keep our inferences empirical, while not denying dream experience — as opposed to (mere) dream report — as the actual object of study. He points out that it was the assumption of unobservable dream experience which facilitated the remarkable discoveries of Aserinsky and Kleitman (1953).

Stoyva and Kamiya (1968) applied some contributions from the philosophy of science and methodological theory (Campbell & Fiske 1959; Garner, Hake, & Erikson 1956) to give a more detailed exposition of the logic of dream research, paying particular attention to the role of physiological indicators in validating inferences concerning private experiences. They argue that the dream should be viewed as an hypothetical construct imperfectly indexed by verbal report, motor behavior, and physiological measures, which themselves are the convergent operations which corroborate inferences we make concerning the dream experience itself. Noting the partial derivation of this idea from Campbell and Fiske's (1959) notion of convergent and discriminant validation, they point out that the various indicators of dream experience — REMs, verbal reports, etc. — are convergent because "they are *not* perfectly correlated and . . . can converge on a single concept [p. 196] ." Inferring that there was a dream experience of a particular quality constitutes a most probable hypothesis to explain the correlation of a verbal report (which, following Rechtschaffen, 1967, we assume to be more or less honest) with various physiological signs. The dream is an event separate and distinct from REM sleep, and from what subjects say; although it is correlated in time with both of these variables.

Stoyva and Kamiya (1968) go on to show that this view of the logical status of dream experience places the study of dreaming right alongside other unobservable phenomena and/or dimensions of private experience which science has long been interested in, such as mood, state of consciousness, and subatomic particles. In each case we use as many publicly observable indicators of the phenomenon of interest as are available in order to corroborate and strengthen the inferences we make. The indicators, or convergent operations, always measure the construct with some variable degree of error. The multidimensional measuring approach advocated by Campbell and Fiske (1959) and Stoyva and Kamiya (1968) aims to lessen this error. Different methods of measurement should tend to cancel each other's error variance out. In this very convincing argument Stoyva and Kamiya (1968) rob the study of dreaming of some of its uniqueness, but also return it and other dimensions of experience to the domain of researchable questions.

After surveying some of the large volume of research which implicitly or explicitly has adopted the methodology advocated by Rechtschaffen (1967) and Stoyva and Kamiya (1968), Hauri (1975) reports that much more traditional pitfalls of human behavioral research have stymied progress.

The first area which Hauri (1975) focuses on as a major source of difficulty is the assessment of verbal reports through the use of rating scales. (See also Chapter 2 of this volume on measurement and design.) Citing a recent survey by Winget and Kramer (in press), Hauri (1975) reports that approximately 150 such scales have been developed in the past 25 years. According to this survey, very often these scales do not provide such basic psychometric information as reliability and validity data. Furthermore, although many of these scales nominally measure the same aspect of dream content, different studies using different scales to measure apparently similar phenomena have produced data going in opposite directions. In order to further investigate the real meaning of some of these scales Hauri (1975) conducted the following study: 10 sleep laboratories provided 10 mentation reports each, of at least 100 words, elicited after at least 10 min of REM sleep, so that a total of 100 REMP reports were used. Researchers, associated with 20 different dream-rating scales, each rated all of the dream reports. The scores thus produced were subjected to factor analysis and placed in a correlation-coefficient matrix. The results of the factor analysis indicated that various scales, which should be expected to overlap because they allege to be measuring similar constructs, did cluster together to form coherent interpretable factors; however, Hauri (1975) regarded these data to be vitiated by the fact that most scales which loaded a given factor correlated with one another in the

.50s. Also, relatively weak correlations were obtained between some scales with similar names. As an example, Hauri (1975) cites Sheppard's (Saul et al. 1954) "hostility" scale correlating .37 with the Gottschalk-Gleser scale of "ambivalent hostility." He interprets this type of finding to indicate that each hostility scale was measuring the construct in "a highly idiosyncratic way."

Although Hauri's conclusion is probably correct, that the scales contain much unique variance, most personality researchers are pleased with validity coefficients which simply reach statistical significance, between scales which are *not* supposed to be measuring exactly the same construct: "hostility" is not the same as "ambivalent hostility." The error, introduced by subjects' idiosyncratic styles of recall and translation, as described by Rechtschaffen (1967), to which these scales may be differentially sensitive, makes the expectation of high intercorrelations between similarly named scales somewhat unrealistic. Furthermore, the Pearson product-moment correlation techniques, which Hauri (1975) used, is designed for interval scale measuring instruments, making it a very stringent test of scales designed to assess the quality of dreaming. Certainly it is unfortunate that different laboratories do not use each other's measuring instruments frequently enough; but this is the inevitable product of the variety of theoretical orientations which influence research. A better way of evaluating the validity and practical use of dream-content scales would be to apply the principle of convergent and discriminant validation. (Campbell & Fiske 1959; Stoyva & Kamiya, 1968). Does a given scale correlate with other indicators of the same construct, and do related types of indicators of different constructs fail to predict as well as does the scale in question? The following data cited by Hauri (1975) exemplifies this type of validity check and supports a more optimistic assessment of one current dream scale. In Hauri's (1975) study Gottschalk-Gleser's "anxiety" measure of dream content correlated .55 with Gottschalk-Gleser's measure of "hostility turned outward." However, in a recent study of the relationship between dream content and length of birth labor in primiparae (Winget & Kapp 1972) the Gottschalk-Gleser measure of "anxiety did predict the length of labor (high anxiety related to short labor) while their measure of 'hostility turned outward' [p. 275]" did not.

In examining studies of dream content from different subject groups Hauri (1975) reports a major deficit in the use of adequate control procedures. Citing Van de Castle's (1967) review of a study by Langs (1966), which contains comparisons of the dreams of hysterics and depressed patients, Hauri notes that most of the hysterics' dreams were twice as long as the depressed patients' dreams, so that the greater incidence of particular types of themes in the hysterics' dreams reported by Langs (1966) could easily be accounted for on the basis of the greater quantity of all types of themes in their dreams.

As Hauri (1975) points out, the solution to this sort of problem is not easy to find, since selecting different patient groups to be comparable on one parameter may create atypical samples, that is, typical depressives may in fact report shorter dreams. Hauri argues that we need empirically derived mathematical formulae which relate dream length to specific scales. The larger methodological point here is the same as for any attempt to compare different subject groups: controls must be matched with patient or experimental groups on as many potentially relevant variables as possible, without excluding the difference factor under investigation.

One aspect of dream research particularly exciting to behavioral scientists is that it produces psychophysiological data, that is, data which correlates a mental or "mind" event with a physiological or "body" event. As Hauri (1975) shows, this feature is also the source of some problems which are relatively peculiar to psychophysiological research. One example of such a problem is what Hauri (1975) calls "individual response specificity," or the fact that "most individuals [manifest] specific and unique [relationships between] psychological and physiological variables [p. 277]." For example, for some subjects, emotionality in a dream may manifest itself in heart-rate variability, while for others its only significant physiological correlate may be lowered GSR. Hauri cites a study by Stegie (1973) that revealed that among six subjects, there were positive (two subjects), negative (one subject) and zero relationships (three subjects) between emotionality of a dream report and respiratory variability in the last 30 sec before awakening. Stegie also reports that an individual's pattern of response specificity during sleep is not the same during wakefulness.

Similar to the problem of individual response specificity is the phenomenon of forgotten content. Many dream scales score such reports as "zero." However, Hauri (1975) notes that Shapiro et al. (1964) reported that when subjects said they were dreaming but had forgotten the content, breathing irregularity during the REMP was always highest. Informally Hauri and Van de Castle (1973b) found that "no content reports" are associated with either very high or very low arousal. Hauri (1975), therefore, recommends that for the present "no content" reports should be eliminated from data analyses.

THE NORMATIVE CONTENT OF DREAMS

What sort of things do people generally dream about in the course of their "garden variety" dreams? Perhaps more than any other investigators, Hall (1966) and Hall and Van de Castle (1966) have carried out monumental systematic content-analytic studies of people of both sexes, all ages, different cultures, under varying conditions and different personality types. The reader is enthusiastically referred to their work. However, their results, though of first rank importance are based upon daytime dream recall. As we have previously said, our chief focus is on laboratory dream study and the amount of work in this area using electrographic technique is not extensive. We have included reviews of content-analytic studies of the dreams of "normal" college students and children, and less detailed reports on dreams of the very young, the aged, the middle aged, and dreams in association with the menstrual cycle. It is of great interest that the findings of

Snyder show resemblances to the overall results of Hall's and Van de Castle's comprehensive work, that is, both indicate that manifest dream content on the whole is "continuous" with daily life and often tends to be prosaic and undramatic.

Snyder (1970) conducted one of the few studies intended simply to determine how dream experience differs from or is similar to waking experience. To do this he collected 635 REMP dream reports from 58 subjects over 250 subject nights and rated numerous aspects of their content.

The subjects were male and female middle-class college and medical students who were studied at two different locations, and consisted of three separate groups. The generality of the results is, therefore, limited. Also, data was not collected in a standard manner, and the exact total number of subjects did not appear in this article.

Mentation reports were classified as dreams only if: (1) the words conveyed some sense of complex, organized perceptual imagery; and (2) the imagery had undergone some temporal progression or change. Isolated images and fragments were discarded. The details of data processing and interjudge reliability were not adequately furnished in this study but it still, in our opinion, provides useful information.

Of REM awakenings 75% produced narratives involving progression of organized and complex visual imagery with great variability in word count and detail (55% were less than 150 words; 32% were between 150 and 300 words; 13% were more than 300 words).

The broadest generalization possible about the nature of dream experience is its more or less faithful reflection of daily life. Snyder (1970) reports, "In almost every instance the progression of complex visual imagery . . . was a realistic facsimile of the visual perception of external reality; . . . it was representational [p. 133]."

Thirty-eight percent of the subjects recognized the physical settings as familiar (one's home or present real-life setting); and 43% had settings which were described but not familiar. Of this latter group, 5% had exotic settings.

One's self rarely appeared alone, distorted or as one was in childhood. Rather, the self pervaded the dream almost always in interaction with others who were people sometimes known, and sometimes not known, to the dreamer. The most usual mode of interaction was by talking (86-100%). Almost as frequently, the content or nature of the conversation was reported with awareness in the dream of tone of voice, subtleties, and frequent actual quotations from dream speeches, which were sometimes lengthy. From this, Snyder (1970) concluded that auditory imagery was almost as common as visual (76% and 100%, respectively). Furthermore, contrary to Freud's description that speech in dreams tended to have only something of the character of waking speech, dream speech tended to be actual and hallucinatory. Other auditory imagery included such items as music, rain, and animal barks.

Contrary to vision and audition, other sense modalities were rather uncommonly represented, that is, taste, smell, touch, and kinesthesia were infrequent or rare. (see Arkin et al., 1975, below for results of a study on pain sensation in dreams.) Snyder (1970) suspected, however, that the incidence of these items would be greater if subjects had been systematically asked about such content at times of awakening.

One of the perennial favorites is the question of dreaming in color. Snyder found that 61% of dreams were in color and that this proportion increased for longer dreams. This figure is consistent with those published in other reports. Thus, Kahn et al. (1962) found that color elements (as distinct from the entire dream being in brilliant "technicolor") were present in 82.7% of REM reports. Also, the incidence of such color was greatest when awakenings were made during an ongoing REMP, intermediate during a body movement and least 1 min after a body movement associated with REMP termination. These results were interpreted to indicate that recall of dream color fades rapidly with time. Berger (1963) similarly reported that the incidence of color in dreams exceeded 70%.

The incidence of cognitive elements is described as a range of occurrence percentage. This range denotes the lowest value found in any one of the three groups of subjects studied and, at the other end, the highest value (figures are approximate inasmuch as they are read from a bar graph):

1. Volition: references to making decisions (either their mere contemplation or actual implementation) were present in 10-50% of subjects' dreams.

2. Inferential reasoning: reasoning processes appeared in about 7-40% of dreams. The quality of such inferential reasoning in almost all cases seemed adequate by waking standards, although there were no "brilliant flashes."

3. Memory processes: references to memory function (like having forgotten to do an errand) appeared in from less than 1% to 10% of dreams.

4. Reflective contemplation: silent observation and detached musing about dream events external to the self appeared in about 17-75% of dreams.

In general, all of these four cognitive elements, volition, reasoning, memory processes, and reflection were least often observed in the group of short dreams and most often seen in the dreams of over 300 words.

Emotion was tabulated in dream content only when clearly identified by the dreamer as such. This occurred in only 35% of one of the three subject groups for which the incidence of emotion in dreams was a matter of special interest to the investigator.

Dysphoric emotions outnumbered pleasant ones by two to one. Fear and anxiety exceeded anger. Of the pleasant emotions, friendliness was the most common; erotic feelings were rare and representations of sexual relations even rarer. Although bathrooms were not uncommon dream settings, acts of waste elimination were rarely depicted. Violent aggressive reaction appeared in less than 4% of the total sample. The most primitive emotions were rare; the most common emotional tone was blandness or a general nebulousness.

Formal characteristics of the dreams could be broken into the following categories:

1. Coherence: relatively few dreams were disjointed or chaotic. Most resembled daytime narratives in coherence, especially in the awakenings from the second half of the night. Of the awakenings, 10% yielded reports of two or three apparently unrelated scenarios. Snyder (1970) thought these came from different segments of the same REMP.

2. Lucidity and detail: the majority of dreams were moderately clear, some extremely lucid and detailed, some quite unclear and vague. Interestingly, subjects often did better on recounting the same dream in the morning, postsleep.

3. Complexity: much variability was observed. One group of subjects, especially prodded for more descriptive detail, provided more complex dreams.

4. Temporal progression: 50% of all dreams showed only slight temporal progression; most of the remainder were moderate in this respect, and sagas were rare.

5. Activity: about half the dreams were "sedentary" and about a third contained active exertion such as sports or fighting.

6. Bizarreness and incredibility: dreams which were "crazy" and impossible, together with dreams which depicted unlikely, but nevertheless possible events, were uncommon but definitely represented in the total sample.

7. Dramatic qualities: for the most part, dream scenarios were mundane and everyday-like.

8. Provocative of interest in the judges: only 25% of the dreams aroused a feeling of interest in the judges.

9. References to the laboratory: occurred in 7-12% of dreams. By way of interesting comparison, references to eating and to automobiles each occurred in 15% of the dreams.

10. Typical dreams: "typical dreams" described in the psychiatric literature were rare ($< .5\%$). Examples of this general category in the psychiatric literature include dreams of examinations, loss of teeth, finding money, death, nudity with a sense of embarrassment, and so on.

The general impression left by this study is that dreams are "not so dreamy after all." The work has many methodological flaws but, nonetheless, a more careful study might not turn up data which is drastically different, judging from experience in our own laboratory with mentation reports. How can one account for the difference between these findings and the general popular impression of dreams as strange and uncanny? Snyder (1970), citing Hacker (1911), believes that most dreams recalled at home have been remembered because they contained some emotion which was intense enough to awaken one and hence left an impression on memory; it is just these REM dreams which have contributed to our popular conception.

While we find these data interesting, in accordance with a theme that has pervaded this chapter, we would like to suggest how such a study might be improved. The actual experience of dreaming can be approached from the point of view of what the manifest content means to each subject as well as the "raw content itself." We suspect that these uncollected data might have been found more interesting and less mundane than the manifest content, upon which Snyder has based his conclusions.

Kramer, Winget & Whitman (1971) were also interested in normative content which they collected using a survey questionnaire on 300 adults in Cincinnati, without electrographic techniques. Their data were not essentially different from Snyder's.

(Material on home versus laboratory dreams and the dream content of male homosexuals may be found in Chapter 8 of this volume.)

Pain in Dreams

Of all earlier laboratory dream-content analyses in the literature, not one refers to the frequency of references to physical-pain sensation in dreams. Therefore, Arkin et al. (1975) attempted to assess this issue on 119 REM reports collected from 20 college students under baseline conditions following 3 days of REM deprivation. The awakenings were performed both proximate to, and remote from, REM bursts 2-4 min after REMP onset. Only *one* of the total sample contained a reference to pain and this was ambiguous. In accordance with other published content analyses, visual and auditory sensory modalities prevailed and the total frequency of other nonvisual, nonauditory sensory modalities was low but definite: 7 reports out of 119 (5.9%), 1 each per 7 subjects contained references to olfaction, taste, touch, and temperature.

The results of this study are not unexpected. The age-old test of whether an event is real is a pain test: "I had to pinch myself to see whether I was dreaming." Pain means reality, and thus, pain sensation tends to be incompatible with dreaming. We say tends, because in a clinical or nonlaboratory population, we *have* observed dreams which involved the experience of pain. Usually, when this is the case, the pain is short-lived and the dreamer awakens. Much more common are dreams in which pain normally would have been felt if the dreamed episode had occurred while awake, but was nevertheless absent. The neural basis of this finding may be related to the close relationship between intracranial self-stimulation systems (reward systems) and REM sleep (Steiner & Ellman, 1972a) which may serve to inhibit aversive experience.

The phenomenon is an interesting example of dissociation between vivid dream-like experience and normally expected (but absent) sensory concomitants. Why a dreamer can sustain the experience of anxiety in a dream without immediate awakening and cannot do the same with painful sensation is an interesting question — both experiences are aversive.

As previously stated, because of space limitations and the chief focus of this volume being on laboratory studies, we only refer the reader to some of the work on dream content based upon daytime dream recall outside the laboratory (Hall 1966; Hall & Nordby 1972; Hall & Van de Castle 1966; Van de Castle 1971; Winget & Kramer 1972). In addition, Cohen has made resourceful use of morning recall of dreams reminding us of the persisting usefulness of this approach in an expensive electronic age. Much of his thought and bibliography can be found in a paper presenting Cohen's (1974) theory of dream recall.

Dreams before Adulthood

Since Freud (1900/1955a) himself regarded his theory of dreaming to be his most important contribution to psychology, it is no surprise that his ideas on this subject have been a prime stimulus and organizer of the new dream research. If we add that Freud's theory of psychosexual development was probably his most provocative and challenged contribution, then it is to be expected that the dreams of children would provide a fertile area for hypothesis testing.

Unfortunately, Freud actually said very little about the quality of children's dream experience. But even this has been the source of some research. Freud argued both from clinical observation and by deduction from theory, that dreams of preschool children are relatively blatant and undisguised expressions of wish fulfillment. Foulkes and his associates (Foulkes, 1967, 1971; Foulkes et al., 1969, 1971) took this and other pre-EEG era generalizations concerning children's dreamlife as starting points for several interesting studies. Before proceeding to examine these studies, one point concerning Freud's statement and a methodological point, are worth noting.

First, as stated, Freud's (1900) assertion is a somewhat overly simplified hypothesis. We presume that he did not mean that young children's dreams would be totally without defensive process or structure; rather he probably meant that they would have significantly less masking of expressed wish fulfillment than adults' dreams. Therefore, we should not expect children's dreams to contain overt pregenital psychosexual material.

The problems of translation and recall in the collection of sleep mentation, so well described by Rechtschaffen (1967), may take on new and special difficulties when children are the subjects. It may be unrealistic to assume that children will assimilate a rather novel experimental situation with the same degree of nonreactivity shown by adults. We explore this important issue more thoroughly in the context of the studies themselves.

It has often been wondered: when do children begin to dream? Or at least give signs of dreaming? Although neonates spend more time in REM sleep than they ever will in later life, there is no proof that they dream in association with it. The following study on 2-year-olds is therefore fascinating and important.

Kohler, Coddington, & Agnew Jr., (1968) studied 6 healthy 2-year-old children in the laboratory. They were selected because of superior verbal ability from a population of 16 on whom normative electrographic measurements were made. The children were awakened a total of 35 times (3-7 times each) at random throughout the night. Four children were accompanied by their mothers, who often assisted in their interrogation on awakenings. Subjects were then asked to describe such things as what they had been doing, what they had seen, and whom they were with. Dreams were defined as any verbal production that was out of context with the experimental situation. Thus, material related to playmates, activities outside the laboratory, animals, and television were considered representative of dreams. The tapes of reports were classified by a child psychiatrist unaware of the electrographic awakening conditions, into dreams and nondreams.

The investigators were unable to get any verbal descriptions from three children regardless of awakening conditions. The other three children consistently reported dream material when awakened from REM and never from NREM sleep. Overall, 30% dream recall was obtained from REM awakenings and 0% from NREM. Of the three recallers, there was dream recall on 3/3, 2/3 and 2/2 REM awakenings, respectively. The authors concluded that 2-year-old children do have nocturnal dreams and that such dream recall, when detectable, is associated with REM sleep. Finally, a nonsignificant correlation was observed between mental age and amount of REM sleep.

In the first EEG study of older children's dreams Foulkes et al. (1967) examined the REMP mentation collected from 32 boys, aged 6-12 years. Immediately after the elicitation of the report, subjects were asked if their dream was a good dream or a bad dream. Later, mentation reports were independently rated by two judges along dimensions such as spatial and temporal extensity, unpleasantness, parental warmth, hostility press, and guilt. Several days before the study, the children were given the Otis quick-scoring mental ability test and the children's apperception test (CAT), so that relationships of intelligence and waking fantasy to dream content could be examined.

The authors described the dream content they collected as mundane, nonbizarre, and dominated by references to current concerns, such as recreation. When subjects were divided by age, Foulkes et al. (1967) noted a trend toward more pleasant, social, and friendly dreams among the older children. The one significant difference which emerged was that 10-12-year-olds had a higher incidence of dreams (25.9%) with female strangers than 6-8-year-olds (10.9%; $p <$ .05). (This value, 25.9%, is similar to that found by Foulkes and Rechtschaffen, 1964, for a group of young adult males.) Foulkes et al. (1967) felt that the actual significance of this finding was enhanced by the facts that there is a decline in maternal dream reference with increasing age and that the oedipal situation is postulated to be appropriately different for these two age groups.

The content ratings of the children's dreams were also compared with analogous data collected from young adult males in an earlier study (Foulkes & Rechtschaffen, 1964). The authors summarized the results of this work as follows: Compared to young adult males, 6-12-year-old boys' dreams were more concerned with nuclear family members; male age mates played a larger role in their dreams, and female age mates a smaller role than is the case with young adult males; the children had fewer dreams with extrafamilial known adults, indoor settings, and social plots. Children's dreams with social plots tended more often to be unpleasant. "Potentially symbolic personnages such as supernatural figures or animals . . ." occurred more frequently in the dreams of children. School-related plots were virtually nonexistent for children and appeared with moderately low frequency for young adult males. The trend for social, friendly, and pleasant dreams to increase with age was also strongly evident in the comparison with young adult's dreams.

Foulkes and Rechtschaffen (1964) had correlated parameters of dream reports with corresponding dimensions of their subjects' TAT scores, and obtained several significant correlations. These relationships were *not* found between the children's dreams and corresponding categories from the CAT protocols, with the exception of one category: omissions. Foulkes et al. (1967) interpreted this to indicate that "styles of mental approach are not nearly so stable or consistent across the sleep-wakefulness border for children as they are for adults [p. 463] ." If this inference is expanded somewhat it might be taken as an indirect confirmation of some Freudian notions concerning development: that is, the lack of correspondence between styles of dream reporting and of waking fantasy during childhood may be one indicator of a general lack of crystallization and full elaboration of defensive and cognitive structures, which lack would be expected before psychosexual maturity.

Interestingly, Foulkes et al. (1967) did obtain modest but significant ($p < .05$) positive correlations between mental age and several parameters of dream reports. These were: word count ($r = .37$), spatial and temporal extensity ($r = .36$), and imaginativeness ($r = .44$). This seems to be consistent with the developmental notion described above.

Foulkes et al. (1967) concluded that earlier reports (e.g., DeMartino, 1955) that described children's dreams as traumatic and populated by bogeymen, were most likely the result of atypical sampling of total dream experience, since only 20% of the dreams they collected were described by the boys themselves as "bad."

The dreams of latency children are not the appropriate data with which to evaluate Freud's (1900/1955a) blatant wish-fulfillment hypothesis, and Foulkes et al. (1967) did not tabulate obviously wish fulfilling dreams separately; however, it was their impression that although such dreams did appear, they were exceptional. In general they found almost no characteristics which clearly differentiated children's dreams from those of young adults.

Overall, Foulkes et al. (1967a) found their data to be as consistent with an Adlerian approach to dreaming, as with Freud's ideas. They describe the former as the position that dreams are continuous with waking experience, while the Freudian position is described as the view that dreams, in some sense contradict waking expression or are complementary to it. We reserve our critical remarks with respect to this conclusion until the end of this section.

Foulkes (1967a) was apparently aware of the criticism often leveled at nomothetic studies of private experience, and responded to it with follow-up case studies of four of the subjects used in Foulkes et al. (1967). Two pairs of brothers were selected by Foulkes (1967a) so that one pair consisted of two boys who were among those who reported the "most vivid and bizarre mental content from REM sleep, while the other 2 brothers had reported relatively everyday and unintense experiences [p. 82] ." Dreams were collected on six weekly nights, approximately four awakenings being made each night. Foulkes (1967a) reports that following the

> "...night's run, the subject was taken to a room where he listened ... to tape recordings of the preceding night's dream reports. He was then asked if he could recall anything else of the experience he had reported during the night, and an unsystematic set of questions was asked to illuminate the connection, if any, between the dream and his waking experience. ... These interviews were not free-association periods in the psychoanalytic sense, i.e., no probes were designed to tap indicators of unacceptable impulses [p. 84] ."

The general purpose of the above procedure was to shed light on qualitative aspects of dream experience, unencumbered by a particular theoretical orientation.

Subject 1, 9½ years old, reported dreams that were predominantly bizarre, frightening, and populated by monsters that underwent unusual transformations (like lilies becoming a charging moose). Common themes were loss of control and danger to the subject's body and family. Foulkes (1967) describes these dreams as highly symbolic, containing abundant references to oedipal situations, also noting that there was some evidence that "much of the bizarre and otherworldly qualities could be traced back to ... pre-sleep experiences [p. 88] ," in that Subject 1 read "scary" comic books on two of the experimental nights.

Subject 2, the brother of Subject 1, 8½ years old, also reported mostly bizarre dreams. However, elements of fear and unpleasantness were generally absent. There was much reification of mass-media fantasy characters. Foulkes (1967) also found these dreams very symbolic and concerned with oedipal issues.

Subject 3, 7¾ years old, reported dreams whose content was much more realistic and generally devoid of fantastic or unpleasant elements. Foulkes (1967a) describes their theme as "the struggle to achieve adult status, with its attendant hazards and competition [p. 91] ." For example, the subject dreams of the Fourth of July. His big brother has a big firecracker that makes a big dent in a tin can, while little brother's firecracker only makes a "sizz." In another such dream, "King," a man who keeps slaves, denies the subject and some of his peers access to picking some cotton. However, the king's daughter intercedes for them. In at least one dream there was reification of a fictional personnage; "Parker," from the television series *McHale's Navy,* appears as a character.

Foulkes (1967a) describes the dreams of Subject 4, 11½ years old, as falling into two main classes: "those of minimal distortion, in which he is actually or vicariously involved in . . . masculine recreational pursuits, and those with more distortion [p. 93]," with some elements of danger. Foulkes (1967) felt that these dreams could be interpreted, in the former case, as rehearsals of adult masculine role behavior, and in the latter case, as fearful anticipation of the reactivation of object-directed sexuality. Examples of the latter include the subject dreaming he is in his family's basement, watching it flood with water, and dreaming of a horse-drawn circus wagon which is tipped over by the forceful pushing of elephants.

Foulkes (1967a) found that the waking styles of the four subjects were continuous with the differentiation he observed in aspects of dream experience. Subjects 1 and 2 were noticeably more emotionally expressive and fantasy-oriented, for example, they were both "addicted" to comic books. By contrast, Foulkes (1967a) reported, Subjects 3 and 4 appeared "somewhat emotionally constricted . . . (particularly [Subject 4] who appeared almost sullen on several evenings); . . . (and) more matter of fact in their approach to the world [p. 95]." Subject 1, whose dreams seemed more anxious and bizarre than any of the other subject's dreams, often provided unreliable information during the morning association periods, when measured against the responses of his mother and brother. He appeared to experience occasional difficulty in speaking during the experiment, sometimes whispering or remaining silent. Foulkes (1967) took these data to be consistent with Foulkes and Rechtschaffen's (1964) finding of an association between vivid and bizarre dream content, and waking personality disturbance in young adults.

From these data (Foulkes 1967a; Foulkes et al. 1967) Foulkes concludes that the dreams of preadolescents are not predominantly of an obviously wish-fulfilling nature and that during REM sleep the latency child does not always think in a highly disguised form; on the contrary, he asserts that realism is an impressive feature of the dreams of the male child, although as the child comes closer to conceiving things he fears, dreams become less straightforward. In support of this assertion, Foulkes (1967) cites the firecracker dream of Subject 3. The case of Subject 1 suggests to Foulkes (1967) that ". . . only [when] a child is overwhelmed by as yet unsolved emotional problems, tracing back to past developmental crises [p. 96]," do dreams lose realism and become more disguised.

We must take issue with the generalization that realism and lack of disguise typify the preadolescent's dream life. Although this may be a fact, the type of data described above do not constitute evidence for inferring it. In order to know if the content which a subject reports is in fact "disguised," i.e., also representing something which is literally not the same, ——it is necessary to know how the subject experiences the content; that is, to know whether the cognitive and affective reactions to the content are consonant with its denotative meaning, or whether to the subject they are not *only* "firecrackers." The ordinariness of manifest dream material is no guarantee that it does not mask very out of the ordinary conscious or unconscious experience. For example, if a racketeer appears in respectable society disguised as a minister, we cannot say that the minister is not a disguise because he seems so ordinary and above suspicion; one has to evaluate attempts to "blow the minister's cover" before we can even tentatively assert that he is not an imposter. It may be the case that some children provide better, that is, more effective, defended, or expressively inhibited disguises than others. The sort of free-association procedure that might address this question was specifically eschewed with the very good purpose that dreams be collected in an atmosphere of minimal theoretical bias. However, the question of disguise is thereby not adequately investigated.

The manifest content of the male child's dreams seems to consist mainly of extended conceptualizations of himself (Foulkes 1967a). The dreams are pervaded by an active wish to become masculine, accompanied in some cases by confidence in that prospect, and in others by fear. Foulkes (1967a) regards this as confirming Freud's theory of psychosexual development, but considers the concerns with mastery and anticipatory socialization as supportive of more contemporary Freudian conceptions such as those of Erikson (1963) or those of Adler (1958).

In contrast to the data collected in Foulkes et al. (1967), the material collected in the four case studies (Foulkes, 1967a), notably lacked mother figures as a central focus, and tended to be dominated by the father's masculine presence as a model and object of identification. This would appear to be further support for Freudian conceptions of postoedipal development. This finding may also be taken as an indicator of the relative superiority of adding case-study methods to EEG techniques of dream retrieval.

As we indicated above, the place to evaluate Freud's (1900/1955) "blatant wish-fulfillment" hypothesis is in the dreams of preschool children. This has been the stimulus for research in two other studies by Foulkes and his associates (Foulkes, 1971; Foulkes et al., 1969). Together these studies examined the REMP mentation collected from 13 boys and 13 girls aged 3½-5 years, the majority of the children being under 5 years of age. In Foulkes et al. (1969) children were also assessed using Laurendeau and Pinard's tests of precausal thinking and the Blacky test. The children's parents were given the Traditional Family Idealogy scale, (a measure of authoritarian attitudes). As part of a larger longitudinal study, Foulkes (1971) collected much additional psychological data (but that material is not reported in this chapter).

The two studies produced data which are remarkably consistent. The most striking finding is the infrequency of recall and brevity of young children's dream reports. The percentages of awakenings with some substantive content were 27 (boys and girls pooled) and 44% for the 1969 and 1971 studies, respectively. Although there was a considerable range among subjects, it is clear that most preschool children frequently do not report anything when awakened from

REM sleep. In Foulkes et al. (1969) the average word count per dream was 21.9 words, while the median word count in Foulkes (1971) was 13.5 words, indicating that when young children do report a dream, the report is very brief compared to reports of older children (median word count for older children = 68 words; Foulkes, 1971) and adults. Here, too, there was much subject variability.

Foulkes (1971) describes these dreams as generally impoverished in motoric, affective, and cognitive content; however, what content there is he describes as realistic with respect to setting and plot, and as usually bearing a demonstrable relationship to the subjects's behavior in the period immediately preceding mentation collections. Foulkes et al. (1969) are careful to add that this material does not consist simply of memories or recreations; rather they clearly are "dreams," that is, "worked over and reconstructed bits of past experience [p. 632]."

The content of the children's dreams was conspicuously lacking in the presence of parents, siblings, or peers, while they were well populated with barnyard-type (as opposed to pets) animals (Foulkes 1971). Foulkes (1971) also points out that the young children's dreams were not so dramatic, traumatic, or dreadful as other observers (Hall, 1966) have stated. He ascribes the discrepancy between the "prosaic" dreams he obtained using EEG awakening techniques (Foulkes, 1971) and earlier reports (Hall 1966, DeMartino 1955), as the result of the more representative sampling of normal children, which the more recent studies have achieved. Foulkes (1971) points out that the spontaneously recalled dreams from any sort of clinical population might be expected to be more intense on a variety of parameters. Noting the possible objection that the laboratory setting may have had an inhibitory effect on the children's dream reporting, Foulkes (1971) responds that there is evidence from young adults, that dreams collected at home and in the laboratory do not differ in intensity (Weisz & Foulkes, 1970), and there is "no reason to believe that youngsters are more facile at situational suppression of their nocturnal fantasies, than are college students [p. 63]." Foulkes (Foulkes et al., 1969) also doubts the likelihood of the possibility that the preschool children lacked the vocabularies and concepts to accurately report the nature of their dream experience, because there was a positive correlation of recall with the adequacy of the concept of "dream" on the Laurendeau-Pinard tests ($r = .36$; n.s.) and the descriptive ability scale of the Blacky test ($r = .61$; $p < .05$). Furthermore, Foulkes et al. (1969), noting that "subjects' stereotyped conceptions of dreams before coming to the laboratory ... were ... that [they] were 'scary', often involving frightening animal figures [p. 641] ," reason that these children do have the ability to report relatively unrealistic dreams, but that such dreams are actually less frequent under representative sampling conditions.

Foulkes et al.'s (1969) and Foulkes (1971) conclusions regarding the dreams of preschool children are as follows: In general they may be regarded as reflecting more the influence of ego processes, than of "destructive id impulses" in normal children, and as such their content is prosaic and realistic, reflecting current waking-life concerns. This reflection of current concerns is incomplete in that certain presumably important concerns, such as parents are omitted from dream contact. Nevertheless the authors feel that dream content is very much continuous with, and mirroring current waking life.

When typically omitted areas of content do appear in young children's dreams, the situation tends to be conflictful or frightening to the child. Foulkes et al. (1969) assert that, in general, preschool children's dreams are marked by "the constructive stamp" of developing ego processes.

We would like to suggest that this conclusion may be a premature neutralization of some, as yet undiscovered, experiential content in the young child's dreams. The actual data sample which Foulkes et al. (1969) and Foulkes (1971) have generalized from is very small and possibly systemically biased. Of the 12 children used in the Foulkes et al. (1969) study, one-third reported *no dreams at all*, while an additional child reported a single dream fragment. Similarly low rates of recall and very abbreviated dream length were evident in the less detailed data presented in Foulkes (1971). The nature of these substantial missing data is unknown. (Unless we are to presume that close to one-third of preschool children have *no* dream experience). That it may be predominantly unpleasant, unrealistic, or anxious material is suggested by our conceptions of what may elicit defensive forgetting or denial in children. Also interesting in this context is that the authors noted that when atypical (that is, usually "omitted") categories of dream content appear, they are in the context of anxiety. Foulkes minimizes the possibility that the absence of unpleasant or bizarre dream content is the product of cognitive inability by citing the fact that before coming to the laboratory, subjects spontaneously reported such dreams, the implication being that reporting frightening dreams outside the laboratory indicated having the ability to report them in the context of experimental dream retrieval. Although this seems to be a reasonable inference, it does not address the issue of how the exercise of this ability is affected in preschool children by being experimental subjects in a sleep laboratory.

Although there is evidence that the intensity of *young adult's* dream reports is not affected by being collected in a laboratory as opposed to at home (Weisz & Foulkes, 1970), no such evidence is available for young children, and in fact some possibly relevant data point in another direction. Wallach and Kogan (1965) found that when creativity tests were presented to children in an unrestricted game-like setting, positive correlations with intelligence tests which other investigators (Getzels & Jackson, 1962) had obtained, completely disappeared, while the quantity and quality of creative production both increased. In this context it is interesting to consider that there are similarities between the psychoanalytic theories of creativity and dream formation, in that they are both said to involve the process of condensation. We are suggesting that at least for some preschool children the laboratory setting and EEG dream procedures may have a selectively inhibiting effect on the reporting of unpleasant or bizarre dream experience. This hypothesis is consistent with the very low rates of recall and dream-report length which Foulkes (1971) and Foulkes et al. (1969) obtained. It seems important to remember that young children neither volunteer themselves, nor are paid, for entering into an unusual environment wherein adult strangers administer a somewhat annoying and novel procedure to them. There is no need to assume active confabulation or conscious withholding to reasonably suspect that what such subjects do *not* say may be as indicative of their private experience as the manifest content of their terse reports. Therefore we feel that the question of whether or not the dream life of young children is more, less or equally popu- lated with fearsome, bizarre, and otherwise "regressive" content is still very much open. If, indeed, dream content reflects wakeful experience, children dis- play a lively interest in the magical, uncanny, and the wish fulfilling during the day and by Foulkes et al.'s (1969) own contentions, this should show up more extensively in children's sleep mentation.

Possible ways of surmounting some of the methodological problems which we believe obscure the meaning of Foulkes et al.'s (1969) and Foulkes (1971) data might be:

1. to collect mentation at the subjects' homes;

2. to have parents participate in mentation collection as much as possible;

3. to secure, if possible, the active consent and understanding of the subjects themselves; and

4. to more thoroughly apply Stoyva and Kamiya's (1968) principle of conver- gent operations; for example, it would be interesting to know if "no reports" in children during REM sleep were accompanied by a consistent electrographic pat- tern.

What the authors have shown is that there are important continuities between styles of waking functioning and patterns of dreaming, extending the findings of Foulkes and Rechtschaffen (1964). An interesting example of this is the signifi- cant negative correlation ($r = .74$; $p < .02$) obtained between Fathers' scores on the Traditional Family Ideology scale (TFI) and their children's incidence of dream recall. On this scale, higher scores indicate more authoritarian attitudes. Mothers' scores did not correlate at all (Foulkes et al., 1969). The authors point out that such negative correlation has also been obtained elsewhere between fath- ers' TFI scores and their children's waking-achievement imagery (Clausen, 1966). This suggests an important connection between children's attitudes toward au- thority and their reporting of fantasy material in both sleep and waking, and also serves to remind us that the child's perception of the experimental situation, cer- tainly as very authoritarian, or hierarchical, (or even more so than for adult sub- jects), may be related in unknown ways to the child's reports of private exper- ience.*

*At the time that this was written the authors were unaware of several relatively recent studies published by Pivik and his associates which addressed some of the questions which we have raised above. While we still feel that most our criticisms are valid, we would like to refer the reader to those studies which space and time do not permit us to discuss here.

Such continuities were also in evidence in data collected by Foulkes et al. (1969) from institutionalized emotionally disturbed male adolescents ($N = 7$) and normal male adolescents aged 13-15 ($N = 7$). The dreams of these two groups differed from one another in that the institutionalized adolescents' dream reports were longer, rated as more imaginative ($p < .09$), more unpleasant ($p < .05$), containing more physical aggression, but less verbal aggression, less heterosexual content, and as being less related to everyday experience. These differences were enhanced when, using a social worker's ratings of parental deprivation, the least deprived institutional subjects were excluded. For all 14 subjects correlations between aspects of dream content and scales of the California Personality Inventory supported the general notion that subjects who were less well adjusted in waking life had more vivid and bizarre dreams.

Another interesting finding of this study was that a large plurality of the dreams reported by these adolescent boys were of hostile social interactions (30.8% for disturbed; 20.5% for normals). This is similar to a finding in 6-8-year-olds (Foulkes et al., 1967), but in contrast to data from older preadolescents.

The firm findings which emerge from the four studies reviewed above are that:

1. Until adulthood recall frequency and dream report length increase with age.
2. Animals play a surprisingly large role in the manifest content of young children's dreams.
3. Waking personality styles are strongly related to individual differences in patterns of dreaming and this correlation increases with age.
4. Unexpectedly, presumably important areas of waking concern are omitted from the manifest content of children's dreams.
5. Case-study approaches to dreaming in combination with EEG techniques may prove very effective methods of examining dream experience in children.

In its simplest form Freud's (1900) expectation of blatant wish fulfillment in children's dreams is given little obvious support. However, psychoanalytic conceptions of development are well represented in the content of dreams. Perhaps new studies, employing methodological considerations of the sort suggested by us, may increase what we know of young children's private experience.

Breger (1969a) has published an interesting case study of a 7-½-year-old boy in the throes of a developmental struggle. An integral part of the study is a series of REM dreams collected over four nights during a 1-month period. The interrelationships between the dream material, developmental history, and the psychosocial problems of the subject are richly illustrative of the process of dream-symbol formation in which the repetitive dream element of a finger endowed with magical properties is related to multiple psychological contexts. For Breger, dreams are viewed as fantasy experiments in which the dreamer attempts to find solutions to pressing psychological problems — a variety of theorizing in which dreams are deemed useful in mastery and problem solving.

Zepelin (1972) studied 321 REM dreams of 58 male alumni of a private university. They ranged in age from 27 to 64, with ages evenly distributed throughout. It was concluded that there was no evidence of "far-reaching age-related change in dream content that would constitute evidence of progressive decline in psychological energy over the age range studied [p. 128]."

Little laboratory work has been published dealing with dreaming in the aged. The most comprehensive study is that of Kahn, Fisher, and Lieberman (1969). In their experiment 27 subjects ranging from 66 to 87 years of age slept one or two nights in the laboratory. There were 19 male (mean age = 76.5) and 8 female (mean age = 74.3) paid volunteers obtained by means of advertisement in newspapers or at senior citizen centers. None had significant health problems and were leading apparently "normal" active lives. All subjects were awakened 5-10 min after each REMP onset yielding a total of 166 mentation reports. Of these, 92 (55.4%) resulted in retrieval of *some* mental content (even if fragmentary), and 75 (45.2%) at least a short but coherent dream. For both categories, the percentage of recall was lower than the 87% recall reported for young adults in the same laboratory ($p < .001$). Women tended to have more frequent recall than men. Earlier reports in the literature, based on dreams obtained from retrospective daytime recall indicated that the elderly have a disproportionately high incidence of content related to loss of resources and increased frustrations (Altschuler, Barad, & Goldfarb, 1963; Barad, Altschuler, & Goldfarb 1961). By contrast, the analyses of REM reports in this study revealed no such trends. Also, a small but nonsignificant correlation was found between the amount of recall and the WAIS memory scale (.31) and the WAIS verbal scale (.24).

Dreams in Relation to the Menstrual Cycle

Given a psychoanalytic approach to female sexuality, it is possible to hypothesize temporal correlations between women's feelings, wishes, and experiences of themselves, and the phases of the menstrual cycle. Insofar as dreams are considered to be related to current personal concerns, in particular those related to sexuality, we might expect them also to show particular content differences during different phases of the menstrual cycle.

Benedek and Rubenstein (1939) conducted a classical study of these issues using 15 neurotic subjects in psychoanalysis. They reported that changes in the menstrual cycle were paralleled by changes in the thematic content of free associations and dream material. For example, they reported that during the pre-ovulative phase, sexual desire was heightened and was more heterosexually active and object-oriented, whereas during menses there was decreased excitability, a predominance of womb and offspring concerns, and a sense of relief. The premenstrual phase was characterized by themes of rebellion against femininity and aggression towards men.

Since other investigators have failed to support some of Benedek and Ruben-stein's (1939) assertions (Davis, 1929; Terman, 1938), Swanson and Foulkes (1968) felt that it was important to attempt a partial replication of their study, using electrophysiological techniques of dream retrieval. In contradistinction to Benedek and Rubenstein (1939), they hypothesized on the basis of informal reports from college women, that overt heterosexual-drive expression in dreams would be greatest during menses. They also felt that this hypothesis was compatible with the notion that wishes which were being frustrated in waking life would find more expression in dreams, since they assumed that menses was a time of relative sexual deprivation for women.

Their subjects were 4 "normal" undergraduate women. Dreams were collected during 1 experimental night per week, sampling several REMPs during the night, for 11 consecutive weeks. Following each experimental night subjects rated their own most recent dream reports on a variety of dimensions, such as distortion, hostile press, sexual press, and sexual need. Hostility, sexuality, and menstrual symbols in dreams were also evaluated independently by raters.

Three of four subjects rated their dreams as most unpleasant on the average during menses ($p < .05$; binomial test). Self-rated unpleasantness of dreams related more strongly ($p < .01$) to feelings of waking depression, which were greatest during menses for the three subjects who had rated their dreams as most unpleasant at that time; and during premenses for the one subject who had rated her dreams as most unpleasant during premenses. Therefore, as the authors conclude, for these subjects inner-experienced reaction to the menstrual cycle was a better predictor of dream unpleasantness than cycle phase itself. The only other significant finding in the self-rating data, was that dreams with the most recent temporal reference occurred during postmenses ($p < .05$).

Judges' average ratings of dreams on a manifest sexuality scale were highest during menses for three subjects ($p < .05$). However, once again a stronger relationship between dream content and subjects' waking reactions to cyclical changes was obtained, than between dream content and cyclical changes themselves. Swanson and Foulkes (1968) wrote that the three subjects whose manifest sexuality dream rating was highest during menses, also "reported decreased waking sexual desire during menses [p. 361]." The one subject whose highest manifest sexuality in dream ratings was during postmenses, also reported decreased waking desire during postmenses, and actually indicated increased waking desire during menses.

Thus the relationship between manifest sexuality ratings in dreams and subjects' reporting a cycle phase to be one of increased waking desire, was stronger than the relationship between manifest sexuality in dreams, and particular phases of the menstrual cycle. That is, the relationship between two psychological variables (sexual dream content and wakeful sexual desire) was stronger than that between a psychological and a physiological variable (dream content and cycle phase.) In addition it is worth noting that these findings are a clear contradiction of Benedek and Rubenstein's (1939) data, albeit collected in a very different way and from a very different subject group of smaller size.

Peak hostility ratings of dreams were highest for three of the four subjects during menses ($p < .05$). For the fourth subject's highest hostility ratings were during postovulation. The authors suggest that this might be a reflection of the unpleasantness, physical discomfort, and activity restrictions generally associated with menstruation. No other rated dimensions of dream content were significantly related to cycle phase.

The authors conclude that their data contradict Benedek and Rubenstein's (1939) assertions of a direct connection between hormonally regulated phases of the menstrual cycle and arousal of the sexual drive in women. This conclusion was based on the postulation of a direct relationship between manifest sexual content of dreams and drive state, a relationship which is not yet established. However, Swanson and Foulkes' (1968) data must be viewed with caution because of the very small sample used and because of the consequently limited statistical analysis they performed.

Nevertheless, their data are very suggestive of an important point which might guide future studies of relationships between dream experience and fluctuating biological conditions. Psychological correlates of organic states may at least mediate, and possibly override the influences of physiological variables which we might intuitively expect to be quite powerful in determining dream experience.

DREAM CONTENT IN RELATION TO PSYCHO-PATHOLOGICAL SYNDROMES

Because of the extensive use clinicians have made of dreams in understanding and treating patients, and also the enormous contribution made by dream investigation to the elucidation of human psychology, it was with great eagerness that researchers sought to study the sleep mentation of people who were psychologically ill. We start with the most puzzling enigma of all: schizophrenia; can dreams tell us something new and valuable?

The Dreams of Schizophrenics

The excitement generated by the discovery of a relationship between a physiological state, REM sleep, and a psychological state, dreaming, partly stemmed from the hope that grounding dreaming in the solid rock of the nervous system would lead to a better understanding of the nature of psychopathology, particularly of schizophrenia. This hope itself is developed from the idea that there are important connections and similarities between the experience of normal dreaming and of waking consciousness in schizophrenia. There are at least two aspects to this hypothesis of a relationship between schizophrenia and dreaming. The first is that the symptoms of schizophrenia and the content of dreams are both reflections of the primary process. They are each seen as behavioral and experiential manifestations of a wish-dominated, nonlogical, nonrealistic subjectivity that is usually inhibited during wakefulness. The second aspect of this hypothesis is that if the quantity of primary-process ideation is more or less constant for a given individual (as Freud, 1900, believed), then an individual who displays relatively more of it, and thereby discharges some of it during wakefulness — as with schizophrenics — would experience less ideation of this type during sleep. In other words, it would be predicted that such an individual's dream life would be relatively less populated with bizarre, blatantly wishful and nonlogical elements than the nonschizophrenic.

To be sure, this is a somewhat simplistic deduction from psychoanalytic theory. For example, it is possible that schizophrenics, as a group, are constitutionally endowed with a larger constant quantity of primary-process ideation pressing for expression, and therefore would not necessarily show any diminution of dream experience, and might even have more bizarre or "primitive" dreams than normals. Nevertheless, it has been the more simplified notion of a compensatory, or complementary relationship between waking and sleeping cognition which has inspired some investigators to attempt to examine the dreams of schizophrenics, using the superior techniques of EEG dream retrieval in the hope of providing evidence for psychoanalytic formulations of schizophrenia and dreaming.

It is worth noting here that Freud's (1900) conception of a reciprocal functional relationship between the contents of sleeping and waking experience was not unique. Although Dallett (1973), in her review of theories of dream function, stresses the differences between Freud's (1900/1955a) and Jung's (1945/1960) theories, it is clear from her exposition of Jung that he, too, saw dream experience as expressing components of the personality which were inhibited during waking, although not in the context of a drive discharge model of mental functioning.

Now we turn to a consideration of some of the data, as well as to the interesting problems that have emerged in the recent investigation of the dreams of schizophrenics. In order to provide some historical perspective and share some of the authors' useful theoretical comments we include some studies which did not use EEG dream-retrieval techniques.

Dement (1955) conducted the first EEG study of schizophrenics' dreams. He collected dreams from 17 chronic schizophrenics (9 men and 8 women, aged 21-53 years) and 17 male medical students (aged 22-32 years) as controls, during periods of sleep with and without rapid eye movements. Two basic findings emerged. During REMs the schizophrenics gave fewer actual dream reports. They produced a dream report for 60% of their awakenings, as compared to 88% for the medical students. One half of the schizophrenics frequently reported dreams of isolated, inanimate objects, devoid of any overt action, while the medical students reported no dreams of this type. Exemplary of this type of dream report is: "I was dreaming of a ripped coat." "Anything else?" "No."

These data seem to confirm the compensatory or hydraulic model of dream function alluded to above. However, Dement's (1955) study is also illustrative of the very difficult methodological problems besetting dream research with schizophrenics, that make such an easy conclusion difficult to support. He describes his schizophrenic subjects as having been selected from a hospital population on the basis of their being manageable and "at least to a slight degree communicative." Further, Dement (1955) notes that "certain of the schizophrenics consistently replied negatively to interrogation [with] a monotonous stereotypy [apparently not] a true verbalization of inner experiences [p. 267]." This would seem to imply that the strangely barren reports of the schizophrenics may as much reflect their negativism and residual symptomatology as their actual experience prior to being awakened. In other words, it may be that the reporting style of chronic schizophrenics when awakened from REM sleep, obscures the experience to which it is supposed to correspond. Dement (1955) felt that this was not so because "some patients described other dreams which seemed quite normal and were able to communicate fairly adequately in the waking state [p. 266]." Implicit in this argument is the assumption that the negativism of chronic schizophrenics does not vary a great deal, particularly between sleeping and waking conditions. This is not consistent with Carrington's (1972) finding that while her schizophrenic subjects would not report dreams after morning awakening, they were prolific dream recallers later in the day. We do not mean to imply comparability between Dement's (1955) and Carrington's (1972) studies, which were very different in many respects. However, there seems to be some evidence that schizophrenics' style of dream reporting is more variable, and possibly much less indicative of their nocturnal experience than that of normals. Nevertheless, Dement's (1955) findings were certainly consistent with the compensation model of dreaming in schizophrenia described above, and made clear the need for more research into these phenomena.

Richardson and Moore (1963) collected dreams from 25 schizophrenic inpatients (15 paranoid, 5 chronic undifferentiated, 2 acute undifferentiated, 2 simple, and 1 schizoaffective) and 25 nonschizophrenic psychiatric inpatients, not using EEG techniques. (Precisely how dreams were collected is not described in the report.) Fifteen psychiatrists blindly rated the dreams as to whether they felt they were from schizophrenics. They were correct 55.7% of the time, which is significantly better than chance expectations (phi coefficient, $p < .01$). The authors also reported that the schizophrenics' dreams had less affect generally, that their expectation of more fearsome and bizarre content in schizophrenics' dreams was not borne out, and that schizophrenics reported more dreams with "cosmic" and strange qualities than did nonschizophrenics. An example of the latter quality that Richardson and Moore (1963) cite is: "Now it seems I have changed. I am seeing myself through the eyes of my wife, or I am my wife. I want to run to kiss myself as I depart [p. 290] ." In addition it is apparent from Richardson and Moore's data that schizophrenics' dreams were shorter than non-schizophrenics' (20 lines versus 28 lines; no statistics presented). Their dreams had fewer changes and lower incidence of fathers than nonschizophrenics. The authors also report that schizophrenics had a higher incidence of sexual dreams.

The authors were most intrigued by the incidence of "strange" dreams among the schizophrenics, as exemplified above. They suggest that this aspect of the dream report may be more a function of ineffective secondary revision, that is, the patient's waking defensive assimilation and presentation of the dream experience, than of the experience itself. This is a more psychoanalytically phrased formulation of the possibility we raised in regard to Dement's (1955) finding of peculiarly empty dream reports in a group of chronic schizophrenics, that the schizophrenic's style of report may exert a powerful influence on what is collected in dream studies. Richardson and Moore's (1963) data have two added complications. Dreams were not retrieved from experimental awakenings, a difference which may certainly affect the influence of wakeful revision, although how we do not know; and their subjects, although all schizophrenics, were diagnostically quite variegated and different from Dement's (1955), who were all chronic schizophrenics. It may be that the depletion of nocturnal primary-process ideation postulated by the compensation model of dreaming in schizophrenia, is a process that requires the time that chronic, but not acute schizophrenia provides. In the light of these considerations it is interesting that Richardson and Moore's (1963) data offer some modest support for the expectation that schizophrenic dream experience may be relatively impoverished. Their schizophrenic subjects' dreams were shorter, had less affect and fewer scene changes than controls. The authors had expected to find uncensored drive material, such as clearly sadistic or mutilatory content. They suggested that the absence of this type of material was possibly the result of repression during sleep requiring less counter-cathectic neutralized energy than it does during waking, making it a task the schizophrenic ego could accomplish.

Langs (1966) collected both recent and temporally removed dreams from 3 groups of female inpatients both without using electrographic techniques (12 paranoid schizophrenics, 12 hysterics, and 12 psychotically depressed patients). He reports various thematic and content differences between the dreams of the 3 groups, but as Hauri (1975) correctly points out their differences are confounded with the length of the dream reports, which varied greatly between the 3 groups. With regard to the compensation hypothesis however, dream length may be a more important variable than manifest thematic content. Langs (1966) reports that while 7 hysterics had at least 1 dream over 60 words long, only 1 paranoid schizophrenic fell into this category, and only 1 depressed patient even had 1 dream over 30 words in length. It seems likely that some impoverishment of dream experience is operating for the schizophrenic and depressed patients; however, let us once again raise the possibility that reporting style, or later-phase secondary-revision processes are exerting their influence. It seems to us most reasonable to argue that this is the case for the psychotically depressed patients, since a significant proportion of patients in this diagnostic category suffer from psychomotor retardation. This is not the case for paranoid schizophrenics and therefore it is reasonable to regard Langs' (1966) data as giving some additional confirmation of the expectation that schizophrenics' dreams may be relatively more barren experiences than those of nonschizophrenics.

Langs does not report dreams of the peculiar varieties which Dement (1955) and Richardson and Moore (1963) described. This may be due to the fact that all of Langs' patients were female paranoid schizophrenics (a different group from either of the other two studies), that he did not collect dreams using the EEG as Dement (1955) did, and that only a small part of his dream sample was "of the previous night" (as was Richardson and Moore's), thus allowing more extensive later-phase secondary revision to operate. Langs' (1966) failure to find comparatively diminished affect in schizophrenics' dreams may be due to the fact that his controls were quite different from either of those studies, and possibly extreme in both directions on this variable.

Carrington (1972) found the kind of morbid, bizarre, and apparently uncensored schizophrenic dreams which Richardson and Moore (1963) were expecting. She did not find diminished dream length or the other signs of impoverished dream experience described above. Particular characteristics of her subject group and procedure may account for these discrepancies. Carrington's (1972) patients were 30 female schizophrenics who were predominantly acute, that is, 70% were first admissions. She reports that her patients were too negativistic and intractable in the morning for dream collection (no EEG was used) and so dreams were collected from them later in the day. Dreams from 30 "normal" college women were collected in the morning only. Besides the fact that this represents a confounding of the dependent variable, it does not seem surprising that subjects in the acute state of waxing psychosis would give midday reports of the quality Carrington (1972) describes. However, such reports may correspond much less accurately to the dream experience they are supposed to represent than do the reports from the patients and conditions in Dement's (1955) and Richardson and Moore's (1963) studies.

Cartwright (1972) used the Foulkes DF scale to assess the REM and NREM mentation of eight schizophrenics and two groups of normals (high and normal scorers on the K-corrected schizophrenia scale of the MMPI, $N = 10$; $N = 14$ respectively). The data she reports seem to support her compensation model and have the advantage of being collected using EEG techniques of dream retrieval. Of the three subject groups the REM dreams of schizophrenics received the lowest DF ratings. Unfortunately the study is beset with several serious methodological problems, which have been carefully reviewed by Pivik (1974). In an effort to minimize the stressing of the schizophrenics Cartwright (1972) did not awaken them as she did the normals. Instead "... content reports were requested ... and tape recorded at each spontaneous awakening" until two REM and two NREM reports were obtained. This might certainly have affected the dream-like qualities of the reports obtained. In addition three "schizophrenic" subjects were later determined to be misdiagnosed as such, although they evidenced waking hallucinatory experiences. We (and Pivik 1974) also note that the statistical analysis was inadequate.

Cartwright (1972) mentions that of 128 reports collected, 25 were discarded because they contained "no recall." From the point of view of the compensation model it would be interesting to know if the number of no-recall reports was different for schizophrenics versus normals. Also, she reports that schizophrenics' dream reports were shorter but that this difference was not statistically significant. If these data could be replicated more rigorously, strong support might be provided for the compensation model of dreaming in schizophrenia.

Okuma, Sunami, Fukuma, Takeo, & Motoike (1970) collected dreams using the REMP awakening technique, from subjects who were more diagnostically similar to Dement's (1955) original group than those in most studies. The authors were interested in both the dream experience and in the reporting and behavioral styles evidenced by schizophrenics. Their subjects were 21 chronic hebephrenic schizophrenics (11 men and 10 women), hospitalized an average of 9.9 years each, ranging in age from 22 to 44 years. These patients were described as communicative, although having delusions and hallucinations. The authors add that their symptoms were well controlled by pharmocotherapy; and so, 10 days prior to the study all subjects were taken off drugs. The 34 normal controls consisted of 20 college students (10 men and 10 women) ranging in age from 19 to 22 years, and 14 male psychiatrists ranging in age from 25 to 42 years.

In several ways the schizophrenic population displayed a style of response to dream collection which might be taken as indicative of a relative diminution of the vividness, clarity, and cinematic qualities associated with REM dreams, *and/or* of the inability or unwillingness of these subjects to spontaneously translate a perceptual dream experience into a verbal report. The authors also note the possibility that a differential level of wakefulness for the schizophrenics might produce the response style they observed. The latency from the experimenters' request to describe their dream to the beginning of a dream report was significantly longer for schizophrenics ($p < .01$). The average amount of time schizophrenics spent in spontaneously reporting a given dream was significantly shorter and less variable than controls (15.9 ± 6.2 sec for schizophrenics; 43.5 ± 31.5 sec for controls; $p < .01$). Not surprisingly the average word count of such reports was significantly lower for schizophrenics (15.0 ± 12.1 words for schizophrenics; 52.8 ± 76.0 words for controls; $p < .01$). It is worth noting here that the average spontaneous dream narrative of a schizophrenic person amounts to barely a couple of sentences, and that schizophrenics had much lower variability on this parameter than controls.

Following the initial dream narrative, subjects were asked a series of supplementary questions to collect information missing from the spontaneous reports. Schizophrenics required significantly more of these questions ($p < .01$) than controls. In the morning, subjects were asked to recall the dreams they had reported during the preceding night. Schizophrenics had a significantly lower incidence of such recall than controls (73% for controls; 53% for schizophrenics; $p < .01$). When the experimenters used suggestion to facilitate morning recall, schizophrenics responded with both a higher incidence of positive recall and of no recall than controls.

The conceptual richness of dreams was assessed by counting the number of independent clauses in each report. Schizophrenics had an average of 1.6 ± 1.0 independent clauses per dream, while controls averaged significantly more ($3.7 \pm 3.6; p < .01$).

As Okuma et al. (1970) point out, the simple and abbreviated dream reports they obtained from schizophrenics may be the product of various interdependent factors, some of which are related to the actual dream experiences of these subjects, and others which are not. For example, the fact that schizophrenics' morning recall of their dreams of the previous night is relatively poor, may be the result of the vagueness or unclarity of the dream itself, or of deficits in waking cognitive functioning. On the other hand, cognitive deficits may be operating to interfere with dream formation as well as dream recall and dream report.

The relatively low variability of the schizophrenics on most of the parameters described above suggests that some stereotyped process is influencing their reporting, although comparison is difficult here, since the controls consisted of two distinct but relatively homogeneous groups, — college students and psychiatrists.

Examination of dream content revealed that schizophrenics had a significantly lower incidence of dreams which could be classified as bizarre, coherent, or complex (chi square, $p < .05$). Bizarre elements in the dreams were identified chiefly by using Domhoff's (1962) scale, which included metamorphoses, unusual acts, and magical occurrences. Dreams which were understandable, unfragmented, and presented a unified story were called "coherent." Dreams were labeled "complex" if they contained more than one person as well as other elements which involved vivid and complex (sic) activities, and in which the narrative was at least two sentences. Dreams whose elements seemed to have been perceived clearly and described concretely were labeled "clear." Schizophrenics had a lower incidence of this latter type of dream report (58.6% for schizophrenics; 74.1% for controls), but this difference was not statistically significant.

These data on the incidence of bizarreness, clarity, coherence, and complexity are difficult to interpret, since in some ways these variables are confounded, that is, correlated, with dream length, which significantly differed between the groups being compared. Snyder (1970, pp. 144-147) has presented some data which suggest that ratings of bizarreness, complexity, and clarity are positively correlated with the length of dream reports. If this is so, then it is possible that the apparent unclarity and simplicity of schizophrenic dream reports are artifactual products of the schizophrenics' tendency to withold a full accounting of their experience. Snyder's (1970) data suggested that the relationship between coherence and dream length is negative in normals, that is, shorter reports tended to be more coherent, and therefore we can feel much more confident in stating that schizophrenics' dreams are less coherent than controls', independently of their other formal characteristics.

Other content differences between schizophrenics and controls found by Okuma et al. (1970) were that schizophrenics had a higher incidence of dreams with family members (22.6% for schizophrenics; 9.9% for controls; $p < .01$) and a lower incidence of dreams with friends (20.4% for schizophrenics; 37.3% for controls; $p < .05$). The two groups did not differ on the number of characters per dream, but schizophrenics had a significantly lower incidence of dreams with crowds (4% for schizophrenics; 10% for controls; $p < .05$). Schizophrenics also had a lower incidence of dreams with no emotional elements (45% for schizophrenics; 70% for controls; $p < .01$).

Okuma et al. (1970) also remark that the incidence of dreams with negative affect (sadness, anger, fear, anxiety) was significantly higher for schizophrenics. However, we notice that this difference seems to be an artifactual result of the schizophrenics having more emotional dreams in general. When emotional dreams are examined alone, we see that schizophrenics have only slightly more unpleasant dreams (61%) than controls (53%).

Schizophrenics had a higher incidence of dreams containing sexual acts, but this difference was not significant. There were no significant differences between the groups with regard to the interpersonal emotional relationship of the dreamer to dream characters, but the authors regard this finding as tentative because of the small dream sample for male schizophrenics in this category.

As we discussed above, Okuma et al.'s (1970) data are generally supportive of the expectation that dream reports of schizophrenics are relatively impoverished compared to normals, a prediction developed from the compensation model of dreaming in schizophrenia. However, schizophrenics' dreams do not seem to lack emotion or human characters as Dement's (1955) early data seemed to suggest.

One of the advantages of Okuma et al's (1970) study is that a relatively homogeneous group of schizophrenics was used and both their behavioral styles and presented dream content were carefully examined. An important disadvantage of their study was the selection of controls, more than a third of whom were male psychiatrists, a subject group whom we can assume a priori to be significantly more articulate, psychologically minded, and intelligent than the average chronic hebephrenic schizophrenic, a fact that might influence dream reporting in unknown ways. In support of this methodological criticism is Okuma et al.'s

(1970) finding that as a group, the psychiatrists had a significantly higher incidence of dreams with experimental elements (like electrodes) compared to other schizophrenics or college students. Also, interestingly within both the college student and schizophrenic groups, females had significantly more dreams with experimental elements.

The most serious difficulty for all dream studies with deviant and/or psychopathological populations is teasing apart the influences of waking cognition from nocturnal dream phenomenology. One way to strengthen the validity of current findings such as Okuma et al.'s (1970), as well as to add to our general understanding of dreaming in schizophrenia would be to pay greater attention to the assessment of waking cognitive deficit in schizophrenics. The results of such assessment procedures should be correlated with aspects of sleep mentation, so that their influence on dream reports might be dealt with using analysis of covariance techniques. Such information could also be used so that schizophrenics with minimal waking cognitive deficits could be compared to normals.

Kramer et al. (1969) collected dreams without using EEG, from 40 male paranoid schizophrenics, 40 male psychotically depressed patients, and 40 male medical inpatients. After independent rating of dream reports, the following differences between the groups emerged: average dream length was highest for schizophrenics, followed by depressed, and medical patients (54, 47, and 31 words, respectively; ANOVA, $p < .01$). (Although the schizophrenics seem to have the longest dreams here, 54 words is much shorter than most normative studies report; Snyder, 1970). The incidence of hostility was greatest for schizophrenics' dreams, followed by depressed and medical patients (78, 55, and 30%, respectively; chi square, $p < .001$). Schizophrenics' dreams were most often rated as implausible, followed by depressed, and medical patients (68, 38, and 15%). The most frequent character in schizophrenics' dreams was a stranger (62%); for depressed patients it was a family member (58%); while for medical patients it was a friend (40%). The authors felt that their main hypothesis of a difference in dreams between different diagnostic groups was confirmed.

Kramer and Roth (1973) compared the EEG collected REMP dreams of 10 depressed patients (5 men and 5 women) to those of 13 schizophrenics (11 men and 2 women; diagnostic subtype not given). Dreams were assessed using the Hall-Van de Castle scoring system. Schizophrenics had a higher frequency of dream recall (71%) than depressed patients (51%). (No statistical analysis is reported for this finding). The most frequent character for schizophrenics was a stranger, while for depressed patients it was a family member (chi square, $p < .01$). Schizophrenics' dreams had a relatively high male/female character ratio, while for depressives this value was closer to 1 (chi square, $p < .01$). For both schizophrenic and depressed patients, groups of characters were more frequent than individuals, but this effect was more pronounced for the depressed patients (chi square, $p < .01$). Schizophrenics' dreams contained more aggressive than friendly or sexual interactions, while depressed patients' dreams were more evenly divided among these categories, exceeding the schizophrenics only for friendly interactions. The most frequent emotion in schizophrenics' dreams was appre-hension, while depressed patients showed a relatively even distribution of different emotions. The least frequent emotion for depressed patients was happi-ness and the most frequent was anger. The least frequent emotion for schizo-phrenics' dreams was sadness.

As Weisz (1975) has pointed out in his review of Kramer and Roth's (1973) study, their work has several important methodological shortcomings. For exam-ple, we are not told what kind the schizophrenics are, and it is not clear that raters were blind to the diagnosis of the patient whose dreams they were judging, al-though they may have been blind to the hypotheses of the experiment. Weisz (1975) also remarked that the predominance of males in the schizophrenic group might account for the increased male characters in the schizophrenics' dreams, as well as increased aggression. The authors replied that the differences they observed were maintained even when subjects were broken down into sex-specific groups.

In spite of these problems it may be instructive to examine Kramer and Roth's (1973) data more carefully insofar as some of their findings bear upon the data reported in earlier studies. For example, as Kramer et al. (1969) reported in a non–EEG study, the most frequent character for schizophrenics is a stranger, while for depressed patients it is a family member. Okuma et al. (1970) also found that the most common character in schizophrenics' dreams was unfamiliar or unknown, but that their frequency was not very different from normal con-trols. Furthermore, although family members did not appear very frequently (22.6%), Okuma and co-workers report that their incidence was significantly greater in schizophrenics' dreams than in controls'. What this seems to suggest is that comparing schizophrenics' dreams to those of depressed patients may dis-tort the differential phenomenology of schizophrenics' dreams with respect to nonpathological subjects.

Kramer and Roth's (1973) finding that apprehension was the most frequent emotion for schizophrenics' dreams, contradicts both Kramer et al. (1969) and Okuma et al. (1970) who agreed that the incidence of anger exceeded fearful-ness; the latter group also found that happy dream reports were more frequent than either fearful or angry ones individually.

Kramer, Trinder, and Roth (1972) report data very similar to Kramer and Roth (1973), comparing male paranoid schizophrenics' dreams before and after drug treatment to normal college males; however, the value of that study is seri-ously flawed by the fact that control dreams were *not* collected using EEG tech-niques, while patients' dreams were.

In his review of manifest-dream studies, focusing on reports from morning recall, Kramer (1970) states "the dreams of schizophrenics may . . . be generally characterized as unrealistic, affectively neutral, openly hostile . . . less blatantly sexual than waking life and with the dream action focused on the dreamer who finds himself most of the time with strangers [p. 154]." Some of these asser-tions, such as the claim that schizophrenics' dreams are unrealistic, have been directly contradicted by new research using EEG dream-retrieval techniques (Okuma et al., 1970). However, what may be a more important point is that even where these generalizations are supported (e.g., dream actions focused on the dreamer) these aspects of schizophrenics' dreams do not necessarily differentiate them from normals' dreams, as these have been characterized by recent research. Snyder (1970) finds that emotions are generally infrequent in manifest dreams of normals, but when they do appear, they are predominantly unpleasant, with fear and anger most common. Unidentified characters (who may be strangers) are also frequent in the dreams of normal young adults, and the dreamer himself is the most pervasive presence in the dream (Snyder, 1970).

We feel that the methodological difficulties, which we have alluded to above, make any generalization concerning the actual dream experience of schizophrenics in comparison to normals, premature. Some support has been given to the expectation, based on the compensation model of dreaming and schizophrenia, that REM dreams of chronic schizophrenics are relatively impoverished and empty, compared to normals. However, this finding needs to be replicated with careful assessment and control of the effects of waking cognitive deficits on dream reporting.

Schizophrenia and "Wakeful Dreaming"

The hypothesis which asserts that schizophrenia represents a breakthrough or spillover of REM dreaming into wakefulness was a continuation of an old traditional clinical belief. Its attractiveness as an explanatory principle has made sleep investigators unwilling to part with it easily despite the amount of opposing or inconsistent experimental evidence. The evidence that breakthrough of REM mentation into wakefulness (whether because of REM deficit or cognitive insufficiency) seems more persuasive in the case of toxic deliria (see Chapters 11 and 14 of this volume), than in a schizophrenia. With the possible exception of Vogel, Barraclough, & Giesler (1972) and Oswald (1962), we may have lost sight of what are probably many more convincing parallels between the hypnagogic state and schizophrenia. The sleep-onset state of mind is noted for its auditory hallucinations of voices, strange word play, bizarre verbal constructions (including neologisms), brief grandiose delusions, catalepsy, and impairment of ability to discriminate between reality and fantasy (Oswald, 1962). To this we may add the common body-image distortions, disturbances of attention, and emotional-cognitive withdrawal from the environment occurring during sleep onset. (See Schacter, 1976, for an excellent review). Instead of insisting that schizophrenia is a breakthrough of REM mentation into wakefulness, it might be interesting to think of ways of testing the hypothesis that many cases of schizophrenia represent a persistent, tenacious, sustained, sleep-onset cognitive-affective state (or ego state) into which the patient has either lapsed or else has self-produced, and from which one has great difficulty in emerging, or extricating oneself, and sustaining typical stage W in an appropriate, autonomous manner (AMA).

Depression and Dreaming

While the general issues of models of dreaming could be raised in relation to depression, we shall not go further into these issues in this section, as we feel they have been adequately discussed in the sections on general theory (see p. 221) and schizophrenia (see p. 230). In addition, the methodological criticisms we have levelled at the studies on schizophrenic dreams (see pp. 164-173) are relevant here as well, and will not be reiterated. In the following section, non-laboratory studies of dreaming and depression will be briefly reviewed, followed by EEG studies. Finally, dreams of patients in treatment and remitted patients will be discussed.

Beck and Ward (1961) studied 287 randomly selected psychiatric patients from a variety of diagnostic categories. Subjects were assessed for depression by a battery of psychological tests, including a depression inventory, as well as being evaluated as to severity of depression by two independent judges. Patients reported their most recent dream; which was scored either positive or negative for masochism by two independent judges. A positive score meant the dreamer was one of the following: deprived, disappointed, thwarted, exploited, disgraced, rejected or deserted, blamed or ridiculed, punished, physically injured or discomforted, lost something, or showed a distorted body image. The 218 patients who gave scorable dreams were ranked according to their scores on the depression inventory and divided into three equal groups. Significantly more masochistic dreams occurred in the most depressed group than in the nondepressed group ($p < .01$). There was a significant overall association between the degree of depression and the incidence of masochistic dreams ($p = .01$). Of the masochistic dreams, 84% were obtained from patients in the mildly to severely depressed range. When all the cases were divided into two groups (one showing masochistic dream content and another group which did not show such content), the differences in the rank of the depression inventory scores between patients in the masochistic dream group and those in the non-masochistic group were significant at the .003 level.

No significant differences were noted in the above two groups as to age, sex, race, IQ, or socioeconomic class. However, almost as many mildly or moderately depressed patients reported masochistic dreams as did severely depressed patients. Thus, masochistic dream content seems to be associated with depression regardless of the severity of the illness. Similarly, masochistic dreams do not seem to be diagnostic for depression, as cyclical depressives continue to have them even in symptom-free periods. Masochism in the dream report is also seen in non-depressed masochistic character disorders (Beck & Hurvich, 1959). Thus, Beck and Ward may have tapped more into an underlying personality trait related to depression rather than identifying a dream style peculiar to depressed patients. This study suffers from using only recalled dreams and scoring all reports with a subject and a verb. Because of the way the dreams were scored, qualitative measures were not taken. Associations to the dreams were not taken and only things done to the dreamer were scored as masochistic, although other characters could represent the dreamer as well.

Lang's (1966) study has been reviewed in the section on the dreams of schizophrenics (see pp. 167-168). Langs found that the depressive group reported the shortest, fewest, and most barren dreams. They had the most dreams with family members ($p < .1$), and lacked nonfamily members altogether ($p < .01$). They were low on eight thematic scores as well, including uses of the mouth ($p < .1$), separation-loss ($p < .05$), and themes of illness, death, and damage. Various role constellations were low, including indications of a person losing control ($p < .05$). Depressive dreams were marked by an absence of movement ($p < .05$). Langs concluded that the dreams reflected a decathexis of the external world, and external objects. The dream environment never appeared as overwhelming or traumatic. Langs' (1966) results are not in agreement with Beck and Ward's (1961) in that he did not find a predominance of masochistic themes. However, the author notes that this may be due to the fact that his control group included women with depressive features who would have been noncontrol depressed subjects in the latter study. Also, he hypothesizes that in the most severely depressed patients, denial and decathexis of the external world are greatest, perhaps resulting in the reduced prominence of masochistic themes and more barren dreams. Problems with the study include the fact that the groups were not age matched, nor were dream reports matched for length.

Kramer et al. (1969) studied the manifest dream in 40 male paranoid schizophrenics, 40 male psychotically depressed patients, and 40 male non-psychiatric medical inpatients. Dreams were rated by 2 raters whose interrater reliability was .90 for the number of words and scores for hostility both towards the dreamer and away from the dreamer, plausibility, and the relationship of the dreamer to other dream characters. The mean word count of the depressives' dreams was midway between that of the schizophrenics and the medical patients (54 versus 47 versus 31). The degree of hostility was also intermediate for the depressed group. It was equally likely to be turned against the dreamer as against others. The dreams of depressives showed only family members 58% of the time, while those of schizophrenics showed mostly strangers (72%) and medical patients' dreams were largely of friends (40%). Dreams of depressives scored midway between schizophrenics and controls on plausibility and were more often plausible than not. The lower than hypothesized degree of hostility present led the authors to conclude that self-esteem rather than hostility is the central issue in depressive illness. The direction of hostility (equally against others and against the dreamer) suggests that this is also *not* a distinguishing feature of depression since the control group had similar results. Finally, the high percentage of family members seems to argue against Freud's (1917/1955b) notion that the world of the depressive is depleted of meaningful others. One serious question about the validity of this study is raised by the atypically low recall of nonpsychiatric medical patients. Their interviewing procedures did not seem to facilitate adequate recall.

Van de Castle and Holloway categorized 97 inpatients as depressed and 337 as non-depressed on the basis of their MMPI profiles. Recently recalled dreams were compared from each group, as well as being compared against the dreams of 200 normal college students. Mean ages for the depressed group 38, for the nondepressed group 35, and for the controls, 21. Education level was slightly higher for the controls. Among the depressed males, dreams had less color, more adjectives describing wrongness and unattractiveness, more parental figures, more changes of one character to another, and less reference to the human body. Depressed females, compared to other female groups, had dreams with less color, more adjectives describing wrongness and unattractiveness, less personal emotion, and the dreamer engaging in less movement. Statistical analysis of these results was not presented.

In general, laboratory studies have been in agreement with nonlaboratory studies. Kramer et al. (1966) studied five male and five female inpatients with severe depressive illness who showed no signs of schizophrenia or organic involvement. Their average age was 40; their average educational achievement was the eighth grade. Patients were put on imipramine placebo and had their dreams collected for two nights in the laboratory. They were then placed on medication and slept one night weekly for three additional weeks, and were clinically reevaluated and retested on a depression inventory. A comparison group of five male and five female nondepressed college students slept in the laboratory one night per week for four weeks. The content of the dreams was rated for depressive themes including low self-regard, deprivation, self criticism or self-blame, overwhelming problems and duties, self-commands and injunctions, and escape or suicide. To control for the differing number of dreams from the two groups, a depressive-theme index was calculated. Frequency counts were made to determine the rate of appearance of each theme in both groups. Dreams were also rated for themes of helplessness (defined as being discouraged, let down, or left out as the result of a change in a relationship and leading one to desire protection from others) and hopelessness (defined as a feeling that nothing is left, or despair eventuating in a desire to do nothing).

After the attrition of one subject, patients produced a total of 177 awakenings from which 91 dreams were reported, with a recall percentage of 51%. The control group had a recall percentage of 85%. Depressed patients averaged more spontaneous awakenings per night (3.7 versus 3.4) and had less dreams per night (1.9 versus 2.8). Awakenings from the depressed group more often failed to yield a dream report ($p < .001$). The total depressive index was higher for the depressed group ($p < .05$). Escape and suicide themes accounted for 40 to 49% of the depressive themes in the patient group, while in the control group, themes were more evenly distributed among different categories. This suggests a certain stereotype of solutions among depressives to their problems. Helplessness and hopelessness themes appear far more often in the dreams of the depressed (31/60 awakenings versus 8/106 control awakenings).

Comparing the first night of dreaming with the last night, there was no difference as to the percentage of recall, depressive theme index, or the frequency of escape themes. There was a nonsignificant trend in the direction of reduced frequency of helpless or hopeless elements. However, all cases showed clinical improvement and a reduction in depression-inventory scores. Thus, it is suggested that clinical improvement precedes intrapsychic change; and the dream content follows after overt change.

There are some methodological difficulties which cloud interpretation of this study. Since the decreased frequency of dream reports does not seem to be accompanied by a decreased frequency of dreaming (REM) sleep by EEG criterion, the authors conclude that there is some difficulty in reporting dreams rather than their lower occurrence. The fact that no single case in the study moves in a positive direction on more than two of the parameters measured (greater recall, lower depressive theme index, less helplessness-hopelessness elements, less escape themes) was interpreted by the authors to mean that they may have had a mixed group of depressive types. This suggests that individual types of depression should be studied separately.

Kramer and Roth (1973) studied 5 male and 5 female depressed patients for 5 consecutive nights in the laboratory and compared them with 2 female and 11 male schizophrenic patients who were each run 6 nonconsecutive nights. Dream reports were scored using scales of the Hall-Van de Castle dream-content scoring system. Depressed patients had 51% dream recall, while schizophrenics had 71%. Depressed patients more often had family members as their most frequent character ($p < .01$). The ratio of male to female characters was about equal. Both patient samples had more individuals than groups in their dreams but was significantly more frequent for depressives ($p < .01$). The ratio of pleasant to unpleasant emotions was about 5:1 in both groups, although sadness is more frequent in depressed patients. In short, this study largely confirms the earlier spontaneous recall study of Kramer et al. (1969). The authors concluded on the basis of these findings that there is a continuity of waking and sleeping life that allows patient groups to be differentiated during both states.

In sum, the literature on dreaming in severe depression has some firm findings, despite methodological problems. Depressives' dream reports are shorter than controls (with the exception of Kramer et al., 1969). They show a greater incidence of family members (Langs, 1966; Kramer et al., 1969; Kramer and Roth, 1974). They seem to have a higher incidence of depressive themes than a comparison group (Kramer et al., 1966) and more masochistic content (Beck & Ward, 1961), although this may be related to a stable character trait, rather than clinical depression.

How does the mentation of depressives alter with improvement? If one accepts Freud's (1917/1955b) hypothesis of depressives' anger turned against themselves, then with improvement one might expect more hostility turned against others. Most studies see the dreams of remitted depressives remaining similar in some respects to that of patients. Miller (1969) hypothesized that improving patients would have more troubled dreams which would consist of the dreamer hurting others. She collected recalled dreams from 16 deeply depressed patients and 13 improving but still partially depressed patients. Dreams were also collected from 38 graduate students and 39 paranoid schizophrenics. The 16 severely depressed patients produced 22 dreams of which 17 were pleasant or bland. Content analysis revealed that 17 dreams showed an absence of conflict, threat from other people or the environment and an absence of inner conflict. The 13 improving patients produced 21 dreams, only 2 of which were happy. There were 3 dreams of death, and 5 in which the dreamer was experiencing or reporting harm inflicted by another. Unique to the improving depressed group were dreams in which the dreamer is stopped from carrying out some activity by other persons. Thwarted action is common. Miller (1969) concluded that when patients improve, their dreams become more troubled and may begin to deal with problems. While improving, the depressed person in dream life is neither alone, self-blaming nor guilty, but rather active and trying to accomplish things. However, many of the things Miller defines as being active, (that is, being thwarted in an endeavor) are identical to criteria for masochistic content of Beck and Ward (1961). The author concluded Beck and Ward's masochistic dreamers correspond to her improving patients; yet, given that many of Beck and Ward's (1961) patients were severely depressed, this seems implausible. A major problem in Miller's (1969) study is that definitions are not clearly stated, thus making comparisons with other literature difficult. Also, a number of her subjects were receiving drugs prior to dream reporting and two had received ECT. Control groups were not age matched, nor was there any control for dream length. Thus, her conclusions that, while improving, the dreamer believes that others are trying to inflict harm, and the dreamer thus becomes angry and anxious, feeling that people act to block and coerce the dreamer's actions, are at best suggestive. However, support for this notion was provided by Kramer et al., 1968; (reviewed in Chapter 11 of this volume), who found that the short-term effect of imipramine on the laboratory-collected dreams of 10 depressed patients was to increase hostility and anxiety. The long-term effects were to decrease both hostility and anxiety, and to increase motility and heterosexuality. As hostile feelings decreased they were replaced by more tender feelings.

Similarly, Kramer et al. (1970) studied 5 male and 5 female patients in the laboratory for 2 nights before and 2 nights after treatment with anti-depressants. There were 38 dreams pretreatment and 32 dreams posttreatment. There were 24 words per dream on the first 2 nights, and 25 words per dream on the two posttreatment nights. Scoring by the Hall-Van de Castle categories, it was seen that following treatment emotions increased in males while in females social interactions decreased and activities increased. Similar to earlier findings (e.g. Kramer and Roth 1974), both sexes always dreamed more about the family than strangers and more about individuals than groups. Following treatment, males dreamed more about females. No statistics are reported.

Hauri (1976), in a well-controlled study, examined the sleep of patients remitted from reactive depression. Ten female and 1 male remitted patients with at least 1 psychiatric hospitalization in the last 10 years and a final diagnosis of severe reactive depression slept in the laboratory for 3 nights. Subjects were awakened 4 to 8 times per night from varying times in both REM and NREM sleep. They were given the Beck depression inventory and Nowlis mood-adjective checklist. Mentation was taken and rated by the experimenters on the Foulkes DF scale. The subjects then rated their own mentation. The 11 control subjects were matched for age, sex, education, and occupation. Awakenings were matched according to time of night, length in a sleep stage, and for roughly the same place in the circadian cycle. These procedures yielded 79 REM dream pairs and 16 sleep onset dream pairs from 7 dyads of matched subject and 20 matched NREM dream pairs from 10 subject dyads. Thus, differences in mentation could not be attributed to sleep-pattern differences.

Remitted patients had more difficulty falling asleep than controls and had fewer REM periods for the same amount of total sleep time. In most respects, their dreams were similar to the controls' dreams. Both felt they had fair recall and dreams from both groups were similar on self-ratings of vividness, amount of color, distortion, intensity of feelings, and overall hedonic tone. Both groups saw themselves as equally involved in their dreams and thought humans and animals exerted equal effort in their dreams. The main differences were as follows:

1. The remitted patients more often had dreams dealing with the past, while controls dreamt about the future and the present ($p = .05$).
2. The remitted patients had more childhood elements in their dreams ($p = .01$).
3. Patients tended to dream of events in the inanimate environment more often ($p < .05$).
4. For both REM ($p = .06$) and sleep-onset mentation, the patients' reports had less words. Sleep-onset narratives were more barren in terms of items as well ($p < .01$).
5. Controls' sleep-onset mentation was more REM-like.

NREM mentation was equal for both groups in length, number of ideas and REM likeness.

After rating the 42 matched pairs of REM narratives of more than 70 words in length, the patient dreams scored higher on the Beck and Hurvich masochism scale ($p = .05$) and on Gottshalk and Gleser's covert hostility out ($p = .03$), which measures hostile acts in the environment not involving the dreamer. Remitted patients had more dreams rated on the middle (neither pleasant nor unpleasant) of a hedonic tone scale.

Thus, Hauri (1976) concluded from their dreams that remitted patients see the world as more threatening, hostile, and violent, although not necessarily directed against the dreamer. Masochism remains high, thus arguing against Freud's (1917/1955b) model of depression of anger turned against the self. One would expect to see less masochistic elements in remitted patients' dreams. However, this may only mean that certain characterological variables remain stable.

Comparing mentation from the three sleep stages (REM, NREM, and sleep-onset) Hauri concluded that depressives might have a cognitive style such that the reporting of both realistic and fantasy-like material would be difficult. This would lead to the conclusion that remitted patients have more material in NREM sleep than controls. Hauri and Hawkins (1971) have shown that the percentage of phasic REM (number of 2.5 sec intervals with an eye movement during REM) correlates with clinical state as assessed by the Beck depression inventory. Thus, the sleep parameters of remitted patients may remain atypical in some ways, as does their mentation.

In sum, the dreams of remitted depressives are similar to normal populations on many dimensions, but retain some characteristics (like more masochistic content) of their still depressed counterparts. Many further comparisons could be made if mentation of depressed patients was taken from a variety of sleep states. In addition, the interesting idea that depressives have more NREM mentation should be examined, especially in the light of their barren REM mentation.

Dreams and Organic Brain Disease

Greenberg et al. (1968) studied the sleep and dreaming of 14 hospitalized patients afflicted with Korsakoff's psychosis. They were interested in two questions: do the lesions involved in the disease have typical effects on electrographic parameters of the sleep cycle? and is there any effect on sleep mentation?

The patients were divided into two groups: acute (ill less than one year), and chronic (ill more than one year). Their age range and degrees of memory impairment were not significantly different. Two patients were on tranquilizers until one week before the study and two patients received chlordiazepoxide during the observation period to help them sleep. The patients, all severe alcoholics, had no alcohol two weeks prior to the study.

After establishment of a stable baseline, seven patients were then studied for another two to three nights, with awakenings from REM and NREM sleep over varying elapsed durations.

In the acute group, with a mean total sleep time of 363.6 min the mean REMP time percentage equaled 29.6 min and the mean latency to the first REMP equaled 47 min. The REMPs tended to be fragmented with frequent Stage 2 REMP alternation.

In the chronic group with a mean total sleep time of 388.9 min, the mean REMP time percentage equaled 19.3 min and the mean REMP latency equaled 74.7 min. (No result of a statistical test of the significance of this difference between 1st REMP latency was given.) Although the REMPs tended to be intact, overall sleep throughout the night was fragmented by frequent spontaneous awakening.

Other findings in both groups included above normal REM density and loss of the usual systematic relationship between REM sleep and minimal chin EMG levels.

With regard to mentation, out of 34 awakenings in 7 patients (2 acute, 5 chronic), only 1 vivid unequivocal dream report and 1 elaboration of a stereotyped kind of mentation given on other awakenings were elicited. Acute patients also reported 2 possible dreams in which confabulation was likely. In the remainder recall was absent. NREM awakening produced either no-content reports or brief thoughts about home.

Kramer and Roth (1975) reported on laboratory studies of 17 hospitalized patients with a chronic organic brain syndrome (CBS), 7 of which were considered mild, and 10 severe. In addition, 4 aged severe CBS patients received separate attention. REM reports were obtained 5 min after each REMP onset. Mild CBS patients recalled some material apparently reflecting previous sleep mentation on an average of 57% of 35 awakenings and severe CBS patients had an average of 35% recall from 42 awakenings. Out of 54 awakenings, the severe aged CBS patients showed an average of 8% recall.

Comparison of the REM reports of the two age-matched CBS groups showed one significant difference: the middle-aged severe CBS patients had more characters in their dreams than the middle-aged patients with a mild CBS ($p < .05$). This result is puzzling, and since the level of significance is marginal the result should be regarded with circumspection. The authors found a number of differences between their subjects' mentation and that of matched normal controls but the comparison norms were based on daytime dream recall rather than laboratory reports and therefore are of limited value.

In general, the results of the above investigations are in accord with that of Torda (1969) for 51 REM reports of 6 patients afflicted with postencephalitic memory loss. That is, organic cerebral syndromes are associated with dream recall which is much less frequent, shorter, simpler, reality bound, and lacking in emotional depth.

To what extent this poverty-stricken state of REM mentation is a result of cognitive deficits secondary to brain-tissue damage, as opposed to loss of affective impetus, is difficult to assess. That the latter factor may play a role is suggested by Greenberg et al.'s (1968) observation that two Korsakoff patients, who had provided mundane laboratory dream reports had intense, affect-laden and dream-like experiences under the influence of nitrous oxide, were able to give detailed descriptions of them and remember them for some time after completion of the experiment. The authors ascribed this to the increase in emotion during nitrous oxide administration, and this was thought to overcome the hippocampal-cortical block to which the memory impairment has been partly attributed.

War Neuroses and Dreaming

Freud (1919/1955a) interpreted the repetitive dreams of patients suffering from war neuroses as belated unsuccessful attempts of the ego to master a prior traumatic episode. Greenberg, Pearlman, and Gampel (1972) suggest that one function of dreaming is "to reconstitute characteristic defenses in relation to recent waking experiences which have stirred up old unresolved conflicts [p. 27]."

They hypothesized that the recurrent nightmares were evidence of dreaming which did not fulfill its function, and that war neurosis patients would have a greater "pressure" to dream. This would be manifested as a shorter REM latency and longer REM time.

Nine patients suffering from war neurosis slept for at least three nights in the sleep laboratory at intervals of about one week. On half the nights, they slept undisturbed and on the other nights they were awakened at the end of each REMP and asked to relate their dreams. A 5-min verbal sample was collected from each subject before sleep and when awakened in the morning, in order to assess the subjects's psychological state. The 5-min samples were scored for defensive strain, a composite score, which was derived from three factors (degree of emergence of traumatic material, the relative prominence of safe versus unsafe interpersonal interactions, and the extent of emergence of threatening ego-alien impulses). On the basis of defensive strain scores, and without knowledge of the REM latencies, the presleep mentation samples of seven patients were ranked as either high or low latency nights. It was predicted that high defensive strain scores would be associated with shorter REM latency.

In the nine patients, average REM latencies were less than 40 minutes in 14 of a total of 29 nights. Sleep onset REM occurred frequently. Such short latencies have previously been found only in adults who were narcoleptic (Rechtschaffen, 1963). Of the seven patients whose depressive strain scores were ranked to predict REM latency, there were four where all three independent judges agreed in their scores and where the four nights were ranked accurately ($p = .005$ for each subject, one-tailed test). Of a possible 87 independent judgments for the 29 nights scored, 71 were scored correctly.

A second prediction was that changes in defensive strain from evening to morning would be related to the amount of total REM time, such that decreased defensive strain would mean that a high percentage of Stage REM had occurred. The changes in REM time with change in defensive-strain scores were not as clearcut as the latency measures and no statistics were given. The authors suggest two reasons: the morning samples were often barren; and it was even more difficult to make predictions based on the difference of 2 scores, as the possibility for error was greater.

Certain features of this study indicate methodological problems. For example, the low incidence of actual nightmares in the laboratory suggests that measuring the phenomenon by allowing subjects the security of sleeping in the laboratory may have altered results. Also, the authors presented no reliability data for the defensive strain measure. As the authors suggest in a later article (Greenberg & Pearlman, 1975), 5 min provide an inadequate sampling of behavior to assess psychological state. However, this remains a suggestive study in that there is some evidence for a psychological parameter being correlated with a physiological variable. Furthermore, the laboratory study of the dreams and electrographic parameters of patients with post traumatic neuroses may help to elucidate the possible functions that dreams and various stages of the sleep cycle may serve. A serendipitous observation from this work is the low incidence of actual nightmares in the laboratory, as opposed to home sleep. If the belated psychological mastery of trauma were an exclusively intrapsychic task, then such a difference would not have been observed. That is, the residue of the trauma would have been relatively insulated from environmental influences, and would have retained their intensity unabated leaving the stress to the psyche unrelieved. These observations are consistent with a model of dream formation, which takes into simultaneous account the interaction between dynamic intrapsychic, environmental and more or less stable cognitive factors.

Dreams of the Subjects with Impairments of Special Senses or of Motor Functions

How do the cruel experiments of nature affect dreaming? A variety of studies are available attempting to relate sensory and physical impairments to dream content. In cases of such impairments acquired in adult life, it is of interest to compare the relative degree of persistence of imagery derived from the pre-impairment period of life to the very short lived persistence of the "red-goggle effect" (an experimentally imposed sustained alteration of afferent input, described in Chapter 9 of this volume). In both instances, the sustained "tonic" background input is drastically altered — one by the impairment and the other by the experimenter. One is followed by relatively tenacious imagery, the other by a fleeting red effect.

Dreams of the Blind

Prior to the era of electrographic research, Blank (1958) extensively reviewed the topic of dreaming in the blind. The dreams of the congenitally blind are devoid of all visual imagery. Should blindness be acquired in childhood, a critical age range plays a role in whether visual imagery persists afterward. That is, with few exceptions, visual imagery was said to remain for varying periods, even into adulthood, when blindness occurred between the ages of 5 and 7 years. However, even among these, the capacity for visual imagery tends to deteriorate with time, so that visual dreams eventually become a rarity. According to Blank, with the exception of the absence of vision, dreams of those whose blindness antedates the critical period do not differ in essential respects from those of the sighted. In line with the incidence of nonvisual sensory percepts in the normal, the dreams of the early blinded contain auditory, tactile, kinesthetic, gustatory, olfactory and temperature sensations in decreasing order. In the early *deaf*-blind, a high incidence of anxiety content with later maturational tapering off was reported, with apparent emphasis on tactile-kinesthetic sensation. Helen Keller, however, reported occasional dreams with apparently vivid visual imagery in adult life.

In general, laboratory studies with blind subjects are in agreement with Blank (1958) on the relative incidence of non-visual sensory material (Amadeo & Gomez, 1966; Berger, Olley, & Oswald, 1962). Berger and co-workers reported on 8 blind adult males. Three (17, 25, and 30 years of age) had been blind from the age of 18 months or earlier, and visual sensations were absent from their dreams. Two additional subjects (ages 52 and 60) had each been blind for over 30 years and stated that they had lost both the ability to picture events and dream visual imagery. Finally, 3 subjects (23, 33, and 40 years old), totally blind for 10, 3, and 15 years, respectively, claimed to still experience visual imagery and visual dreams. A quoted example shows intensity and color: the subject, blind for 15 years, described a vivid REM dream in which the subject was swimming, did the "crawl" rapidly to the other end of the pool, and could see the white skin and black costume of a friend's wife, and splashed water over her teasingly.

The electrographic sleep findings on blind subjects had occasioned an interesting controversy. REMs were not detectable in five of eight subjects studied by Berger et al. (1962) and in one subject observed by Offenkrantz and Wolpert (1963). Their REM periods were otherwise apparently "normal." In both studies, absence of REMs and absence of visual dream imagery coincided and this finding supported the hypothesis that REMs were essential to and closely corresponded to visual dream events.

By contrast, Amadeo and Gomez (1966) reported that seven of eight subjects (three adults and five children) with various types of congenital blindness consistently showed REMs during "REM" periods albeit at a lower frequency and amplitude as compared to sighted subjects. "REM" awakenings yielded reports of elaborate nonvisual dreams. Accordingly, they concluded that REMs and visual dreaming were not related in a one-to-one manner and that REMs were merely the expression of the increased neural activation associated with REM sleep. In support of the latter notion, they described experiments on three blind subjects in which, while awake, REMs were twice as frequent during experimentally produced states of increased attention in contrast to wakeful rest.

These discrepancies were apparently resolved when Gross, Byrne & Fisher, (1965) demonstrated, by visual inspection of the eyelids of 5 sleeping blind subjects, and also by means of ceramic strain gauge recording of eye movements, that those blind subjects who seemed to lack REMs had a great deal more REM activity than was revealed by standard EOG recording. That is, certain of the blind subjects were afflicted by diseases that destroyed the retina (such as retrolental fibroplasia); and this, in turn, resulted in the loss of the corneo-retinal potential — the necessary basis of the EOG signal. In the absence of the corneo-retinal potential, subjects may have REMs which are recordable by a ceramic strain gauge (activated by physical deformation produced by eyeball movement) but not recordable by the EOG.

Thus, it appears that with suitable techniques of detection, all blind subjects with intact extraocular muscle systems will have abundant REM activity, though possibly reduced in amplitude; and such REM activity may occur independently of visual imagery.

Extensive coverage of the dreams of the blind and blind deaf may be found in Kirtley's (1975) study.

Dreams of the Deaf

Mendelson, Siger, & Solomon (1960) reported on the dream content of 26 deaf male and female adults between the ages of 18 and 24, without using electrographic technique. The analyses were based upon "daytime" dream recall. The population consisted of three groups: the congenitally deaf (N = 12), those whose deafness was acquired before the age of 5 (N = 8) and after the age of 5 (N = 6). Both the congenitally deaf and the deaf-before-5 group were reported as high in dream occurrence frequency, color content (primary colors, saturation and intensity), vividness on recall, and three-dimensional quality. By contrast, the deafness-after-5 group was strikingly lower in these categories. In all deaf subjects, the perception of motion in the dreams, other than movement involved in communicative signing, was described as low. It is of interest that the language of signs was their usual means of communication in dreams but in those accompanied by intense anxiety, there was a striking prevalence in the congenitally deaf of primitive signs (gestural communication employed by parental figures in early childhood before the standard language of signs was learned; gestures of this sort usually conveyed such strong affective qualities as anger, disapproval, warning, fear, and occasionally approval and praise). Such primitive signs did not appear in the anxious dreams of the other two groups. Other less marked differences were observed across groups in the frequency with which sign language, nonverbal, primitive signs, and amorphous sounds were used for communication in the event sequences of anxious, pleasant, and neutral dreams. The suggestion was made that the greater vividness and color representation in the dreams of the deaf served a compensatory function.

The main detraction from this work is its lack of a control group, making adequate comparison with normals difficult. Nevertheless, the study is intriguing and the dreams of such a subject population have rich potential for integrated psychophysiologic, linguistic, and developmental research. Such opportunities would be further enhanced by comparative laboratory dream studies on the blind, and matched normal controls.

The only laboratory study of the dreams of the deaf is that of Stoyva (1965). This work was instigated by an earlier classic report that in deaf subjects, a close relationship exists between EMG potentials of the arm and finger muscles and subsequent recall of dreams (Max, 1935, 1937). On 33 occasions of such EMG bursts, 30 instances of dream recall were observed upon immediate awakening; whereas in 62 awakenings following intervals of EMG quiescence, only 10 reports of dreams were obtained. It was concluded that in the deaf who use sign language, finger-EMG activity was associated with high dream recall. By contrast, no such association was found in 11 hearing subjects during 33 similar observations.

Stoyva (1965) deemed it valuable to repeat this work with the benefit of improved electrographic technology. He was interested in two questions. Does the EMG activity associated with finger movements of the deaf indicate NREM mentation? Are the deaf different from hearing controls with regard to finger-EMG activity in relation to frequency of episodes, their nightly distribution, or association with specific sleep stages?

In two experiments (one with seven deaf male subjects and four hearing controls and a replication with six deaf and six hearing controls), essentially the same results were obtained. (The total deaf sample regularly communicated in sign language; seven were congenitally deaf and six had acquired deafness before two years of age. Specifically:

1. The rates of dream recall from REM sleep were similar in the deaf and hearing groups.
2. Finger-EMG activity in NREM sleep was not associated with mentation.
3. In both deaf and hearing groups, a consistently accelerated rate of finger-EMG activity was observed during REM as opposed to NREM sleep.
4. Contrary to expectation, rates of finger-EMG activity were similar among the deaf and the hearing subjects.

Stoyva explained Max's (1935, 1937) findings by assuming that, because EMG activity is highest during Stage REM, increased finger-EMG activity and REM sleep and decreased finger activity and NREM sleep were overlapped. This situation could have resulted in Max's findings because of higher recall in REM as opposed to NREM sleep — variables unknown at the time of the early work. Stoyva (1965) concluded that his findings, contrary to those of Max, do not support the motor theory of thinking (Jacobson, 1932).

Dreams of Subjects with Physical Disabilities

We are unaware of any systematic laboratory studies of subjects with major motor paralysis. Newton (1970) has published his observations on 27 quadraplegic and paraplegic men based upon post sleep-period dream recall as recorded in writing for 4 successive days. A control sample of 29 normal males similar in age, education, and occupational status was employed.

The chief focus of interest was on the amount of physical activity present in the dreams of each group; and the results were to be used to test Lerner's (1967) hypothesis (based upon Rorschach's work) that dreams are kinesthetic fantasies serving to maintain the body image, versus an alternative hypothesis that dreams may serve an emergency repair function, shoring up the body image only when the latter is in flux. The former hypothesis would predict that the physically disabled, because of a threat to the integrity of the body image, have more than normal physical activity of the self in dreams by way of compensation. The latter hypothesis, by contrast, views dreaming kinesthesis as having an emergency repair function for a disrupted body image, and predicts an increase of physical activity immediately following the disability and dropping off below normal when the new body image becomes stabilized and kinesthesis is no longer necessary for its maintenance. This latter hypothesis predicts an inverse relationship between the amount of dreamed physical activity and the duration of the disability.

The mean proportion of dreamed self-propelled physical activity for disabled and normal subjects was not significantly different; nor was there any correlation between dream physical-activity scores (Hall & Van de Castle content-analysis method) and a Rorschach index of body-image integrity (Barrier score on the Holtzman inkblot test). On the other hand, it was found that immediately after the onset of the paralysis there was an upsurge of dreamed physical activity in excess of that of the normal controls and that with the passage of time, its level decreased and remained stable at lower than normal levels. Thus, the emergency repair hypothesis was supported.

PSYCHOPHYSIOLOGICAL PARALLELISM

People often experience themselves as "arrested" when viewing some daytime event. Particularly in the theater, one becomes absorbed; individuals often "lose themselves" and participate in the illusion vicariously. Under such circumstances, various physiological measures will respond accordingly, as if our vicarious participation were verging on the real. To the extent that appropriate concordance and patterning exists between the content of the psychic experience engendered by being engrossed in the play and changes in physiological measures, we speak of a psychophysiological parallelism. To what extent does this occur when we are immersed in our dreams and momentarily "live" within them?

The answers to this question have strong, more moderate, and weak forms. The strong form is excellently expressed by Roffwarg et al. (1962):

> . . . the dreamer is almost totally immersed in his dreaming consciousness. But he participates in the dream with both emotional and physiological responses as if it were a waking experience. In placid dreams, his pulse and breathing are fairly regular, and he lies motionless. When he is under emotional stress or is physically active in the manifest dream, his pulse appears to quicken, his respirations become irregular in rate and depth, he exhibits attenuated motion of those muscles being called into action in the dream, and he gazes sharply about at the dreamed visual imagery that he clearly 'sees' [p. 252].

The moderate form of the hypothesis of psychophysiological parallelism is well expressed by Fisher et al. (1970) in their laboratory study of REM nightmares. Of 20 subjects, only 8 showed increased respiratory, cardiac, and eye-movement activity just prior to awakenings from intensely anxiety-infused REM nightmares; the other 12 showed no significant change despite experiencing comparable amounts of dreamed anxiety. Fisher et al. (1970) hypothesize a dissociation of subjectively experienced anxiety from its usual physiological concomitants. They suggest further that the REM dream has a mechanism for reducing and modulating anxiety through a desomatization process.

Comments on the Relationships between Eye-Movement Activity and Sleep Mentation

The relationship between eye-movement activity and dream content may be seen "from two perspectives, one suggesting a very precise correspondence between the two variables, and another noting a general, nonspecific association [Pivik, p.   , this volume]." The precise correspondence perspective has been referred to in the literature as the "scanning hypothesis," and Pivik cited Rechtschaffen (1973), who extensively reviewed this topic, as concluding that "the issue is still in doubt." That is, many studies have produced inconsistent and inconclusive findings lending themselves to alternate interpretations. Actually, Rechtschaffen went on to state, as did Pivik, more or less, that in one sense, the precise correspondence hypothesis may not be subject to a crucial test because of formidable methodological problems.

But what about the current status of the hypothesis of a *nonspecific* relationship? Exemplars of this line of through are the studies of Dement and Wolpert (1958b), Berger and Oswald (1962), and Molinari and Foulkes (1969), which indicated that there was a significant association between eye movement patterns and dream events. We wish to cite the most recent literature pertaining to this hypothesis.

Keenan and Krippner (1970) elicited 97 dream reports from a single subject during 20 all-night sessions. A content analysis was attempted using the Hall-Van de Castle "activities"-content category. The mean number of activities per dream was 4.73; all reports containing 5 or more activities were termed "high-activity" reports and those with 4 or less were categorized as "low activity." Each REMP from which the report had been elicited was categorized as possessing high- versus low-REM density in accordance with a predetermined rule. When the data were entered in a chi-square table (high activity, low activity, high density, low density) significant results were obtained ($X^2 = 12.7$; 1 df; $p < .01$). Thus far, the results were in accord with those of the earlier studies cited previously. However, upon observing that the night's first report was usually a low-activity dream and also associated with a low-REM density REMP, the data were reanalyzed after elimination of the 20 first REMP reports. Recomputation of the statistics on this basis yielded *nonsignificant* results. Although this finding was based on only one subject, it nevertheless suggested to the authors as well as to Hauri and Van de Castle (1973b) that what seemed initially to be a demonstrated association between REM activity and dream activity may actually have been an artifact reflecting a time of night effect.

Specifically, previous studies had demonstrated that early REMPs have lower REM density (Aserinsky 1969b, 1971; Goodenough et al., 1965), and dreams elicited from these REMPs contain less activity (Foulkes, 1966). The earlier conclusion that REM density and dream activity were positively correlated was based upon data collected *throughout* the night; and when the time of night was held constant — when dream reports with high and low activity were correlated with REM density from REMPs occurring at the *same* approximate time of night — results were no longer statistically significant. Thus, the earlier conclusions seemed to have derived from a correlation between dream activity and time of night such that earlier dreams tend to be less active; and because the first REMP usually contains a low-REM density, the correlation between the latter and dream activity previously reported may have been spurious.

In their own experiments, Hauri and Van de Castle (1973) carried this work forward using 15 adult male subjects. Each slept in the laboratory for 1 adaptation night and 3 nonconsecutive experimental nights. Awakenings for mentation reports were carried out only after 3.5 hr of undisturbed sleep was allowed. These occurred twice during REMPs (the third or fourth) usually 15 min after REMP onset, except with those occasional subjects when, because of a tendency to short REMPs, awakenings were made after 10 min of REM sleep. NREM awakenings were made either about 4 hr after initial sleep onset, or 20 min after a previous awakening. Sequences of REM/NREM awakenings were counterbalanced between subjects. Each mentation report was blindly rated by a single experienced judge on 3 global 7-point scales, measuring the dreamers' emotionality, physical activity in the dream, and the dreamer's involvement as an actor in dream events.

The study entailed continuous measurement of a number of physiological variables including eye-movement activity. Relationships between the sleep-mentation ratings and eye-movement activity for the total preceding interval of REM sleep, preceding 6 min and 1 min were assessed. The only positive finding was a weak association ($p < .05$) between the mean eye-movement count during the last minute of REM sleep prior to the awakening, and the ratings of the involvement of the sleeper in his dreams. (Additional positive findings were obtained with respect to some of the other physiological variables as detailed elsewhere in this chapter).

Further attempts were made to assess other types of relationships between eye-movement activity and mentation content. These included comparisons based upon sorting dreams into "active" and "passive" categories (similar to the procedure of Berger and Oswald, 1962); into dreams which involved active looking around versus those which did not; and attempts to relate emotionality, "active" dreams and "active looking" dreams to the peak number of eye movements obtained during any 1-min period of the preceding REMP. *None* of these relationships reached significance at the .05 level. Hauri & Van de Castle (1973b) concluded that "the amount of eye movements during REM [sleep] does not relate in any major way to the . . . dream [content] dimensions [p. 304]" measured in their study.

This work is of obvious importance, and one therefore regrets that ratings were not carried out by more than one judge and with attendant reliability data.

The most recent attempt to reassess whether REM profusion and dream activity are related is that of Firth and Oswald (1975). This report is based upon data collected by Firth (1974) in an experiment dealing with the effects of amylobarbitone and nitrazepam on dream content (the schedule and results of which are presented in Chapter 11 of this volume pp. 17-22). Briefly, 20 subjects provided 256 mentation reports (128 each from the second and fourth REMPs) during an experimental schedule allowing for placebo (baseline), drug, and drug-withdrawal conditions. All reports were elicited after 7.5 min of the REMP had elapsed. Of the 256 reports, 116 from the second REMP and 117 from the fourth REMP (total of 233) contained some item of specific content and only these were used in the data analysis under discussion.

REM density (or EM profusion) was assessed by counting the number of 1-sec epochs with eye movements in the last 5-min and the last 1-min prior to each awakening. A point-biserial correlation was calculated to determine the extent to which "active" dreams were associated with REM profusion. The results were as follows:

1. Results from all awakenings from both REMPs 2 and 4 analyzed together disclosed a trend for passive dreams to have been elicited from REMPs with fewer REMs; but, notwithstanding, a large proportion of active dreams came from low-REM profusion REMPs. The point-biserial correlation between active or passive dreaming and REM profusion was .16 and .17 (last 5 min and last 1 min prior to awakening, respectively.) This relationship, though weak, was nevertheless statistically significant (Wilcoxon matched-pairs signed-ranks test T 20 = 37.5; $p < .05$).

2. Results from REMP 2 and 4 analyzed separately (awakenings from all conditions) revealed a correlation of .20 and .21 for the second REMP and .12 and .11 for the fourth REMP; but in this situation statistical significance was achieved for the second REMP only, (T 20 = 43), and not the fourth REMP, (T 18 = 43.5).

3. Results from nondrug nights analyzed separately revealed:

a. The correlation between REM profusion in the last 5 min prior to awakening and active or passive dreaming was .15; and the coefficient for the second and fourth REMP were .12 and .19 respectively.

b. The corresponding correlation for the 1 min prior to awakening data was .12; and for the second and fourth REMPs, .07 and .12 respectively. (In summary, *none* of the correlations obtained from the placebo nights was statistically significant.)

c. Correlations between REM profusion for the 5 min-prior-to-awakening interval and the subject's statement as to whether he had been thinking or dreaming were negligible and insignificant.

The final conclusions of Firth and Oswald (1975) are that their study, using numerical measures of the profusion of eye movements and ratings of visual activity versus passivity in dream reports, demonstrated that:

the magnitude of the association between visually active dreaming and eye movement is only slight, so that prediction of active dream content from eye movement activity will be poor. This association moreover only exceeds possible chance effects when a wide range of eye movement profusion exists in the data. With a more restricted range of eye movement profusion (data from placebo conditions only, or from the fourth REMP only), the strength of association between visually active dreaming and eye movement did not even prove greater than possible chance effects [p. 604].

In effect, they stated that the positive relationship between REM profusion and active dreaming previously repeated by Berger and Oswald (1962) is not demonstrable with REMP or time of night controlled.

There seems to be only one possible factor that might make their interpretation of the findings slightly questionable: the interjudge reliability regarding visual activity and passivity was not as high as one might hope. Agreement between two judges was 75% for 24 dreams rated independently by a second judge. Although Firth and Oswald (1975) state that "the reliability of these ratings is not low enough for the low correlations reported to be ascribed merely to poor reliability of the measures [p. 604]," no computational data was presented in support of this assertion (even though it seems to possess face validity). As with the Hauri and Van de Castle (1973a) study, in view of the crucial nature of this measure in the experiment, and the fact that the results were cited as reversing a previous influential conclusion from older studies, one would welcome a replication of this work, or else a reprocessing of the data with a new set of trained, blind judges rating all of the mentation reports. Such a recommendation seems all the more worthwhile in view of the statistically significant but weak association found between REM bursts and more dream-like mentation by Ellman et al. (1974). (See Editors' Foreword to Chapter 8 of this volume). This modest but significant result should be considered along with other modest but significant results of the subanalyses of data from similar studies (Foulkes & Pope, 1973; Hauri & Van de Castle, 1973; Firth & Oswald, 1975). These taken together with the minor methodological flaws mentioned above indicate that the hypothesis of a relationship between REM activity and dream activity is not dead; we are dealing with a subtle, unimposing but nevertheless real finding.

Other Physiological Variables

Hauri and Van de Castle's (1973b) report, which we discussed above, for its data on REMs, seems to be among the better evaluations of the hypothesis of a general, nonspecific association between physiological variables and dream experience for several reasons:

1. Their procedure avoided the possibility of confounding with time of night effects by making all awakenings after at least 3.5 hr of undisturbed sleep.
2. Several different physiological parameters were assessed, each during three different time intervals within the REMP.
3. Mentation reports were assessed along three dimensions.

In addition to REMs Hauri and Van de Castle (1973b) recorded: heart rate, phasic vasoconstrictions, breaths per minute (using a strain gauge attached to the subject's mattress), and rapid fluctuations in skin potential (measured from the left hand). During REM sleep mean values of each of these were obtained: (1) during all of the REMP prior to awakening (2) during the last 6 min of REM sleep prior to awakening; and (3) during the last 1 min of REM sleep prior to awakening. Variability for each physiological parameter during these intervals was computed using Hotelling's T for 1 and 2 and the absolute difference between the second and the last 1-min epoch [sic] for 3. During NREM sleep these variables were assessed only during the last 6 min prior to awakening.

Mentation reports were rated by one judge along three seven-point scales of the following "global" dimensions: (1) total emotionality (emphasizing sexual and aggressive impulse expression); (2) physical activity of the dreamer (the output of physical energy which would be involved if the dreamer were engaged in these activities during wakefulness); and (3) involvement of the dreamer as an actor in the events of the dream (how much the dreamer apparently tried to influence the dream events, rather than being a nonparticipant observer). Ratings on these three scales intercorrelated significantly (.59-.73).

Mentation and physiological variables (from REM sleep) were dichotomized around each subject's median value and placed in 2 X 2 tables which were then combined across subjects using Cochran's method. Dream reports with higher total emotionality were significantly associated with higher heart-rate variability during the last 6 min ($p < .005$) and the last 1 min ($p < .05$) prior to awakening; with the number of skin potential fluctuations ($p < .005$) and its variability ($p < .05$) during the last 1-min; with respiratory rate during the last 1-min ($p < .05$), and with vasoconstriction variability during the last 6 min ($p < .05$). As the author's note, emotionality of dream reports was not significantly related to any aspect of the total REMP prior to awakening.

Dream reports with greater physical activity of the dreamer were significantly associated with higher heart-rate variability during the last 6 min ($p < .01$) and with higher skin-potential fluctuation variability during the last 1-min ($P < .05$).

The active involvement of the dreamer with dream events was significantly associated with mean heart rate during the total REMP ($p < .005$) and during the last 6 min ($p < .01$); with heart-rate variability during the last 6 min ($p < .05$) and with the mean number of phasic vasoconstrictions during the 6 min ($p < .01$).

Citing Hauri, Sawyer, & Rechtshaffen (1967) and Foulkes (1966) the authors (Hauri & Van de Castle, 1973) assert that general "dream intensity" is an important "distinguishing factor" between different dreams, and that emotionality, physical activity, and involvement are all correlated with it. Therefore they summed their three global ratings of each dream to produce general intensity scores. These scores were significantly associated with heart-rate variability during the last 6 min ($p < .005$) and 1 min ($p < .05$); with skin-potential fluctuation variability during the last 1 min ($p < .01$), with the mean number of skin-potential fluctuations during the entire REMP ($p < .05$) and with mean respiratory rate during the last 6 min ($p < .05$).

During NREM sleep the only relationship which reached significance was between heart-rate variability and general dream intensity ($p < .03$).

Hauri and Van de Castle (1973) begin their discussion of their data by noting that some of the weaker but statistically significant relationships may be spurious since so many individual statistics were computed (120). Therefore, they confine their discussion to the findings which were at least at the .01 level of significance. This leaves 8 significant psychophysiological relationships, of 120 assessed. The authors regarded 4 of these as highly significant ($p < .005$). Hauri and Van de Castle (1973b) conclude that dream content can be related to physiological variables during REM sleep which, they add, is no surprise considering the dense interconnections of the human brain. Indeed, we echo this lack of surprise. Why should relationships between psychological state and autonomic arousal which obtain during waking, cease during REM sleep? Nocturnal psychophysiological parallelism is only interesting, it seems to us, insofar as its pattern suggests something concerning the mechanisms or function of dreaming and REM sleep. In this regard, Hauri and Van de Castle (1973b) speculate that the apparently differential development of different REM dreams from the same time of the night, somewhat correlated with higher levels of autonomic activity and irregularity, may be the product of differential rates of PGO spike discharge, that is, "causing *both* a more rapid succession of dream images and more autonomic arousal [p. 304]."

The authors note that this speculation encounters some difficulties. For example, Baust and Engel (1970) reported a significant *negative* relationship between heart-rate variability and dream intensity. Hauri and Van de Castle (1973b) suggest that this reversal of their own data may be due to "individual response specificity." By this they refer to Lacey et al.'s (1963) findings, that individuals respond to different kinds of stress with relatively stereotyped patterns, differing from person to person with respect to intensity, direction, and organ systems involved. Hauri and Van de Castle.s (1973b) data are consistent with such an interpretation; they report that only nine subjects showed a clear positive relationship between dream emotionality and heart-rate variability, while five showed no association and one showed a reverse trend. The authors conclude that their subject sample may have had an unusually high number of heart-rate responders. They felt that this was additionally supported by the fact that their subjects also produced a significant association of heart-rate variability with emotionality during NREM sleep, a finding which is specifically *not* obtained elsewhere (Shapiro et al., 1964; Verdone, 1965).

In spite of these restrictions on the meaning of their data, Hauri and Van de Castle (1973b) conclude that dream emotionality is at times related to physiological variables, while physical activity in the dream is not, (since they found virtually no association between this aspect of subjects' dreams and the physiological variables). If this is correct it may certainly bear upon our understanding of the psychological functions of dreaming and REM sleep, insofar as it specifies the importance of emotional processes. However, it is precisely in the assessment of psychological variables that this study is seriously flawed (cf. Baldridge, 1974, for other criticisms). Ratings on the three mentation scales intercorrelated with one another substantially (range = .59-.73). When this is coupled with the fact that only one judge with unestablished reliability rated dreams, it becomes totally unclear as to what these scales assess. If the intercorrelation of the scales exceeds the reliability of the judge — a logical possibility from the data presented — the ratings may indicate more about the measurement process than about the mentation itself. Although it may be the case that emotionality, involvement and physical activity in dreams in fact covary, it is necessary to establish the independence of these respective measures in order to make any specific statements concerning their differential association with physiological parameters. Just such statements are what this sort of study might usefully provide. For example, if Hauri and Van de Castle's (1973b) data indicated primarily a strong relationship between heart rate and emotionality, but not with vividness of imagery, and it was found that following REM sleep deprivation REMP heart rate increased, it might suggest that an important functional psychological component of REM sleep was some form of emotional process, rather than, for example, a perceptual or cognitive process. A phenomenological mapping of the psychological correlates of the different types of autonomic arousal during REM sleep, including the burgeoning population of phasic events (MEMA, PIP and so on), coupled with their systematic variability under different conditions in different subject groups, may go a long way toward furthering our understanding of the functions of dreaming and of REM sleep.

As Hauri and Van de Castle (1973b) correctly point out, individual response specificity must be examined and may seriously complicate such a research program. But let us hope that nature is not quite so unparsimonious as first glances may seem to indicate.

Older studies on relationships between respiratory measures showed mixed results. Thus, Shapiro et al. (1964) found that intense respiratory irregularity rather than rate was significantly associated with greater REM dream reporting. Hobson, Goldfrank, & Snyder (1965), found with 10 adult subjects that awakenings immediately following intervals of high respiratory rate or high variability were more likely to yield reports of dreaming from both REM and NREM sleep, than were awakenings associated with low or moderate levels of these respiratory measures. A negative relationship prevailed between respiratory measures and "non-dream mental content" reports. A further relationship was demonstrated by pooling mentation-content ratings for emotion, physical activity, and vividness to form a single total-content rating (the single-category ratings alone did not reach significance). The clearest correlation between specific items of mentation reports was observed between apnea and respiratory-dream content, like content involving speech or laughter on choking followed apneic patterns, almost twice as often as with other respiratory categories (32.8% versus 17.9%).

Penile Erections

Freud (1900/1955a) in *The Interpretation of Dreams* wrote:

> The more one is concerned with the solution of dreams, the more one is driven to recognize that the majority of the dreams of adults deal with sexual material and give expression to erotic wishes .... From no other instinct are so many and such powerful unconscious wishes left over, ready to produce dreams in a state of sleep [p.396].

Thus, it is not surprising that the observations of Ohlmeyer, Brilmayer, and Hullstrung (1944) of a cycle of penile erections during sleep acted as a spur to further research in the hopes of elucidating Freud's theory. A cycle of penile tumescence and detumescence would seem to tie the hypothesized sexual meaning of dreams to a measurable biological event.

Fisher, Gross, and Zuch (1965) were the first to publish results of systematically studied penile erections coterminous with the REM period. Using four methods of observation (phalloplethysysmograph, direct observation, strain gauge, and strain gauge plus thermometer) they studied 86 REM periods in 17 subjects over a period of 27 nights. Fisher noted that 60% of the REM periods contained full erections, 35% partial erections, and 5% showed no erections. Erections occurred 2.5, ($SD \pm 3$) min before the beginning of the REM period. Maximum erection was reached 5.4 ($SD \pm 3.9$) min after the onset of the REM period, while full detumescence occurred 12.4 ($SD \pm 2.0$) min after the termination of the REM period. Fisher saw no indication of erection during NREM sleep, although there were slight episodes of tumescence in association with NREM body movements, and 1-2 min during Stage 2 preceeding the onset of the REMP. Once erection was attained, it was generally sustained without much fluctuation throughout the REMP. Erections took place independently of the recency of sexual gratification. In short, more than 90% of the REMPs seemed to be associated with some degree of erection, and misses occurred most frequently during the unstable first REM period of the night.

Karacan et al. (1966) examined the relationship between erections during the REMP and anxiety in the content of the dream. Given the clinical evidence that anxiety may cause impotence during waking, they hypothesized that anxiety in the dream would also prevent erection from occurring, and that when subjects were awakened from REM periods with full erections, they would be less anxious than when awakened from REM periods with irregular or no erections.

Sixteen subjects slept in the lab for six nights each. The first night served as an adaptation night; on the second night erections were also recorded and on Nights 3-6 a film of either an exciting or a neutral character was shown to the subject as well. They were awakened 5-15 min after the beginning of the REMP. They then gave dream reports and completed mood adjective check lists adapted from Nowlis. The check lists measured seven variables: aggression, anxiety, surgency, social affection, depression, distrust, and quiet. The emotional content of the dreams was assessed by scoring dream transcripts for anxiety, hostility inward, and hostility outward, by Gottschalk's (1967) method.

Of the 237 Stage REM periods, 80% were accompanied by erections. Steady or regular erection accompanied 42%. Irregular erection (fluctuating amplitude or one in which detumescence occurred befor awakening) comprised 37% of the awakenings. Like Fisher (1965), Karacan et al. (1966) found that erections generally began at the same time as the onset of the REM period. However, on rare occasion erections began as much as 30 min before Stage REM and sometimes followed REM onset by some minutes. Also 19 erections occurred during NREM sleep. Three of these occurred between REM periods and the others occurred either early in the night during an absent first REM period, or late at night after an awakening (when an erection would occur immediately after the subject returned to sleep). The difference between Karacan et al.'s (1966) data and the Fisher et al. (1965) study might be accounted for partly by the fact that Karacan and co-workers were waking their subjects for mentation reports and probably slightly REM depriving them in so doing. Hence, there might have been a slight deprivation effect, thus causing the erections to "intrude" into NREM sleep. Also, although Karacan et al. (1966) claim that the neutral film condition was not significantly different from the exciting film condition, we cannot assess the effect that any presleep stimulus would have on the penile erection cycle; for example, it may have contributed to the lower reported incidence of erections. To test the hypothesis that anxiety will interfere with nocturnal erection, REM periods were separated into those showing irregular and full erections. The mean of the subjects' Gottshalk anxiety score was significantly greater for dreams from those REM periods with irregular or no erections than for those showing regular erection ($p < .01$). For the adjective checklist, the trend was in the same direction, but did not reach significance. This was attributed to the fact that many subjects who seemed to be anxious rated themselves as depressed in their self-reports. Hostility outward, hostility inward and the other Nowlis mood clusters showed no difference between REM periods with full or irregular erections.

REM periods were also divided into high and low activity on the basis of the number of eye movements in the last 3 min before they had been awakened to give a dream report. The sum of relevant Nowlis clusters was then computed and a mean of the total-affect score obtained for all low-activity and high-activity periods for each subject. Total affect was significantly higher following high eye-movement activity ($p < .01$). In addition, there was more eye-movement activity with regular erection than with irregular or no erection. Finally, 95% of all awakenings following REM periods with regular erections yielded reports of preawakening experience with some content as compared to 85% of awakening following irregular or no erection ($p < 0.1$).

Thus, anxiety dreams do tend to accompany REM periods with irregular or no erections. However, as Karacan et al. (1966) conclude, anxiety may be only one of many factors responsible for the absence or irregularity of erections. Some REM periods usually early in the night have a low rate of eye movements and yield no content reports. Absence of erection during these REM periods may be physiological as well. Finally, Karacan et al. (1966) suggest that dream reporting may be related to erections more than the REM period per se.

Fisher, (1966) attempted to test the idea that erections during the REMP were related to sexual content (in the broad psychoanalytic sense including both genital and pregenital aspects) and could be viewed as examples of the discharge of mobile instinctual energy. Six college student volunteers in the 20s were observed for 15 nights. They were awakened from REM periods during a particular state of penile tumescence (during the initial flaccid phase, after abrupt rapid tumescence, during sustained maximal erection, or after abrupt rapid detumescence). Detailed accounts of dreams were then elicited. Fisher then attempted from a study of the 58 dream accounts to make blind predictions of the fluctuations of erections in any given direction.

Fisher's most successful predictions were in instances in which there were sudden sharp detumescences. In seven or eight instances predictions made on the basis of marked anxiety in the manifest dream prior to awakening were correct ($p < .001$). In five or six instances a sudden increase of tumescence was predicted correctly ($p < .001$) on the basis of overtly or symbolically sexual elements.

Dreams with no or slight erections were compared to those with full erections. Of the 17 records with no, slight, or inhibited erections, there was not a single instance of the presence of erotic content in the manifest dream, and there was no physical contact between the dreamer and any other person in the dream. Among the 30 dreams with full erections, 8 had erotic feeling in the manifest dream. This is by no means a striking correspondence; especially if one had expected that on the basis of the correspondence between the REMP and erections, that at least 80% of the dreams would have some sexual elements. Fifteen of the 30 dreams with moderate to full erections, and 7 of the 17 dreams associated with flat records showed latent erotic content. Combining figures for manifest and latent content, we see that 23 of 30 dreams with moderate to full erection showed sexual content, as opposed to 7 of 17 dreams with minimal erection ($p = .02$). However, if erections are caused by the sexual content of dreams, any theory would have to explain why the 7 dreams showing latent erotic content did not evoke erections. Dreams with minimal erections contained much more aggressive content, anxiety and other negative affects, such as jealousy, shock, resentment, or rejection. Ten of 17 flat records were associated with such content, while only 5 of the 30 showing full erection were associated with such content.

This is roughly in agreement with the data of Karacan et al. (1966), that anxiety will inhibit REM erections.

From his data, Fisher (1966) concludes that where there is erotic content (either manifest or symbolic) free from anxiety, there will be erections. If there is a shift to marked aggression in the dream content, there will be rapid detumescence. Also, if aggressive content is present from the onset of the REMP, erections will be inhibited.

Several questions arise in connection with Fisher's (1966) study. It is clear that there is nowhere near the high percentage of unambiguous sexual content in dreams that could have been hypothesized. This is confirmed by Hall and Van de Castle (1966) whose male subjects showed overt sexual activity in only 12% of their manifest dreams. As Rechtshaffen (1973), in an excellent review of this literature has pointed out, Fisher's (1966) claim that erection may be associated with disguised, latent, and symbolic erotic content, even though there is no erotic feeling in the manifest dream is based on a theoretical assumption – namely that there is something intrinsically sexual about dreaming. In order to correctly test this notion one would have to have set up prior criteria as to what one would consider a sexual act in the dream. This might require extensive interviews with each subject as to what represents sexuality to each subject symbolically. One could then rate dreams for sexual content on the frequency with which these elements appear.

Fisher assumes that there are certain symbols which represent discrete sex related acts. Clinical research certainly supports the notion that such relationships are quite frequent. Thus, castration is represented by being bitten by an animal. Intercourse is represented by a dreamer going up an elevator with several girls, as well as climbing up a flight of stairs. But it is also true that often classic psychoanalytic symbols appear in dreams referring not to an unconscious element but to a real day-residue item, that is, the dreamed staircase may represent a real staircase climbed the day before the dream en route to a bookstore; usually the subject's associations are required in order to make the necessary distinctions. Although Fisher is careful to make the conceptual distinction between manifest and latent content, when judging the dream report he affords them equal weight. Yet, undoubtedly there is some psychological difference between a blatantly represented sexual act, and its disguised equivalent. Again, the problem is primarily one of defining clearly what is to be considered sexual. Although Freud, in *Three Essays on the Theory of Sexuality* (1905/1953b) claims, "that all comparatively intense affective processes, including even terrifying ones, trench upon sexuality [p. 203]," it does not mean that one can equate the two for the purposes of a research paradigm. This comment should not be construed as an attack on psychoanalytic theory. Rather, it is a point of methodology.

Fisher's (1966) interpretation of his findings is influenced, in part by his assumption that dreaming is coterminous with the REMP and does not occur outside of REM sleep. He conducted a REM-deprivation study to show that erections could occur outside of REM sleep. Two subjects were REM deprived by forced awakenings and two by Nembutal and d-amphetamine plus forced awakenings. With REM deprivation erections occurred between awakening and Sleep Onset Stage 1 and were often sustained through several awakenings. Fisher's (1966) rationale is that "the sexual excitation which began with the REMP, if not permitted to develop during it, continued on into NREM sleep, thus becoming dissociated from it, and indicating that erection was even more difficult to suppress than other manifestations of REMP activity [p. 552]." One would predict, from this, that the psychological quality of sexual excitation would be transmitted to NREM dreams as well. However, mentation was not elicited and the notion could not be tested. Similarly, mentation has never been taken from normal NREM erections, although the infrequency of their occurrence suggests dreaming can go on in the absence of penile erections as well.

Both Fisher (1965, 1966) and Karacan et al. (1966) use grouped data. Because of their bias that REM and NREM sleep are completelely unique and discontinuous entities, they tended not to look at the continuum of individual differences in degrees of penile fluctuation throughout REM and NREM sleep.

Thus there is suggestive evidence from Fisher (1966) and Karacan et al. (1966) that penile erections are related to dream content. The "firm" findings are as follows:

1. There is a fairly constant cycle of penile erection coterminous with the REM period in the sleep of normal male subjects.
2. Rapid detumescence can be associated with dysphoric dream content, that is, mentation associated with anxiety or aggression. This is supported by Karacan et al.'s (1966) finding that dreams with partial or no erection contain more anxiety related elements than those with full erections.
3. Rapid tumescence is associated with erotic material in the manifest content of the dream.
4. There is better recall of mentation from REM periods with full erection than those with partial or no erection.
5. The presence of penile erections as such is not predictive of sexuality in the manifest dream content.

Overall, the results seem most consistent with the earlier interpretation of Fisher et al. (1965) that normally REMP erections are more a reflection of general REMP activation than of sexual ideation. This accords well with the observation of REMP erections in subhuman mammals and human newborns, presumably unburdened by a sophisticated tripartite psychic structure. The pattern of relationships between REMP activation, the associated REMP erections, and sleep mentation must be seen as the varying outcome of a complex, mutually interactive process. For example, in some cases, psychological processes derived from current wakeful tensions and unconscious factors may prepotently influence the events of sleep mentation, REMP activation and associated penile-erection patterns. The sleep-mentation content itself may in turn introduce an added modulating influence. As a result REMP activation and its associated penile erection may be enhanced leading to nocturnal emission, in the case of overtly sexual dreams, or inhibition of erection, in the case of dysphoric dreams.

In other more usual cases, psychological processes may be in varying equilibrium and the degree of penile erection may vary primarily with REMP activation levels and patterns. In such instances, minimal erection might reflect low-intensity tonic physiological rhythmic (for example, the first REMP), rather than inhibitory psychological influences. And the less intense associated sleep-mentation content might likewise be prepotently determined by such factors intrinsic to REMP physiology.

The most important consideration is to recognize the need for a complex, interactive-factor scheme to account for all the observations. A view which considers activation levels, penile erections and sleep mentation as related, interactive but quasi-independent phenomena possesses the added advantage of taking into consideration the relative infrequency of penile erection during NREM sleep when, as it is now accepted, an impressive amount of dreaming occurs.

Future research would hopefully incorporate the previous methodological criticisms, as well as examine individual differences in the relation between penile erections and dream content.

In the main, the results favor a moderate to weak version of psychophysiological parallelism in dreams.

BODY MOVEMENTS AND SLEEP MENTATION

Large Movements

An early study which attempted to look at differences between mentation from 2 points in the REMP was that of Wolpert and Trosman (1958). They believed that a gross body movement signaled a change in dream activity and betokened a completed dream episode. Ten male subjects were observed for a total of 51 nights. Awakenings were made during ongoing stage REM sleep, during stage REM sleep followed by a gross body movement, during Stage 2 within 5 min after REMP termination, and during Stage 2 at least 10 min from the last eye movement. Dream-recall data were divided into detailed, and single or fragmented recall.

They found dream recall high from Stage REM and low from periods of spindling brain waves. But the amount of recall from ongoing Stage REM awakenings was 82.5% as compared with 69.1% from Stage REM followed by a gross body movement. NREM recall was higher from the 5, as opposed to the 10-min post-REMP awakenings. Although in both REMP conditions recall was quite high, the authors did not discuss if awakening after a gross body movement was associated with recall of a more complete dream episode; that is, they did not present specific data which indicated clearly that a gross body movement was associated with the "natural end of a dream scenario." Rather, it seems that the lower incidence of REMP recall succeeding such movements was understood by the authors to be a sign of completion of a previous dream event sequence, and their very rapid memory decay.

These results and their interpretation are partly consistent with earlier observations of Dement and Wolpert (1958b). Fourteen men and 2 women provided 46 dreams which were long and continuous, and 31 containing 2 or more apparently unrelated fragments. The latter sample was associated with electrographic evidence of body movements, whereas the former was associated with their absence. Also, dream narratives after 10-20 min of REM sleep tended to be equal to or shorter than those elicited after 4-5 min of REM activity, provided that a gross body movement had occurred several minutes prior to the awakening. Finally, 10 REMP awakenings were performed just after a gross body movement with the following results: 3 yielded no content; 3 provided usual REMP dreams; and 4 contained spontaneous comments very suggestive of completion of dream episodes, like, "I had just come to the end of a dream," "The dream seemed to be over," or "The dream had reached its natural end." Dement and Wolpert (1958b) concluded that body movements during dreams tend to signal a change in dream activity or termination of an event sequence. It is a fact that body movements are more frequent in intervals immediately preceding and following REMPs and the question was left open as to whether the body movement interrupts the REMP and its associated dream, or whether with REMP termination, tonic muscular inhibition ceases permitting a "released" body movement concurrent with the end of a dream. The authors favored the latter interpretation.

Similarly, the diminished recall from NREM sleep 10 min, as opposed to 5 min post-REMP found by Wolpert and Trosman (1958) is consistent with findings of Dement and Kleitman (1957b). Specifically, the incidence of dream recall dropped steeply following REMP termination. Of 17 NREM awakenings performed before 8 min post-REMP, 5 dreams were recalled (28%); and of 132 such awakenings after 8 min, only 6 dreams were recalled (5%).

Small Movements

REM sleep is accompanied by much fine-muscle activity, some, but not all of which, is related to concurrent dream activity. Also, dreamed motor activity need not be reflected in the EMG. (We have described the pioneer work of Max, 1935 and Stoyva's, 1965, attempt to replicate elsewhere in this chapter). Wolpert (1960) found, in some subjects only, that there was an impressive relationship between specific EMG patterns and specific dream content just before awakening. An example is the dreamer's use of a hand in a dream and concomitant EMG activity over the appropriate wrist. Dement (1972) has mentioned observing his wife twitching her legs during REM sleep, upon awakening from which she reported a dream of doing an energetic dance. Also, McGuigan and Tanner (1970) reported a relationship between conversation content of REM dreams and increased chin and lip EMG activity in one subject.

The most systematic attempt to study this issue has been made by Grossman et al. (1972) and a comprehensive review of motor patterns in human sleep has been published by Gardner and Grossman (1976). Ten young adult subjects who were good dream recallers were observed 4-8 nights in the laboratory during which REMP awakenings were carried out and mentation reports were independently judged for dreamed muscular movements. The movements of each upper and lower extremity were separately monitored. When both upper and lower extremities were active, the mean number of movements was 2.15; when either upper or lower extremity girdle was active, the mean was 1.16 and when none were active, the mean was 0.89. The last value indicates that many false positives (EMG activity without concomitant dreamed movement) occurred. An analysis of variance revealed, however, that despite the false positives, the above results were significant ($p < .05$).

In a second analysis, with 8 or 10 subjects, more upper than lower extremity dreamed actions occurred after upper extremity preawakening movements; and the converse was true with 9 of 9 subjects with lower extremity movements ($p < .05$). It was concluded that a significant relationship exists between actual and dreamed action with respect to amount and girdle location.

SLEEP-STAGE CORRELATES

One method that has been used to clarify the relationship between physiological and psychological events is the study of mentation collected from different sleep stages. It was hoped that this would shed light on the process of dream formation as well. The following section reviews the literature on sleep-stage correlates of mentation and the sequential relationship of mental activity in one sleep stage to another with and without experimental manipulation.

Stage W

For purposes of comparison in sleep research, the waking state has generally been assumed to provide a baseline index for rational-reality-oriented non-dreamlike mentation. Foulkes and Fleischer (1975), impressed by surprising results from an earlier study (Foulkes & Scott, 1973), attempted to systematically look at cognition during relaxed wakefulness. Ten male and 10 female subjects were questioned during 45-60-min sessions on their last mental experience at selected intervals from 1-9 min. Using questions from previous sleep studies, Foulkes and Fleischer asked them about the prevalent modality (auditory or visual) of their thought, and whether they believed the experience was really happening or if they realized at the time that they were just thinking. They were also questioned as to whether they were aware of being in the laboratory, and if they were voluntarily controlling the nature of their thoughts, rather than having an experience that seemed to be spontaneous and devoid of efforts to control. Finally, subjects evaluated how accurate they believed their recall to be, and if they were asleep or awake. They were monitored on EEG and EOG during the sessions, half of which occurred in the morning and the other half in the afternoon.

Reports were judged for regressivity of content, based on the following six criteria: (1) if they consisted of a single isolated image; (2) an incomplete or fragmented scene; (3) inappropriate or distorted imagery; (4) bizarre sequencing or superposition of images; (5) dissociation of thoughts from images; or (6) magical thought content.

The amount of mental activity during waking was striking. Of 120 arousals, 118 yielded reports of content. Of these, 68% yielded some type of visual imagery present prior to interruption and 16% involved auditory imagery experiences. Endogenous imagery was reported as having hallucinatory qualities in 19% of the "awakenings." Following Vogel et al. (1966), Foulkes and Fleischer (1975), quantified the regressive quality of the reports. They evaluated two ego functions: maintaining contact with reality, and maintaining nonregressive content. Neither ego function was found to be invariably present in waking mentation. One quarter of the reports were judged to be regressive (on the basis of questions and content assessed by judging procedures) and about 50% of the reports showed a lack of reality contact.

Of the 118 reports 38% showed full reality contact. Twenty percent were classified as mindwandering, in which the subject was not controlling his thoughts, but was simultaneously aware that he was in the laboratory. Twenty-two percent of the reports showed a "lost-in-thought" pattern, in which the subject might have been controlling thoughts, but was aware of being in the laboratory. Fifteen percent showed no reality contact at all. Regressive reports were most often associated with the lost-in-thought pattern, and least often associated with full reality contact. Forty-two percent of the lost-in-thought reports were regressive, while only 20% of the reality-oriented reports were regressive. Mentation was seen to be either hallucinatory or regressive, but rarely both at the same time. Hallucinatory ideation and regressive ideation were thus relatively independent report characteristics.

EEG activity and EOG patterns were examined in relation to the mental content of the reports. All EEG and EOG patterns indicated that subjects were awake, except for one EOG pattern with slow eye movements, which can be seen at sleep onset. However, this pattern was quite rare, and except for 3 of the

120 awakenings, subjects were unequivocably awake. Hallucinatory and regressive mentation were likely to occur in a variety of EEG-EOG patterns, with the exception of a low-voltage random EEG accompanied by REMS.

In a recent review of this study Singer, (1976) suggests that the subjects were oriented toward regressive and hallucinatory mentation by being told that this was a sleep study. Kripke (1972) has shown that the 10-20-cycle-per-day oscillations expressed during sleep by the cyclic occurrence of REM periods may be present during waking. Lavie and Kripke (1975) reported periodicity of daytime fantasy and it is therefore possible that the Foulkes-Fleischer (1975) data reflected ultradian rhythmic effects in interaction with other wakefulness factors.

However, if it can be replicated, this study has important implications for how we view further research on sleep-stage correlates of mentation. The idea of waking mentation as a baseline measure must be questioned, as there is a high percentage of waking thought which shows characteristics similar to dream mentation when assessed by identical scales. There is, of course, some difference in sleeping and waking cognition but it is possible that this difference is primarily quantitative, rather than qualitative. Thought in the waking state is, thus, only momentarily regressive or hallucinatory. The lapses into primary-process modes of thought are fleeting, and change rapidly. They are not so clear-cut as those found during REM or sleep onset mentation. Also, the relative independence of regressive mentation and hallucinatory thought can be taken as evidence that subjects show some control over their mentation. Also, the sharper dichotomy of primary-and secondary-process thinking does not seem to be applicable. Reality testing seems rather to be a continuous process which can be sustained for longer or shorter periods of time in sleep or wakefulness. Dreams could merely be the end point on a continuum, and the "dream state," mentally speaking, could be tapped in a variety of ways, including meditation, hypnosis, introspection and relaxed wakefulness. Thus, what we know as primary process thinking may go on at all times and may anticipate the events of the night's dream. This latter idea is similar to Freud's use of the "day residue." Of course these speculations would have to be tested experimentally.

REM and NREM Mentation

Much of the material relevant to this topic is covered in other sections of this volume (sleep-onset mentation in Chapter 6, NREM mentation in Chapter 3, and the dichotomy between REM and NREM sleep in Chapter 7). However, a short summary of findings, and some recent research not covered elsewhere are reviewed here.

Originally, NREM sleep was thought to be without any mental activity that could meet Dement and Kleitman's (1957b) criterion of "detailed dream description." Mentation elicited from NREM sleep in their original study was attributed to recall of previous REM dreams. Stage REM was believed to be the unique state in which meaningful psychological activity could take place during sleep. However, later studies, which used recollection as criteria (i.e. Kamiya, 1961) found much greater percentages of NREM recall, and were able to demonstrate that NREM recall of prior REM dreams did not account for NREM recall values.

The qualitative differences between REM and NREM reports have since been well documented in the literature, and summarized by Foulkes (1966). NREM reports are less elaborate than REM reports. NREM reports show a greater incidence of more conceptual thinking, whereas REM reports tend to be more perceptual in quality. NREM reports have less content involving emotional processes especially, anxiety, hostility and violence. There is less visual activity and less physical involvement than in REM reports. REM narratives more often had more than one character and take place in more than one scene. NREM reports tended to make use of more recent events in the subject's life, and tended to represent a continuation of material reported on a previous awakening. They were more likely than REM reports to be a realistic recreation of some recent event. What was most striking about NREM reports was their everyday quality; they were much more likely than REM reports to "make sense." In Freudian terms, the REM report is more like primary-process thinking, more unrealistic and subject to processes of displacement and condensation. NREM reports are more like secondary process ideation.

However, in many ways NREM and REM reports were undifferentiable with regard to average length, the subject's awareness that the content was not real, and the time of occurrence relative to the awakening stimulus. By way of summary, Foulkes (1966) has said:

> It is important not to overestimate the difference between REM and NREM mentation, however, even though all these points of statistical differentiation have been established. Although most undistorted memory processes occur in NREM sleep, most NREM reports are not undistorted memory processes. Although most themes derived from an everyday routine of work or school occur in NREM narratives, most NREM awakenings do not produce such reports. Although REM reports are rated as more distorted than NREM reports, most of the latter contain some distortions. Although most "thinking" reports come from NREM sleep, most NREM reports are of "dreaming" (a visually hallucinated, dramatic episode). And although the typical NREM report is less dreamlike than the typical REM one, some NREM narratives get very dreamlike indeed [p. 110] . . ."

In addition, individual differences in mentation must be taken into account, inasmuch as the dream-likeness of mentation reports differs among subjects. Therefore, it is possible that using grouped data, the NREM report of a subject which is more dream-like than average would be indiscriminable from a less than average dream-like report from another subject. Similarly, time of night must be controlled for, as mentation becomes more intense later in the night.

Tracy and Tracy (1974) concerned themselves with the question of mentation differences between NREM Stages 2 and 4 by studying the extremes of this range. Eleven male and 10 female subjects spent 3 nonconsecutive nights with continuous EEG, EOG, and EMG recording. The majority of awakenings were from 5-min samples of descending Stages 2 and 4 sleep, but some 20-min samples of Stage 4 sleep were taken as well. For the first data analysis 103 report pairs, of a 5-min Stage 2 and a 5-min Stage 4 report each, were matched within subjects for night, and for time of night; and for the second analysis, 20-min Stage 4 reports were paired with 5-min Stage 4 reports similarly matched as before. Thus, by these analyses, it was possible to compare Stage 2 mentation with Stage 4 mentation with controls for elapsed time of sleep stage, time of night, night and subject; and also Stage 4 mentation following short prior intervals of Stage 4 sleep with Stage 4 mentation following long prior Stage 4 sleep intervals. Each report was rated by 2 independent judges on the Foulkes DF scale (reliability coefficient = .96).

The results of the first analysis were:

1. mean recall: Stage 2 = 54%; Stage 4 (5 min) = 50%;
2. mean DF-scale values: Stage 2 = 2.83; Stage 4 = 2.43;
3. percentage vivid dreams (DF scale   5.5): Stage 2 = 27%; Stage 4 = 20%;
4. mean word count of reports: Stage 2 = 48; Stage 4 = 38.

None of the foregoing differences were significant (Wilcoxon test). Of 35 content-category comparisons, only one showed a significant difference: Stage 4 reports were more often described by subjects as vague as opposed to clear ($p = .01$).

The results of the second analysis were:

1. mean recall: Stage 4 (5 min) 41%; Stage 4 (20 min) 32%;
2. mean DF-scale values: Stage 4 (5 min) 2.64; Stage 4 (20 min) 1.67.

The difference in mean recall values was not significant; the statistical significance of the mean DF-scale-value differences were $.05 < p < .01$.

The results show, therefore, that when time into sleep stage and time of night are controlled, Stage 2 and Stage 4 mentation show few differences. The data also contain a trend suggesting that mental activity levels of early Stage 4 slightly exceeds that of later Stage 4. It was concluded that the intensity of mentation cannot be explained as only a monotonic increasing function of EEG cortical arousal as reflected in conventional sleep stages.

The mentation correlates of elapsed time into sleep stage is an important area as it provides clues concerning the temporal organization and tendencies of the components of the sleep cycle. Perhaps with a larger sample over a greater number of nights some additional mentation items would have reached significance. Also, time since the previous REM period could not be controlled in this design, a factor shown to have some influence on NREM recall (Wolpert & Trosman, 1958). Finally, Tracy and Tracy (1974) used group data, which might tend to mask significant individual differences.

CHANGES OF DREAM CONTENT WITH ELAPSED TIME
INTO REMPS

Czaya, Kramer, and Roth (1973) attempted to study the pattern of the development of a REM dream at 6 different points in time. They woke 4 male subjects at intervals of 30 sec, 2.5 min, 5, 10, 20, and 30 min into their second REM period and fourth REMP of the night. Subjects rated 12 aspects of their dreams: recall, activity, emotion, anxiety, clarity, pleasantness, violence/hostility, degree of distortion, how frightening, how related to personal life, and sensibleness, all on a 5-point scale. Of these categories, emotion, recall, anxiety and pleasantness showed significant linear increases in intensity as a function of time ($p < .05$), as did clarity ($p < .10$). For emotion, anxiety, and pleasantness, in addition to a linear trend, there was a leveling off and decline in intensity of the dream at 20 min, followed by an increase at 30 min. In an extension of their 1973 study (Kramer, Czaya, Arand, & Roth, 1974) all dream reports were rated by two independent judges on the aspects of the report listed above. Content was scored for characters, descriptive elements and activities using Hall and Van de Castle (1966) categories. Results were essentially the same, showing that the development of psychological parameters in the REMP is the same whether defined by subjects' rating of their experience, judges' ratings of content, or manifest scoring of content categories. Unfortunately, the small subject sample limits the degree to which we may generalize from these findings. In addition, no measurement of interjudge reliability was presented.

In summary, recent research has shown that there are significant differences in the development of certain parameters of dreams during the course of the REM period, while NREM dreams do not seem to undergo similar intensification over the course of Stages 2-4 (Tracy & Tracy, 1974). Thus, time into a sleep stage is a crucial factor in assessing REM dreams. It may reflect the amount of phasic activity that accrues during the course of the REM period. This evidence and the work of Foulkes and Fleischer (1975), suggest that the dreamlikeness of mentation is a quality influenced partly by state of arousal, and partly by attention focus. No state of arousal is inextricably tied with a single mode of thinking (that is, primary or secondary process) but rather that modes of thinking persist for differing amounts of time in varying arousal states.

DREAMING AT DIFFERENT TIMES OF THE NIGHT

It is not immediately obvious why we should be interested in variations in dream experience in relation to time of night. However, there are several empirical and theoretical reasons for this concern. One of these is that various physiological parameters of sleep reliably covary with time of night. Among these are REMP length, REM density (as well as other phasic events associated with REM sleep), quantity of delta sleep, and body temperature; the latter two variables being negatively related to time of night. Since relationships between these physiological variables and dream content have been hypothesized, it is important to know how time of night independently relates to dream content in order to assess its possibly confounding effects.

A more theoretically based concern with dreaming at different times of the night is given us by Freud (1900/1953a). He argued that the cessation of sensory input during sleep permitted the revival of early memories in the form of images. The obvious corollary to this notion is that more regressed memories would be experienced with greater or more prolonged blocking out of external sensory input; hence, dreams that occurred later in the night would be expected to show temporal regression, and possibly formal regression as well.

It was this latter idea which formed part of the basis for Verdone's (1965) study of intraindividual variations in the temporal reference of manifest-dream content, with respect to the amount of time subjects spent in bed; physiological variables, such as body temperature; and other aspects of dream content, such as vividness and emotionality.

Using 4 young adult subjects (3 men and 1 woman), Verdone (1965) made 210 REMP awakenings in the course of 40 nonconsecutive subject nights. These awakenings were divided into 2 groups: 1 subset 5 min, and a second subset, 12 min after REMP onset. One hundred ninety-six usable mentation reports were elicited which the subjects self-rated at the time of awakening, using Likert-type scales on the following dimensions: goodness of recall, plausibility, actual temporal distance of dream elements (like a character actually seen one week ago, one month ago, and so on), the oldest temporal distance for a single dream element, and emotionality. Measures of body temperature and heart rate were recorded every 2 min during REM sleep, and every 10 min during NREM sleep. Dream reports whose elements were relatively recently encountered by the subject in reality, were labeled contemporary reference (CR), while reports whose content corresponded to real events more remote from the present were labeled noncontemporary reference (NCR). NCR versus CR status was also evaluated with respect to the "age" of the single oldest element in a dream.

Ratings of all variables (including time in bed) were dichotomized around each subject's median, so that NCR reports did not represent a "qualitatively unique entity." In fact, the general median for all four subjects which divided NCR from CR reports was one month, so that dream reports containing elements encountered in reality more than one month prior to the experiment were called NCR reports. Twenty-eight percent of the reports referred to events which took place within the last day before dreaming, while 10% of the reports referred to events from over five years before.

The relationships among the dichotomized ratings of sleep and dream variables were assessed using the Cochran test, which is a method for combining individual chi squares. Significantly more NCR reports were elicited later in the night ($p < .001$). There was a significant relationship between NCR reports and lower body temperatures. This relationship was stronger when NCR was evaluated using overall temporal reference ($p < .001$), than when the age of the oldest dream element was the criterion for NCR ($p < .01$). NCR reports were also significantly related to goodness of recall ($p < .001$), vividness ($p < .001$), implausibility ($p < 0.5$), emotionality of dream reports ($p < .001$), total amount of REM activity in the REMP ($p < .05$) and in the last 2 min of the REMP.

Prior duration of REM sleep within a specific REMP was not significantly associated with temporal reference. Significantly more well-recalled ($p < .001$), vivid ($p < .01$), and emotional ($p < .05$) dreams were elicited relatively later in the night. These variables were also significantly associated with more REM activity ($p < .001$; p H .05; p H .001) longer intervals after REMP onset (12 versus 5 min) ($p < .001$; p H .05; p H .001) and lower body temperature. REM activity was significantly related to time of night ($p < .001$), and lower body temperature ($p < .05$). There was no relationship observed between body temperature and time of night; however the authors note that this may be the result of body temperature being measured only during REMPs, since the first 1-2 hr of the night typically show the greatest decline in body temperature, and is largely responsible for the overall negative relationship between body temperature and time in bed. This period is minimally represented in Verdone (1965) since the only data used are from REMPs which do not occur until 1-2 hr of sleep have elapsed.

We might summarize these results by saying that dreams that were reported relatively later in the night were more regressed with respect to temporal reference, and more dream-like in the sense that Foulkes (1966) has used this term. Verdone regarded noncontemporary reference in dreams as a component of experiential regression in that it manifests a disregard of objective reality and historical time. He noted, however, that these results must be regarded with some caution since only four subjects were used, and only intraindividual variations were analyzed, that is, correlations between variables across subjects did not influence the outcome of statistical tests. This produced the following anomaly: Subject 4 reported dreams with older temporal references than the other subjects, but had a higher median body temperature. In addition, although awakenings were made after two different durations of the REMP had elapsed (5 min or 12 min), both of these intervals are relatively short, so that the average amount of REM sleep that had elapsed before the final awakening of the night was only 50 min. Therefore these data represent a relatively selective REMP sample. It is possible that if only the middle or end of REMPs were sampled, the increase in phasic activity (REMs) which takes place with time into the REMP, might have had an effect on mentation which could have washed out the effects of differences across the night.

Furthermore, it is worth considering the possibility that the REMP awakenings made "later" in the night may have been preceded by some REM deprivation, which has been shown capable of enhancing dream-likeness of REMP reports within the night (Pivik & Foulkes 1966).

Verdone (1965) also notes that because of the dichotomizing of variables it is not possible to assess the linearity (or lack thereof) of the relationships obtained. We feel that this is a particularly serious problem: it is possible that the median "time of night" value for a given subject may be relatively early, for example, after as little as 17 min of REM sleep (following Verdone's paradigm), so that "early" reports would be preceded by only a very few minutes of REM sleep. Therefore the obtained relationships would not represent change across the night, but rather differences between reports that followed a REMP and those that did not. In itself this may be very important, (cf. Pivik & Foulkes, 1968), but only indirectly related to temporal aspects of the sleep cycle.

Responding to this problem, Verdone (1965) reported that when curves for temporal reference were plotted against time in bed, the following trends were visible: during the first 3.5 hr of the sleep period dream reports referred to elements encountered in reality in the last week; during the next 4 hr, temporal reference moved back in time toward more remote events following a negatively accelerated curve, until approximately 7.5 hr of the sleep period had elapsed, when a reversal of this trend occurred toward more recent temporal reference. These trends suggest that a more thorough data analysis might reveal greater complexity in these relationships than are now apparent.

As part of an effort to better understand the sources of differences between REM and NREM mentation, Pivik and Foulkes (1968) conducted a total of 158 NREM awakenings beginning 30 min after sleep onset, from 20 young adult male subjects on 2 nonconsecutive nights, so that there were 4 awakenings per night per subject. Subsequent awakenings (Awakenings 2, 3, & 4) were each made 30 min after the first, second, and third REMPs respectively, during any NREM stage. Reports from retrieval interviews were rated using the Foulkes dream-like fantasy (DF) scale. Also, latency from experimental awakening to subjective orientation was computed. Scores from the MMPI Byrne repression-sensitization scale, Barron's ego-strength scale, California Personality Inventory, and some TAT scales were obtained for all subjects. The authors reported the following results: 64.6% of the awakenings produced "recall," defined as a DF rating of at least 2, which is a mentation report with some substantive content. Both recall and DF ratings, the authors assert, increased with time of night. Mean DF ratings for Awakenings 1, 2, 3, & 4, respectively, were: 1.71, 3.30, 3.60, and 3.74. Recall for these 4 awakening positions was 45, 70, 70, and 73%, respectively. No statistical analysis is presented for either of these findings.

Among the correlations with personality measures that the authors report was a significant positive relationship of the MMPI schizophrenia scale with mean DF scores ($r = .47; p < .05$) and a negative correlation of TAT stories' word count with mean DF scores ($p < .05$). There were also negative correlations of sleep-mentation word count with CPI psychological mindedness ($r = -.49; p < .05$), and ego strength ($r = -.45; p < .05$), and a positive correlation-of-mentation word count with the MMPI schizophrenia scale ($r = .48; p < .05$).

Pivik and Foulkes (1968) interpreted some of these results as indicating that subjects whose fantasy production during waking was relatively constricted, tended to produce more fantasy when awakened from sleep.

The authors conclude that late-night NREM mentation reports are not very different from early-night REMP reports. However, since no REMP reports were collected from these subjects, we feel that such a conclusion cannot be drawn and since no statistical analysis of the relationship between mentation quality and time of night is presented, it is difficult to assess the meaning of these data with respect to the issue of progressive or continuous changes in mentation quality with time into the sleep cycle. Furthermore, as Rechtschaffen (1973) has pointed out, the possible effect of time of night is confounded with sleep stage in Pivik and Foulkes' (1968) study, in that Stage 4 awakenings predominated for the first NREM aawakening of the night, and were virtually absent from Awakenings 2, 3, and 4, in which Stage 2 and Stage 3 awakenings predominated; that is, of the 40 first awakenings only 7 were from Stage 2, while of the 38 fourth awakenings, 28 were from Stage 2, with none from Stage 4, and only 10 from Stage 3. Although, as Pivik and Foulkes (1968) point out, this seems not to have produced the lowered DF ratings and recall which were evident for the first awakening, insofar as the first Stage 4 awakenings of the night were no lower on these variables than the first Stage 2 awakenings, it is nevertheless a systematic difference between two experimental conditions and may have operated in unknown ways. For example, the 7 first Stage 2 awakenings may have been from subjects whose latency to delta sleep was longer (since they were still in Stage 2, 30 min after sleep onset, when other subjects had reached Stages 3 or 4) and there is evidence that variations in quantity of delta sleep are associated with important subject variables (Feinberg 1969; Mendels & Hawkins 1967, 1968).

However, let us put aside these problems to examine what these data may suggest. The only eye-catching difference in mentation is an increase in "dreamlikeness" and recall from the first to the second awakening of the night. Aside from the fact that the first awakening is preceded by less uninterrupted sleep than the second, as Pivik and Foulkes (1968) point out, these two awakenings are differentiated from each other in that Awakening 1 is not preceded by REM sleep while Awakening 2 is. The authors noted this as well and suggest that the first REMP may have a stimulating effect on subsequent NREM dreaming. It is also possible that the first REMP triggers physiological processes which take place during NREM sleep and influence mentation.

Data are available, from an independent source which support Pivik & Foulkes' 1968 conclusion that Stage 2 mentation reports from the latter portion of the night are more dream-like than those elicited earlier. Using 40 adult subjects, Arkin and Antrobus have reported on the effects of REM deprivation on Stage 2 mentation. For this purpose, part of the procedure entailed awakening subjects for Stage 2 reports during REM deprivation and NREM-control-deprivation conditions, during the first and second halves of the night. Throughout, regardless of deprivation condition, Stage 2 reports elicited during the second half of the night were significantly more dream-like than those from the first half. (See pp. 21-22 of this volume for full details). This finding may serve to reduce doubts about purported increases of Stage 2 dream-like qualities later in the night in that it tends to weaken objections based upon the possibility of a slow-wave sleep confounding factor.

Since significant correlations have been obtained between personality measures (notably the MMPI schizophrenia scale) and the quality of NREM mentation, (Pivik & Foulkes, 1968), we think that it might be interesting to see if personality factors interact with time of night in relation to changes in the quality of mentation. Perhaps, just as it has been reported that certain personality measures (MMPI, Sch K, field-dependence measures) differentiate subjects who respond to REM deprivation with increased "REM pressure" from those who do not (Cartwright et al., 1967; Cartwright & Ratzel, 1972; Gillin et al., 1974), it is possible that such measures may also differentiate subjects who increase dream-likeness across the sleep cycle from those who do not.

A recent report from Cartwright (1975) in which she attempted to collect REMP mentation early and late in the night without confounding later awakening with the effects of some REM deprivation, indicates that the difference between mentation collected from the first and fourth REMPs are quite weak across 10 subjects, if one pair of mentation reports from each subject is used.

In summary, we feel that little firmly can be said about the changes in mentation quality across the night, except that the first awakening, be it REM or NREM, produces less dream-like mentation than the second. However, this is clearly an area with much potential for providing better understanding of psycho-physiological relationships.

THE TIME INTERVAL IN DREAMS

How long does a dream take? Until modern electrographic research, the generally accepted answer was that what was experienced as an extended time interval in dreams corresponded to an actual process that was completed almost instantaneously. Incredibly, this opinion was largely based upon a hoary anecdote related by Maury (1861) about one of his own dreams that had occurred in his early youth. In abbreviated form, he had been watching condemned people being guillotined during a dream. His turn came to mount the scaffold and at the moment of feeling the blade on the back of his neck, he awoke in terror only to find that the top of his bed had fallen, struck him on the back of the neck, exactly as had the blade in the dream, and awakened him. He inferred from this that the entire lengthy dream had been initiated and completed between the time the falling bed top had struck his neck and the time of his awakening – a fraction of a second.

Maury's conclusion found support in work by Schjelderup (1960) in experiments on hypnotic dreams. Somewhat lengthy dreams were induced during a period of purportedly 1-2 sec of hypnotic sleep.

Not until the work of Dement and Kleitman (1957b) was there solid evidence of a positive relationship between the length of actual dream experience and the length of electrographic evidence of dream experience. Specifically, five subjects were awakened either 5 or 15 min after REMP onset and asked to decide from their dream experience whether they had been awakened after 5 or 15 min of dreaming. Four out of five subjects were able to guess correctly with highly significant accuracy and the one unsuccessful subject made systematic errors. Furthermore, there were consistent, strong, highly significant correlations in all five subjects between the word count of the dream narrative (an index of dream duration) and the 5-versus 15-min REMP-awakening categories.

More recently, Koulack (1968) performed an experiment on 10 adult male subjects in which attempts were made to determine the frequency with which percutaneous, subawakening-threshold electric shocks to the median nerve were incorporated into REM dream experience. Part of the procedure entailed stimulating the sleeper either immediately after or else 3 min after the first REM. The subjects were then awakened either 30 sec or 3 min after the stimulation and a mentation report was elicited. On its completion, if there was clear evidence that the stimulus had been incorporated into the dream events, the subject was then asked to estimate if the dream-incorporated event had occurred 30 sec or 3 min prior to the awakening buzzer. (This experimental procedure is described in detail in Chapter 10 of this volume).

There were 12 instances obtained from 5 subjects in which the presence of the stimulus in the dream could be clearly identified. Of the subjects' judgments, 92% (11 of 12) correctly corresponded to the actual time interval between stimulation and awakening.

Thus, the evidence points to the conclusion that the time sense in dreams corresponds to time intervals in reality over a considerable temporal range.

SEQUENTIAL DREAMS AND ORGANIZATION OF PSYCHOLOGICAL CONTENT DURING SLEEP

To what extent are the contents of dreams of the same night or across nights related? This question has certainly been of interest to such clinicians and investigators as Freud, Alexander (1948), French and Fromm (1964), and Hall (1966). (See Jones, 1970c, for an excellent review.) In keeping with our major interest, however, we shall focus on laboratory studies. As Offenkrantz and Rechtschaffen (1963) point out, one would expect some degree of consistency between sleeping and waking adaptations and defenses, since the same individual who is producing both the dream and the waking fantasy is monitoring any ongoing action. Yet, a number of questions remain. If a night's dreams do indeed have the same meaning or center around a psychological conflict, why would one choose to represent them in such a variety of differing contexts? And why are certain contents chosen over others? These and other theoretical problems have plagued the development of research on the sequencing of dreams across the night.

Dement and Wolpert (1958b) collected 4 to 6 REM dreams from 8 subjects on each of 38 nights; a total of 38 dream sequences. Their criteria for relatedness in dreams was "the appearance of identical or similar characters, plots, actions, environments, or emotions." The overall incidence of dream recall was 80%.

In the 38 sequences, no single dream was ever duplicated exactly by another dream, nor did the dreams of a sequence ever form a perfectly continuous narrative. Rather, each dream seemed to be a relatively self-contained production, somewhat independent of its precedent or consequent dream. Nevertheless, the manifest content of nearly every dream showed some obvious relationship to one or more dreams on the same night. In 7 of 38 dream sequences (18%), all of the dreams seemed united by a common theme, but in the majority of cases only contiguous dreams were obviously related. For example, in any particular sequence, Dreams 1 and 2 would have elements in common, while Dreams 3 and 4 would share different ones. Individual items appearing in different dreams varied widely, ranging from single, apparently trivial details to instances in which the plot, setting, and action sequences were the same. Consideration of each dream content on an individual basis may not reveal a common underlying theme which yet emerges when the entire sequence is examined.

Despite the considerable degree of relatedness observed among members of many dream sequences, the authors were careful to state that one may not conclude that this relatedness is the natural state of affairs outside the experimental situation. They considered several alternative hypotheses including the possibility that the mentation report offered at one awakening provides "day-residue" material for the next dream.

Trosman et al. (1960) studied REM dreams of 2 subjects obtained over a total of 32 experimental nights. Subjects were given psychological tests and clinical interviews. In addition, associations were obtained at the time of the experimental awakenings. They examined 12 parameters of dream content including: hedonic tone, excitement, activity, clarity, vividness, spatial expanse, observer-participant, interpersonal involvement, thematic coherence, plausibility, elaboration, resolution, and success. Based on this material, the following conclusions were drawn:

1. Within nights, unambiguous relationships among the contents of mentation reports were rarely observed (once in 32 nightly sequences).

2. Across nights, the appearance of unique features at similar points in a sequence, lateral similarities (so-called lateral homologies) between events from

one night to the next, and the combination of similar qualitative dimensions, all suggested an organization of REM mentation into regular patterns; for example, on two successive nights, one subject observed an athletic event in the first dream, experienced rejection by a friend in the second, and freed a buried object in the third.

3. Assessment of "latent" dream content by means of psychological test findings, subjects' associations following REMP awakenings, manifest-dream content and the investigators' psychodynamic inferences also suggested cyclic relationships thought to be generally characteristic of sequential dreams. Specifically, the early dreams of a nightly sequence reflect accumulation of "need pressures" which are "discharged in a pitch of excitement either directly or by a highly dramatic visual representation" in subsequent dream events, and which are followed finally by a period of "regression or quiescence". Thus, this regularly recurring nightly sequence indicated that the latent content of dreams mirrors cycles of tension accumulation incident to psychic conflict, discharge, and attempted conflict resolution. It should be remembered, however, that these conclusions are the results of post hoc analyses, not tests of experimental predictions, and accept the validity of methods of dream interpretation which themselves have not been vigorously tested.

Offenkrantz and Rechtschaffen (1963) examined the dreams of a patient who was seen for 83 hours in the laboratory. It was hoped that the greater amount of information available about the subject from the therapy hours would aid in discovering previously elusive continuities among the dreams of a night. As did Trosman et al. (1960), they found a tendency for specific manifest dream elements to occur in similar positions in the nocturnal sequence of dreams. For example, on 11 of the 15 nights the second dream was concerned with the experimental situation, while no later dreams dealt with the laboratory in the manifest content. Second, they found the manifest dream was located in a geographical setting of childhood or adolescence in 9 dreams occurring after 4:30 AM on 8 different nights, whereas childhood scenes never occurred early in the night. (See the section on time of night and dreams in this chapter).

Offenkranz and Rechtschaffen (1963) record the patient's descriptions of his dreams:

1. Dreaming about his own experimental methodology and misgivings about the validity of his method. This was accompanied by fear and a spontaneous awakening.

2. Dreamt about receiving news that his rival had killed himself after the dreamer remarked to a third dream character that the suicide had options other than taking his life. This served to exculpate him in playing a causative role in the suicide.

3. Dreamt about being in a physics laboratory in his hometown and working on some mathematical problem. The experimenter was employed in the dream to carry out the menial work of looking up squares of numbers for him.

4. Dreamt about being in a library talking with a girl who likes to ride horses. His is displaced by a larger more aggressive male who together with the girl behave in a demeaning manner toward the dreamer.

From their interpretations of the patient's dreams, the authors arrived at a number of conclusions about the interrelationship of mental content during the night. These conclusions were based conceptually primarily on the work of French and Fromm (1964). First, all the dreams of a night tend to be concerned with the same conflict, or a few different conflicts. There was a parallel between the sequence of defensive adaptive-waking behavior and the sequence of the same ego functions in the dreams of a night. Finally, the tension accumulation, discharge, and regression sequence noted by Trosman et al. (1960) is "correlated with a psychological sequence in which the organization of a particular dream seems to depend upon the results of the dream work of the preceding dream; for example, increasingly bolder gratifications will be visualized until suddenly reactive motives predominant [p. 500]. As in the Trosman et al study (1960) analyses were done post hoc—no real experimental predictions were made before the dream sequences were collected.* Also, the dream interpretation was done *with* the knowledge of the sequence from which the dream came. This is clearly a confounding factor. Ideally, the dreams would have to be interpreted separately, and then the order of conflict and resolutions noted.

Rechtschaffen, Vogel, and Shaikun (1963) studied the interrelationships of mental content throughout the night, including NREM content. Two subjects who were known to have good NREM recall were studied for three nights each. Six to nine awakenings were made per night from both REM and NREM sleep. The authors sought to look at only obvious relationships among the manifest content — identities or repetitions of manifest themes or elements. As they noted, appropriate statistical procedures were impossible, as there was no way to assess the baseline occurrence of certain elements in dreaming. Such procedures would have provided an index for judging the likelihood of specific dream elements or their combinations on the basis of chance. They were compelled, instead, to rely on a common-sense judgment of whether the probabilities of co-occurrence of elements exceeded that which one expects on the basis of randomness.

They found that identical or closely related content elements were often repeated in reports from NREM awakenings throughout the night and throughout all NREM stages. Importantly, specific manifest elements from NREM awakenings were reported in accounts from REMP awakenings and vice versa. Moreover, the identical or closely similar elements appeared in different contexts, and thus

---

*From a strict scientific point of view the validity of such a finding is questionable. However, judicious *post hoc* analysis should not be brashly condemned. It may be the only type of analysis to which such complex data is susceptible.

cannot be dismissed as recall of previous reports since they were not part of a continuous story. Finally, an element might have appeared initially in pre first REMP NREM reports — further evidence that NREM images need not be recalled from previous REMPS.

In a second experiment, Rechtschaffen et al. (1963) compared the quality of REM and NREM mentation. Seventeen subjects selected without regard for efficiency of NREM recall, slept in the laboratory for 1 to 3 nights for a total of 30 experimental nights. They were awakened according to an unsystematic schedule. In reports of 8 nights, elicited from 6 subjects, there were instances of unique NREM manifest elements which recurred in different contexts at different times of the night. However, these were not so striking as in the first experiment, possibly because the subjects were not specifically chosen on the basis of their having good NREM recall. Nonetheless, one subject provided a sequence of 8 mentation reports with alternating REM and NREM awakenings which contained repeated references to boats, school exams, parked cars, sunshine, and the like. Instances of repetition of elements across consecutive nights were also observed.

In summary, the results show that specific manifest elements and thematic units appearing in NREM reports are sometimes repeated in a striking way in consecutive or nonconsecutive awakenings spanning the entire night. Speaking against the possibility of recurring elements merely being recollections in sleep mentation of earlier reports are: the wide differences in mentation contexts of each item repetition; and that dreams referring to the subject actually rendering aloud a mentation report are rather rare in the laboratory, and yet it is an invariant, repetitive, prominent occurrence in the sleep experiments described. If incorporation of reporting material was likely, then one should see quite often laboratory dreams in which the subject is specifically speaking into a microphone. Certainly, a great deal of striking discontinuity from one dream to the next is the more prevalent finding. Yet, without associations of the subject and methods of assessment of personal meanings of the dream material, it is difficult to say how much such discontinuity is only apparent.

In conclusion, Rechtschaffen et al. (1963) state that the manifest structure of sleep mentation:

> is marked both by an apparent lack of observable connections between different episodes of mental activity on some nights and by the repetition of elements in varying contexts in different episodes on other nights. On those nights when themes and images persist through both NREM and REM periods, the dreams do not arise *sui generis* as psychologically isolated mental productions, but emerge as the most vivid and memorable part of a larger fabric of interwoven mental activity during sleep [p. 546].

We can only hypothesize that manifest elements tend to be repeated during a night on occasions when preoccupations of the recent past remain so intense that they "press" for discharge throughout the sleep period. Furthermore,

NREM elements that are later repeated in REM suggested to the authors that these elements were conscious representations of preconscious day residues during sleep. NREM elements, being more secondary process in nature, are seen as being more apt to be derived from preconscious processes than REM elements.

Thus, the literature on sequential mental content through the night shows that there is some continuity among manifest elements, and a greater continuity when latent dream thoughts are taken into account. However, a number of general criticisms of the methods that most of these studies used severely limits their generalizability. All but one study used very small samples, and only two attempted to integrate NREM recall. None of the studies tested predictions, and all of the analyses were post hoc, and depend on the interpretation that the authors give to the material. Still it is of interest to cite the impressive studies of Breger et al (1971a) dealing with the effects of stress on REM dreams collected within and across nights. In agreement with the general trend of the foregoing studies, Breger and co-workers state "The (nightly) sequences suggest a course in which the early dreams display the currently aroused information and later dreams work it over, bringing in more and more early memories including earlier 'solutions' and defenses [p. 91]." (These studies are described at length in Chapter 10 of this volume.)

DREAM SEQUENCES AND DREAM MEANING

Kramer et al. (1975, 1976) and Roth et al. (1976) took up the problem of empirical demonstration that dreams have meaning, that is, possess some kind of orderliness and are not merely a collection of random events. They reasoned that if dreams have meaning for the individual, they should be distinguishable among individuals within a group (trait-like component), within an individual at different times (state-like component), and that dreams should be psychologically relatable to the individual's current wakeful concerns.

Attempts were made to test these hypotheses in several studies by providing judges with randomized series of REM dreams obtained from several different subject populations including young adult male college students and middle-aged male hospitalized schizophrenics. The judges were asked to carry out various sorting tasks which entailed:

1. Arrangements of the REM reports in a sequence corresponding to their actual sequence of occurrence both within and across nights.

2. Sorting of REM reports by individual subject from which they were obtained, on the basis of cues in common appearing in mentation content across dreams.

The results in the main indicated that it was possible to correctly sort dreams in accordance with the subject who produced them; and that it was possible, within subjects to correctly sort dreams by night of occurrence in a sequential series. The finding of orderliness of dreams in relation to the individuals who dreamt them implied that dreams had stable trait-like features; and that orderliness of an individual's dreams in relation to night of occurrence within a series implied that dreams reflect day-to-day changes within subjects, i.e., had state-like features.

In another study, the experimenters demonstrated positive correlations between content ratings of REM mentation and those of contiguous wakeful mentation. This implied that dreams were related to wakeful life in an orderly manner. Taken together the findings of orderliness in the data as described indicated that dreams possess psychological meaning.

These results are both intriguing and puzzling. The foregoing work on sequential content of dreams (see previous section) showed that while relationships were often discernible across nights, this was by no means as regular an occurrence as the studies mentioned here suggest. Perhaps, if Kramer, Roth, et al. had provided us with the specific cues judges utilized in making their discriminations, the apparent inconsistency could be resolved and important additional information be obtained about the ways in which dreams have meaning.

Dream Interruption and its Relationship to Dream Meaning

Among the experimental approaches to the issue of meaning in dreams, an interesting technique has been to measure dream content changes if the dreamer were repeatedly frustrated in his attempts to complete his fantasy. This question has been thoroughly treated in Chapters 12, 13, and 14 of this volume, but here the emphasis is on dream content as the expression of unconscious dynamic psychological conflict rather than the vicissitudes of manifest fantasy *per se.*

In an early pilot study, Rechtschaffen and Verdone (1964) reported that in a series of REM-dream fragments, obtained by repeatedly awakening sujects 3 min after REMP onset, there was evidence of "mounting frustration, hostility and paranoia" about not being permitted to complete "tasks" recurrently depicted in dreams. While rarely observed in REM dreams which were permitted completion the investigators were impressed by the much greater tendency for interrupted REM-dream sequences to affectively depict striving toward overcoming obstacles to dream-event completion. They were nevertheless cautious to state that dream sequences of this type are uncommon overall even with partial REM-deprivation schedules, and cited the importance of individual differences as factors in outcomes. No statistical data were given.

More recently, Fiss, Klein, and Schollar (1974) studied two adult subjects for 13 consecutive nights in the laboratory: 4 baseline nights, 4 REMP-completion nights, 4 REMP-interruption nights, and 1 recovery night. On interruption nights one subject was awakened approximately 8 min, and the other 12 min after REM onset. They remained in the laboratory until they had accumulated their normal amount of REM sleep to control for the possible effects of REM deprivation. Life history and clinical data were collected to provide a brief idea of the subjects' focal conflicts.

Dream reports were rated for length, affect intensity, vividness of imagery, and bizarreness. Each 3-sec interval was scored for the presence or absence of REM, and REM percentage calculated. Judges were given a summary of the subjects' focal conflicts and asked to sort the dreams as to whether they showed evidence of this conflict.

The authors report the following results: dream reports following interrupted REMPs were, on the average, equal in length to dream reports after completed REMPs but interrupted dreams were different in important and consistent ways: they were more vivid, dramatic, emotional, conflictful, and seemed to facilitate the emergence of unconscious material. In addition, they were less bizarre, narrated with greater articulate clarity, and were accompanied by more intense REM activity, less frequent body movement, Stage 2 "intrusions," and alpha bursts. To a lesser degree than the above differences the dreams from interrupted REMPs showed greater evidence of themes of adaptation and effectance than REMP-completion dreams.

Fiss et al. (1974) concluded from their data that REM sleep and dreaming are two functionally dissimilar organismic states. Because the interruption in REM time was slight, they assumed that the experience of dreaming was what mattered most, and that the dream was squeezed into a shortened REM period. Results were interpreted as indicating a need to complete a psychological task, and that we may dream periodically to work out some sort of solution to what troubles us most. However, Fiss and co-workers' assumption that dream physiology and psychology are independent is unwarranted. Their interrupted REMP procedure clearly led to more physiologically intense REM periods as well. For example, there were fewer intrusions from other stages, and phasic activity was more intense. One might easily hypothesize that it was the alteration in physiological patterning that influenced the dream's intensity and not the reverse. Thus, it seems that an interactional model, rather than a primarily psychological one, would be required to interpret data of this sort. This remains a most interesting study, and the interruption versus completion paradigm seems an important experimental approach.

COMMENTS ON THEORIES OF DREAM FUNCTION AND DREAM FORMATION (AMA)

Jones (1970b) has drawn attention to crucial distinctions between the psychology of dream interpretation, the psychology of dreaming processes, and dream formation including conceptualizations regarding the function of dreams. He points out that these are separate domains of discourse and investigation and much scientific discussion has not been sufficiently mindful of their distinctness.

In earlier years, the most influential body of scientific thought concerning these matters arose out of clinical observation, and in more recent times newer viewpoints have received stimuli from laboratory research. Some theorists have attempted to arrive at new integrations of both sources of knowledge and have sought to test aspects of clinical theory in the laboratory. It is to issues arising from these endeavors that we addresss some remarks in the light of Jones' caveats.

First, we wish to introduce certain terms which have been frequently used in the scientific literature for the purposes of discussion. Cartwright (1969) has proposed that most current dream theory can be usefully classified in accordance with two types of relationships between dream content and the conscious waking behavior preceding the dream: a compensatory-complementary relationship and a continuity relationship. The former, Cartwright (1969) identified as the basis of the Freudian viewpoint, predicts that "the order of relationships between the fully conscious, ego-controlled, wakeful mentation and the preconscious, less controlled projective test behavior be low and positive, and the correlations between [wakeful] consciousness and dreaming be moderately negative [pp. 366-367]." That is, Freud is said to have believed that dream mentation bears a compensatory-complementary relationship to wakeful mentation, being more concerned with disguised gratification of instinctual drives rather than coping with reality. By contrast, the continuity hypothesis, identified by her as the basic Adlerian (1958) viewpoint, predicts that the above relationships be all moderately positive. (Briefly, she concluded that the evidence for the continuity hypothesis was "quite mixed.")

In discussing Cartwright's (1969) paper, Beck (1969) felt that the compensatory-complementary versus continuity subdivisions cut across several different important variables and suggested certain reformulations. We present these below with amplifications and modifications so as to broaden the perspectives even further. The assumptions of contemporary dream theory are best presented in terms of two categories.

The Functions-of-Dreaming Category

Dreams serve the function of *attempted* wish fulfillment (Freudian view) and if one broadens "wish" to include "drive or uncompleted task-tension reduction," this proposition is consonant with the thought of Klein (1967) and Fiss et al. (1974).

Dreams play a role in adaptational processes as follows:

1. Dreaming is derived from or represents attempts to cope with or solve current emotional problems from waking life. This proposition is consonant with the thought of clinicians such as Maeder (1916), Adler (1936), Erikson (1954a), Fromm (1957), Bonime (1962), Ullman (1962), French and Fromm (1964), Hall (1966), and others.

2. REM dreaming is intimately involved in information processing of inputs from the external world, especially inputs which are novel and pose a threat to psychic equilibrium. This proposition is a corollary to the previous one but with greater emphasis on the newer concepts of information theory. That is, adequate information processing is essential to adequate coping and problem solving. This proposition is consonant with the views of Shapiro (1967), Breger et al. (1971a), Hawkins (1966), Gaarder (1966), Greenberg et al. (1970), Dewan (1970), Peterfreund and Schwartz (1971), and others.

3. Dreaming plays a role in the development, regulation and/or maintenance of cognitive, self, or ego systems. This proposition is consistent with the views of Piaget (1951), Erikson (1954), Lerner (1967), Jung (1945/1960), Breger et al. (1971a) and others.

4. The function of dreaming is the preservation of sleep. Freud and many of his clinical followers are perhaps alone in this belief.

5. Dreams do not serve any function but are simply phenomena that occur during sleep and are the expression of psychic activity during sleep. As such, sleep mentation shows the influence of established cognitive schemata and reflects wakeful behavior. This is consonant with Beck's (1969) views.

The Continuity-Discontinuity-between-Dreaming-and-Wakeful-Mentation Category

1. Dreams are continuous with waking mentation and behavior. This proposition is held by most of those authors who subscribe to lines of thought linking dreaming and adaptation, including the information-processing theorists.

2. Dreams are discontinuous with, or reciprocal to, wakeful behavior and mentation.

In Beck's (1969) discussion, contrary to Cartwright (1969), no statement appeared relating continuity-discontinuity specifically to Freud or Adler.

We should like to state our opinion that Freud's model of dream formation quite nicely allows for both continuity *and* discontinuity between dreams and wakeful mentation as well as manifest-dream events which deal with problem solving, coping, and adaptation. We quote in full one of Freud's (1960b) comments pertaining to the subject:

> Dreaming has taken on the task of bringing back under control of the preconscious the excitation in the *Ucs.* which has been left free; in so doing, it discharges the *Ucs.* excitation, serves it as a safety valve and at the same time preserves the sleep of the preconscious in return for a small expenditure of waking activity. Thus, like all the other psychical structures in the series of which it is a member, it constitutes a compromise; it is in the service of both of the two systems, since it fulfills the two wishes in so far as they are compatible with each other [p. 618].

This is a concise statement of his views concerning *dream function*. In a footnote to this passage, added in 1914, Freud then states:

Is this the only function that can be assigned to dreams? I know of no other. It is true that Maeder [1912] has attempted to show that dreams have other, 'secondary,' functions. He started out from the correct observation that some dreams contain attempts at solving conflicts, attempts which are later carried out in reality and which thus behave as though they were trial practices for waking actions. He therefore drew a parallel between dreams and the play of animals and children, which may be regarded as practice in the operation of innate instincts and as preparation for serious activity later on, and put forward the hypothesis that dreams have a *'fonction ludique'* ['play function']. Shortly before Maeder, Alfred Adler [1911, 215 *n.*], too, had insisted that dreams possessed a function of 'thinking ahead.' (In an analysis which I published in 1904 ['Fragment of an Analysis of a Case of Hysteria,' Part II (1905e)], a dream, which could only be regarded as expressing an intention, was repeated every night until it was carried out. [Cf. above, p. 222.])

A little reflection will convince us, however, that this 'secondary' function of dreams has no claim to be considered as a part of the subject of *dream-interpretation.* [our italics] Thinking ahead, forming intentions, framing attempted solutions which may perhaps be realized later in waking life, all these, and many other similar things, are products of the unconscious and preconscious activity of the mind; they may persist in the state of sleep as 'the day's residues' and combine with an unconscious wish ... in forming a dream. Thus the dream's function of 'thinking ahead' is rather a function of preconscious waking thought, the products of which may be revealed to us by the analysis of dreams or of other phenomena. It has long been the habit to regard dreams as identical with their manifest content; but we must now beware equally of the mistake of confusing dreams with latent dream-thoughts [p. 618-619].

We have included this material, not by way of defending the scientific validity of Freud's (1900) model, but rather to draw attention to a neglected passage. Thus, if in laboratory studies of dreams, we find much material related to current life, problem solving, adaptational stresses, and an absence of items which on the face of it seem "not to sound like wish fulfillments," we cannot take such results as disconfirmation of the Freudian models of dream formation. The above passage clearly makes provisions for such matters. On the other hand, the complexities of Freudian theory and the difficulties of disconfirming Freudian interpretations in general, as noted in the literature, are probably so formidable that critical, predictive tests of Freudian dream theory are well nigh impossible. The theory arose in the course of clinical work and will thrive or perish in proportion to its usefulness in the clinic. (Further discussion of dream theory may be found in Chapters 10, 13, 14, and 17 of this volume.)

Some Further Aspects of Dream Theory (DGS)

As Foulkes (1964) has pointed out, there are at least three questions which may be addressed by theories of dreaming: What is the meaning of dream content? What psychological functions does dreaming perform? How do dreams form and develop? Although the answers to these questions may be logically independent of one another, the tendency of theorists (Freud, 1900; Adler, 1936, 1958;

Jung, 1945) has been to provide theories which bear upon several of these issues at once. Previously in this chapter, in relation to schizophrenia, we have discussed a theoretical controversy which works in this way, that is, the issue of
whether dreaming is continuous with waking life and thought processes, or is in
a complementary or compensatory relation to contemporaneous waking functioning. To some degree, whichever of these two positions we adopt, we may be
saying something about all of the above three questions. For example, if we argue that dreams are psychologically complementary to waking experience we
may imply that their meaning or significance to the individual is in some way opposite to current waking concerns; or that dreaming accomplishes psychological
processes which are currently not being carried out in waking life; or that their
structure reflects aspects of personality not currently evident in waking.

It seems to us that this ambiguity of dream theories has served to obscure the
implications of electrophysiological dream research and falsely dichotomize the
opinions of pre-EEG-era theorists (particularly Freud 1900) in relation to their
own contemporaries (e.g. Adler), and in relation to current research findings.
Therefore we devote some discussion to an examination of how current data
bears upon the continuity-complementarity controversy with respect to each of
the three aspects of dream theory mentioned above.

Put in terms of the continuity-complimentarity controversy, our first question is: Is the psychological significance or "meaning" of dreams to the individual a reflection of current waking life concerns — the continuity position — or,
on the other hand, are the dream themes of an individual representative of issues
which we presume are not contemporaneously consciously salient, like infantile
sexual concerns? The former point of view is strongly endorsed by Adler (1958)
and Foulkes (1964), while the latter statement is usually taken to represent
Freud's (1900/1955a) position, though much less precisely. Freud asserted that
while the manifest content or literal elements of a dream were frequently the
residues of recent experience, the latent content, that is, the "meaning," was always a conflictful theme from early in the life of the dreamer.

If we accept Freud's distinction between the manifest and latent content of
dreams — and we, as well as the vast majority of clinical opinion do — then we
must regretfully note that there is virtually no experimental data to confirm or
refute Freud's (1900/1955a) or Adler's (1958) point of view on this issue. This
is so because in order to assess the latent content — the meaning — of a dream, it
is necessary to know the idiosyncratic rules of translation from the manifest content to the underlying meaning and experience for a given individual. This might
be done using psychoanalytic free-association, or other techniques, but no EEG
study has (although one such pilot investigation is underway with fascinating
initial results; Vogel, personal communication, 1975). Foulkes (1967a) observed
evidence of continuity between current waking life and the REMP dreams of
four preadolescent boys, but he specifically avoided the subjects' free associations to their dream reports and drew his conclusions from clinical observation

and manifest content coupled with parental interviews. Furthermore, this issue should ideally be examined in adults to whom Freud's (1900) and Adler's (1958) hypotheses are most relevant. The continuities which many observers have reported between dream material and recent events in the dreamer's life are consonant with Freud's notion of the role of the day residue in dream formation, but do not speak to the larger issue of dream meaning.

One reason appropriate studies of this question have not been conducted is the technical difficulty in reliably assessing the meaning of dreams. One possible way to attack this problem might be to record subjects' free associations to their own dreams, and have them, in conjunction with manifest content, rated independently. Such rating could then be matched with subjects' and judges' characterizations of subjects' current-life concerns to see how well they fit each other. (See Roth et al., 1976, for an approximate attempt at such work.)

The second aspect of the continuity-complementarity debate that we consider is the question of what psychological function dreaming serves. We do not mean "psychological function" in the very broad sense of how dreaming contributes to adaptation, but rather: of the multitude of psychological processes taking place in an individual, which are the stuff of which dreams are made? The continuity theorist might reply, that for a given individual dream process is analogous to current waking process, that is, when waking is characterized by the experience of frustration, for example, then so will be dream content: the complementary or compensatory point of view (Freud, 1900) argues that with respect to psychological experience the functional relation between dreaming and waking process, is reciprocal, that is, when waking is characterized by frustration, dreams will be of wish fulfillment. Another prediction which would follow from the compensation theory of dream function, is that when waking cognition is most bizarre, nonlogical and uninhibitedly wish-dominated — primary-process-like — dream experience will be impoverished, or at least relatively devoid of these elements. Since, as we discussed previously in this chapter, primary-process-like waking cognition is more characteristic of schizophrenics than of normals, a comparison of the dreams of these two groups would speak directly to this issue, and in fact does offer some modest support to the complementarity or compensation point of view. For example, the study of Okuma et al. (1970) indicated that the dream life of schizophrenics was relatively impoverished compared to controls.

Foulkes (1971) finds some support for the continuity position in his studies of the dreams of preadolescent boys, in that their dream life seemed preoccupied with the issue of masculine-role assumption, and developing social mastery, just as was their waking life, so Foulkes presumed. Here again, we feel it is important to distinguish between the manifest-dream report of the subject, and how the subject reacts to the dream, especially since we are considering the question of psychological function or process. The continuity position should predict that if a child is experiencing conflict around the assumption of male-role behaviors, then dream experience of this issue should reflect conflictful or ambivalent process as well, that is, should *not* contain experiences of the self as easily displaying masculine characteristics such as aggression and strength. In order to evaluate this prediction it is necessary to record the child's subjective reactions, such as free associations, to the dreams which manifestly display these issues. Since Foulkes (1971) avoided such a procedure his data only support the continuity position in the very general sense of what issues dream life is concerned with, rather than in the sense of what psychological processes it reflects, such as conflict resolution or wish fulfillment.

The best way to evaluate the continuity-complementarity controversy with respect to psychological function would be to independently manipulate the waking state of subjects to see if subsequent changes in dream experience were in the direction of the manipulation or away from it. For example, if the amount of sexual gratification experienced by a subject were diminished relative to baseline, the continuity model would expect more dream experience of sexual frustration, while the compensation model would predict dreams whose content the subject associated with sexual gratification. This sort of paradigm is superior to those used with schizophrenics, children, and women during menses, because it operationalizes the waking life of subjects and makes fewer unvalidated assumptions concerning the actual waking experience of different subject groups. The technical difficulties of such paradigms with humans may leave this question in its ambiguous state for some time.

The third question we consider to which the continuity-complementarity controversy can be applied is that of the nature of the structures and processes which control dream formation. The continuity position would argue that waking cognitive structure and style should be reflected in nocturnal dream formation, while the complementarity position (advocated by Jung, 1945; cf. Dallett, 1973), contends that styles of an individual's thought which are not evident in waking behavior, will be manifested in dreaming styles. It should be noted that for this aspect of the continuity-complementarity controversy, Freud (1900) is not at all clearly on the side of complementarity. In fact we feel that a correct reading of his theories of defense and dream formation are quite congruent with the idea of continuity between waking and sleeping thought style.

On this issue some evidence exists and it appears to support the continuity model, in some ways, albeit not simply. Foulkes and Rechtschaffen (1964) and Pivik and Foulkes (1968), find that for both REM and NREM mentation, subjects who report dreams which are more "dream-like" — vivid, bizarre, perceptual, emotional, dramatic, and so on — score higher on clinical scales of the MMPI, (that is, significant rhos between ratings of dreams and test scores). Furthermore, they report that this relationship appeared to be stronger for NREM mentation than for REM mentation, although it was significant for each. This can be understood as representing a structural continuity in that the characteristics of mentation which are regarded as making it more "dream-like" when transported to waking cognition are generally taken as indicators of neurosis and/or psychosis. In other word, the psychopathology of everyday life finds its parallel in the psychopathology, or "dream-likeness" of nocturnal mentation. Further, we might infer from this that there is at least some overlap, that is, continuity, between the structures which form dreams and those which organize waking functioning. These conclusions, from Foulkes and Rechtschaffen's (1964) and Pivik and Foulkes' (1968) data, rest on the premise that scoring higher on clinical scales of the MMPI, among "normal" volunteer subjects is associated with pathology; and this, in fact, is the interpretation the authors give to such scores, which they support with anecdotal observations. However, it should be noted that there is no controlled data to support such an interpretation of MMPI scores among normals, (although it appears to have face validity) and recent reanalyses of MMPI subscales (Messick, 1971) suggest that they may relate more to general tendencies to endorse socially disapproved self-descriptions than to the specific psychopathologies for which they are named. Our point here is not that there is no continuity between patterns of dreaming and waking functioning, but that this continuity is not clearly of pathology versus adjustment, as Foulkes and Rechtschaffen (1964) and Pivik and Foulkes (1968) suggest, but may be of other psychological factors common to dream formation and waking cognition.

Foulkes and Rechtschaffen (1964) note that such a factor might be reporting style, rather than an aspect of the dream experience itself. They argue that this is suggested by their finding that REM density, which they assumed to be more closely related to experienced dream-likeness than subjects' reports, was not nearly as well correlated with MMPI scores as was subjects' and judges' ratings of dream reports. Aside from the fact that recent data (Firth & Oswald, 1975; Hauri & Van de Castle, 1973b; Keenan & Krippner, 1970) has seriously questioned the strong association of eye movements with qualitative aspects of mentation, we feel it should be remembered that a necessary assumption of psychophysiological dream research is that the content as well as style of the subjects' verbal report are largely a function of their dream experience, unless some unusual circumstances lead us to believe that this is not the case (as with patients with psychomotor retardation or special aphasias; cf. Rechtschaffen, 1967).

A recent report by Starker (1974) suggests that some particular aspects of waking experience may tie together nocturnal mentation and waking functioning. After administering the Marginal-Processes Inventory (IPI; an inventory of Likert-type items designed to assess daydreaming habits, e.g. "I often daydream of becoming very rich") to 55 "normal" males, he selected subjects who scored high on the 3 factors which factor analyses have indicated influence scores on IPI subscales (Singer & Antrobus, 1963). These factors are positive daydreaming, negative daydreaming (guilt ridden, conflictful, frightening) and anxious distractible daydreaming. The latter defines subjects for whom daydreaming is an intrusive distraction from ongoing mentation, often emotional and negatively toned. Starker selected 3 high-scoring subjects for each of these factors, and obtained their nocturnal mentation by having them fill out a morning dream log for 14 consecutive nights. Two independent judges rated these reports for number of idea units, emotionality, bizarreness, and affective polarity, that is, positive versus negative affect. The results generally indicated that anxious distractible daydreamers reported night dreams which were significantly more bizarre, emotional, and rich in idea units, than positive and negative daydreamers, as well as containing significantly more affectively negative content than positive daydreamers. Furthermore, of 8 reported instances of subjects being awakened by nightmares, 6 were reported by anxious distractible daydreamers, while 2 were from negative daydreamers and none from positive daydreamers ($X^2 = 30.3$; $p < .001$). These data suggest that in subjects for whom daytime-fantasy processes are unusually intense and possibly negative, to the extent that ongoing objective cognition is somewhat displaced by such fantasy, nocturnal imagining is likewise more dreamlike and disrupting. Since these data come from very few subjects and EEG techniques were not used, they must be interpreted cautiously. However, they suggest a continuity between the structuring of waking and sleeping experience which may include and go beyond the issue of pathology.

Further nuance is added to these phenomena by the TAT data (an indicator of actively structured waking fantasy) which Foulkes and Rechtschaffen (1964) and Pivik and Foulkes (1968) obtained. While Foulkes and Rechtschaffen (1964) found a significant relationship between the imaginativeness of REM mentation and the imaginativeness of TAT stories ($p < .05$), they found no such relationship for NREM mentation. Pivik and Foulkes (1968) found a negative correlation between the dream-likeness of NREM mentation and the word count of TAT stories ($p < .05$). The authors interpreted this finding as indicating that subjects with constricted waking fantasy produced the most dream-like NREM mentation, and therefore as supporting their notion that more dream-like NREM mentation is associated with waking pathology. In the absence of data to indicate that apparent constriction on the TAT is associated with pathology, we do not find this inference compelling. However, the fact that a continuity between waking structured fantasy, TAT stories, and REM dreaming, fails to be paralleled for NREM dreaming, while other indicators of waking process, MMPI subscales, do correlate with NREM dreaming, certainly requires some conceptualization of these phenomena.

Assuming these findings are valid, one possibility is that the TAT demands that subjects perform a task in a way that mentation collection and personality inventories do not, suggesting that while waking *styles* of functioning are continuous with REM and NREM dreaming, waking *abilities* are only continuous with REM dreaming. In other words, patterns of NREM dreaming are influenced by cognitive structures which only partly overlap with those which control REM dreaming. Such a notion of stage-specific continuities between waking and sleeping fantasy formation is given some support by Foulkes, Spear, Symonds' (1966) findings that subjects who reported more dreamlike mentation from the sleep onset period — descending alpha and descending Stage 1 NREM — were also subjects who by virtue of their scores on the California Personality Inventory were more self-accepting and socially poised (though less "socialized"), a finding apparently quite different from the data obtained using REM and ascending NREM mentation. We discuss this study in more detail in the personality-and-dreaming section of this chapter.

In our brief consideration of three aspects of a current theoretical controversy — continuity versus complementarity — three points seem to have emerged:

1. To properly investigate the meaning of dreaming it is necessary to thoroughly explore the phenomenology of dreaming using more than just the objectively described dream report. This has not yet been done experimentally.

2. The question of what psychological functions are involved in dreaming additionally requires experimental manipulations which may be very difficult to carry out.

3. The relationship between waking and sleeping cognitive processes appears to be quite complex, differing in ways dependent upon what stage of sleep is sampled and how cognition is assessed. This fact, if thoroughly investigated, may contribute greatly to our understanding of the psychological nature of different stages of sleep.

Looming over our consideration of a few aspects of theories of dreaming is the most influential and broadly conceived theory of dreaming of all; Freud's (1900). Following current dream-research trends, this chapter has been oriented toward questions either raised or stimulated by Freud's extraordinary contribution. Therefore we would like to propose several caveats as they have been suggested to us in the course of reviewing numerous attempts to prove and disprove Freud's mettle on the EEG battleground:

1. It is important to test Freud's model rather than his aphorisms. For example, although Freud says that children's dreams are blatantly wish fulfilling, this is not the best deduction from the larger model which clearly implies that defense is involved in dreaming even during childhood.

2. If we are interested in assessing dream experience we must go beyond manifest content and using either traditional or "new-fangled" techniques, determine how the subject experienced the dream report, that is, what it meant to the subject. One person's wish fulfillment may be another's counterphobia.

3. The most efficient way to assess the relationship between waking and sleeping psychological functioning is to independently manipulate the one and watch the other. However the exigencies of human social life make such a research program impractical to say the least. Therefore we may be better off if we do not set out to demonstrate the truth or falsity of Freud's theory, but rather are satisfied to see if the intercorrelations of the characteristics of people with their dream-lives fit with his model, or if it needs modification.

Personality and Dreaming

We have already discussed several studies of correlations between patterns of dreaming and personality in other portions of this section (Foulkes & Rechtschaffen, 1964; Pivik & Foulkes, 1968; Starker, 1974). Therefore at this point, we focus on only one study in order to illustrate some problems in this area.

Foulkes et al. (1966) collected 3 REMP and 4 sleep-onset (descending alpha- and Stage 1 NREM-) mentation reports during 1 night of recording from each of 16 young adult males and 16 young adult females. Mentation was rated using the Foulkes DF scale and subjects were given the California Personality Inventory and asked to make up stories for 2 TAT cards. DF ratings of sleep-onset mentation correlated significantly with CPI social presence ($r = .35; p = .05$), CPI self-acceptance ($r = .37; p = .05$), and negatively with CPI socialization ($r = -.57; p = .001$). The authors interpreted these data as indicating that subjects who report more dream-like sleep-onset mentation seemed to have greater social poise, to be more self-accepting and less rigidly conforming to social standards than "hypnagogic nondreamers." They also found that the dream-likeness of sleep-onset mentation was positively associated with TAT word count ($r = .42; p = .05$), TAT aggression ($r = .51; p = .01$), TAT sex ($r = .39; p = .05$), TAT hedonic tone ($r = .44; p = .05$), and TAT imagination ($r = .40; p = .05$).

The dream-likeness of REMP mentation was negatively correlated with the CPI paychological-mindedness scale ($r = -.40; p = .05$), and positively associated with TAT aggression ($r = .45; p = .01$), and TAT hedonic tone ($r = .42; p = .05$).

The dream-likeness of sleep-onset mentation correlated significantly with the word count of REMP mentation ($r = .47; p = .01$), but its correlation with the dream-likeness of REMP mentation was nonsignificant ($r = .20$).

Foulkes et al. (1966) suggested that "one might conclude that hypnagogic fantasying is under the same kinds of ego-controls as predominate in the TAT, but that neither share as much in common with . . . [REMP dreaming] as they do with one another [p. 283]." In other words, the authors tend to see sleep-onset mentation as an ego function, becoming more dream-like with increasing ego strength and expansiveness while REMP dreaming (and NREM dreaming by the same reasoning) is seen as a defensive response to tensions outside the ego (cf. Vogel, Foulkes, & Trosman, 1966), becoming more dream-like with less adequate ego functioning. Briefly, the authors concluded, in confirmation of an earlier study (Foulkes & Vogel, 1965), that healthy ego functioning in wakefulness is positively associated with more dream-like mentation during sleep onset. Specifically, hypnagogic dreamers tended to have greater social poise, be more self-accepting, less rigidly conventional and more adept than hypnagogic nondreamers at producing voluntary waking fantasy. This finding was contrasted with the suggestions from the Foulkes et al. (1966) study and more impressive evidence from elsewhere (Foulkes & Rechtschaffen, 1964) that indications of psychopathology in wakeful responses are positively linked to dream-like qualities of REMP mentation.

This sort of interpretation rests upon particular assumptions concerning the meaning of scores on the CPI scales and the TAT-scoring categories, similarly to the interpretation Foulkes and Rechtschaffen (1964) and Pivik and Foulkes (1968) made of their data. Foulkes et al. (1966) were not insensitive to this issue and attempted to illuminate it further by examining those CPI items which were most successful in discriminating subjects rated high in hypnagogic dream-like fantasy, (that is, the DF rating of sleep-onset mentation) from subjects rated low in hypnagogic DF, and in discriminating subjects rated high in REMP DF from subjects rated low in REMP DF. There was little overlap among these four subject groups. Foulkes et al. (1966) noted that the CPI items which were most successful in discriminating high- and low-hypnagogic dreamers seemed to be related to characteristics of the "authoritarian personality" syndrome (e.g. rigidity and intolerance), with hypnagogic nondreamers closely approximating the authoritarian syndrome. The authors felt that the CPI items which discriminated high- and low-REMP dreamers were less apparently homogeneous (like "I am fascinated by fire;" "I have strange and peculiar thoughts;" "Police cars should be especially marked so that you can always see them coming;" "A person should adapt ideas and behavior to the group that happens to be around at the time"); however they noted that all these items were keyed "false" on several CPI scales of social adjustment. They also noted that seven of the eight items which discriminate high- from low-hypnagogic fantasizers were keyed so that endorsement of the item was typical of low-hypnagogic fantasizers. Foulkes et al. (1966) interpreteted this item analysis as indicating that

> ... while the low-hypnagogic fantasizer exerts rigidly successful control over ... impulse life, the high ... [REMP] fantasizer shows fascination with impulse life (as symbolized for example, by fire) in conjunction with weakened ego-control mechanisms (as indicated by the presence of strange and peculiar thoughts and by the concern with evading detection evident in the police car response and in the strategy of adopting the protective coloring of conformity to the environment in which one finds oneself) [p. 285]."

While this is an interesting interpretation of these data, others could be made. For example, we find it noteworthy that high-hypnagogic fantasizers say "no" to authoritarian or conventional self-descriptions, while high-REMP fantasizers say "yes" to socially disapproved ("impulsive") self-descriptions. Perhaps the high-REMP fantasizers are relatively less distant from their waking fantasy and unreflectively endorse atypical self-descriptions, while high-hypnagogic fantasizers are more careful and reflective about how they depict themselves, making a finer distinction between who they are and what they think, than do the high-REMP fantasizers. This speculation is not meant to contradict Foulkes et al.'s (1966) suggestion, but rather to make a methodological point concerning the attempt to conceptualize individual differences in dreaming in a very differentiated way. Personality must be assessed in as many ways as possible in order to minimize the number of alternative possible interpretations of data (cf. Campbell & Fiske, 1959). The use of only the CPI and TAT does not allow us to rule out any of the numerous factors which influence scores on these tests. Measures of variables such as response style and reflectivity, would add greatly to our understanding of the processes involved in producing variations in dreaming, hence the processes operating in different stages of sleep and of their physiological correlates.

SLEEP MENTATION AND AUDITORY-AROUSAL THRESHOLDS

Zimmerman's (1970) study of sleep mentation and auditory-arousal thresholds (AAT) showed the relevance of examining individual differences in relation to both the amount of, and qualitative differences in, NREM mentation. Sixteen subjects were assigned to a light-sleeper group (LSG) based on previously determined auditory arousal thresholds, and 16 subjects were assigned to a deep-sleeper group (DSG). They each spent one night in the laboratory being allowed to sleep the first 3.5 hr undisturbed, and then awakened for mentation reports twice during REM sleep and twice during NREM sleep. Upon completion of each mentation report, the experimenter elicited the subjects' responses to a questionnaire designed to measure 16 dream-content dimensions. The 2 groups did not differ in the distribution of their awakenings, and time of night of the awakenings was comparable.

Two independent judges made ratings of the mentation reports from an expanded questionnaire based on the one the subjects answered. The questionnaire included measures of aggression, sexuality, and imaginativeness. Interjudge reliability was adequate.

The results were as follows:

1. Differences in the REM mentation of the LSG versus DSG were negligible.

2. All subjects after all NREM awakenings claimed to have experienced prior mentation.

3. LSG subjects reported dreaming after 71% of their NREM awakenings, whereas DSG subjects reported dreaming after only 21% of NREM awakenings ($p < .02$).

4. Among LSG subjects, REM and NREM mentation were not statistically different on the dimensions of dreaming versus thinking, perceptual versus conceptual, volitional control, awareness of presence in bed, belief in the reality of the sleep experience and distortion of dream content. By contrast, the REM-NREM differences on each of these dimensions among DSG subjects were significant at levels ranging .02-.002. Thus, the NREM mentation of LSG subjects seems more nearly identical to their own REM mentation, that is, both are equally dream-like; whereas, the DSG data does conform to the older view that "thinking" is more prevalent during NREM sleep than "dreaming."

5. The judges' ratings were consistent with those of the subjects.

As Zimmerman (1970) notes, not all of the LSG-DSG differences in the NREM mentation reports were statistically significant; and one could not even claim that a greater-than-chance number of differences reached the .05 level because the 16 questionnaire items were not sufficiently independent, one from the other. Yet, the typical NREM mentation of LSG subjects was experienced as "dreaming," and that of the DSG the more commonly accepted "thinking."

To account for his results Zimmerman proposed that dreaming is a function of cerebral arousal in the absence of reality contact; and dream-like mentation occurs whenever cerebral-arousal levels exceed a certain critical point in the absence of contact with the external world. Arousal levels below this critical point are deemed sufficient to produce thought-like mentation. Although both kinds of sleep entail loss of reality contact, Stage REM is more conducive to dreaming than NREM sleep because of its much more intense cerebral arousal, plus greater occlusion of reality, whereas arousal levels of NREM are generally lower, more variable and produce less intense dreaming or thinking by turns, depending upon the fluctuations of cerebral arousal. In this scheme, sleep-onset dreams are explained as follows: in the hypnagogic state, arousal levels are moderately high because of proximity to wakefulness while contact with reality is faltering and tenuous.

Is there any evidence form Zimmerman's (1970) study to support this compelling notion? Indeed, baseline arousal levels of LSG subjects seem significantly higher than those of the DSG. This is betokened by their low auditory-arousal threshold, greater frequency of spontaneous awakenings in undisturbed sleep, greater frequency of gross body movements, faster resting heart and respiratory rates, and higher body temperatures (Zimmerman 1967). And it is precisely in the LSG subjects that one sees strikingly more and vivid NREM dreaming than in the DSG. Among the subjects of Zimmerman's (1970) study, if one tried to make a prediction as to whether a report was from REM or NREM sleep, significantly better results would accrue by taking the LSG versus DSG criteria into account, than on the basis that REM equals dreaming and NREM equals not dreaming ($p = .02$). AAT thresholds were higher in Stages 3 and 4 than in Stage REM or Stage 2; thus, a reliable stage correlate. However, there was an interaction with a subject variable. Only by taking this interaction into account can predictions be made as to which sleep stage mentation comes from. In addition, there is evidence in the literature of other relevant individual difference parameters which influence mentation. For example, Cartwright (1972) and Pivik and Foulkes (1968) have suggested that personality variables may be related to the dream-likeness of NREM mentation. Finally, it would be interesting to look at the distribution of phasic activity in the LSG subjects. One possibility is that the heightened cerebral arousal, postulated by Zimmerman (1970) as necessary for dreaming, may be due to the arousing effects of a greater frequency of phasic activity in NREM sleep in the LSG in comparison to the DSG.

LABORATORY STUDIES OF DREAMS OF PATIENTS
IN PSYCHOTHERAPY

The technique of dream interpretation and interest in dream mentation has historically been tied to clinical therapeutic work. It is surprising that the therapeutic enterprise has not made more use of the techniques of the sleep laboratory in order to augment the amount of dream collection and to test hypotheses about dream formation. This section is a short review of the available data.

Rarely in psychotherapy are more than one or two dreams reported per session. Yet laboratory findings have shown that people dream much more than this. To see which dreams the patient recalls in the morning and to examine whatever systematic biases exist Whitman, Kramer, and Baldridge (1963) performed a study in which one male and one female subject spent two nights a week, for eight weeks in the laboratory. Subjects were allowed 5 min of REM sleep and then awakened for a dream report. Associations to the dreams were elicited. After the dream night, the subject was interviewed by a psychiatrist, alternatively either 1 hr after the subject awakened or a full day after the night of dreaming.

The male patient reported only 7 dreams to the psychiatrist out of the 34 recalled on 46 awakenings. In part this was due to the fact that the psychiatrist did not, in this case, ask for dreams. However, many of the dreams not told to the psychiatrist dealt with homosexual themes, which were a major area of conflict for the subject. The female subject (who was specifically asked for dreams) reported 54 dreams from 60 awakenings, and retold 41 of these to the psychiatrist. At first, dreams of a sexual nature were told only to the experimenter. Later, as fantasies began to develop about the experimenter, certain types of dreams were told only to the psychiatrist.

The authors concluded that the accuracy of the retelling of most of the reports indicates that ordinary forgetting plays only a minor role. The amount of dreaming recalled 1 hr after awakening differed only slightly from that recalled a full day later. Whereas during the night, dreams were fragmented, undergoing a great deal of organization by the time they were told to the psychiatrist, and included a greater degree of thematic coherence. The nature of the subjects' relationship to the experimenter or the psychiatrist largely determined who was told what for both major changes such as omission of one or more dream scenes, change of situation, or omission of prominent details, as well as partial omissions. The authors' findings suggested that the unreported dream may be the one containing evidence of major interpersonal conflicts that the patient is struggling with.

In sum, a number of factors were seen to have relevance to what is recalled in therapy. Besides dream content, the process of awakenings, the stated interest of the therapist in the dreams, the therapist-patient relationship, and the time of night are all relevant in decreasing order. In addition, the process of being awakened and asked to give mentation reports must influence the amount of remembering which occurs — a kind of rehearsal effect.

Another approach has been to correlate REM time with the contents of a single psychotherapeutic session. Freedman, Luborsky, and Harvey (1970) studied a single patient seen in therapy for 2 sessions a week over a period of 19 weeks. The patient slept in the laboratory on the night between a Friday evening and Saturday morning session. The therapy sessions were assessed by 3 judges on 20 variables, which included some factors individual to the patient (like menstrual tension) and more common assessment parameters (e.g. the amount of depression/elation, anger toward others, and body-image dissatisfaction.) Objective session variables (the number of words used in the session by the patient and the therapist, average speech rate, session number) were also scored. The subject's dreams were collected only if she awakened spontaneously. The subject gave a total of 13 dreams on 8 experimental nights. Dreams were scored on the Gottshalk anxiety scale, as well as scored for objective parameters such as the number of words and number of people in the dream.

The mean REM percentage, 13.5%, was lower than the average value of 25.23% (Williams, Karacan, and Hursh, 1974). The hypothesized correlations between "dream time" and anxiety, pressured feelings, and oral needs were nonsignificant. There was a .46 correlation between depression ratings of the Saturday session and REM-time percentage ($p = .05$; one-tailed test). REM-time was unrelated to the number of dreams reported, the number of words used in reporting the dream, the number of the people in the dream, or the objective session variables. Examination of the dream transcripts showed a slight relation between anxiety in the dream report and a longer than average REM time ($p = .035$; one-tailed test). The authors then correlated the length of the fourth REM period with the session variables of self-satisfaction, wish fulfillment, depression/elation, control and anxiety, on both the Friday and the Saturday sessions. The higher the rating for these variables for the Friday sessions, the longer the fourth REM period. However, these positive correlations were opposite and shifted by the Saturday session. The patient then became more anxious, more depressed, and less self-satisfied.

The authors hypothesized that the combination of a late and long REM period which preceded the dramatic negative shift seen in the Saturday session, was an example of a failure in the dream mechanism. But the authors did not control for the total sleep time of the patient. Since most REM sleep occurs later in the night, the low REM percentage may only indicate that the subject was waking up early. Thus, we have no way of knowing what factors are responsible for the mood shift. It could be total sleep time, an augmented fourth REMP, or greater total REM time in general. Another serious flaw of this study was that the subject was taking a number of drugs at the time that may have affected the amount of REM sleep experienced.

An additional attempt to correlate REM parameters (REM latency, REM time) with stress in the psychoanalytic session is that of Greenberg and Pearlman (1975). A patient in psychoanalysis was seen in the sleep laboratory on 24 separate nights, one night a week, with a month between each group of 4 nights. The laboratory session was scheduled on the night after an evening analytic hour, which was then followed by a morning analytic hour. While in the laboratory, the subject alternated nights undisturbed sleep and nights awakened to give mentation.

A measure of defensive strain was utilized to score the analytic sessions. This included three separately scored subsections (the degree of emotional disturbance produced by the material in the hour, the relative prominence of safe and threatening self-other fantasy constellations, and the flexibility of defensive functions) which were then summed to produce the defensive-strain score. It was hypothesized that a high defensive-strain score would indicate a need for REM sleep or a pressure to dream, which would show itself in a shortened REM latency. Changes in strain from the evening to morning hours were rated with the prediction that low REM time would be associated with increase in strain and high REM time with decrease in strain. All ratings were done by the authors.

There was extreme variability in the physiological parameters. REM latency ranged from 39 to 174 min, with about half the nights distributed on the extremes of high and low latency. REM time varied from 22 to 78 min. In contrast, a control subject showed a relatively consistent REM latency. Clinical scores also showed great variability.

A Spearman rank order correlation showed that there was an inverse relationship between the defensive strain measure of the Friday session and REM latency. As the authors predicted, higher defensive strain scores were followed by shorter REM latencies. This relationship was significant at the .05 level for one rater and at the .10 level for the other. For the hours in which the rater's defensive strain scores were in closest agreement the correlations between strain and REM latency were more specific. The examiners were able to predict which eight nights would have the most REM time and which eight nights would have the least REM time on the basis of changes in the defensive strain scores ($p < .03$ for one rater; $p < .05$ for the second). For the nights on which there was the greatest agreement between the raters about the amount of change in defensive strain, correlations with REM time were even higher.

In conclusion, the small amount of work done, using patients in psychotherapy as sleep laboratory subjects, has yielded interesting data and observations but attempts to relate the content of therapy sessions and REM parameters remain merely suggestive. As Knapp et al. (1975) state, "Psychoanalysis allows in some ways a more complete knowledge of a human being than any other form of encounter, but its very comprehensiveness militates against structuring a simplified model for testing its conclusions [p. 420]."

DREAMING AND THE NONDOMINANT CEREBRAL HEMISPHERE

In recent years with a growing body of knowledge of lateral cerebral specialization, it has been proposed by several investigators that dreaming experience is intimately connected to nondominant hemisphere (NDH) processes (Ehrlichman & Antrobus, 1974; Bakan, 1975; Galin, 1974). Perhaps the most extensive theoretical presentation of ideas relating REM dreaming and the NDH is that of Bakan (1975), who cited the following evidence in favor of this concept:

1. Evidence of a relatively greater activation of the right hemisphere during Stage REM was found (Goldstein, Stolzfus, & Gardocki, 1972). More specifically, the method of integrative EEG analysis was used to establish ratios between the amplitudes in the left and right cerebral hemispheres during the sleep of seven normal adult human males, four female cats, and five male rabbits. The data indicated that with each occurrence of a shift from a period of slow-wave sleep to a REMP, a reversal of the deviations of the individual ratios from the overall mean ratio established for the whole period of recording took place. These shifts indicated relative greater NDH activation in comparison to the DH.

2. Evidence of greater independence of cerebral-hemispheric processes resulting from markedly reduced commissural activity during Stage REM was found by Berlucchi (1964, 1966).

3. Association of right hemisphere lesions with loss of ability to produce imagery and to have dreams (Bogen, 1969; Humphrey & Zangwill, 1951).

4. Association of dream-like epileptic aurae with seizures originating in the right hemisphere, and instigation of dream-like experience in some epileptics by right-temporal lobe stimulation was demonstrated by Arseni and Petrovici (1971).

5. Improved stereopsis is found at the conclusion of REMPs, and stereopsis appears to be mediated by the right hemisphere (Berger & Walker, 1972).

6. There are marked similarities between dream experience and the kind of mentation associated with right-hemisphere function (Nebes, 1974).

Bakan (1975) added a few additional speculations not cited here. At any rate, he concluded by putting forth the notion that ". . . REM sleep provides an opportunity for the exercise of the right hemisphere while it is functionally disconnected from the left hemisphere as a result of reduced callosal transmission [p. 17]." The relative ascendance of the NDH during REM sleep is deemed adaptive.

THE PÖTZL PHENOMENON AND RELATED ISSUES

In his original and exciting work on peripheral stimulation, Pötzl (1917-1960) showed pictures tachistoscopically to subjects and found that there is a delayed entry into consciousness of those parts of the picture not consciously perceived at the time of stimulus reception. Furthermore, these originally unconscious elements will usually arise in an altered state of consciousness (like dreams) or a pathological one (hallucinations). Pötzl claimed that 3 factors determine later dream formation: a sensory factor, which is the unconscious registration and fragmentation of the percept; a motor factor dealing with the role of incomplete eye movements; and a symbolic factor, similar to Freud's (1900/1955) concept of an unconscious wish.

Fisher (1957), in a partial replication of Pötzl's work, exposed simple pictures (geometric forms, four-digit numbers, or words) at a speed of .001 sec to a collection of friends, patients, and children. After exposure, subjects were given a period of free imagery, during which they drew their images. Subjects were then asked to make comparisons between their drawings and the percepts. Some were also given suggestions to dream.

Basically, the drawn images had one of three characteristics. 1. They were occasionally photographic or distorted representations of the preconscious percepts resulting from tachistoscopic presentation of the figure or number. 2. Images could be condensations of a recent memory image with the exposed percept, or 3. They were condensations of a childhood memory with the exposed figure. Fisher concluded that both the visual raw material for later dreams, as well as the latent dream thoughts, were present in the imagery period after the stimuli were shown.

On the basis of his findings, Fisher expanded Freud's original notion of day residue to include not only preconscious thoughts, but sensory events and environmental stimuli as well. While Freud (1900) believed that an unconscious wish cannot emerge into consciousness unless it is covered by day residue, Fisher added that visual scenes associated with the unconscious wish will fuse with the preconscious visual percepts associated with the day residue. The day residue percepts are not repressed in the classic sense, as they were never capable of entering consciousness.

Fisher, then, slightly amends Freud's (1900) theory of dream with the suggestion that it does not explain how the dream makes contact with day residue. His revised model is as follows: During the day, in temporal association with the day-residue thoughts, there are percepts. Some go through and immediately attain consciousness. Others are retained in the preconscious, incorporated as memory images. Still other percepts attain consciousness, lose attention cathexis, and fall back to the preconscious. Simultaneously the unconscious wish makes contact with the day-residue thoughts, and the surrounding subthreshold or peripheral imagery. The intensity of the unconscious wish is transferred to these images and they undergo distortion. During sleep there is a second activation of the unconscious wish, and an arousal of some of the same memory images associated with the wish during the day. These images are the raw material for the sensory structure of the dream and are fused and condensed with infantile-memory images. They attain consciousness in a delayed and fragmented manner when they reach hallucinatory intensity. Thus, Fisher (1957) concluded, the postulation of backward regression in Freud's (1900/1953c) dream theory is unnecessary, and the problems this causes are eliminated.

This intriguing area of dream research and theorizing cries out for replication and extension by means of the new electrographic techniques. (Some such preliminary studies are described in Chapter 10 of this volume.)

DREAMS AND ESP

Freud (1922) had made observations on patients in treatment that strongly suggested the possibility that telepathic phenomena could become manifested in dreams. The new electrographic techniques have made it possible to design experiments permitting experimental evaluation of this issue. In a series of studies, Ullman and Krippner (1974) have published positive findings in support of the hypothesis. Briefly, the typical experimental design has involved 2 subjects: an agent and a receiver. The receiver sleeps in the laboratory in the standard manner. The agent, isolated in a separate room 12 m away, selects one of 12 sealed envelopes each of which contains a small reproduction of a well-known painting — the "target." The agent then gazes at the picture for about 30 min, writes down personal associations and attempts to influence the receiver's dream content accordingly. The experimenter, unaware of the specific target selected by the agent, awakens the receiver 5-10 min after REMP onset and obtains a mentation report in the standard manner. The method of assessing the degreee of correspondence between the target and the receiver's dreams involves the ranking of all 12 potential targets against the REMP mentation reports, separately by the subject, and the three independent judges.

The findings have repeatedly demonstrated that such rankings are correct to a statistically significant degree. Furthermore, there are many anecdotal examples of striking correspondences between target and dream, for example, one target was Dali's "The Sacrament of the Last Supper," portraying Christ at the center of a table with his twelve disciples. A glass of wine and loaf of bread are on the table, and a body of water and a fishing boat are in the background. A corresponding dream contained references to fishing boats, the Sea Fare Restaurant, and "about a dozen men or so pulling a fishing boat ashore". Another dream on the same night with the same target referred to Christmas.

This work, like so much other research in the area of the paranormal, is intriguing and exciting but requires careful replication in other laboratories and by other investigators with positive results before it can begin to compel belief. Two attempts to replicate this work have not been encouraging. Globus et al. (1967) stated that they could find no substantial evidence in favor of ESP manifesting itself in dreams but also indicated that the hypothesis cannot be summarily discarded because post hoc analysis revealed some slightly suggestive evidence in favor of it. Belvedere and Foulkes (1971), on the other hand, reported an outright failure to replicate the findings of the Ullman and Krippner (1974) research.

Part III

PSYCHOPHYSIOLOGICAL MODELS OF SLEEP MENTATION

EDITORS' FOREWORD TO CHAPTER 7

Pivik has astutely traced the development of psychophysiological research in terms of how physiological models have influenced researchers in their approaches to studying sleep mentation. The essential question that is posed in his review is how good are the correlations between physiological models and sleep mentation, and the answer he comes up with is that the most recent physiological model, that is, the phasic-tonic model, does *not* correlate well with the type of sleep mentation a subject will report. Perhaps this conclusion is stated too baldly but it accords well with the introductory sentence to Pivik's final remarks, "The early notion of sleep as a relatively uncomplicated state where mind-body relationships might be profitably studied inbred an oversimplified view of sleep psychophysiology. . ."

Why hasn't the phasic-tonic model produced better correlative data? Pivik suggests several alternatives that get to the heart of the matter and rather than reproduce his alternatives we will briefly focus on one alternative that he mentions in passing that seems particularly germane to us at this point in sleep research.

One of the striking aspects of this chapter is that it contains virtually no psychological hypotheses. This does not reflect a bias of the author's point of view but rather is an accurate reflection of the state of affairs in the field. Most of the research in this area attempts to correlate mentation data with physiological conditions that are assumed to be established by one or several physiological generators. It is rarely if ever discussed why one would assume dramatic or even subtle differences in mentation because different types of physiological generators are being activated. The basic hypothesis that seems to have governed this type of research is a simple notion that if there is more neural activity of one sort or another, it will be reflected directly in increased activity in events depicted in sleep-mentation reports. Thus, if there are more eye movements there will be more visual activity in the dream report (separate-generators hypothesis) or more sensory events in the dream report (single-generator hypotheses). The idea that endogenous stimulation will be directly translated into mental imagery is one that should demand close scrutiny but until recently it has been accepted virtually without question. The implication of Pivik's review may be that we will have to seriously consider how a person actively processes endogenous stimulation rather than simply attempting to formulate research questions in terms of how types of endogenous stimulation are impressed on a passive receiving instrument. This point is highlighted by the fact that two studies have recently appeared that have even questioned the relationship of eye-movement density (or number of eye movements per unit time) and activity in the dream report. Thus, Hauri and Van de Castle (1973), Keenan and Krippner (1970), and Firth and Oswald (1975) report that they failed to replicate earlier studies that showed a positive correlation between density of eye movements and amount of activity in REMP mentation reports.

On the other hand, Ellman et al. (1974) have found that eye-movement awakenings during REMPs yielded reports significantly more dreamlike than awakenings made during ocular quiescence. In addition, either type of REMP awakening yielded mentation reports that were significantly more dreamlike than reports from NREM awakenings. This study was significant in that it was designed to control for two factors that were not well controlled in a previous study (Molinari & Foulkes, 1969), namely time of night of awakenings and time into the REMP before awakenings. It was expected that with these variables controlled, there would be no difference between mentation reports gathered from ocular activity (phasic) and ocular quiescence (tonic) awakenings. The fact that a difference was found argues that these variables do at least affect the "dreamlike" quality of sleep mentation. However, the amount of variance that eye movements uniquely account for is relatively small. One could conclude on the basis of these results that differences in mentation associated with phasic and tonic conditions are small; or one could conclude alternately that the small differences observed were due to the possibility that conditions defined as tonic had, in fact, contained phasic events. This is probably symptomatic of the difficulty in the "phasic-tonic model;" there are no clear-cut predictions except for the hope that physiological conditions will be translated directly into mental events. The history of sleep research seems to belie this hope.

S. J. Ellman

7

Tonic States and Phasic Events in Relation to Sleep Mentation

R. T. Pivik
University of Ottawa

Research fields often progress by a reconceptualization of known facts. Before sleep research embarked upon a new era in the early 1950s, sleep had been viewed as a unitary state. As data from the new research gradually accumulated, it became apparent that this monistic legacy would have to be discarded and replaced by a dualistic view of sleep. By the early 1960s sleep was seen as the cyclic alternation between two states which were physiologically and neuroanatomically distinct entities — rapid-eye-movement (REM) and nonrapid-eye-movement (NREM) sleep periods (Dement, 1964b; Hawkins, Puryear, Wallace, Deal, & Thomas, 1962; Jouvet, 1962; Snyder, 1963). Yet another manner of viewing sleep events was to emerge which took concrete form in Moruzzi's (1963, 1965) distinction between the long lasting, sustained *(tonic)* and short-lived, sporadic *(phasic)* events of REM sleep in the cat — a distinction which was subsequently expanded to include NREM sleep events as well (Grosser & Siegal, 1971).

   In this chapter I review the development of sleep psychophysiology in the context of the state and tonic-phasic models with the intention of imposing some historical perspective on the empirical developments and providing a current view of progress made in the attempt to understand the mesh between the psychology and physiology of sleep.

THE REM-NREM DICHOTOMY

The new sleep research began in the spring of 1953 when Aserinsky and Kleitman announced their discovery of periods of physiological activation during sleep. Although this activation was evident in several physiological measures, its most striking manifestation was in the occurrence of peculiar rapid eye movements. This eye-movement activity was so prominent and characteristic of these episodes that they soon came to be called REM periods, and the remainder of sleep

NREM periods (Dement & Kleitman, 1957b). In the initial publications (Aserin-sky & Kleitman, 1953, 1955; Dement, 1955), the physiological measures differ-entiating REM from NREM sleep apart from eye movements included a low-voltage EEG, and increased heart and respiratory rate. Over the course of the next several years the physiological distinctions between the two kinds of sleep were more highly accentuated and the state boundaries more emphatically drawn. Thus, in contrast to NREM sleep, REM sleep showed marked activation in several systems, including changes in heart rate and regularity (Snyder, Hobson, Morrison, & Goldfrank, 1964), respiration (Aserinsky, 1965b; Snyder et al., 1964), blood pressure (Snyder, Hobson, & Goldfrank, 1963), brain temperature (Kawamura & Sawyer, 1965; Rechtschaffen, Cornwell, & Zimmer-man, 1965; Reite & Pegram, 1968), and blood flow (Kanzow, Krause, & Kuhnel, 1962). In association with these signs of activation was a condition of tonic muscular and reflex inhibition (Berger, 1961; Hodes & Dement, 1964; Jacobson, Kales, Lehmann, & Hoedemaker, 1964; Pompeiano, 1966, 1967). Notable ex-ceptions to the apparent static characterization of NREM sleep are the greater activation of the electrodermal response in the human during NREM Stages 3 and 4 relative to REM sleep (Asahina, 1962; Broughton, Poire, & Tassinari, 1965; Johnson & Lubin, 1966), and the episodic occurrence of sleep walking and talking (Jacobson, Kales, Lehmann, & Zweizig, 1965; Kales, Jacobson, Paulson, Kales, & Walter, 1966; Rechtschaffen, Goodenough, & Shapiro, 1962), and night terrors (Broughton, 1968) during these NREM stages of sleep.

Among the early studies which served to strengthen the REM-NREM dicho-tomy, one weighing most heavily was Dement's (1960a) dream-deprivation experiment. This study demonstrated that curtailment of REM sleep eventuated in the partial recuperation, or rebound, of the apparent REM sleep debt incurred by the deprivation procedure, thereby suggesting a need fulfilling role for REM sleep.

The consensus of these data, bolstered by neuroanatomical evidence from animal studies (Jouvet, 1962; Jouvet, Dechaume, & Michel, 1960; Jouvet & Jouvet, 1963), was to overwhelmingly endorse a two-state tonic model of sleep, the full implications of which might be appreciated in the following characteriza-tion by Snyder (1966), "The physiological characteristics of this phenomenon prove so distinctive that I consider it a third state of earthly existence, the rapid eye movement or REM state, which is at least as different from sleeping and waking as each is from the other [p. 121] . . ."

MENTAL ACTIVITY AND TONIC SLEEP PHENOMENA

The psychological differences between REM and NREM sleep proved to be as dramatic as the physiological distinctions. The early studies (Aserinsky & Kleit-man, 1953; Dement, 1955; Dement & Kleitman, 1957b; Dement & Wolpert, 1958b) found a high incidence of dream recall from REM sleep awakenings (greater than 70%), and a relative mental void in NREM sleep (consistently less than 10% recall). Even during this first wave of studies, however, some reports surfaced which suggested a considerable amount of NREM mentation (Goodenough, Shapiro, Holden, & Steinschriber, 1959). These reports continued to mount, so that by 1967, Foulkes was able to cite data from nine studies subsequent to 1959 across which NREM recall ranged from 23 to 74%. Part of the discrepancy in NREM recall values between the early and later studies could be attributed to differences in what investigators were willing to accept as a dream. Dement and Kleitman (1957b) demanded a coherent, fairly detailed description, whereas Foulkes (1960, 1962) and the majority of subsequent investigators have been willing to admit more fragmentary, less clear impressions of mentation as dreams. However, despite the consistency and strength of the NREM recall results, the reluctance of investigators to accept these data at face value remained widespread (Foulkes, 1967). The reasons for this hesitancy were not without apparent empirical bases. For example, comparisons between REM and NREM mentation with respect to amount of recall and qualitative characteristics seemed to indicate an absolute, even fundamental, REM-NREM distinction. In addition to the quantative data already cited, the greater degree of subject variability in the incidence and quality of NREM reports appeared to attest to the ephemeral nature of NREM mentation. However, REM-NREM differences in recall are usually presented in terms of average recall values which mask intersubject variability. A closer examination of the data reveals that there has always existed a great deal of subject variability in recall of mentation from both REM and NREM sleep. The early Dement and Kleitman (1957) study had a range of REM recall values extending from 57.1 to 90%, with a median value of 80%. Subsequent studies have reported variability of comparable magnitude for REM recall, for example, Foulkes (1962) and Pivik (1971) have reported median recall values and ranges of 85%, 64-100%; and 94.5%, 62.5-100%, respectively. With respect to NREM mentation, the latter two studies reported median recall values and ranges of 71%, 44-100% and 44.3%, 19-90.9%, respectively. These figures suggest that recall from REM sleep is not much less variable than that from NREM sleep. Although such variability was overlooked for REM recall, it served to emphasize the unreliability of NREM reports, thus contributing to the characterization of such reports as capricious or artifactual events.

Qualitative distinctions between REM and NREM reports do exist, and those differences which Foulkes noted in 1962 have been upheld by subsequent investigations (Foulkes & Rechtschaffen, 1964; Pivik, 1971; Rechtschaffen, Verdone, & Wheaton, 1963a):

> Reports obtained in periods of REM activity showed more organismic involvement in affective, visual, and muscular dimensions and were more highly elaborated than non-REMP reports. REMP reports showed less correspondence to the waking life of the subjects than did reports from spindle and delta sleep. The relatively frequent occurrence of thinking and memory processes in spindle and delta sleep was an especially striking result [Foulkes, 1962, p. 24-25].

Although, as Foulkes (1962) indicated, NREM mentation is relatively more thoughtlike than that elicited from REM sleep, NREM reports of dreaming are as frequent (Goodenough, Lewis, Shapiro, Jaret, & Sleser, 1965) or more frequent (Bosinelli, Molinari, Bagnaresi, & Salzarulo, 1968; Foulkes, 1960, 1962; Pivik, 1971; Pivik & Foulkes, 1968; Rechtschaffen, Vogel, & Shaikun, 1963b; Zimmerman, 1968) than NREM thinking reports. Nevertheless, the differences between reports from the two kinds of sleep are of sufficient magnitude that judges can discriminate between them, given that a method of paired comparison is used (Bosinelli et al., 1968; Monroe, Rechtschaffen, Foulkes, & Jensen, 1965). Exclusive attention to this REM-NREM discriminability neglects the degree of variation in incidence and quality which has been demonstrated among NREM sleep stages (Pivik, 1971; Pivik & Foulkes, 1968; Zimmerman, 1970). Most neglected in this respect is NREM sleep onset mentation, which compares favorably in incidence, hallucinatory dramatic quality, and length of report with REM mentation (Foulkes, Spear, & Symonds, 1966; Foulkes & Vogel, 1965; Vogel, Foulkes, & Trosman, 1966). Moreover, REM and sleep onset Stage 1 reports share specific perceptual and emotional qualities which considerably blur the discriminability between them (Vogel, Barrowclough, & Giesler, 1972).

Investigators impressed with the differences between REM and NREM mentation offered various explanations for the latter, the most reasonable of which suggested that NREM reports were: recollections of mental activity from a previous REM period; artifacts of arousal, that is, hypnopompic experiences; or reports confabulated by subjects in an effort to please the investigator. In his review, Foulkes (1967b) was able to effectively counter each of these claims with empirical evidence which had been previously available. What, then, might be the reasons these data were ignored or slighted? Foulkes (1967b) listed three probable reasons which grew out of the then prevailing theoretical thinking:

1. While the low-voltage, random EEG of REM sleep is compatible with the existence of ongoing thought processes, the high-voltage, low-frequency EEG of NREM is not.

2. A report of a mental experience is not credible unless supported by public behavioral or physiological observation.

3. REM sleep is so vastly different physiologically from NREM sleep that there must also be a vast psychological difference between the two, such as vivid dreaming versus little or no mental activity.

It would seem that the first two statements could be considered variants of the third, suggesting that the REM physiology, perhaps in conjunction with the early reports indicating a unique relationship of REM sleep to dreaming, had been the primary restraining force behind the hesitancy of investigators to accept the reality of NREM mentation. In support of this notion, and of most direct relevance to the need for a public event to which Foulkes referred, is the observation that the most convincing arguments for the authenticity of NREM mentation come from situations in which the presence of preawakening stimuli, either naturally occurring (e.g., sleep-talking, Arkin, Toth, Baker, & Hastey, 1970b; Rechtschaffen et al., 1962) or experimentally induced (e.g., incorporations, Foulkes, 1967b; Foulkes & Rechtschaffen, 1964; Rechtschaffen et al., 1963), in postawakening NREM reports provides an event to which the mentation can be time locked.

The demand that observational psychological data conform to observable physiological events forced psychophysiologists to sift through the physiology of sleep in search of public physiological events with which to correlate and validate the already observed psychological data. One bonus which resulted from this search was a more complete and extensive description of the physiology of sleep.

PHYSIOLOGICAL CORRELATES OF MENTATION

The great variability in both incidence and quality of sleep mentation within sleep stages prompted investigators to look for physiological variations within sleep stages which might covary with the mentation. An extensive review of the current status of these psychophysiological correlations has been completed recently (Rechtschaffen, 1973), and it is more to the point of this chapter to concentrate on the distillates of that review than to duplicate the effort.

At a very general level, the EEG can be used as an index of both recall and quality of mental activity during sleep. Specifically, the more desynchronized the EEG, the greater the recall and the more dreamlike the recalled material. Thus, awakenings from low-voltage, mixed-frequency EEG (Stage 1) are productive of the greatest amount of recall and recall of the most vivid and bizarre quality (Dement, 1955; Foulkes & Vogel, 1965; Vogel et al., 1966). Furthermore, with EEG slowing and increased voltage there is a corresponding decrease in recall (Pivik, 1971; Pivik & Foulkes, 1968) and the quality of the recalled material is generally less dreamlike (Pivik, 1971).[1] The positive correlation between degree of EEG activation and recall squares well with other work indicating increased recall across the night (Foulkes, 1960; Goodenough et al., 1959; Shapiro, Goodenough, & Gryler, 1963; Verdone, 1963), since there is a considerable reduction in the amount of slow-wave, high-amplitude activity in the second half of the night. This intrinsic confounding of sleep stage and time of night presents an enduring obstacle to attempts to arrive at independent correlations of either with sleep mentation.

At a more detailed level of analysis the deficiencies of the EEG correlation with recall and quality of sleep mentation are evident. As already pointed out, there is much variation in both the incidence and quality of mental activity within a sleep stage where a given EEG pattern is essentially constantly maintained.

---

[1]Tracy and Tracy (1974) have recently found, however, that differences in recall and qualitative differences in mentation between Stages 2 and 4 become negligible when time within the stage prior to the awakening is controlled.

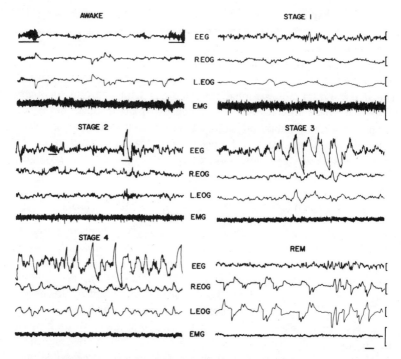

FIG. 7.1. Representative samples of awake, NREM, and REM sleep EEG patterns with accompanying eye movement (EOG) and electromyographic (EMG) activity. The wakefulness pattern in this case consists of a low-voltage, mixed-frequency EEG upon which bursts of 8-12 cps alpha activity (underlined) are periodically superimposed. Rapid eye movements and highly activated EMG are typical of wakefulness. Stage 1 is also characterized by a low-voltage, mixed-frequency EEG, but the accompanying eye-movement patterns consist of slow, pendular movements. EMG activity may be at a level comparable to that of wakefulness, but generally undergoes a slight reduction at sleep onset. Prominent characteristics of Stage 2 are the occurrence of 12-14 cps sleep spindles (underlined) and generally high-amplitude, biphasic K complexes (underlined). The EOG tracings of Stages 2, 3, and 4 do not represent eye movement activity, but rather are reflections of EEG activity. The EMG patterns of these NREM sleep stages are subject to much variability, but their general reduction relative to that of wakefulness is typical. Outstanding in the EEG tracings of Stages 3 and 4 is the occurrence of high-amplitude, slow (1-2 cps), delta-wave activity. The EEG and EOG patterns of REM sleep are similar to that of wakefulness, but the tonic EMG inhibition is unique to this stage of sleep. Calibrations: 1sec; 50μv.

Likewise, where marked differences in EEG pattern exist, relatively slight differences in recall may be obtained. For example, two recent studies (Pivik, 1971; Pivik & Foulkes, 1968) report recall differences of only 6.3 and 7.3 percentage points, respectively, between Stage 2 (spindles and K complexes on a low-voltage, mixed-frequency background EEG) and Stage 3 (spindles and K complexes on a high-voltage, low-frequency background EEG). Conversely, marked similarities in EEG patterns, as is the case for sleep onset Stage 1 and REM sleep, may result in discriminable content reports (Vogel et al., 1972).

Apart from the EEG, two major classes of physiological measures have been studied in relationship to mental activity during sleep; namely, autonomic variables and motoric phenomena. Several autonomic variables have been examined in this regard and, in general, tonic levels of such activity during REM or NREM sleep have proven to be poor correlates of mental activity. Of the studies correlating heart rate (Fahrion, Davison, & Berger, 1967; Hauri & Van de Castle, 1970a; Knopf, 1962; Shapiro, Goodenough, Biederman, & Sleser, 1964) or respiratory rate (Kamiya & Fong, 1962; Knopf, 1962; Hauri & Van de Castle, 1970a; Hobson, Goldfrank, & Snyder, 1965; Shapiro et al., 1964) with REM sleep mentation, only respiratory rate was found to relate to qualitative (Kamiya & Fong, 1962; Hauri & Van de Castle, 1970; Hobson et al., 1965) or quantitative (Shapiro et al., 1964) aspects of the mentation. It is notable that the positive relationship observed by Hobson et al. (1965) obtained for both REM and NREM mentation. Although cardiac and respiratory rate do not relate well to ongoing mentation, variability in these measures does relate positively to dream emotionality (Fahrion et al., 1967; Hauri & Van de Castle, 1970a).

The most dramatic autonomic display in NREM sleep is provided by the "storms" of electrodermal activity that occur during Stages 3 and 4 (Burch, 1965). Despite the intensity of this activity, Hauri and Rechtschaffen (1963) found no relationship between spontaneous or evoked electrodermal responses and mental activity during NREM sleep. The only positive relationship between mental activity and GSR that has been reported was obtained during REM sleep. Hauri and Van de Castle (1970a) found that GSR activity in the last minute preceding content awakenings related positively to dream emotionality. These authors emphasized, however, that, unlike NREM GSR storms, REM GSR potentials consisted of small, unipolar, isolated deflections which are more like waking reactions to emotional stimuli.

Penile erections occur regularly during REM sleep and only rarely during NREM sleep in man and monkey (Fisher, Gross, & Zuch, 1965; Karacan, Goodenough, Shapiro, & Starker, 1966). If a strict psychophysiological parallelism obtained, the data from these studies would suggest that 80-95% of REM dreams would contain overt sexual elements. This is clearly not the case. Hall and Van de Castle (1966) found overt sexual interactions in only 12% of the dreams they examined. Nevertheless, some variations in tumescence during REM sleep relate to variations in both recall and specific qualitative aspects of dream content. Karacan et al. (1966) obtained significantly greater recall from REM-period awakenings accompanied by sustained erections than from those associated with partial or no erections. Fisher (1966) was able to show a strong relationship between highly erotic sexual content and sudden increases in tumescence. When Fisher examined the relationship between presence and degree of tumescence and corresponding presence and intensity of sexual content, he found the strongest relationship to be between highly erotic sexual content and sudden increases in tumescence. This latter observation points to a general principle to be derived from these autonomic studies, that is, a better psychophysiological correlation is obtained when periods of rapid physiological change have been related to sleep mentation, than when correlations are attempted between tonic levels of these variables and such mentation. Better relationships are found between mental activity and cardiac and respiratory variability, sudden GSR deflections, and sharp increases in tumescence than between mental activity and tonic activity of any of these autonomic measures. In the discussion of motoric events and sleep mentation which follows, we will find that this observation continues to hold true.

Except for twitches and body movements, the tonic activity of trunk and limb muscles remains essentially constant during sleep (Jacobson, Kales, Lehmann, & Hoedemaker, 1964). The muscles of the face and neck, however, undergo significant tonic inhibition which begins prior to and extends throughout REM sleep (Berger, 1961; Jacobson et al., 1964). The question of whether the pre-REM decrease in facial and submental muscle activity reflects the onset of REM sleep-like mental activity has been examined with some rather surprising results. Contrary to expectation, awakenings from low-EMG pre-REM periods yield not only less recall than those from NREM sleep associated with high EMG levels (Larson & Foulkes, 1969), but the recalled material is of a less dreamlike quality (Larson & Foulkes, 1969; Pivik, 1971).

The psychophysical correspondence improves when more discrete muscle activity is considered. For example, some, but not all, discrete twitches of peripheral musculature have been appropriately related to specific dream content (Grossman, Gardner, Roffwarg, Fekete, Beers, & Weiner, 1971; McGuigan & Tanner, 1970; Stoyva, 1965a; Wolpert, 1960). Much greater success has been obtained in studies relating another index of discrete motor activity, namely, eye movements, to REM sleep mentation. These studies have described the eye-movement-dream-content relationship from two perspectives, one suggesting a very precise correspondence between the two variables, and another noting a general, nonspecific association. The former, more specific, view is embodied in the scanning hypothesis, that is, the notion that the eye movements are elaborated in the service of scanning the dream imagery. The development and current status of this controversy, which has endured for years, are extensively reviewed by Rechtschaffen (1973) who concludes that the issue is still in doubt. The second, nonspecific view is supported by data relating the presence of eye movements to the vividness and emotionality (Hobson et al., 1965; Verdone, 1963) of the dream, and to activity within the dream (Berger & Oswald, 1962; Dement & Wolpert, 1958b; Pivik & Foulkes, 1968).

Apart from the strong nonspecific relationship of eye movements to dream content, it is important to note that many measures which have been related to mental activity in REM sleep have also been shown to occur in close temporal contiguity to the eye movements. These measures include cardiac and respiratory variability (Aserinsky, 1965b; Baust & Bohnert, 1969), penile erections (Karacan et al., 1966), GSR activity (Broughton et al., 1965), and changes in muscular and reflex activity (Hodes & Dement, 1964; Pivik & Dement, 1970). This confluence of physiological activity highlights the necessity to seek out instances where these measures are dissociated in order to establish specific, unconfounded psychophysiological correlations — an effort which is yet to be realized.

Fortunately, in scientific research the best predictor of future results is not always past results, for the efforts to determine physiological correlates of sleep mentation had been largely negative or inconclusive. Although much had been learned about the descriptive physiology of sleep, the strongest psychophysiological association remained that between eye movements and dream content in REM sleep, with only frail hints of possible physiological correlates of NREM mentation. The situation was not very different from that which existed just after Aserinsky published his initial (1953) report. The need for revitalization and redirection was apparent, and the beginnings of such changes became evident in Moruzzi's (1963, 1965) tonic-phasic distinctions for REM sleep. Moruzzi (1963), on the basis of observations derived from the descriptive physiology of sleep in the cat, suggested that REM sleep be considered not as a homogeneous entity, but as the irregular alternation between periods of sustained (tonic) activity and periods of activity upon which are superimposed "sudden [eruptions] of an ensemble of phasic events [p. 291-292]." Moruzzi's notion served as a conceptual focus for the ongoing stream of European animal research (Gassel, Marchiafava, & Pompeiano, 1964a, b; Jeannerod, 1965; Jouvet, 1965b), whereas the earliest explicit expression of such a distinction on this side of the Atlantic was in terms of both animal and human research (Aserinsky, 1965a, b; Dewson, Dement, & Simmons, 1965). The real surge of research utilizing these concepts began in the late 1960s with the appearance of several papers applying the tonic-phasic distinction to both physiological and psychophysiological studies of sleep (Aserinsky, 1967; Ferguson, Henriksen, McGarr, Belenky, Mitchell, Gonda, Cohen, & Dement, 1968; Molinari & Foulkes, 1969; Pivik & Dement, 1968; Pivik, Halper, & Dement, 1969a).

Although the tonic-phasic distinction was originally confined to the REM period proper, it became apparent that phasic variations also occurred during NREM sleep. In the human, such variations have been noted in vaginal-blood flow (Cohen & Shapiro, 1970), penile tumescence (Fisher et al., 1965; Karacan & Snyder, 1966), respiration (Hobson et al., 1965), and vasoconstriction (Johnson & Karpan, 1968). Even eye movements have been observed during "NREM" sleep (Jacobs, Feldman, & Bender, 1971). In the cat, transient increases and decreases in brain temperature during slow wave sleep have been reported (Rechtschaffen et al., 1965), and limited amounts of ponto-geniculo-occipital (PGO) spike activity occur regularly outside the definitional confines of

REM sleep (Dement, 1965a; Michel, Jeannerod, Mouret, Rechtschaffen, & Jouvet, 1964; Thomas & Benoit, 1967). This latter event, the PGO spike, has been singled out for intensive study during the past few years. When first described (Jouvet & Michel, 1959), PGO activity appeared to be merely one more sleep event among many which were useful in differentiating REM sleep from NREM sleep. Data soon accumulated, however, suggesting that this event deserved special attention. For example, during REM sleep this activity was prevalent throughout the visual system (Bizzi & Brooks, 1963; Michel et al., 1964; Mikiten, Niebyl, & Hendley, 1961; Mouret, Jeannerod, & Jouvet, 1963), and was present in the pontine region designated by lesion studies as necessary for REM sleep (Jouvet, 1962). Moreover, PGO spiking occurred sporadically throughout NREM sleep and regularly anticipated REM sleep onset by 30-40 sec (Michel et al., 1964) of intensified activity. As demonstrated below, PGO activity has assumed a major role in studies attempting to elucidate the nature of tonic and phasic processes during sleep.

THE TONIC-PHASIC DICHOTOMY

What was the importance of Moruzzi's (1963) suggestion? Was his tonic-phasic terminology merely a descriptive clarification of the differentiation of sleep events based on their temporal extensity? If so, then it did not represent anything new, for the terms are common ones in descriptive physiology, and, within psychophysiological sleep research, investigators had long been looking at correlations between relatively long-lasting events (EEG defined sleep stages, autonomic levels) or short-lived changes (autonomic variability, muscle twitches) and sleep mentation. Clearly then, at the empirical level the basis for a tonic-phasic distinction could be traced back to the early Aserinsky-Dement and Kleitman studies. However, Moruzzi was postulating more than a descriptive differentiation; he was suggesting that, along tonic dimensions, REM-NREM differences were largely ones of degree and not of kind, and, furthermore, that the episodic intrusions of phasic events within REM represented activity which was fundamentally different from the tonic background upon which it was superimposed. Although at the time the proposal was initially made it was lacking a solid empirical foundation, the primary demand upon the model was clear, that is, that a dissociation between events defined as tonic and phasic be demonstrated. More a plea for physiological parsimony than an intended corollary to the model was Moruzzi's further hope that the phasic events of REM sleep be unified under the workings of a single system.

Evidence in support of both of Moruzzi's propositions was forthcoming from investigators employing a variety of experimental approaches including lesioning techniques, pharmacological intervention, and behavioral manipulation. Lesions of different brain stem nuclei, for example, were shown to result in the selective elimination of either tonic or phasic components of REM sleep. Bilateral destruction of the nucleus locus coeruleus eliminated the tonic muscular inhibition of REM sleep leaving PGO spiking and eye-movement activity intact (Jouvet & Delorme, 1965). Conversely, after complete ablation of the medial and descending vestibular nuclei, the integrated bursts of PGO spiking, eye movements, transient EMG and reflex inhibition, and autonomic changes were no longer present in REM sleep (Morrison & Pompeiano, 1970; Pompeiano, 1967). The only evidence of phasic activity remaining after this lesion was the sporadic occurrence of isolated PGO spikes and eye movements.

The results of these vestibular lesion studies were important in demonstrating the separateness of tonic and phasic events, but were also relevant to Moruzzi's second proposal that the widespread phasic activity might originate from a single, common generator. The tendency for phasic activity to occur in clustered bursts during REM sleep in both the human and cat suggested this might be the case, and the comprehensive elimination of such bursts of activity through selective vestibular lesions indicated a fundamental role for these nuclei in the generation of these events. It was postulated, however, that the primary source of phasic activity was located in the pontine reticular formation, and that this pacemaker normally interacted with the vestibular nuclei to trigger the intense, integrated bursts of phasic activity. The isolated PGO spikes and eye movements which survived the vestibular lesioning were thought to represent the activity of this pontine center.

Further proof of the independence of tonic and phasic events was provided by studies demonstrating that phasic events could be displaced from REM sleep. It was observed that the suppression of REM sleep, by means of either forced awakenings at the onset of each REM period (Dusan-Peyrethon, Peyrethon, & Jouvet, 1967; Ferguson & Dement, 1968; Ferguson et al., 1968) or the administration of biochemicals (Delorme, Jeannerod, & Jouvet, 1965; Dement, Zarcone, Ferguson, Cohen, Pivik, & Barchas, 1969b; Ferguson, Cohen, Henriksen, McGarr, Mitchell, Hoyt, Barchas, & Dement, 1969) resulted in the enhancement of PGO spiking during slow wave sleep. The latter studies using biochemical methods of intervention reported a displacement of spiking not only into slow wave sleep, but into wakefulness as well. Dement and his colleagues (Dement, 1969; Dement et al., 1969a; Ferguson et al., 1968, 1969) made use of these results to take another look at the REM deprivation-compensation phenomenon. Typically, the suppression of REM sleep is followed by partial compensation of the REM sleep loss. However, by behaviorally or pharmacologically manipulating the number and distribution of PGO spikes, these investigators were able to regulate and even obviate the compensation phenomenon. For example, by making awakenings at the onset of spike intensification preceding REM onset, thereby depriving the animal of a few seconds of NREM sleep in addition to the normal curtailment of REM effected during REM deprivation, it was possible to enhance the amount of rebound over that produced by the classical REM deprivation procedure.[2] In another procedure, animals were gently aroused but not fully awakened during the pre-REM period of intensified spiking. This manipulation deprived the animals of REM sleep while potentiating NREM spiking, and was not followed by a rebound. Furthermore, a count of the number of PGO spikes elaborated during the deprivation procedure and recovery period revealed a nearly exact quantitative compensation for PGO spikes prevented by the experimental manipulation. These studies, by showing the intimate relationship between PGO spike activity and REM deprivation phenomena, imparted a functional significance to the PGO spike independent of the tonic processes of REM sleep.

Although these data provided an especially powerful justification for a concentrated study of the PGO spike at the physiological level, the intuitive appeal of this event as an investigatory tool for the study of the psychophysiology of dreaming seemed equally compelling. Specifically, in addition to being concentrated in REM sleep where reports of dreaming are most prominent, PGO spikes are strongly identified with the visual system, occur in association with quite generalized increases in unit activity (Hobson & McCarley, 1971), and have been observed in the presence of hallucinatory-like behavior during wakefulness in cats (Dement et al., 1969b; Jouvet & Delorme, 1965) — observations which are in harmony with our conception of dreaming as an hallucinatory mental experience of a highly visual nature occurring during sleep. Psychophysiological correlations such as these, together with the physiological data suggesting that PGO spikes represented a primary triggering process for phasic events in general and were crucially involved in the REM deprivation-rebound phenomenon, prompted investigators to view the feline PGO spike as the standard phasic event against which all others were to be evaluated. This concept has constituted the explicit basis upon which much of the research into the psychophysiological processes of dreaming has been conducted for the past six years. This hypothesis that the PGO spike is an intimate correlate of dreaming in the human is based largely on general similarities between the two in distribution and intensity within the sleep cycle, as well as the shared accentuation upon the visual modality. A more empirical test of the correlation would be an examination of the correspondence between known properties of PGO spike activity and reported results from investigations of sleep mentation.

Setting aside for the moment the obvious pitfalls involved in suggesting cross-species analogy in distribution and function between a little understood physiological event and an even less well understood psychological process, let us

---

[2] For reasons which are unclear, the enhanced rebound after spike deprivation could only be obtained in animals on scheduled cycles of sleep and wakefulness. When the manipulation was applied to animals sleeping ad libitum, the rebound was similar to that obtained after classical REM deprivation procedures.

examine five possible points of correspondence which lend themselves to comparative analysis, all having to do with distributional patterning of PGO spikes and sleep mentation:

1. PGO spikes are highly concentrated in REM sleep, a time when dreaming is most prominent.

2. Measured at the pontine level, spikes increase in amplitude and frequency within a REM period (Brooks, 1968), a pattern which finds a parallel in the increased intensity of dreaming as a function of REM time (Foulkes, 1966; Takeo, 1970). Interestingly enough, if the measure of spike activity were taken at the level of the lateral geniculate nucleus, the correlation would be reversed since LGN spikes decrease in frequency and amplitude as a function of REM time (Brooks, 1967).

3. Spiking during NREM sleep is most intense in the 30-60 sec preceding each REM period, but mental activity is not suddenly enhanced during ascending Stage 2, which temporally corresponds to this time of increased spike activity in the cat (Larson & Foulkes, 1969; Pivik et al., 1969a) and may suffer qualitatively and quantitatively relative to post-REM Stage 2 (Pivik et al., 1969a) which would correspond to a time marked by the virtual absence of spike activity in the cat.

4. Deprivation of REM sleep in the cat increases the density of spiking within REM sleep during the ensuing rebound, and increases the incidence of NREM-spike activity during the deprivation manipulation (Dement, 1969; Dement et al., 1969a; Dusan-Peyrethon et al., 1967; Ferguson et al., 1968). Correspondingly, it would be expected that REM deprivation in the human would intensify REM dream content during the recovery period and enhance NREM mentation during the deprivation procedure. With respect to the former, both negative (Antrobus, Arkin, & Toth, 1970; Carroll, Lewis, & Oswald, 1969; Firth, 1972; Foulkes, Pivik, Ahrens, & Swanson, 1968) and positive (Greenberg, Pearlman, Fingar, Kantrowitz, & Kawliche, 1970; Pivik & Foulkes, 1966) results have been reported. Studies looking for the postulated intensification of NREM mentation during REM deprivation have been few, and the results negative (Antrobus, et al., 1970; Arkin, Antrobus, Toth, & Baker, 1968; Foulkes et al., 1968), but these results are based upon either small numbers of awakenings or did not sample from all NREM sleep stages and are accordingly limited in their generality.

5. PGO spikes are virtually absent at sleep onset, whereas several reports (Foulkes & Vogel, 1965; Foulkes et al., 1966; Vogel, et al., 1966; Vogel et al., 1972) are consistent in demonstrating a great deal of very dreamlike activity occurring at this time in the human.

Considering the impressiveness of the animal physiological data, this preliminary review of psychophysiological correspondence is disappointingly unimpressive. The lack of a strong relationship between the spike and content data might reflect a true noncorrelation of the two variables, or indicate a need to refine our method of dream collection and analyses, or point to the need for a better physiological measure. However, the five general comparisons listed above constitute at best a once-removed and largely inadequate test of the spike-content relationship, or the tonic-phasic model as it applies to sleep mentation. A more direct test of the model as it applies to REM sleep (Aserinsky, 1967) suggested that a comparison among content reports elicited from intra-REM awakenings made during periods of ocular motility (phasic), ocular quiescence (tonic), and NREM sleep might reveal greater qualitative similarity between the REM tonic and NREM reports than between those from REM tonic and REM phasic arousals. This suggestion is a more explicit statement, presented in terms of human psychophysiological research, of what Moruzzi (1963) proposed for animal physiology, and, like the latter proposal, it totally disregards any possible distinctions within NREM sleep or between REM and NREM sleep deriving from the presence of phasic activity in NREM sleep. In both cases the disregard did not represent an oversight of available data, but a real absence of data, that is, no consistent, discrete physiological measure of phasic activity during NREM sleep. It is this reason too that prevented application of the tonic-phasic model to NREM mentation.

THE TONIC-PHASIC MODEL AND REM SLEEP MENTATION

All of the investigations which have sought to differentiate phasic from nonphasic periods in REM sleep (see Table 7.1) have relied upon the presence or absence of eye movements for such differentiation, sometimes in conjunction with additional measures (Foulkes & Pope, 1973; Watson, 1972). Several additional physiological measures have been affiliated with the feline PGO spike and examined as presumptive NREM PGO analogues, and a complete cataloguing of these measures, together with pertinent literature and relevant descriptive information is presented in Table 7.2. In some instances the strength of the PGO association is enhanced by direct observation of the event in both man and cat (MEMA, PIP, EMG, and spinal-reflex inhibition; see Figures 7.3 and 7.6), but in all cases there is a basis for the association through correlational inferences, that is, distribution in sleep, response to experimental manipulation, or association with other known PGO correlates.

The tendency toward the use of ever more temporally discrete physiological indices and recognition of the moment-to-moment variability of the dream experience prompted the use of a more microscopic methodology in the collection of dream reports in which attention was focused upon the last experienced preawakening mental event — a technique which had been used extensively in tests of the scanning hypothesis (Roffwarg, Dement, Muzio, & Fisher, 1962). Also, being cognizant of the experimental demands upon the subject (rapid arousal from sleep, attentiveness to the mental experience with special emphasis upon detail and temporal relationships), some investigators have taken to careful preselection of subjects (Foulkes & Pope, 1973; Molinari & Foulkes, 1969; Watson, 1972).

TABLE 7.1

REM Recall as a Function of Phasic (Eye-Movement-Rich)
and Tonic (Eye-Movement-Poor) Conditions

Investigator	Number of subjects	Percentage recall, number of arousals		P-T percentage recall differences
		P	T	
Pivik et al. (1969a)	9	100, 18	79, 29	21
Molinari and Foulkes (1969)	10	80, 20	100, 20	−20
Medoff and Foulkes (1972)	2	81.8, 22	55, 18	26.8
Pivik (1971)	10	90.5, 42	82.5, 40	8
Foulkes et al. (1972)	14	74.1, 81	66.7, 81	7.1
Watson (1972)	4	96.3, 48	90, 48	6.3
Foulkes and Pope (1973)	14	95, 78	87, 54	8
Bosinelli et al. (1973)	10	95, 40	87.5, 40	7.5

Conceptually and methodologically the field was ready for testing the viability of the tonic-phasic model, at least for REM sleep, and the first studies explicitly directed toward this purpose began appearing in the late 1960s (Molinari & Foulkes, 1969; Pivik et al., 1969a) and have continued to mount. The single most important variable left to be determined was the dimension or dimensions along which the tonic-phasic differentiation would be expressed. From the data tabulated in Table 7.1 it is clear that at least in REM sleep this expression is not in terms of incidence of recalled mentation, although the presence of phasic activity does seem to somewhat enhance recall. Among the several qualitative features of mentation that have been examined, the list of those which have proven to be nondiscriminating is extensive, with some surprising entries. For example, the presence or absence of phasic activity is not a strong predictor of the hallucinatory (Molinari & Foulkes, 1969; Pivik, 1971; Pivik et al., 1969a) emotional (Pivik, 1971) quality of mentation, or felt bodily presence or subjective depth of sleep (Molinari & Foulkes, 1969; Pivik, 1971). Furthermore, all the studies listed in Table 7.1 agree that the presence of visual or auditory imagery does not differentiate between "tonic" and "phasic" reports, although "phasic" reports are associated with a greater incidence of both kinds of imagery. The absence of a significant positive correlation between the presence of phasic activity and visual imagery is especially surprising in view of the concentration of such activity in the visual system. It should be noted that the relationship between auditory imagery and phasic activity in the auditory system (MEMAs; see Figures 7.2 and 7.3) is currently undergoing detailed scrutiny, with strong positive preliminary results (Roffwarg, Adrien, Herman, Lamstein, Pessah, Spiro, & Bowe-Anders, 1973).

On the positive side, content elicited subsequent to "phasic" arousals contains significantly more hostility (Pivik, 1971; Watson, 1972), movement (Bosinelli et al., 1973), and self-participation (Bosinelli et al., 1973), but less

TABLE 7.2

Catalogue of Presumptive PGO Analogues in the Human

Investigator	Event[a]	Recording source	Duration	Distribution
Medoff and Foulkes (1972) Foulkes and Pope (1973) Pope, 1973	Theta burst	Frontal EEG	2-3 Hz trains	REM-NREM
Pivik et al. (1969a) Weisz (1972) Antrobus et al. (1973)	K complex	Central EEG	500-700 msec	NREM Stage 2
Pessah and Roffwarg (1972a) Pessah and Roffwarg (1972b) Roffwarg et al. (1973)	MEMA[b]	Compliance of tympanic membrane	500-1000 msec	REM-NREM
Rechtschaffen and Chernik (1972) Rechtschaffen et al. (1970) Rechtschaffen et al. (1972a) Rechtschaffen et al. (1972b)	PIP[c]	Periorbital region	20 msec	REM-NREM
Watson (1972) Wyatt et al. (1972)				
Pivik and Dement (1968) Pivik et al. (1969b)	EMG inhibition	Submental musculature	$\leq$ 100 msec	REM-NREM
Pivik and Dement (1970) Pivik (1971)	H-reflex inhibition	Soleus muscle	7-10 msec	REM-NREM

[a]Refer to Notes to table for a more complete description of these events.

[b]Middle ear muscle activity.

[c]Periorbital integrated potential.

Notes:

Theta bursts: See Figure 4 legend.

MEMA: Middle-ear muscle activity is reflected in movement or variations in compliance of the tympanic membrane which alters the existing baseline sound-pressure level in the external auditory canal. This change is detected by a probe fitted into the canal and translated into an impedance change which is registered on a paper writeout.

PIPs: Periorbital phasic integrated potentials are fast potentials, probably of muscular origin, recorded using integration techniques from surface electrodes placed around the eye.

Reflex inhibition: Electrical stimuli delivered to the tibial nerve through surface electrodes placed over the popliteal fossa elicit action potentials in musculature of the lower leg both directly and through a monosynaptic spinal pathway. The direct response is altered only by peripheral movements, whereas the reflex response is altered by central excitatory and inhibitory influences on controlling motoneurons.

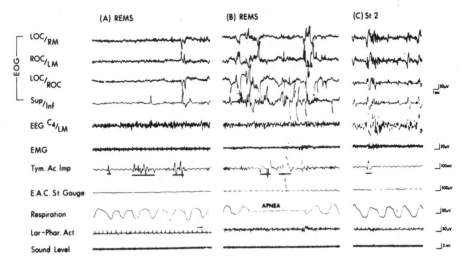

FIG. 7.2.   Polygraph sections containing representative appearances of MEMA in REM and NREM sleep. (A) REM sleep: MEMA with and without concurrent rapid eye movements. (B) REM sleep: MEMA associated with a period of apnea. (C) Stage 2 sleep: MEMA simultaneous with a K complex and slight laryngeal activation. Electroculogram (EOG) horizontal leads: LOC/RM, left outer canthus referred to right mastoid; ROC/LM, right outer canthus to left mastoid; LOC/ROC, left outer canthus to right outer canthus. EOG vertical leads: SUP/Inf, supraorbital ridge referred to infraorbital ridge. Electroencephalogram (EEG) leads: C_4/LM right central to left mastoid. Electromyogram (EMG) leads: masseter muscle referred to submentalis placement. Tympanic acoustic impedance (Tym. Ac. Imp.) deflections underlined, 100 mv = 12.5 acoustic ohms. External auricular canal strain gauge (E. A. C. St. Gauge) mounted on ear mold. Laryngopharyngeal activity (Lar. Phar-Act.) recorded from laryngeal prominence of thyroid cartilage. Sound level monitored from sleep room (2 mv = 7.7 dB). Activity from possible sources of MEMA-like artifact is absent during acoustic impedance deflections, indicating that they represent true MEMA. Reprinted by permission from M. A. Pessah and H. P. Roffwarg (Spontaneous middle ear muscle activity in man: A rapid eye movement phenomenon. *Science,* 1972, *173,* 773-776). Copyright 1972 by the American Association for the Advancement of Science.

conceptual, thoughtlike material (Bosinelli et al., 1973; Foulkes & Pope, 1973; Molinari & Foulkes, 1969; Pivik, 1971). Molinari and Foulkes (1969) found they could differentiate between content elicited from REM phasic and tonic arousals by classifying the reports as primary visual experiences (PVE) or as secondary cognitive elaborations (SCE). Reports were scored for PVE when the very last experience consisted of passively received, nonintellectualized, "thoughtless" imagery (like, watching a clock), and for SCE when this experience included evidence of active conceptualization, cognition or verbalization (like, watching a clock, but considering the indicated time; or thinking about time in the absence of any imagery). REM phasic reports were found to be associated with PVE, whereas the content from REM tonic awakenings and from three categories of NREM sleep (ascending Stage 2, and sleep onset Stages 1 and 2) were characterized by mental activity of the SCE type. This initial study concentrated upon

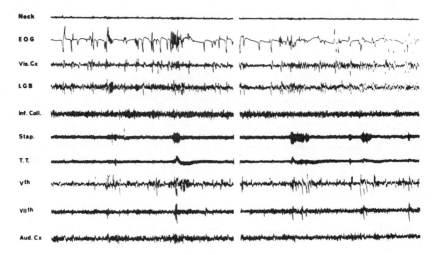

FIG. 7.3.   MEMA during REM sleep in the cat. Middle-ear muscle activity recorded from tensor tympani (T. T.) and stapedius (Stap.) derivations occurs in conjunction with spiking in visual and auditory cortices, lateral geniculate body (LGB), motor nuclei V and VII, and "bouffee" type clusters of eye movements.

the last experience related in subjects' spontaneous reports. The within-REM findings were subsequently replicated (Foulkes & Pope, 1973), but it was also found that if, following the spontaneous report, subjects were specifically asked about the presence of SCE-type material, the response was generally affirmative (Foulkes & Pope, 1973; Medoff & Foulkes, 1972). In other words, although PVE was a very prominent aspect of REM phasic content, conceptual activity was nevertheless present at this time and could be elicited upon direct questioning.

In the latter two studies a third awakening category within REM was included consisting of periods of frontal EEG sawtooth waves [2-3 Hz notched waves generally preceding eye-movement bursts (Berger, Olley, & Oswald, 1962)] in the absence of eye movement activity (see Figure 7.4). Content elicited in association with sawtooth waves was similar to REM phasic awakenings in terms of incidence of PVE ratings, but, unlike the latter, was found to be more discontinuous with respect to the preceding content (Foulkes & Pope, 1973).

Watson (1972), like Foulkes and his collaborators, also made use of three different awakening conditions within REM, but employed a different measure of phasic activity in conjunction with eye movements; the periorbital integrated potential (PIP) (see Figure 7.5). Arousals were made when PIPs were present with and without eye movements (PIP-REM and PIP conditions, respectively), and in the absence of both kinds of activities. Subjects rated the last experience on both PIP and PIP-REM awakenings as very or moderately bizarre significantly more often than they did the last experience on control awakenings. Furthermore, compared to control conditions, the last experience on both phasic conditions was found to be more discontinuous and more bizarre relative to the

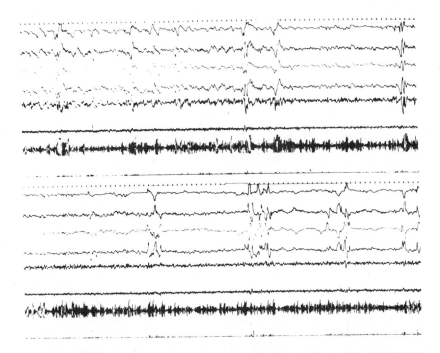

FIG. 7.4.   NREM and REM polygraphic tracings indicating band-pass filtered EEG theta-wave (5-6 Hz) activity and its relationship to other psychophysiological variables. In both the upper (NREM Stage 2 just preceding Stage REM onset) and lower (Stage REM) records, polygraph channels are as follows: time marker (small blips are second indicators); Channel 1: right horizontal electrooculogram (EOG); Channel 2: left horizontal EOG; Channel 3: right infraorbital vertical EOG; Channel 4: left infraorbital vertical EOG; Channel 5: unfiltered F_4 EEG; Channel 6: submental electromyogram (EMG); Channel 7: filtered F_4 EEG; Channel 8: periorbital phasic integrated potentials (PIPs). Note the concordance of theta bursting in ascending Stage 2 with PIPs and EEG K complexes and that the EMG suppression heralding REM onset (at the large minute mark on the time marker) is initiated (almost invariably in our experience) concurrently with a theta burst. In the REM tracing, theta bursts precede and/or accompany other phasic events – REM bursts and PIPs.

immediately preceding experience. Watson interpreted his results as indicating that PIPs, with or without eye movements, "are associated with bizarreness and discontinuity in the stream of dream mentation [p. iii]." The Foulkes and Pope (1973) study discussed above included analyses for bizarreness and discontinuity but did not corroborate Watson's findings on either scale. These differences might be the result of the two studies having used different measures of phasic activity (PIPs versus REM bursts and sawtooth waves), but it is unlikely since PIPs and sawtooth waves have been related to each other (Rechtschaffen, Molinari, Watson, & Wincor, 1970), and both have been related to eye movements.

The inconsistencies may reflect a combination of methodological and analytical differences (for example, clarification and extension of spontaneous content

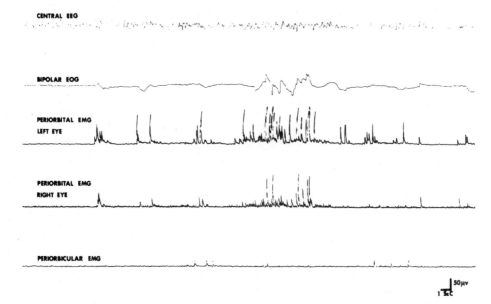

FIG. 7.5.   Illustration of PIP activity during REM sleep. Note the occurrence of PIPs with and without eye-movement activity, and the relative asynchrony between PIPs and integrated phasic muscle activity recorded from the periorbicular (lip) region.

reports in Watson's study were not conducted by an interviewer blind to the awakening condition; many of the quiet awakenings of Foulkes and Pope may have been contaminated by PIPs; interrater reliability on the bizarreness scale in the Foulkes and Pope study was less than that achieved in the Watson study) or, perhaps indicate more fundamental difficulties, such as the reliability of the psychological scales used.

THE TONIC-PHASIC MODEL AND NREM SLEEP MENTATION

The observation that PGO activity occurred intermittently during NREM sleep in the cat spurred the search for analogous measures in the human. It was hoped that a positive correlation between such activity and NREM sleep mentation would obtain, thus providing the "public physiological" landmark needed to lend crdibility to, and promote more efficient study of, such mentation. Apart from the previously cited studies using autonomic variability as the physiological index, another measure which received considerable attention was the K complex (see Figure 7.1). K complexes are most easily detectable during Stage 2 sleep, and are by definition (Rechtschaffen & Kales, 1968) absent from REM sleep. Nevertheless, the distribution of these events before the REM period (Dement, 1967) and their response to experimental manipulation (Pivik & Dement, 1968) suggested they might reflect PGO spike activity. Pivik et al.

(1969a) reported that high K-complex frequencies (determined on the basis of preawakening 3-min counts) were associated with either the absence of recall or with recall of the most dreamlike quality, whereas the lowest rates of K complexes were associated with "conceptual mentation, both mundane and bizarre, and perceptual mentation of a nonhallucinatory quality [p. 215]." Later, Weisz (1972) conducted a study in which awakenings were made in ascending Stage 2 following a single K complex or sleep spindle; he found no significant differences between the two classes of awakenings although a variety of variables were examined, including recall, SCE, PVE, distortion, and active participation. More recently, Antrobus, Ezrachi, and Arkin (1973) made Stage 2 awakenings after REM and after sleep onset and found no relationship between a dreamlike rating on several scales and incidence of K complexes.

If these largely negative K-complex findings are discarded, the case for the feasibility of the tonic-phasic distinction for NREM sleep mentation is reduced to three lines of work, each using a different presumptive PGO index (PIPs, phasic reflex inhibition, and theta bursts) and overlapping only slightly in the portions of NREM sleep sampled.

It has already been indicated that PIPs occur in both REM and NREM sleep (see Table 7.2), and it is notable that the initial sleep mentation-PIP studies were conducted in NREM sleep (Rechtschaffen et al., 1972a, b). In these studies Stage 2 awakenings were made under four conditions: (1) control, consisting of the absence of PIPs or tonic periorbital EMG activity for 1 min; (2) phasic-tonic (P-T), a mixture of PIPs and tonic activity; (3) tonic (T), brief burst of tonic activity without PIPs; and (4) phasic (P), 3-5 sec of PIPs alone. The two studies were consistent in finding that, relative to control conditions, there was an increased likelihood of recall under P-T conditions, and that phasic reports (P and P-T) were more lengthy and more highly distorted.

Another test of the NREM tonic-phasic model made use of transient inhibition of the spinal monosynaptic H reflex as the index of phasic activity (Pivik, 1971; see Figures 7.6 and 7.7). Awakenings were made during all NREM sleep stages except sleep onset Stage 1 under phasic (inhibition of a single-reflex response) or tonic (absence of such inhibition for at least 2 min) conditions. Of a considerable battery of variables (visual, auditory, or kinesthetic imagery, recall, hallucinatory quality, and sleep depth among others) only two — auditory imagery and hostility — significantly discriminated between phasic and tonic reports, with higher scores on both variables under phasic conditions. However, an unexpected clustering of variables emerged from the analyses. With respect to amount of recall, tonic-phasic distinctions obtained for NREM Stages 3 and 4, but not for NREM Stage 2 and REM sleep. Recall in the former NREM stages, generally the worst among all sleep stages, was markedly enhanced under phasic conditions, that is, Stage 3, phasic, 55.6%, tonic, 40.6%; Stage 4, phasic, 58.1%, tonic, 38.3%. Qualitatively, there was a reversal of the tonic-phasic correlates which, however, preserved the above sleep stage groupings. NREM Stages 3 and 4 tonic and REM and Stage 2 phasic awakenings were characterized by content having more visual imagery, movement, higher dreamlike fantasy ratings and being more hallucinatory, whereas NREM Stages 3 and 4 phasic and REM and Stage 2 tonic arousals were rated more thoughtlike, with Stage 4 phasic arousals receiving the highest percentage of such ratings. Although these results need to be cross validated, the internal consistency of the pattern would suggest that they are not capricious fluctuations. Remarkable too, is the fact that these NREM differences

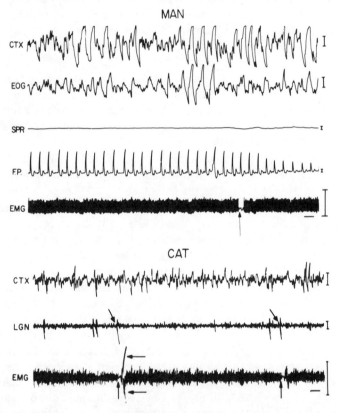

FIG. 7.6. The occurrence of phasic EMG suppressions in man and cat. In the upper tracings the single vertical arrow indicates the occurrence of a relatively long sustained phasic EMG suppression during non-REM Stage 4 sleep in man. CTX, monopolar central (C_3/A_2) EEG; EOG, bipolar horizontal electrooculogram; SPR, spontaneous skin potential; FP, finger plethysmograph; EMG, bipolar submental electromyogram. In the EMG tracing of the cat, two phasic suppressions can be seen (vertical arrows). A biphasic muscle twitch (horizontal arrows) occurs near the end of the first suppression. Note the close temporal correlation between geniculate spiking (arrows, LGN derivation) and phasic EMG suppressions. CTX, visual cortex; LGN, lateral geniculate nucleus; EMG, electromyogram recorded from the posterior cervical muscles. Calibrations: 1 sec; 50 μv. Reprinted by permission from T. Pivik and W. C. Dement (Phasic changes in muscular and reflex activity during non-REM sleep. *Experimental Neurology*, 1970, *27*, 115-124).

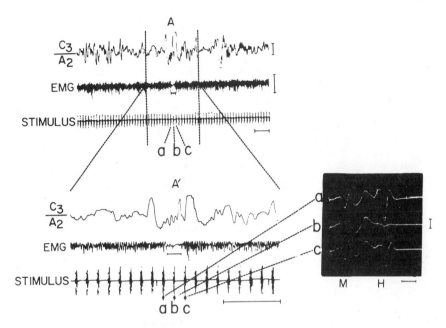

FIG. 7.7.   A phasic EMG suppression (underscored) and associated EEG recorded at standard (A) and enhanced (A') speeds together with the muscular responses elicited by the three consecutive stimuli (a, b, c) overlapping the suppression. The muscular responses (a, b, c) pictured to the right of A' correspond, respectively, to the lettered stimuli in A' directly under the suppression. In the tracings of the muscular responses, note the stability of the direct response (M wave) and the inhibition of the H reflex in tracing b, the stimulus for which occurs coincident with the phasic EMG suppression. Calibrations: A and A', 1 sec, 50 μv; oscilloscope tracings, 10 msec, 500 μv. Reprinted by permission from T. Pivik and W. C. Dement (Phasic changes in muscular and reflex activity during non-REM sleep. *Experimental Neurology*, 1970, *27*, 115-124).

in recall and qualitative characteristics are based on the occurrence of a single observable phasic event lasting only 7-10 msec.

Although PIPs and phasic EMG inhibitions occur at sleep onset (Rechtschaffen et al., 1970; Pivik et al., 1969b), the only study which has attempted to relate a measure of phasic activity to mental activity at this time is one by Pope (1973), using theta bursts as the phasic index (see Figure 7.3). In keeping with previous reports of sleep onset mentation (e.g., Foulkes & Vogel, 1965; Vogel et al., 1966), all three categories of awakenings: 1: 15 sec following EEG alpha loss; 2: theta burst following alpha loss; and 3: 15 sec following a theta burst produced a high incidence of recall (93-100%). Moreover, theta-burst awakenings contained significantly more PVE than pretheta reports and substantially, but not significantly, more than posttheta reports. As the sleep-onset period progressed from pretheta through theta and posttheta conditions, mentation became increasingly more discontinuous in nature. Although these three conditions did not differ significantly with respect to this variable, a declension of theta into high- and low-amplitude categories proved to be discriminating, with high-theta reports being significantly more discontinuous.

OVERVIEW AND SPECIAL CONSIDERATIONS

Ideally, models endure only so long as they sustain a heuristic influence; but it is often the case that such concepts linger on far beyond their use, hindering rather than stimulating, finally dying from neglect, without public or official recognition of their demise. One of the reasons models or theories persevere in the face of glaring inadequacies is the apparent necessity of having something "better" with which to replace them. The 2-state model — the limitations of which were clearly evident even 5 years ago — had been languishing in a state of depreciated heuristic usefulness, and has only recently been laid to rest (Dement, 1973). The continuing influence of the heir-apparent tonic-phasic model is undeniable, but the value of singling out phasic events for study at the psychophysiological interface is as yet unclear. The work that has been completed provides some guidelines that are clearly indicated, and others which are suggestive at best. It is clear, for example, from the measures that have been taken, that phasic activity is not the determinant of sleep mentation per se. Phasic activity does appear to facilitate recall (see Table 7.1), especially during slow wave sleep (Pivik, 1971) but recall is relatively profuse under tonic conditions. In the only study to date in which tonic-phasic distinctions in recall have been examined in REM and the bulk of NREM sleep in the same subjects (Pivik, 1971), only 1 subject out of 10 exhibited a significant tonic-phasic recall difference across all sleep stages, with greater recall under phasic conditions.

With respect to phasic-tonic discriminators at the qualitative level, the results are meager and sometimes conflicting, with suggestions toward a concentration upon discontinuity, SCE, auditory imagery and hostility in NREM sleep, and discontinuity, bizarreness, and PVE in REM sleep. However, even under the most optimal of conditions, that is, during REM sleep when recall and detailed elaboration are at their best, the presence of phasic events proves distinctive only part of the time. The increased bizarreness of PIP-associated REM reports observed by Watson (1972) is experienced on only 55% of such reports, which, although significantly greater than comparable control values, still leaves 45% of PIP and PIP-REM reports of apparently nondistinctive quality. Similarly, Watson's discontinuity effects were present on less than 40% of PIP or PIP-REM awakenings. Pivik's (1971) results indicating auditory imagery and hostility as significant tonic-phasic discriminators are likewise based on the presence of these characteristics on less than half of the phasic arousals. The results of Foulkes and Pope

(1973) suggesting PVE as a REM tonic-phasic discriminator are on more solid footing, with the median-subject PVE value being 100% on REM-burst arousals relative to 63% on control arousals. Except for the latter data, we appear to be dealing with a rather weak effect.

Before concluding that phasic-tonic distinctions apply even to REM sleep mentation, a reassessment of the validity of the bases for our expectations regarding the relationship between presumptive PGO measures and sleep mentation might be useful. The major expectation was for dramatic differences to obtain at the psychological level to match those indicated physiologically and anatomically in the cat. In point of fact, the bases for the latter differences are not clearly established. The separate anatomical mediation of tonic and phasic events (Pompeiano, 1966, 1967) has been questioned (Perenin, Maeda, & Jeannerod, 1972) and the notion of the PGO spike as a unitary event (Bizzi & Brooks, 1963; Malcolm, Watson, & Burke, 1970) — an idea which would fit well with the impression of spikes as intrusive or disruptive events — may be open to review (McCarley, Hobson, & Pivik, 1973). However, from a psychophysiological standpoint, the synaptic processes underlying PGO-spike generation may not be as important a determinant of the resultant effect of such activity as is the *intensity of phasic activity relative to the existing level of background activity.* Reasonable expectations regarding possible measurable effects of phasic activity must consider both the amount of activity and the physiological context within which these events occur. For example, relative to their occurrence in REM sleep, phasic events in NREM sleep occur with vastly diminished intensity and against a dramatically different background in terms of both gross EEG activation and level of unitary activity. It should not be surprising, therefore, that significant REM-NREM differences in both amount and quality of mentation are observed (Foulkes, 1962; Pivik, 1971; Rechtschaffen et al., 1963a).

Many factors contribute to the makeup of the physiological background against which phasic events are elaborated; EEG sleep stages constitute what might be called predictable sources of variation in background activity — predictable because there is a regularity to their occurrence within and across subjects. A less predictable determinant of background activity which is only infrequently considered (Hauri & Van de Castle, 1973; Monroe, 1967; Pope, 1973; Pivik, 1971; Zimmerman, 1970) is that originating from individual differences in physiological stability. The degree to which this factor may influence experimental outcomes is not well defined; but its potential for doing so may be illustrated by considering data from two subjects in a recent experiment utilizing reflex inhibition as the measure of phasic activity (Pivik, 1971). Subject A exhibited a spinal reflex the amplitude and waveform of which in NREM sleep remained virtually unchanged for periods of time ranging from 15-45 min, whereas these measures of reflex stability in Subject B underwent such constant fluctuations that tonic-phasic distinctions were rendered nearly meaningless. At one level of analysis these physiological differences were apparently meaningful, that is, Subject B had 100% recall from REM arousals and 84% recall from NREM arousals, while Subject A had recall percentages of 62.5 and 19..9% for REM and NREM, respectively.

Another intensity related aspect of phasic activity especially evident in the human is the apparent asynchrony of the presumptive PGO analogues. The lack of a tight temporal linkage among MEMA, PIPs, theta bursts, and phasic EMG and reflex inhibition has been commented upon only in passing fashion in the literature (Rechtschaffen, Michel, & Metz, 1972; Roffwarg et al., 1973). This lack of concurrence — least prevalent within REM sleep during bursts of eye movements and most evident during NREM sleep — raises the possibility of multiple phasic-event systems driven by separate generators which become jointly active only during intense bursts of activity. Differentially active phasic-event systems might find expression at the psychological level as variations in salience of event-specific qualitative correlates, and such an interpretation can be easily applied to existing data. For example, at sleep onset, theta bursts correlate with mental activity characterized by PVE and discontinuity; during slow wave sleep, and Stage 2 to a lesser extent, phasic reflex inhibition indicates thought-like, auditory imagery; and during REM PIPs and theta bursts are related to mentation that is relatively bizarre and distorted. The resulting mélange of event and state-specific content correlations, although not an implausible possibility, certainly lacks parsimonious appeal. Pessah and Roffwarg (1972b), in dealing with the apparent problem of a lack of synchrony between MEMA and PGO spikes in the cat, present a cogent discussion of considerations permitting the maintenance of a single generator theory in the face of asynchronous phasic events. They suggest that the partial asynchrony:

> . . . does not necessarily indicate that the primary brainstem discharges, which originate activation in the different systems, are not synchronous. It indicates only that the end motor responses recordable with our transducers . . . are not simultaneous. It is conceivable that impulses transmitted in parallel from a unitary generator into several neuronal channels may eventuate as *apparently* asynchronous peripheral phasic events as a result of a mixture of partial and complete inhibitions variously affecting different motor pathways . . . [Pessah & Roffwarg, 1972b, p. 776].

Attributing these asynchronous phasic manifestations to the activity of a single master generator does not clarify the existing confusion in the psychophysiological data. A situation of event-specific, state-specific content correlations might still obtain if the psychological concomitant of generator activity was a function of the most highly activated end organ. On the other hand, if the psychophysical link is to activity of the generator itself there should be some unique, enduring psychological characteristic which would clearly differentiate "phasic" content from "tonic" content. Such a characteristic is yet to be demonstrated.

CONCLUSION

The early notion of sleep as a relatively uncomplicated state in which mind-body relationships might be profitably studied inbred an oversimplified view of sleep psychophysiology which, although perhaps useful in terms of stimulating interest and promoting popularity in those initial years, was found to be inadequate to the task of answering questions raised by the data. It was replaced by a view which fractionated sleep into tonic and phasic components and made use of the microscopic dream report in conjunction with microphasic physiological measures. The yield from this new view with its new methodology has not been as fruitful as hoped. Perhaps, as Bosinelli et al. (1973) suggest, we may be approaching a physiological limit in this kind of research where, in attempting to match the temporal discreteness of our physiological measures, we are demanding an impossible degree of introspective precision from subjects. Perhaps there is a qualitative aspect of dream phenomenology which is the phasic-event correlate par excellence (Bosinelli et al., 1973; Rechtschaffen, 1973; Watson, 1972); or it may indeed be as Foulkes (1973) portends that "what differences may emerge between phasic and non-phasic moments . . . will have to be relatively subtle, and revelatory of a slightly different 'mix' of dream functions, rather than any kind of qualitative alternation [p. 25-26]."

Research utilizing the tonic-phasic model of sleep mentation has reached a point of diminishing returns. Whether this situation represents a temporary condition or is a signal of the impending demise of the model is a question for time and discerning research to answer.

ACKNOWLEDGMENTS

Preparation of this paper was supported by Grant MHO4151 from the United States Public Health Service and Grant 448-13-RD from the State of Illinois, Department of Mental Health. The author gratefully acknowledges Figures supplied by Drs. David Foulkes, Allen Rechtschaffen, and Howard Roffwarg. The author also acknowledges the helpful comments given by Drs. Rechtschaffen and Foulkes on earlier drafts of this paper.

Part IV

EFFECTS OF EXPERIMENTAL VARIABLES ON SLEEP MENTATION

EDITORS' FOREWORD TO CHAPTER 8

Cartwright nicely highlights one of the critical issues in sleep and dream research, that is, the effects of the subject's environment on mentation reports and the manner in which the environment is represented in them. It is clear from her findings and the studies she cites that one cannot simply predict from a laboratory situation which specific aspect of its content will appear in a given mentation report. She also makes clear that personality traits of the individuals being studied may affect not only the content of mentation reports but even the number of dreams reported in a given situation. What she has done in this chapter is to show us how both state and trait variables may affect the dream report. Although this may seem like an obvious point to some, the fact that it is being studied explicitly is certainly a step forward in experimental studies of sleep mentation.

Cartwright also points to how little we understand about the interaction of presleep stimuli (or daytime experience) and REMP mentation. It is clear that the complex interactions implied by the material in this chapter will keep sleep researchers well occupied in the future.

S. J. Ellman

8

The Social Psychology of
Dream Reporting

Rosalind Dymond Cartwright
Alfred Kaszniak

University of Illinois

It is still a matter of concern to those in the field of EEG monitored sleep research whether the dream reports collected from rapid-eye-movement (REM) sleep periods under laboratory conditions constitute a representative sample from which to generalize about dream life as it occurs under more usual conditions. Studies comparing samples of home and laboratory dream reports from the same subjects have pointed out a number of differences. Dreams collected in the laboratory have been reported to be less aggressive and sexual, less characterized by either success or misfortune; in other words, less dramatic than those dreamed at home, (Domhoff & Kamiya, 1964; Hall & Van de Castle, 1966). Dreams collected in the laboratory differ also in that they often include the laboratory situation itself which is clearly not a usual dream topic (Dement, Kahn & Roffwarg, 1965; Domhoff & Kamiya, 1964; Snyder, 1970; Whitman, Pierce, Maas, & Baldridge, 1962). These findings raise a number of issues: what accounts for these home-lab differences, can they be overcome, and do they matter? Does the experience of coming into the laboratory, with all its attendant novelty and feelings of anxiety, affect not only what is dreamed, but how it is dreamed? If the nature of the process itself is changed this might well invalidate these reports as a basis for understanding dream function and content as they occur more typically. Perhaps, though, the lab may affect only the manifest dream content, and that only temporarily, in terms of providing different grist for the same dream-process mill. If the process itself is not affected but works on these data in its characteristic way, inferences based on these dreams should not differ from inferences based on home dreams.

One possibility is that the reported differences are not due to any basic difference in the dreams that are dreamed but are the result of comparing noncomparable samples. A typical night of content awakenings in the lab involves three to six REM periods being interrupted with all, or all but one, of these yielding a report of a dream. These are then compared to home reports which are usually based on dream diaries written on awakening. Most often these yield only one dream per night and this is most likely to be the final one from which the awakening occurred. Since this dream is characteristically the longest, most bizarre, and exciting (Snyder, 1970), as well as the most recently occurring one, it is also the one most easily recalled (Meier, Ruef, Ziegler & Hall, 1968; Trinder & Kramer, 1971). It is, though, an unrepresentative sample against which the larger sample of lab-collected dreams appears pale by comparison.

In addition to the difference in the nature of the dreams sampled under home and lab conditions, there are differences in the method and circumstances of their retrieval which may have affects of their own. The context for laboratory subjects is that they are sleeping "in public." The environment is strange and the conditions of being wired for EEG recordings unique. On top of this they are awakened unexpectedly and intermittently throughout the night by a voice over an intercom requesting them to report their dreams orally from their bed into the dark. These are then tape recorded remotely. At home these subjects are "in private;" surroundings are familiar; awakenings are spontaneous, or, at a time preset under the subject's own control. The dream reports are usually written, which involves much more formal language structure than is typical of oral speech, particularly when one is sleepy. Perhaps the findings that home dreams are more sexual, aggressive, and dramatic mean only that the last dream of the night, when written out, in private, and in narrative form has these qualities. To test this possibility, Weisz and Foulkes, (1970), undertook a well-controlled study to compare home and laboratory dream reports when they were collected under uniform sampling and reporting conditions. If under these circumstances the differences in reports were negligible, the question of representativeness would be settled. Their subjects were given the same reporting instructions under both circumstances. Each had an alarm clock with which to make their own awakenings, and a tape recorder to report to, for two lab and two home nights of dream-report collections. The alarm was set for 6:30 AM for all occasions and the oral report was made in privacy. The order of the nights was counterbalanced with six subjects sleeping first at home and then in the lab, and the other six sleeping in the lab first. Under these circumstances the dreams were found not to differ in the level of their vivid fantasy. This factor is the one found by Hauri, Sawyer, & Rechtschaffen (1967), to account for most of the variance in dream ratings. It is made up of two components: the unrealisticness or imaginativeness of the reports; and their intensity or dramatic quality. Weisz and Foulkes (1970), concluded that the laboratory-collection method does not alter the basic nature of the cognitive process of dreaming. However, they did support the earlier studies of Domhoff and Kamiya (1964) and Hall and Van de Castle (1966) by finding that even under these conditions home dreams were significantly more aggressive in content than those the subject recorded in the laboratory. Although this study gives a partially affirmative answer to the question: "Are the dreams dreamed in the laboratory equally dream-like to those dreamed at home?" this may hold only under these atypical reporting circumstances in which the social elements of the reporting situation are minimized. Ordinarily these are prominent so that the report must be looked at as a social communication. Subjects often remark before sleep that they hope they do not shock us or dream embarrassing dreams, and they often demonstrate that they feel uncomfortable about being "caught in the act" in a way they have no chance to prepare for or experience beforehand.

The power of the particular subject-experimenter relationship to affect the REM-period content reports has been demonstrated in a study by Whitman, Kramer, and Baldridge (1963). Here, two patients, who were in psychotherapy as well as participating in a sleep lab as subjects, reported their dreams to both the experimenter at the time and to their psychotherapist later in the day. Whitman et al. (1963) report that these subjects unconsciously selected the dreams reported to these two different recipients to be appropriate to the situation as they saw it. To the male therapist, the male subject told the dreams that cast him in an admirable heterosexual light and omitted those reported during the night which had homosexual connotations. The female subject did not report to her male experimenter competitive dreams that she had about him but did report them later to her therapist. She did, on the other hand, report to her experimenter dreams which included some erotic feelings about her therapist although she omitted these when reporting to the psychiatrist. It appears that the subject-experimenter relationship may well have an impact on the dreams themselves as well as on their availability for retrieval. If this is a replicable finding it raises the further issue of whether this is a temporary effect subject to adaptation.

This question has been addressed by Dement, Kahn, and Roffwarg (1965), who reported evidence that adaptation to the laboratory occurred both within the first night, from the first to the last awakening, and progressively over subsequent nights. Dreams which involved direct incorporation of the laboratory dropped from 43% of those recalled from the first REM period of the first laboratory night to 16% of those reported from the sixth awakening on Night 1. Comparing nights, the first yielded lab incorporations on 25% of the occasions and the sixth only 7%. Whitman, Pierce, Maas, and Baldridge (1962), on the other hand, reported no reduction in the anxiety about laboratory sleeping, as expressed in the dreams of 10 subjects over 4 nights of dream reporting. Their analysis was more clinically interpretive whereas the Dement et al. (1965) data was based on an objective scoring of the manifest elements. In a later paper, (Fox, Kramer, Baldridge, Whitman, & Ornstien, 1968), the authors conclude that "since the experimental situation includes an affective human relationship. . . adaptation in any meaningful sense may not occur. . . attempts must be made to control this variable and to account for its influence in any dream content material being evaluated [p. 701]."

In a study reported in 1969, Cartwright, Bernick, Borowitz, and Kling, attempted to influence the amount of sexual dreaming taking place in the lab by exposing heterosexually oriented males to an erotic movie as a presleep stimulus. They reported that no directly sexual dreams were recalled by any of the 10 subjects studied for the next 4 consecutive nights. The fact that there were other changes in the dream content reported by these subjects showed that the film did have an impact on the dream reports if not the one anticipated. There was a significant decrease in the number of REM awakenings from which dreams were recalled in comparison to the number retrieved on the night before the film. There was also a significant decrease in the percentage of dreams involving opposite sex characters and an increase in the proportion of dreams involving only one character. All of these results were seen as pointing to an increase in the strength of the usual defense against the expression of sexual fantasy in the laboratory following the experimental manipulation designed to enhance it. At what point this censorship operated, and how consciously, it was not possible to say. Whether it prevented these dreams from being formed at all; whether once dreamed there was an inhibition on their retention; or whether having dreamed and recalled, it was only the reporting process that was affected. In any case, fewer dreams were reported; those that were, had a different character after the exposure to the film than before, and the change was in the direction of fewer heterosexual situations appearing in the reported sleep fantasy.

The possibility of using these data as a basis from which to gain some further insight into the variables affecting lab dream reporting occurred some three years later when a group of homosexual males agreed to participate in a study of the psychological and physiological concomitants of their sexual arousal response. This made it possible to collect data comparable to the heterosexual sample and look into the effects of the lab on dream reporting in two groups for whom different predictions would be made about their response to the same social situation. If the homosexual subjects, equally sexually aroused before sleep, also show an absence of sexual dreams and an increase in the failure to recall, it could be concluded that the laboratory exerts a general dampening effect on more primitive dreams and that this is exaggerated when impulse levels are heightened. If, however, the inhibition on sexual dream reports was related more specifically to the embarrassment of the heterosexual subjects in reporting to a sexually attractive female experimenter, the homosexuals would be expected not to show this effect. To test the influence of the sex of the experimenter, in relation to the sexual orientation of the subject, on the amount and kind of dream reports collected before and after sexual stimulation, half the homosexual subjects were assigned to a male and half to a female experimenter for their five nights of REM-report collections.

It was predicted that the homosexual subjects assigned to the female experimenter would be less embarrassed to report to her than to a male, and less than the heterosexual subjects had been, and so would not show the reduction in reporting rate after the exposure to the film. It was also predicted that if sex of experimenters contributes to the variance in dream reports those homosexuals assigned to the male experimenter might show effects parallel to those observed in the first group with the female. In addition to testing for a general lab effect across both groups, and a specific within-group sex-of-experimenter effect, there was another variable involved which might lead to some between-group differences. This was a difference in the definition of the role of subject in relation to experimenter of what constitutes appropriate behavior in that interpersonal context.

The subjects in the first study had all been medical students drawn from the institution where the study was being conducted. All were heterosexual in identity and practice, as established by a detailed psychiatric history interview conducted by a senior faculty member of the department of psychiatry. Those in the second sample were selected to match the subjects in the first group in age and educational level, but none were medical students nor had they any connection with that university. Their primary identity as far as the study was concerned was their sexual not their occupational role. All were drawn from the same chapter of the Gay Liberation Front at another university whose president had agreed to participate in the study and who guaranteed the support of his group members. These subjects were also interviewed by the psychiatrist who established them to be homosexual in identity and practice. Both groups were given the Minnesota Multiphasic Personality Inventory (MMPI), and the results shown in Table 8.1 demonstrate that aside from being somewhat more anxious and feminine, these subjects did not differ significantly from the heterosexuals on the other scales.

To the medical-student group the experimenters occupied the complimentary role of faculty menbers in the same institution, and as such had other actual, or potential, relationships with these subjects that might affect their careers. This reinforced the saliency of the subjects' role in the study to be "students" and no doubt created a demand for them to watch their step and look like good prospective doctors in our eyes.

To the homosexual subjects the experimenters had only a passing importance as members of the straight society and researchers in the area of sexual identity. The study provided them an opportunity to educate some potentially influential people and to help change the image of the homosexual from that of despicable pervert to sexually liberated, and even nobly misunderstood, person. Evidence of this view came from the buttons worn to the lab reading "Gay Is Good" and the like, the small talk instigated during the presleep preparation period, and the dream reports themselves. For them the demand characteristics might be phrased: "tell it like it is to show the straight folks what it means to be gay." In other

TABLE 8.1

MMPI Scale Means for Heterosexual-Homosexual Groups

Group		L	F	K	HS	D	HY	Pd	MF	Pa	Pt	Sc	Ma	Si	T. Anx.	W. Anx.	ES	R-S
Heterosex	M	48.0	55.0	58.6	51.7	53.6	56.4	60.2	61.4	51.2	50.9	55.1	60.7	43.0	8.7	5.2	54.1	20.0
$N = 10$	SD	6.0	9.5	7.2	6.8	11.1	5.0	9.5	6.3	7.1	8.2	8.7	5.7	5.9	4.5	3.6	4.6	12.9
Homosex	M	49.6	63.5	58.8	51.7	57.3	62.3	65.1	81.2	58.8	56.8	60.2	67.5	48.6	13.2	10.2	50.9	26.0
$N = 10$	SD	4.9	8.5	4.3	5.7	12.0	7.3	12.4	8.6	7.7	8.1	6.8	12.6	6.4	9.3	5.3	5.2	15.0
Het-Hom t									5.841*							2.442**		

*$p < .01.$
**$p < .05.$

words, the subject role behaviors elicited in response to the lab were potentially different for the two groups. For the first group there may have been some conflict between the student and the subject role behaviors since both were associated with the same persons and place. While expressing sexual fantasies is clearly appropriate behavior for a subject in a sex study, it is not appropriate for a medical student to professors in the hospital context. For those in the second group, who were not known to the experimenters except in their homosexual identity roles, expressing their sexual fantasy material was appropriate, expected behavior.

If these inferences are valid and the groups are both sexually stimulated by the film, the motivation to report fully should be greater for those in Group 2 than Group 1, particularly after being exposed to the movie. The amount of dreaming directly involving sex should be increased for the homosexuals and decreased for the heterosexuals. Also, the amount of dreaming in which the subject is in an occupational versus a sexual identity role should differ with the heterosexual subjects producing more occupational and the homosexuals more sex-role-related dreams.

The question whether the two groups were in fact equally aroused by the movie is a valid one in light of the fact that the same movie was used for both groups and it involved only heterosexual activity. Both groups were monitored before, during, and after the film for their response to it in terms of a number of physiological measures; heart rate, plasma levels of 17 hydroxycorticosteroids, pupilary dilation, and penile erection. For the erection response, each subject was asked after seeing the film if they had experienced an erection and to estimate its extent on a 4-point scale in which zero equalled no response and 3 a full erection. Nine of the heterosexual males and 8 of the homosexuals reported erections above the level of zero. Of the 10 homosexuals, 8 wore a penile plethysmograph. This more objective measure showed 7 of the 8 in Sample 2 to have moderate to full erections (Kling, Borowitz, & Cartwright, 1972). The relation of the verbal to the phethysmographic report showed the verbal to be, if anything, an underestimate for those where the two measures could be compared. When asked to what scene or act their erections took place the homosexuals differed from the heterosexual subjects in the reported stimuli. They most often ignored the female and responded to the male only in the movie and in this way redefined the stimulus as appropriate to them.

What are the effects of this arousal in the dream reports? Can observing a heterosexual interaction stimulate a homosexual dream expression? Two dreams illustrate that this does in fact occur.

Homosexual Subject D

Night 3, REM 4:

I was back in that room, or that sort of garden and Hefner was there... Hefner and I had been talking philosophy... we wandered back into that restricted court-

yard and then we went through the door there, and there was this man sort of fid-
dling around with this young girl and the other young girl looking on. I thought: He's
so jaded this is what he has to do to amuse himself. And there are two guys who
eventually started giving each other blow jobs and I, I joined in, finally.

Homosexual Subject I

Night 4, REM 6:

I was talking to some people, I think it was around Dearborn St. and they were
sitting there. There was a beautiful blonde boy who was sitting with a very fat girl
who was actually very interesting. And I don't know if I was coming by on my
bicycle or if I was just walking along, but anyway, they said hello and I said hello and
we started to chat. . . and the girl asked me which I would rather go to bed with and
I said, "Well probably your friend." And she just sort of smiled. . . All of a sudden
the boy was in my arms. The girl didn't seem to mind at all, and he was kissing me
very violently, no, passionately, and sort of arranging himself in various positions.
Finally he turned over on his back and I started to lick his back, very sensuously. I
did that for a while and he really seemed to like it. He was sort of in my power.

Does the homosexual group follow the heterosexual in having a reduction in
the amount of recall following the film? The most commonly accepted figure for
the percentage of REM-period awakenings leading to a report of a dream is
83.3%. This was derived by Dement (1965), who pooled the samples from several studies to obtain a total of 200 subjects awakened from over 2,000 REM
periods. In this study each REM report for the 20 subjects was individually coded and rated blindly by a judge naive to the study hypotheses. Table 8.2 reports
the pre, and postfilm recall for the 2 samples and shows the heterosexuals to
have a prefilm recall rate almost exactly at the norm quoted above. The decrease
in recall following the film for the heterosexual subject group reporting to a female experimenter was not observed in the second group. The homosexuals
showed a higher rate of recall both before and after the movie regardless of the
sex of their experimenter. The difference between the 2 groups in recall rate on
Night 2 was significant, and within the homosexual group the Night 1 to Night 2
difference was not. Thus the dampening effect on recall following an increase in
sexual stimulation was not replicated showing this not to be a general lab effect
for all subjects.

The best baseline data on the number of sexual dreams occurring in the lab
and home dreams of the same subjects are those reported by Domhoff and Kamiya (1964). They report that 12 males, who slept in the lab once a week for a
total of 10 nights and wrote down any home dreams recalled during that period
had only 2 sexual dreams (2%) in the lab, in contrast to 11 (9%) at home. This
difference, while small, was significant. The 10 medical student subjects reported
only 1 sexual dream out of the total of 31 collected on their first night of awakenings before seeing the film. This gives a 3% figure comparable to the Domhoff
and Kamiya lab rate quoted above. The dream itself demonstrates the fear of
being caught by authority figures while responding to a sexual situation.

TABLE 8.2

Percentage of REM Awakenings Yielding Dream Recall
before and after Film

	Night 1	Night 2
Heterosexual		
Mean	83.00	69.33
SD	31.44	23.40
Homosexual		
Mean	92.22	89.68
SD	17.15	14.35
Homosexual: male experimenter		
Mean	95.00	92.69
SD	10.00	10.38
Homosexual: female experimenter		
Mean	90.00	86.66
SD	22.36	18.25

Note: Het-Hom Night 2. $t = 2.343$; $df = 18$; $p < .05$

Heterosexual Subject J

Night 1, REM 2:

This time there was music in the living room of our apartment and I had my girl friend there, and, I had undressed her and we were just about to make love when there was a knock at the door and it turned out that it was her parents, of all people. . .

For the homosexual sample the prefilm number of directly sexual dreams was identical, 1 out of 39 awakenings that yielded some content, or 2.5%. However, the nature of the dream is much more matter-of-fact.

Homosexual Subject D

Night 1, REM 4:

I was making love. It's hard to remember the details. I remember I was right on top at the same time. . . there is nothing I can add right now.

Following the movie both groups of subjects slept for 4 more consecutive nights of REM awakenings. Of the 157 reports with some content from the heterosexual sample, none of them contained any overtly sexual content. Of the 190 postfilm dreams of the homosexual subjects 6 of them dealt with direct, unambiguous sexual activity, contributed by 5 of the 10 subjects. All of these occurred, however, within the subgroup of subjects who had the male experimenter to report to. This made the comparison 5.4% for the homosexuals reporting to the male compared to 0% for the heterosexuals, and 0% for the homosexuals reporting to the female. These results are rather meager but suggest that, contrary to expectation, the potential sexual element in the experimenter-subject relationship has opposite effects for the 2 samples. Heterosexual subjects suppressed reporting sexual material to a female and Gay Lib homosexuals suppressed to the female but expressed more freely to a male.

More evident was the amount of homosexual content which was not directly sexual in nature but identity defining. The dreams of all subjects for all nights were categorized according to the primary social role of the dreamer in each dream. The differences in the frequency with which these categories were used by the two samples can be seen in Table 8.3.

The three differences which had been anticipated were all found to be significant. The heterosexual subjects define themselves in their lab dreams most frequently occupationally, as students or doctors. This is particularly true in situations which might hold sexual potential. The homosexuals present themselves more often than do heterosexuals as "friends" to other males, or as "sexual," in this case, gay people. Many of the "friend" dreams involved others known to be Gay Lib members. The role-frequency analysis confirmed the saliency of the occupational role of the medical students and the sexual-identity role of the homosexuals across all the nights.

A few examples will illustrate this difference. The first two, from medical students demonstrate how they employ the identity as professionals to deny

TABLE 8.3

The Role of the Dreamer to Others in the Dreams for Five Nights

Role	Heterosexual Subjects		Homosexual Subjects		
	F	Percentage	F	Percentage	Z
Alone	22	12.4	29	13.4	–
Family member	16	9.0	25	11.5	–
Friend	19	10.7	43	20.1	2.76*
Onlooker	16	9.0	10	4.6	–
Sexual identity	9	5.0	28	13.0	2.82*
Sports player	16	9.0	4	1.8	3.27**
Stranger	19	10.7	17	7.9	–
Student or student doctor	34	19.5	15	6.9	3.21**
Subject in experiment	8	4.5	24	11.1	2.45
Victim, escapee	11	6.2	10	4.6	–
Employee	8	4.0	11	5.1	–

*$p < .05$.
**$p < .01$.

sexual curiosity, whereas the next two illustrate the motivation of the homosexuals to be known as gay in order to educate others. In the first dream the subject goes through a patient's room while she is in bed and she protests that he has no legitimate reason to be there. In the film a young man is taken to a prostitute's bedroom, In the dream the subject denies the similarity and says: " I am not staying. Just passing through."

Heterosexual Subject S

Night 5, REM 7:

> I was walking through a patient's room in order to get to another one and she had just returned from the operating room and had on one of those little short robes. She was indignant because I had gone through her room and made some remark about it not being a thoroughfare.

The second dream can be read as a response to watching the movie in which a couple are "making a baby." Again this subject says, "my interest in observing this is legitimate".

Heterosexual Subject J

Night 4, REM 4:

> I had just walked into a room where a young man and a young woman were changing the diapers on a new baby. I don't know whether I was supposed to be a doctor but it was obviously a hospital. She wasn't, you know, in bed or anything, you know. She was standing up. Neither one were in hospital robes but they did have a new kid and I seemed to be very interested in the, in the, kid, you know, the way it looked and the fact that it was healthy and so forth.

The role of the dreamer as doctor appears to be used defensively to prevent the sexual interests being recognized by others whereas the role of the dreamer as homosexual is expressive of their wish to be known.

Homosexual Subject P

Night 1, REM 3:

> It was a really dramatic scene in which, I don't know what doctor, some doctor I haven't met here, well it's like I had already finished the experiment or something like that and this doctor was a lady doctor who was terribly scandalized by the fact that I was homosexual. And she said, "If I had only known what you were for," and I said "That's not true and that's not the approach you should take and, uh, you don't understand what it's all about." And I was very gentle and kind and all that, and she sort of broke down and started crying. And I just explained the way things were, just pointing up the fact that some people make money the center of their lives, and some people make intellect the center of their lives, and some make taking care of their children the center of their lives. And in the end a lot of them make this some sort of monomania. And with homosexuals oft times the center of their lives

can just be sex. But at the same time they might be quite intelligent, and they may be intelligent as far as money matters are concerned, and so on and so forth, but they can never forget, never, never, never, [very dramatic] uh, that they are homosexual and that sort of broke both, broke both of us up.

Homosexual Subject M

Night 3, REM 1:

It was sort of a press conference. And we were talking about the fact that Gay Liberation was trying to do something good for the community with regard to a certain person. And we weren't getting any support. In fact members of the community were trying to destroy the organization. I was standing in front of a large machine of some sort which reminded me a lot of these newspaper racks that they have in libraries where the newspapers are on poles and hang like flags. Anyway, we were in front of a rack and we were illustrating various points of the press conference by pulling out the rack and there were pictures on there. This was after there had been some bloodshed and a lot of trouble. And people were saying things like "Oh what a shame it was, you know, that we didn't see these events sooner so we could have prevented them . . .

The impact of the film in making the homosexual subjects more self-revealing in the research context and the heterosexual subjects less so was also evident in the role analysis. The combined use of the three anonymous categories, alone, onlooker, and stranger, did not differ for the two groups on Night 1. Of the homosexuals', 25%, and 26% of the heterosexuals' dreams fell into these categories. On Night 2, following the movie, the homosexuals' use of these categories was reduced to 15% and the heterosexuals' increased to 46%, a significant difference in proportion.

Three content analysis scales, adapted from those developed by Whitman, Pierce, Maas, and Baldridge (1961) were applied by the rater to each REM report. These 6-point scales measured the degree of homosexuality between two or more men, the degree of heterosexuality, and the degree of intimacy. The mean score for each subject on each night was obtained and the group means of these scores. These scores, (see Table 8.4) appear to confirm the changes from pre- to postfilm nights to be in the opposite direction for the two samples. The heterosexual subjects reduce their scores on all three scales showing the dream interactions to be less intimate with both opposite- and the same-sex characters while the homosexual subjects move toward higher intimacy and closer relations following the film. This was particularly true for those reporting to the male experimenter.

The number of subjects being very small and variances large, few of these differences reached statistical significance. All the evidence, though, is consistent in pointing to a similar interpretation: the dream reports of the two groups of subjects were affected by the experimental situation quite differently and these differences were congruent with what they felt to be approvable behavior in their lab role. The demand characteristics of the laboratory were clearly different for these two groups and their dreams were shaped in response to these. For

TABLE 8.4

Homosexual, Heterosexual and Intimacy-Scale Ratings for Two
Samples before and after Erotic Film

	Night 1			Night 2		
	Homosexual	Heterosexual	Intimate	Homosexual	Heterosexual	Intimate
Heterosex ($N = 10$)						
Mean	1.32	.61	2.69	.96	.43	1.98
SD	1.14	.77	1.70	1.25	.42	1.33
Homosex ($N = 10$)						
Mean	1.05	.43	2.21	1.49	.49	2.99
SD	.71	.59	.89	.73	.35	.89
Male experimenter ($N = 5$)						
Mean	.97	.44	1.89	1.54	.78	3.09
SD	.82	.40	1.14	.83	.20	1.06
Female experimenter ($N = 5$)						
Mean	1.14	.43	2.54	1.44	.19	2.48
SD	.66	.79	.49	.72	.13	.93

Note: Het-Hom Night 2. Intimacy, $t = 1.989$; $df = 18$; $p < .05$, one tailed.

the first group the demand to report to professors was met with a need to hide their sexuality from these authority figures. For the second group the demand to report to straight researchers was met with the need to help us understand them. Two examples illustrate this difference. Both dreams take place in a bathroom adjoining a bedroom and involve an older woman. This was the actual situation in the sleep lab at the hospital where these subjects were seen. The subjects' rooms had been converted from cubicles which had originally housed bath tubs in an old ward bathroom. The bathroom itself was still in use and the subjects entered their bed rooms through this bathroom. The director of this lab was the senior author, a woman older than the subjects. In the first dream the subject, having been standing erect but innocent all night, is caught by an older authority figure.

Heterosexual Subject G

Night 3, REM 3:

> I had been to see my old girl friend, the one from New York. She was living at a dorm at − −, and we often had a habit of staying too late. Well in this case I overdid it and the ladies closed the door and for some reason instead of asking to get out I went with her upstairs and stayed in the bathroom of the little, you know, cubicle she was living in with another girl. The other girl didn't know I was there so apparently I just slept in there standing up all night long. The next morning there was an inspection of the room and I was caught. Ah, L− −, the girl I was going with, was gone and I had no explanation of how I got there so I was in kind of a tough spot. The lady who was doing the inspection was very nice about it. In fact she wasn't the least surprised when she opened the door and found me standing there. And that was it.

In the second dream the subject cooperates and is helpful to the older woman's interests in male sexuality.

Homosexual Subject D

Night 2, REM 3:

> A bathroom has some "male enlightenment." There was this old lady going through some things of her father who had died, and she was looking for a book called *Male Enlightenments*. The room looked like the master bedroom of my mother and stepfather. She was cute but real old and was trying to get this book *Male Enlightenments* in order to learn some sex techniques. It was funny because she was too old for that sort of thing. I liked her and found some things for her that she was looking for.

The findings do not support the interpretation that the laboratory has any general dampening effect on intimate dreaming or dreams with strong affects, nor that there is a sex of experimenter effect on these dreams that can be interpreted outside of the interpersonal context. Whether the lab has the effect to reduce or heighten certain types of dreaming and whether the sex of the experimenter reduces or increases reporting depends on how the experience is defined as a whole and how the possible responses to it are valued by the subject. Dream reports in the laboratory tend to support one's waking motivations and enhance a sense of self-worth in that context.

These data are supportive of the position taken by Whitman, Kramer, Ornstein, and Baldridge (1970), that the interpersonal situation in the sleep laboratory cannot be ignored. How then to respond to the original questions we asked? Are these reports representative of dreaming under home conditions, and if not what can be done about it? The best analogy may be to the behavior elicited in psychotherapy. In that situation as well, the material is responsive to the interpersonal context of patient and therapist and so differs from that observable under more neutral everydayish conditions. Dreams collected in the laboratory must be understood as behaviors in their own right, not as pale shadows of the more "real" home dreams. All dreams have both trait and state characteristics and as such must be interpreted in the light of the particular emotional context which preceded them and the motivations operating at the time. This makes the manipulation of the laboratory factors a fruitful field for research into dream processes as yet almost completely untouched.

ACKNOWLEDGMENTS

This work was carried out at the Department of Psychiatry, University of Illinois College of Medicine as part of a collaborative study with Marjorie Barnett, Gene Borowitz, and Arthur Kling. It was financed by Grants MH 18124 and MH 23450 from the U.S. Public Health Service. The authors are indebted to Nancy Chiswick, Linda Kamens, Sarah Labelle, Harvey Lucas, Frances Morowski, and Phyllis Walesby all of whom acted as laboratory assistants and judges.

EDITORS' INTRODUCTION TO CHAPTER 9

A chapter of this sort poses special difficulties for an editor because he can find little to add or to criticize. The reader will encounter a description of an experiment which is basically simple in concept — the effects of sustained alteration of color in the visual world of subjects during wakefulness on dream content. But this very simplicity leaves the reader a trifle unprepared for a *tour de force* of elegant experimental design, richness of result, thoughtful discussion and graceful prose.

9

The Effects of Sustained Alterations of Waking Visual Input on Dream Content

A PRELIMINARY REPORT[1]

Howard P. Roffwarg*
John H. Herman*
Constance Bowe-Anders
Edward S. Tauber

Department of Psychiatry, Montefiore Hospital
    and
Medical Center Albert Einstein College of Medicine

It is well known that the experiences of waking life may appear in the manifest content of dreams. Individuals can frequently trace elements of their dream content to both the perceptual and emotional experiences of the previous day or days (Freud, 1900/1953c). However, the visual percepts of waking life, when they appear in dreams, are not usually represented without change. Rather, they are transformed in varying degrees. Numerous unanswered questions concerning the sources, formation, and structure of dreams intrigue the dream researcher. It would be of considerable interest were the researcher able to determine, for example, what portion of the dream experience represents incorporated, stable perceptual input from the awake state, and in what part the dream functions as an indicator of the individual's endopsychic reflection and unresolved needs.

Though much has been uncovered about the physiology of dreaming, there have been relatively few attempts mounted to determine the processes underlying the modeling of the dream hallucinations themselves. For example, what

[1]This chapter is not a final report of these investigations. Additional data analysis and statistical evaluation will be published elsewhere. However, firm directions in the data and a preliminary discussion of their implications will be included here.

*Presently at the University of Texas at Dallas

factors govern the introduction of perceived material into the dream? Studies by other investigators have previously demonstrated that a variety of sensory stimuli applied during REM sleep may be "incorporated" into a dream in progress (Dement & Wolpert, 1958b; Berger, 1963). Other studies have examined the manifold ways in which bland or provocative cinematic material (Foulkes & Rechtschaffen, 1964; Witkin, 1969a; Cartwright, Bernick, Borowitz, & Kling, 1969), posthypnotic suggestion administered just prior to sleep (Stoyva, 1965; Tart & Dick, 1970), and group therapy and presurgery interviews engaged in before bedtime (Breger, Hunter, & Lane, 1971b) all may find expression in the night's dream production. However, these experiments have mainly utilized short-term stimulation by a finite stimulus, or by a structured or delimited situation, frequently with strong emotional counterparts.[2]

Though puzzling, it is nevertheless accepted that stimuli, be they inconsequential or deemed important, and paid close attention to by an individual during waking hours, may be entirely avoided in manifest dreams. On the other hand, as Fisher and co-workers have shown, exposure to stimuli of a fleeting and even subliminal nature can strongly affect dreaming (Fisher & Paul, 1959). Perhaps we are simply unaware of the ineluctable perceptual core of all the material in our dreams because memory fails us either in the recall of all dream images or of their sources in the many sensations we receive in waking life. What we can say with certainty is that, frequently, components of daytime experience, especially recent experience, are repeated in dreams. Freud (1900/1953c) contributed numerous convincing examples of this phenomenon in the *Interpretation of Dreams,* and daily confirmations of the phenomenon abound in all our lives.

Freud believed that the choice of a particular piece of recent experience for appearance in a dream was the function of a selective process. A perceptual element has a high likelihood of manifestation in dreaming to the degree that it proves to be a usable vehicle for the expression of basic drive in the operations of condensation, displacement and symbolic transformation. There seems to be considerable logic in this inference because, as has been pointed out, transient daytime percepts will frequently return in a dream, yet items that are daily represented to our senses rarely enter our nocturnal imagery.

Or do they? Perhaps these observations give short shrift to the myriad of sensory materials that may be equally as common in our dreaming as in our waking existences; the miraculous quantities of largely taken-for-granted sensory experiences, the enormous stores of sense data that, by functioning as perceptual building blocks, give the dream its amazing capability of seeming to revivify the actual world while we sleep. Considerable doubt must remain, then, as to whether the bulk of our perceptual experience is truly ignored in our dreams.

---

[2]See Chapter 10 of this volume for a detailed review of this literature [Eds].

Wherever the truth with respect to this issue lies, it appears likely that the natural laws of higher functioning that determine the selection of sense data and their transpositions into dream representations will not be fully elucidated for some time to come. Clearly, we are still at the very beginning of the road to understanding the relationship between our awake and dream existences.

AN APPROACH TO THE STUDY OF PERCEPTUAL INPUT AND DREAMING

The design of the studies we describe is aimed at increasing our knowledge concerning the influence of perceptual input in waking experience upon dreaming. Specifically, we wish to generate a base of elementary information in regard to whether constancies exist when the sensory exposures of waking life are processed in sleep by the central nervous system (CNS). Though our dependent variables are drawn from the content of dreams, this is not a primarily psychological study but rather an investigation into the "physiology" of dream content. In effect, we are looking for the *when, how,* and *how much* that describe the ways sense data appear in dreams.

A number of strategies are available with which to approach a study of this kind. For reasons that are taken up later, we elected to deal not with the foreground of visual information but with its background, which we believe can lay claim to constituting a relatively neutral setting for visual interactions with the environment. In our experimental procedure, we pervasively and continuously altered the coloration of visual perception. By such means, we sought to examine the ways in which dream-mentation processes an identifiable but indifferent perceptual input that, because of its continuousness and background character, would be largely free of associations to the particularities of time, place, person, and emotional change within the experimental period.

Furthermore, modification of the perceptual field solely in terms of color allows avoidance of other perceptual, proprioceptive, and perceptual-motor adaptations. No motor-response changes are required from the subjects except for a diminution of large eye movements. Accordingly, the subjects are not affected by the significant psychological processes inherent in spatio-motor relearning and adaptation. In effect, our goal was to study how the brain processes sensory stimuli of the least possible complexity that are received and registered in the least active manner.

We have followed up several questions in the form of control experiments that have emerged in regard to separation of the perceptual effects upon dreaming from other possible influences (like cognitive, subject and experimenter expectation), some of which could not be avoided. A number of these subsidiary studies are described below.

At this point, we turn to a further discussion of the rationale of this study, as well as to the theoretical issues it addresses.

STABILITY OF PERCEPTUAL MATERIAL IN DREAMING

Whatever else they may represent and functions they may serve, dreams contain the ordinary perceptual data of our everyday lives; that is, contained in our dream hallucinations we recognize, for example, familiar people, objects, and colors, as well as sounds, smells, kinesthetic and vestibular sensations: the routinely experienced contributions of all our other senses. These "perceptions" are sharply defined in dreaming and eminently retrievable by report in spite of the simultaneous examples of distortions, condensations, absurdities, and bizarre recombinations woven into the dream content.

It is a truism, but necessary to mention, that the sense data of dreams are composed of perceptual materials that accrue in our waking interactions with the environment. However, do these registrations function like raw materials, so that many forms and utilizations can be rendered from them? From many reports, perceptual materials appear to be quite plastic as they reemerge in dreaming. Our focus of interest, then, is on the processing principles, and the qualities of the systems of fabrication. Can the latter simply add and subtract dissimilar elements, or is it possible to mix elements and combine them, in the chemical sense, into wholly new compounds? For example, if in his visual experience an individual sees only yellows and blues, will he ever dream green? Or, in his dreams, would he be capable merely of constituting different yellow and blue designs, of interlacing, however finely, but never truly mixing the colors. To put it another way, is it possible that we may be able to reexperience in memory or in dreams only those perceptions that we have known, whereas we acknowledge the likelihood of considerably more creativity in relation to emotional and psychological phenomena? In the latter realms, we seem to be able to have experiences that are truly different from all that was known before.

With this distinction in mind, perhaps we can wonder whether perceptual "givens" are relatively nonpsychologically modifiable parts of the dream and, in a sense, more constitutional. Accordingly, the structural and perceptual building blocks of the dream may be under the predominant influence of the neurophysiological processes associated with perception, whereas the affective, situational and cognitive phenomena in dreams are probably regulated by a more complex interplay of forces. Stated more generally, our hypothesis is that the dream experience may follow the model of perceptual experience in the awake state in that certain aspects of perception such as color responses, depth responses, and all the other elements in the great variety of perceptual constancies are, in the main, quite stable.

Of course, perceptual material, found in fantasy and dreams, may also act to convey sensory realization of psychological meanings and emotional needs. It is possible that certain "sensa" may be stored for later use in representing particular affective and psychological purposes at particular times. If, for example, specific perceptual material were screened for a period of time from access to the CNS, might it nevertheless show up in dreams along with consciously or unconsciously associated recollections of singular experiences, thoughts or affects? Notwithstanding the phenomenon of perceptual reproduction in the workings of broader psychological processes, the question we pose is: *May the sense data themselves exert any influence on when and how they are employed?* In other words, do the sense data, owing to the attributes of quantity or immediacy of registration, take some part in determining their return in dreams? Or is the latter chiefly a function of their messenger potential?

Our experimental method used a quantitatively describable, loosely "tagged" visual input. We systematically monitored the timing and extent of appearance of this identifiable input into dreams, which were retrieved nightly under laboratory conditions. Our studies, then, have goals similar to studies that have attempted to use computer models of the brain in order to investigate information processing and dream material. But rather than attempt to test a favored "program" or "processing" model of our own, and then testing its validity, we have taken an alternative route; namely, of challenging the CNS with a retrievable input and looking at the effect of this input upon ensuing dreams. Thus, our aim is for the mind to "tell us" how it works. To put it another way, we hope that this type of experiment will help towards the development of information essential to the ultimate construction of more accurate models of the relationship of waking mental experience to dreams.

WHAT ELSE MAY BE GAINED FROM FOLLOWING PERCEPTUAL MATERIAL INTO DREAMS?

Also inherent in these experimental pursuits was the desire to add a bit to one of the long-term goals of sleep research: elucidation of the function of dreaming. Does dreaming actually serve as a safety valve for perceptual (and for perhaps other types of) overloads? It is conceivable that the brain may *use* dreaming in order to "junk" direct representations of overloads of perception, or to expel them in a modified or neutralized mode by means of some sort of active processing. Alternatively, it is possible that yet a different capacity may be observed: the capacity to regulate perceptual representation so that dreamlife may eschew excessive or noxious perceptual input. With this capability, the mind has the means to "escape" through dreaming to perhaps more varied or familiar types of stimulation from memory stores.

Possible, too, in these studies is the opportunity to gain information about memory function as it relates to the dreaming process. To what degree are recent and remote memories employed in dreaming, and how resistant are dreams to new experiential inputs? Are the latter taken up quickly in dreams or comparatively neglected in favor of earlier experience? And should dream content show a strong tie to recent input, is it possible that specific kinds of dream imagery associated with past events will break through and find dream expression?

Method

In view of the curious selectivity of the dream process in relation to daily experience, we decided, as discussed above, to study stimuli of a neutral yet unrelenting variety, applied over long periods of time; perceptual alterations that cannot be physically avoided. The "new" visual world of the subject is created through the continuous wearing, during all waking hours, of snugly fitted goggles containing special lenses. The subject thereby is situated in a visual milieu that is inescapably altered, but solely in terms of the color characteristics of the perceived imagery. No effects are induced on the spatio-temporal aspects of the visual field. We have described some early pilot work on these alterations (Tauber, Roffwarg, & Herman, 1968).

Characteristics of the Goggle Filters

In this color alteration study, filters (Kodak, No. 29, Wratten) were employed that interfere with the passage of all wave lengths save the red band. With these filters, entry of light begins only at 605mu, and by 640mu transmission is 88% of total luminosity. The wave length considered to be dominant is 632mu.[3] Total illumination is cut to a level equivalent to that of a cloudy day. No adaptation to these filters is possible, in the usual sense of a uniform shift of color identifications to different points in the color spectrum, because they allow entry of no other wave lengths. Inability to see any of the blue and green hues is complete until the lenses are discarded. Accordingly, this filtering results in perception of color exclusively in the red-orange band, though it should be noted that, in actuality, no red is added; rather, colors other than the transmitted wave lengths are occluded, leaving only the red band.

The goggle frames are designed for welders and are made of lightweight plastic. They are somewhat larger than eyeglass frames and have an aperture that permits 50 mm glass lenses to be mounted 0.75 in (19 mm) in front of the eyes. Though they are worn constantly during the day, they cause the subjects little discomfort because they were individually fitted to the contours of each subject's nose and zygomatic arch, cushioned at points of contact, and extensively ventilated. Peripheral vision was reduced somewhat (72° visual arc) by the opaque side frames.

The Visual Effect

Inasmuch as the appreciation of conventional lighting and color is precluded, the subjects experience a unique visual effect. Phenomenally, the visual surround seems blanketed in a monochromatic hue similar to red but slightly different. By day, the lenses give a light reddish cast to indirectly illuminated space, such

[3] 1931 CIE standard colorimetric and luminosity data (Crowell, 1953).

as the sky. However, circumscribed sources of light appear in stronger shades of true red, depending on the intensity of the light source and the level of proximate illumination. Outdoors at night, everything is seen as black except for light sources, which under these circumstances are vivid red.

The goggle filters induce a "washing out" of object color. Even reds appear strangely bleached owing to the fact that white and red objects are seen as virtually the same. This is so because the lenses allow only the red wave lengths emanating from the white and red objects to impinge upon the retina. In the absence of any contrast, both appear as "goggle color," a term that subjects have routinely used to describe the distinctively altered color coming through the filters. This hue is also variously called salmon, beige, and rose. When contrast is increased; for example, if a white or red object is placed against a large black object, a somewhat redder color is perceived. The size of the lens also makes a difference in the resulting effect; that is, a large "wrap around" lens increases the "washed out" quality, whereas a lens with a small diameter will cut down the input of light, increase contrast and, consequently, increase red coloration.

Since none of the color wave lengths in the yellow, blue, and green range pass through the filters, only the achromatic *value* (the relative whiteness or blackness, in Munsell color-chart terms) of an object in these color groups is perceived, accompanied by an amount of "goggle color" relative to the value of the object. White or lightly colored objects appear as weak red, whereas darker colored objects, or dark grey and black objects, appear achromatic.

Within the first few days, probably due to fatigue of the red-ON receptors, the environmental background seems less reddish. In effect, both foreground and background take on an appearance quite similar to the one that is created if a black and white movie is bathed in red light. As a consequence of the experimental procedure, the subjects are supplied with a continuous, pervasive, memorable, and novel effect.

Data Retrieval

In order to describe the whole range of their color perceptions in standardized and quantifiable terms, the subjects learned the Munsell system of numeric scales for designating hue, saturation, and value. All color types and shadings can be communicated in a highly reliable fashion with this system, and, though the appreciation of color is a private experience, the Munsell system provides objective dimensions for accurate intersubjective communication.

As an additional assist, the subjects memorized over 60 color names that were devised by us to denote singular and frequently encountered hues. (Some examples are "pigskin" brown, "Coca-Cola" sign red, and "Interstate Highway" green.) Though making use of the commonplace, the appellations provide a surprisingly precise means of verbal transmission of color experience. Added to the Munsell language, these names helped to achieve synchrony, and a sense of

TABLE 9.1

Red-Goggle Visual Effects

Atmospheric red tint
Loss of all vivid coloration, including red by day ("washed-out" effect)
Specific block of all greens and blues
No adaptation with time to permit return of filtered wavelengths
Prevalence of goggle color (salmon, melon, beige, rose, and so on)
Effect by day: much like a black-and-white movie bathed in red light
Effect by night: a black surrounding with bright reds from sources of light

shared validation of experience, in the task of communication between subject and experimenter.

Nightly dream production was analyzed for color with the help of a comprehensive dream-color interview schedule that we improved frequently in the course of our long period of trial experimentation. With this schedule, each scene (a single view, or the visual setting seen from a particular point of reference) of every dream was scored for its color content (see Appendix for the dream-scene questionnaire).

In the baseline period of the experiment, the normal color "profiles" of each subject for sleep onset (SO), REM, and NREM were developed from content awakenings. As a result, each subject's ensuing changes in dream color can be analyzed against baseline pattern by stage, as well as against normative data from other subjects. The dream scene interrogation schedule, which is employed with only slight modification in reference to questions about the goggles during all phases of the experiment, aims at designating background and object colors; presence or absence of atmospheric tints or casts; levels of saturation and illumination; prevalent, striking, and abnormal colors; determination of "how long ago" an object was seen in reality; and other items related to emotion and the sense of being in the "goggle world." These data are all retrieved directly from the dreamer at the time of each awakening and coded, quantified, and prepared for computer analysis. (See Appendix for the dream-scene data-entry sheet. The numbers correspond to those on the dream-scene questionnaire; Items 1-35 contain the independent variables, and Items 36-80 (2 sets) contain the dependent variables such as object and background color.)

The approach to the subject in terms of eliciting the desired data requires the important standardized-information schedule, but also the interrogator's "feel" for the credibility of responses, and some skills in elicitation. This is indicated in the admonitions not to bias the subject and in the other suggestions listed as part of the interrogator's "bible." A portion of it is included below. Of course, no interrogator becomes truly expert without many training sessions and pilot night work:

How to Approach the Interrogation of the Red-Goggle Subject

1. You never mention the purpose or reason for the study. Ask the subject to reserve questions until after participation has terminated. Refer to this investigation only as the "goggle study," not the "red-goggle study."

2. Rapidly get the subject to mention briefly the last two or three scenes remembered before being awakened. This will help to fix them in the subject's memory. More details can be elicited later about each one.

3. A scene consists of a single visual "situation" or "view." For example, if the subject describes that after turning around, seeing a different setting, the second setting is to be treated as an additional scene. Thus, if a subject is looking out a window and then turns to look inside a room, this is scored as two separate scenes. The colors, illumination, and so on, of the two views may be entirely distinct.

4. There is a *minimum* criterion for a scene or a single scene dream. The view must contain at least one object in a visual surround. Objects should be asked about for the presence of color and, if present, saturation. All objects have value (white, grey, black). Achromatic objects have no color and are, of course, not ranked for saturation. The assertion by the subject that an object is colorless has to be differentiated from the possible meaning that the subject doesn't know what the color was. The former is an achromatic response; the latter, a "don't-know" response.

5. After you take note of the scenes the subject reported, mention each in turn, allowing the subject to go through the questionnaire. (Use one questionnaire for each scene.)

6. For each scene, allow the subject a period to describe the colors and details in his or her own words. A good question to begin the unstructured portion of the interrogation is, "Let's go back to the scene about . . . ," or "What did the scene look like and what colors did you see?" You must always try to elicit all the required information in the dream-scene questionnaire, and keep the time the subject is kept awake to no more than 25 min.

7. If the description of a scene seems intellectualized or foggy, ask the subject if what is described was really seen. Can the subject picture it as you are being told about it, and as pictured in the dream? For example, if the subject says, "We were at the airport discussing the wingspan of an airplane," further questioning may reveal that during the discussion, the participants were not actually visualizing the plane. The point always is not where the subject was, or what the subject was doing, but what the subject *was looking at.*

8. Try yourself to picture the scene the subject is describing. Imagine what might be in such a scene that has not been mentioned, so that you can draw the subject out. For instance, if the subject speaks of seeing people, ask about their clothing. This is usually a good source of color. If the scene is indoors, ask about floors, furniture, windows, walls, ceiling, and so on. If outdoors, ask about ground covering, sky, trees, water, shrubbery, buildings, roads, and so on. Frequently, questioning the subject about a possible item that turns out not to be in the scene, will elicit the memory of another element of recall.

9. Don't push the subject. Allow time to think about what is being said and allow the subject to get some irrelevant things about the dream out of the way if it seems like they must be said.

10. While you are questioning the subject, scan the questionnaire form to make sure all data points have been covered.

Subjects and Procedures

Nine subjects were run with the No. 29 Wratten filters in the main study and others in control experiments. They were all students between the ages of 18 and 28 and were paid for their participation. Six were women and three were men. All had normal vision and color vision, and all were good dream recallers, as established on pilot nights.

In recruiting subjects for a 15- to 25-day consecutive experiment in which they would be wearing goggles by day and sleeping in the laboratory by night, we found that it was impossible to expect agreement from the subjects to serve if they were not told something about the conditions of the study. Accordingly, they were informed that the goggles contained filter lenses that altered color. The subjects were allowed to look *at* but not *through* some filters on one occasion before the study, but were told that the particular color of the lenses they would wear in the study proper would only be revealed to them on the first day they had to be worn. The frames, without filters, were fitted earlier. The subjects were also told that they would be awakened at intervals during the night and asked to describe the details of their dream imagery, when they recalled it.

The goggles were worn by the subjects during every waking moment. Procedures were worked out so that black occluders were worn, or eyes were closed, during washing, and companions were arranged for traveling in the evening. At first, we attempted to prevent any daylight from leaking in around the edges of the goggle frames. However, in the course of our work, we discovered that after several days with the goggles on, the subjects showed a tendency to become increasingly enmeshed in the new coloration of the goggle world in the awake state. They professed a growing lack of clarity when "visualizing" the screened out colors (yellows, blues, and greens) in their "mind's eye" for the purpose of making comparisons to goggle-transmitted colors during dream interrogations and testing. Though it was critical that the subject be able to distinguish and describe the differences between the induced dream colors and normal colors in their dreams, as the experiment proceeded, they found it increasingly difficult to be certain of differences. In an effort to stem this troublesome tendency, we began to be less rigorous about the small amount of peripheral "leakage" of ordinary light. Though the subjects were, at times, aware of this light at the margins of their visual fields, they could not focus on it foveally. Nevertheless, it provided them with a ready and helpful referent of normal light and coloration. We are aware that the light leakage may have affected our results to some degree. But the problem of inchoate subject inability to distinguish "goggle" color from true color as the experiment proceeded, we felt, represented the greater danger insofar as the critical raw data came exclusively from the subject's differentiations of color in dreams. In terms of the experimental consequences, we made the assumption that any "leakage" of old color would tend only to reduce, not enhance, the effect of the filters.

At night, the subjects slept with black patches over their eyes in an absolutely dark room and were polygraphically monitored. The next morning, before the lights were turned on, the goggles were reapplied by the subjects. Subjects were awakened five or six times nightly for interrogations at points of sleep onset and in REM and NREM sleep.

An attempt was made to achieve a representative number of awakenings from each stage throughout the night so that a time-of-night analysis of the dream reports could be carried out. The data was grouped into early, middle, and late cycles by early, middle, and late nights of the experimental phase. Except for the NREM awakenings, which were actually all from Stage 2, and, consequently, were not adequately represented in the first cycle, the data were collected into three time-of-night groupings: first NREM-REM cycle; second and third cycle; and fourth and later cycles. Unfortunately, because of "skipped" first REM periods, some failures of recall in the first cycle awakenings, and the single-cycle composition of the first grouping, the number of REM scenes is small in the first group. The data groupings across nights were first night, second and third nights, and fourth and fifth nights. Care was taken (by skipping REM periods) that at least 90 min of REM sleep was allowed each night.

In order to avoid REM-deprivation effects, interrogations were kept to a maximum of 30 min though the mean interrogation time was 15-20 min. The total of time asleep averaged about 7 hr per night. (Additional details of awakening criteria for each stage will be provided in another report of these studies.)

Each subject was studied for a period ranging from 12 to 22 days, following upon several adaptation nights. This period of investigation was broken up into several phases. Within each phase the nights were consecutive. There was no break between the baseline, experimental and recovery phases. All subjects went through the phases in the same order:

1. color-baseline period: 4-5 days; no goggles, or goggles with clear glass lenses (clear glass goggles as a control for restriction of peripheral vision);

2. illumination control period (optional): 3-5 days; goggles fitted with neutral-density filters (an opportunity to control for reduction of illumination and restriction of peripheral vision before color alteration);

3. altered-color period ("red-goggle" period): 5-8 days; goggles fitted with No. 29 Wratten filters;

4. return to normal-vision period (recovery period): 3-4 days no goggles, or goggles with clear glass lenses.

During the study period the subjects did not nap. They generally were able to continue in their typical routines of study, recreation, exercise, interpersonal and social contact, and travel during all phases of the study. Every attempt was made to encourage maintenance of daily activities and variation in visual environments.

During the altered-color period, subjects, when queried, spoke of having a great desire to see blues and greens. In the daylight of the first recovery day, when for the first time the red filters were removed, almost all subjects, if asked to gaze at a white screen, reported a green-blue tint. This effect lasted a few hours.

On certain key change days in the study sequence, the subjects were examined in several ways under the conditions of the period they were in (with no goggles in baseline and recovery; with red filters in the altered-color period):

1. During each day the subjects went for a walk with an experimenter. One outdoor and one indoor scene were selected, and the subject was asked to describe them so that a (dream) scene questionnaire could be completed for each one. This test checked on the stability of the waking "goggle effect," and its relationship to any alterations in the visual content of dreams. The purpose of this check was to learn whether an effect of the goggles, reflected in dreaming, was the same or perhaps different from their effect when the subject was awake.

2. During each day a brief interview was given to elicit a description of daily activities, reaction to the experiment, mood level, sensitivity to the comments and opinions of others (during "red goggle" period, particularly), and level of anxiety.

3. Before retiring the task was to put Munsell color patches of various saturations and values in the order the subject thought correct on red, blue, yellow, and green Munsell value and saturation grids; also, a white patch had to be identified in terms of tint, if any. Every night of the baseline period and on the last night of the altered-color period, a red-to-blue continuum of patches was displayed quickly to the subjects' naked eye, and designation of the single achromatic patch was required. A complete (dream) scene questionnaire was completed for several selected vivid-color magazine plates.

Nightly testing of subjects indicated a uniform inability to tell one hue from another in the altered-color period, and an absence of any evidence of adaptation in terms of color perception (that is, the subjects could not identify goggle-occluded colors). In other words, the type and extent of errors in color identification made by subjects wearing the goggles generally remained constant over time. Notwithstanding, in the latter days of red exposure, subjects occasionally noted that an object that they knew to be green (like a head of lettuce or a traffic light) looked green.

The subjects used several methods of trying to enlarge the range of their unyielding, narrowed perception of color. For example, they flirted, though usually unsuccessfully, with the attempt to identify colors by utilizing the value scale, an available but misleading clue. In addition, subjects frequently made attempts during the red-goggle period to surmise the actual color of an object by noting the degree of its visual similarity to another object color, when a memory of the pregoggle color of the latter was still retained.

The visual distortion caused by the goggles seemed to evoke a feeling of social isolation in some subjects. Though all subjects continued to function in their normal daytime routines, they occasionally reported a sense of "separation" from the real world, feeling at times more like observers than participants. They were interested in this experience, rather than alarmed by it, and they exhibited no affective changes of note during the study.

Perceptual Influx-Dream Efflux: Analysis of the Experimental
Effect

As must be already clear, we have employed in this research an experimental paradigm roughly parallel to a metabolic input-output design, or pharmacokinetic study. In terms of this approach, we follow the "excretion" into dream content of the perhaps unchanged or degraded "metabolites" of the new input. The different parameters of analysis of the dream scenes, which were collected night by night and REM period by REM period were utilized to provide the following types of information:

1. the latency time from the first expsoure to the altered perceptual environment to the first changes in the visual appearance of dreams;
2. the degree of alteration or penetration of the hallucinations of sleep by the goggle effect; that is, the "increase over baseline" in the concentration of the new input in response to each "dose," each daily perceptual exposure. (The data are expressed in terms of the average nightly degree of effect of the infusion on successive days.),
3. the intranight, or time-of-night, changes in the "excreted" constituents after termination of each day's dose; and
4. the rate of elimination, or rate of return to baseline, in the concentration of new input in the days (recovery period) following the last exposure.

Outcome Hypotheses

One of the strengths of this design is that each subject is an individual control, so that assessment of individual differences in direction or size of the main effects is possible. Before we began this experiment, and in its early phases, we tried where possible to construct predictions in regard to the effects of a visual red load upon the color and illumination qualities of the dreams. These hypotheses were based on an analysis of preliminary data from pilot subjects. The data-coding and data-quantification system allow us ultimately to reject or confirm these predictions statistically in relation to the experimental outcome in the population studied after their formulation.

An abbreviated list of "goggle effect" hypotheses is listed below, followed by predictions of several general and resultant effects.

Components of the Goggle Effect in Dreams

(Note: "goggle" phase period refers to the experimental period when color alteration goggles are worn; "goggle" color refers to the spectrum of "goggle-"transmitted colors.)

1. (a) There will be an increase in the proportion of tinted scenes in the goggle phase. The increase will be directly proportional to the number of goggle nights until the number of tinted scenes reaches an asymptote.

(b) The color of the tint will reflect the goggle color.

2. The illumination of scenes will become darker (that is, it will reflect the level of the illumination with the goggles) with a progressive increase in illumination as the night continues.

3. (a) On goggle nights, in contrast to control and neutral-density-filter nights, the degree of saturation will be inversely related to the illumination of the scene.

(b) There will be a general decrease in saturation with the goggles and a progressive increase in saturation as the night continues.

4. As to the proportion of individual object colors, there will be:

(a) a decrease in the proportion of *true* object colors during the goggle period;

(b) an increase in the proportion of high value achromatic objects;

(c) an increase in the proportion of goggle color objects, and a decrease in the proportion of nontransmitted colors; and

(d) a general decrease in the reported saturation of all colors.

5. (a) There will be an increase in the proportion of scenes containing a *prevalent* color.

(b) The prevalent color will be a goggle color.

6. There will be an increase in the proportion of *abnormal* colors reported during the goggle phase. (*Abnormal* color is defined as an inappropriate color, neither seen without, nor with, the goggles; perhaps indicating a "symbolic" transformation such as, for example, bright red money.)

7. As to the goggle effect on sources of light, there will be:

(a) an increase in the proportion of tinted light sources; the increase will be positively accelerated as the number of goggle nights increases; and

(b) the tint of the light source will reflect goggle color.

Temporal and Interactional Effects

1. The characteristics of dream coloration in the phases of the experiment will be found in equivalent degree in the hallucinatory material from REM, NREM, and sleep onset awakenings.

2. There will be a progressive increase in the "goggle effect" (components 1-7 above) as the number of goggle days increases.

3. All strengths of the goggle effect will diminish serially with the ordinal period of the awakening in the night.

4. The recovery time (the number of days before the goggle effect has worn off) will be directly related to the time spent in the goggle condition, or to the intensity of the goggle effect.

5. During the recovery phase (period of return to normal vision), the deprived colors and tints will be in greater proportion than in the baseline phase; "goggle effect" colors and tints will be in lesser proportion than in the baseline phase.

6. Waking experiences, occurring during the goggle period and incorporated into the dreams, will have a greater likelihood of showing the goggle effect than will waking experiences occurring prior to the goggle period and present in goggle-phase dreams; the latter will display more nontransmitted colors and true colors than the former.

7. There will be a correlation between particular emotions and particular tints or prevalent colors.

As pointed out earlier, we decided to study a distinctive but hopefully neutral change in color perception with the aim of gathering data about whether it would provoke a shift in dream color. The *direction* of change was secondary in our interests. When trying to guess the results before the pilot experiments, the members of our group differed in their opinions; some took as a guide the frequent expression in dreams of daily experience and sensation in near to original form; others were influenced by the idea that the overwhelming and inescapable nature of the perceptual load would force an active neutralization into compensatory (opposite) forms. They buttressed their view with information that the effects of color overload are not limited to the retinal receptors but occur also at higher levels of the CNS. DeValois, Abramov, and Mead (1967) have demonstrated a diminution in the firing of red-ON receptor neurons and a lowered firing threshold of the blue-green-ON units in the lateral geniculate nucleus after chronic exposure to red light. It might also be that the cortex is similarly affected. In terms of these findings, it was argued that the increased nocturnal firing of the "ready" blue-green-ON cell, and the corresponding reduced nocturnal discharge of the fatigued red-ON cells, would result in an internal "input" to the visual cortex and a relative increase in hallucinatory appreciation of the unseen (by day) color. A perhaps somewhat too simply drawn wish-fulfillment view also prompted others to the conclusion that deprived colors would be increased during the dreaming of the goggle phase. In sum, when these experiments were being formulated, the weight of opinion within our group tilted slightly to the view that predicted compensatory color dreaming (active processing) in the goggle phase, and away from the passive transfer (red effect) view.

Of course, many different outcomes could be hypothesized. For example, why not expect an initial take-up of the red world in the early days of the goggle period, and a reversion to earlier inputs in the latter days? Or, perhaps an oscillating predominance of new and old inputs. Another point of view was that with the advent of goggle color vision, all color in dreams would temporarily increase in proportion to noncolor elements, and that this effect would soon wear off, even though vision is still altered in the waking state.

During many presentations of this experimental design to scientific gatherings and to color perception experts, we polled the audiences as to their prediction of the result. Generally, the group that expected red-type results and those predicting blue-green results shared approximate pluralities. However, a smaller, though sizable group, has always asked to be counted for a no-effect result. The latter view sees the dreaming process as able completely to avoid the new input and rely on longer-term memory storage.

Sampling our own earlier views and those of sophisticated experts has made one conclusion plain: though our experimental manipulation was uncomplicated, and the phenomenal experience of the subjects quite uniform, prediction of the outcome on dreaming proved difficult. Neither the operations of common sense nor the sifting of theoretical models fostered universal agreement with respect to the main effect. Unitary and sweeping, the red-goggle condition tempted easy predictions. But rarely were the reasons for particular choices unquestionably superior to the logic of other predictions.

Some Conceptual and Methodological Issues

We have taken the liberty of interpreting the goggle-color entry-dream output concept as an analogy to a pharmacokinetic paradigm. Naturally, the parallel is inexact in many respects. One important difference, which must be understood before the issue of data significance is resolved, is that in drug studies, little, if any, concentration of the agent will be present in body products before its interpolation. In our research, however, the degree of goggle effect is scored from a grouping of red and red-related colors in a variety of forms. Though the effect is at times distinctive, it is at times partial, and the proportion of this group of colors in relation to the proportion of nontransmitted colors becomes the critical variable. Inasmuch as red-related colors are present in normal vision, the goggle colors are not qualitatively new. In other words, there is a goggle-color level in baseline and recovery.

The task in this study is, therefore, not the discovery of something wholly new in dreams against the standard of its prior nonexistence, but the identification of an increase or decrease in a set of materials in dreams, measured against their, fortunately, fairly stable baseline dream levels. For this reason, the significance of the color ratios in the goggle period can only be decided relative to the values in the baseline period.

Another question is why we chose to impose the color red and not another color on the visual terrain. The reason is empirical; we would have been equally happy with green or blue, and delighted to examine for selective penetrance of several colors. However, no filters are made that are as exclusive for these colors as the sharp cutoff filters for red. Hence, blue and green rapidly lost their saliency for the subject in the awake state. Perhaps also because of the greater representation of blue and green in the background coloration in nature (e.g., vegetation, sky), when the subjects wore blue or green lenses in strengths that would not make all imagery exceedingly dark, the world did not look sufficiently unusual or idiosyncratic to stand out for identification and comparison purposes. This specific methodological finding hints at a general problem with dream recall data in this experiment: differences between standard and altered imagery *must* be remembered; what is not poignantly identified as atypical imagery is presumed to be standard. It could thus be claimed that if experimental changes in dream content are found at all, their true magnitude in dreams may be greater than we will be able to ferret out of subjects's reports.

Experimental Bias and Subject Set

In the evolution of this project, we have become aware of the many possibilities for bias, and the necessity for controlling, or at least partitioning off the variance due to such factors. This study required exposure of the subject to: (1) a distinct and identifiable change in perception; and (2) a concentration on the color characteristics in dreams (because of awakenings for dream content in the laboratory). Therefore, we had to contend with the almost inevitable likelihood that the subject would make a connection between the two. The subject is propelled into native theories probably, but not exclusively, concerning the effects of the new surround, or contact with the laboratory upon dream life. The subject might also become concerned with other "purposes" of the research and other "directions" of effects.

As a matter of fact, the subject is affected by at least two categories of suggestion: the first, growing out of compliance with, or negativism towards, what the subject speculates are the laboratory's "expected" results, may affect the veracity of dream reporting; and the second, *attention to* rather than *perception of* redness during waking life, is more occult and may actually affect the nature of the dream perceptions themselves. Whatever the prior expectations about the goggle effect, the subject begins to "think" about redness when the goggles are first seen, and certainly when first donning them and having the initial red effect.

For the purpose of differentiating between an effect in the dreams as a result of the subject's *perception* of red or as a result of *attention* to red, we must at least acknowledge the possibility of a *cognitive* "input" (or "output," if you will) in addition to a *perceptual* input of red. Of course, in a given individual the conscious awareness of redness may set up even a countervailing subject expectation. For example, a student, who came to the pilot experiment as a subject, had previous knowledge about "after-image" phenomena. After experiencing the "goggle" effect, the subject swiftly drew the conclusion that flashes of complementary color would soon be expected in dreams, as often experienced during "after-image" experiments at the university.

In view of these contingencies, a group of control experiments, designed to test the power of various sources of suggestion and bias, were carried out. (They are described following the Results Section of this chapter.) The experimental team, in pilot work, gradually became aware of the demand characteristics of this experiment upon the subject's expectations. We attempted to keep in mind the possible influence and significance of the demand characteristics throughout the several phases of each "run." Towards this same end, we also asked the subjects to record their initial ideas and impressions about the purposes of the study, as well as any later shifts in their belief system.

Although several additional sources of contamination are possible by virtue of experimenter suggestion, we attempted to be aware of them and minimize them (as well as to test for them in control runs). We paid close attention to our experimental contacts with the subjects, and kept our casual conversations, as well as our dream-scene interrogations, as free as possible from the kinds of comments and responses that might transmit real or fancied expectations.[4]

However, because we never could be certain that we had not dropped "clues" in regard to our experimenter expectations, or put unwitting or unconscious "pressure" upon the subject to perform in line with an expectation, we attempted to account for these possibilities by encouraging the subject to be sensitive to our presumed cues or slips. The subject knew that, following the study, we would allow a discussion about if and how the subject had been influenced. In these rather extended "debriefing" sessions, we checked on such items as the subject's beginning- and end-of-the-run theories about the experiment; the hints the subject felt he or she received from the experimenters; the colors, if any, in the dreams, which the subject thought were most favored by the experimenters; the responses given that the subject sensed aroused the most experimenter "interest," as well as other sources of suggestion.

Of course, as mentioned above, most subjects harbored the idea through the course of the study that the investigators' interests pertained to the relationship between perceived color in the awake state and color in dreams. It was encouraging, however, in terms of our wish that subject expectation not influence the results, that the range of these expectations spanned all the theoretical possibilities about color shifts in dreams. A minority of subjects had divined, or were in agreement, with the laboratory's postpilot hypothesis in comparison to the majority who entertained inaccurate suppositions about our expectations. However, certain subjects became convinced, as the study proceeded, that finding out about color in dreams *could not* be the purpose of the 24-hr-per-day, multiday investigation. Rather, they speculated, the study was designed to test their psychological reactions under certain circumstances. On the basis of cursory analysis, there was no correlation between subject expectation and experimental outcome.

Another methodological problem is that the optimal design of a "red-goggle" study would have the dream interrogators experimentally blind to what phase of

---

[4] In retrospect, it is clear that several items on the dream-scene questionnaire potentially biased the subject's dream reports towards the visual effect seen with the goggles during the day. They did so by virtue of asking the subjects to compare the coloration of the dream scenes against that of the appearance of the world when subjects were awake and wearing the goggles. The subjects were not asked to reference the dream scenery to the opposite coloration or to any other standard. In view of this skew, it is fortunate that the data elicited from the inquiries in question were very much in line with the data observed in response to other items for which no standard of comparison to the dream imagery was required. (Of course, it could still be contended that the *few* items that presented a comparison to the waking state visual effect could have biased *all* responses.)

the experiment the subjects were in at any time. Ideally, all members of the experimental team who had communication with the subjects should have been unaware of the objectives and possible hypotheses of the investigation. Superior though such a design would be, it was not practicable to do a series of "runs" that each could take up to several weeks under such circumstances because of lack of adequate personnel and difficulties in control over laboratory communication for such long periods of time. In terms of maintaining interrogators "blind" as to phase of experiment, one obvious problem is the great potential for a subject, when being interrogated about comparative-color appearances in dreams, to divulge what is currently being seen through goggles by day. As a matter of fact, several of the interrogator's questions required comparative information about the waking goggle effect.

The possibility of experimenter influence over the subject's responses was reduced owing to the interrogator's use of a semiquantified interrogation system that was designed to eliminate subject and experimenter judgements as to the responses. The questions are standardized; the scales are dichotomous, or numerical rankings; the subject is trained to make independent choices in all cases; the data flows virtually direct from subject to sheet, leaving the interrogator little room to make decisions and interpretations. Further, the interrogators were encouraged to see themselves only as prompters of responses to the questionnaire items, and to be concerned only with the flow of data, not with its nature.

We by no means wish to argue that our procedures obviated the possibility of subtle cues and encouragements coming from the experimental team. However, it is our belief that the procedures were of considerable protection. We have an additional opportunity to learn about interrogator pressure by obtaining the ratings of independent judges on the subjects' free narrative of the dream — a portion that is collected before questioning by the experimenter — in order to compare the spectrum of its color references to the subjects' questionnaire responses.

Preliminary Survey of Experimental Results

A recapitulation of the main procedural facets of the study: after a baseline period in which data were accumulated for individual baseline-color profiles, the subjects wore the red goggles, which blocked out all light except in the red wave lengths, all day long for a period of five to eight days. The subjects, who were excellent dream recallers, were awakened from REMS, NREMS, and SO periods. Their dreams were systematically collected and were later analyzed for the types and intensities of foreground and background color.

Goggle Effect in Dreaming

There can be no question that the perceptual alterations that the subjects experienced in waking hours were reflected in their nocturnal dreams. Every subject who wore the goggles, like the earlier pilot subjects, had a strong, phenomenal "goggle effect" in dreams. This effect rendered the visual imagery scarce for blues and greens. It significantly increased the proportion of object colors in the red-orange band, and tinted sources of light and the atmosphere in the same shades. No subject increased dreaming of blues, greens, and other deprived hues.

A critical finding was that the reddish-tint effect in dreaming was precisely the type seen in the waking state. Though it did not affect all dreams, when present the color experience of the whole scene or parts of it was typical of the appearance of the goggle world. The presence of a reddish tint in their dream views of open atmospheric space was considered by the subjects to be a prime feature of the daytime alteration of the visual milieu. An analysis of the data in our first five subjects indicated a more than fivefold increase over baseline in the number of red-related, tinted scenes in REM dream awakenings during the goggle phase of the experiment (see Figure 9.1). The entire population of subjects showed a 3.5 multiple of enhancement in this dimension. And, though baseline tints of other colors were not numerous, a decided trend to fewer tints in all other (goggle-filtered) colors was evident under interference filter conditions. The latter finding indicates that the red-goggle period did not provoke a general increase in all dream color; rather the increase seemed to be selective to the goggle-permitted wave lengths.

Several specimen examples follow of the opening, unrestricted narratives of dreams, which were collected in the goggle phase (first two) and baseline phase (last dream). Extensive questioning followed each of these uninterrupted beginnings.

The first dream was well recalled and was considered to have a strong goggle effect.

Subject MS
4th REMP, 3rd goggle night

"Yeah, yeah, I really remember this . . . . Just as you woke me up, a girl named Chris was saying, 'This creep is going on national TV, advertising himself.' She was talking about a guy we were looking at. He was dressed in a forest green shirt. He was sitting on a bench, outdoors. The man had just said, 'My dancing could be improved . . . you don't have to be so great looking.' There were faded autumn leaves all over the ground. The setting was like Central Park by the Sheep Meadow. The whole scene was kind of dim, sort of like later afternoon, and all the colors were very washed out. His green shirt was almost black, the way things that I know are green look through the goggles. This whole scene was like a movie I went to see the other day with the goggles on. Everything was sort of red and white (laugh). On the scene there was a pervading amber tint but it wasn't all black around, like in the movie house. The sky was a dark, reddish brown. This is similar to the way things look through the goggles, but not exactly the same."

The following specimen was less well recalled. Nevertheless, the restricted range of color and the emphasis on "goggle" colors is clear.

Subject MH
2nd REMP, 4th goggle night

"A crowd of blacks was having some kind of a ritual ceremony on the main street of a small southern town. Rows of low wooden buildings made up the sides of the street. They were really dilapidated! As you were waking me up, this guy was admonishing me for not showing respect by standing when I should have been sitting down. His skin was black with a hint of amber wherever light was reflected. His clothes were nondescript, but they looked something like what light colored objects look like through the goggles in the daytime; you know, kind of shades of grey, but all faintly reddish. The sky and the walls of the building were that amberish, reddish, brownish, orange type of color (goggle color) that I see outdoors through the goggles, at about six or seven PM when I look at the sky. In this dream I must have been wearing the goggles because — I think I was — because I experienced a sense of restricted vision at the sides. I know you're going to ask me some questions now, but I want to tell you that I felt awe and confusion about the ceremony. I was really embarrassed because I messed up their program . . . ."

The final example, by contrast, is from a baseline period.

Subject SJ
4th REMP, 2nd baseline night

"I was sitting with a little boy I know in a room I never saw before. I used to baby sit for him. There were flowers all over the room. He was saying, 'The only way you can communicate is through writing.' Then I said he was lucky because he had somethig of the new world and something of the old. That's when you woke me up. The room was well lit. It was paneled in walnut wood, sort of a light brown color, and the furniture was also light brown wood. Let me tell you about the rest of the room. There were flowers all over the room; lots of vases just filled with them. There were white mums, pink roses and sky blue petunias. On the right was a light green radiator cover and the windows were covered by egg shell colored blinds. The boy was wearing a white t-shirt with yellow elephants on it and green pants. I think there was a light gray carpet on the floor. On the left was a maroon chesterfield couch . . . ."

As pointed out earlier, the color effect in the altered-color condition is inferred from differences in the parameters of tint object color types, and so on, between the experimental and baseline conditions. Though these parameters are obviously components of a goggle effect, they do not define the actual totality

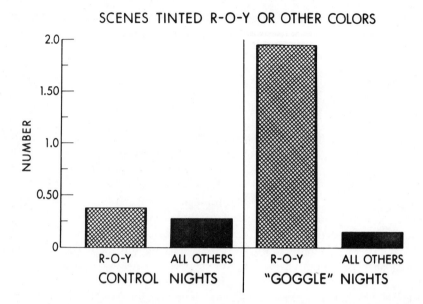

FIG. 9.1   Preliminary count of tinted dreamed scenes per night in the first five subjects. R-O-Y: red-orange-yellow band of colors, equivalent to "goggle," or transmitted, colors, as defined in the text (orange-yellow is at the border of the red band). Control nights: baseline-period nights; "goggle nights: nights in the goggle phase of the experiment.

of impression (goggle effect) that the subject experiences in viewing the surround during the awake state with the red goggles on. Another item in the questionnaire, "goggle-world appearance," probes specifically for the subject's sense of the total effect. This measure reveals that more than half of *all* dream scenes in the goggle phase (60% on Nights 4 and 5) had wholly or pervasively incorporated the goggle-altered daytime experience. This effect is actually quite rare in baseline conditions, but we have conservatively estimated its presence in baseline, during which it cannot be asked about, at 22%.

In each dream scene recalled, the subject had an opportunity to report up to 10 objects visualized in the panorama. The percentage of all objects in each scene comprised by particular color bands was calculated. Figure 9.2 is based on the data from our first 5 subjects. In the first 5 nights under altered-color conditions, a sharp, serial increase occurred simultaneously with a progressively descending, albeit undulating, course taken by the nontransmitted colors. The highest proportion of the achromatic or white-grey-black group of object colors, was found during the illumination-control period prior to the red-goggle phase. Their lowest percentage was posted on the fifth night of the goggle period. This set of successive whole night, object-color proportions also reveals a surprising finding: the apparent return to virtual baseline values on the very first night after goggle-altered vision was terminated. The data concerning object colors has been subjected to somewhat different analyses as part of the data from our total group of subjects. Absolute percentages for each group are subject to some revision, but the relative proportions among color groups across the phases of the experiment are entirely representative.

The same data has been grouped to look for different effects through the course of each night's sleep. We examined mean dream-scene data in each of the baseline (precontrol, in Figures 9.2 to 9.3), neutral density, red-goggle and recovery (postcontrol, in Figures 9.2 to 9.3) phases along a vertical continuum in three blocks, essentially tantamount to thirds of the night (REM Periods 1, 2 and 3, and 4 and 5).

When the results are surveyed this way, the striking finding emerges that the increase in goggle-color objects and the decrease in nontransmitted-color objects is an early-night effect primarily, all but disappearing after the third REM period (see Figure 9.3). The effect is sufficiently strong in the early REM periods to endow the total-night means (see Figure 9.2) with the effect. The presumption would be that the effect must gain in strength primarily in the early REM periods as the experiment proceeds.

The specific data for the chromatic groups in each of the more than 15 scene-color variables are too numerous to be included here and will be described in future publications. However, the findings first noted for object colors (see Figures

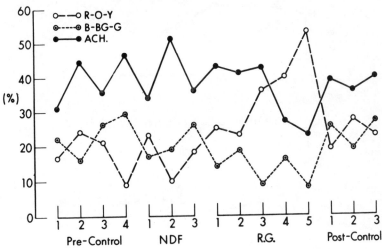

FIG. 9.2 Preliminary data on object colors represented in the dream scenes of the first five subjects. R-O-Y: as in Figure 9.1; B-BG-G: blue, blue-green, green object colors; ACH: achromatic objects; Pre-Control: baseline period; NDF: neutral-density-filter period; R.G.: red-goggle period; Post-Control: recovery period.

OBJECT COLORS
FIRST REM PERIOD

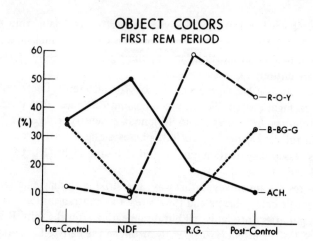

SECOND AND THIRD REM PERIODS

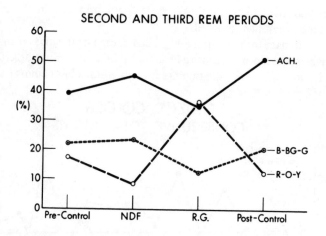

FOURTH AND SUBSEQUENT REM PERIODS

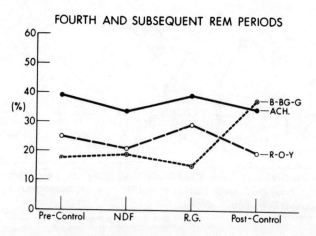

9.2 and 9.3) are in harmony with the data in other goggle-effect parameters as well. Two-way tables of incidence of each parameter were prepared for the duration of time (days) in the goggle phase and for the duration of time (REM periods) in the goggle nights. Such data displays (see Tables 9.2 and 9.3) make it even clearer that the goggle effect was observed chiefly in the early REM periods and the later nights of the altered-color period. Accordingly, two vectors of activity, one showing a gain in activity with increasing number of nights, the other showing a loss of activity in the course of nights, combine into a resultant hypothetical vector that predicts the weakest goggle effect in the last REM period of the first goggle night and the strongest effect in the first REM period of the last goggle night. This prediction was largely borne out (Roffwarg, Bowe-Anders, Tauber, & Herman, 1975).

The reverse of this picture expresses the goggle effect for the nontransmitted colors, which are, in effect, the complementary colors of the red band. Among this group, the first REM period of Goggle Nights 4 and 5 fell to about 11%, and the fourth and fifth nights showed a total reduction of 50% in baseline representation of the colors. Because the goggle effect wears off in the latter portion of the first night, the proportion of nontransmitted colors, like goggle colors, is about normal.

The Recency Phenomenon

Though total period data made it appear that the effect was almost exclusively in the first two-thirds of the night (see Figure 9.3), it became clear that the effect extended later into the night in direct proportion to the number of nights in the goggle condition. Figure 9.4 is an attempt to illustrate the several temporal and intensity components of the goggle effect. The data strongly suggest what we have come to call the recency phenomenon in relation to the effect of perceptual change upon dreaming; that is, recent perceptions tend to be dreamed in the first REM periods of the night, and with increasing longevity of the input, their expression in dreaming penetrates into the later REM periods.

It should also be pointed out that, though prominent, the goggle effect in the subjects' dreams, except in certain scenes, never completely obliterated the appearance of other colors. Blues and greens sharply fell off, yet even in the latter nights of the goggle period, dreams were reported that still were composed of nontransmitted colors. These could only have been preserved in memory. Only in the first REM period of the last nights in the goggle condition did goggle-effect penetrations become almost exclusive. Mean dream-penetration incidences for whole nights did not exceed 60%.

An unexpected and theoretically significant finding is the "recasting" in goggle colors of some imagery in dreams that had been observed in waking

FIG. 9.3 a, b, c.   Same data as in Figure 9.2 broken up by REM-period groupings, with the value of each color rubric presented as the mean value of the nights in the phases of the experiment. Abbreviations are the same as in Figure 9.2.

TABLE 9.2

Percentage of Goggle Colored Objects

	Baseline			Experimental Phase				Recovery		
	All but last two nights	Last two nights	Total baseline	First night	Second and third nights	Fourth and fifth nights	Total Experiment	First night	All but first night	Total recovery
First REM/NREM period										
N scenes	3	15	18	3	4	10	17	4	4	8
% goggle objects	34.4	41.2	37.8	56.7	37.5	85.2	60.4	26.1	32.8	28.3
% of baseline total	88.5	105.8	97.2	145.6	96.4	219.0	155.3	67.1	84.2	72.8
Second and third REM/NREM periods										
N scenes	37	43	80	19	39	18	76	18	8	26
% goggle objects	44.9	44.3	44.6	43.0	58.4	44.0	49.5	48.6	41.1	46.1
% of baseline total	115.4	113.9	114.7	110.4	149.9	113.1	127.3	124.8	105.6	118.4
Fourth and later REM/NREM periods										
N scenes	26	47	73	27	44	23	94	15	7	22
% goggle objects	26.7	41.9	34.3	37.7	41.8	53.1	45.5	40.6	33.8	38.4
% of baseline total	68.6	107.7	88.2	96.9	107.3	136.3	116.8	104.4	86.9	98.6
Total for night										
N scenes	66	105	171	49	87	51	187	37	19	56
% goggle objects	35.4	42.5	38.9	45.8	45.9	60.8	51.8	38.4	35.9	37.6
% of baseline total	90.9	109.1	100.0	117.6	117.9	156.2	133.1	98.8	92.3	96.6

TABLE 9.3

Percentage of Scenes with a Goggle-World Appearance
(Among all scenes with recall)

	Experimental Phase				Recovery		
	First night	Second and third nights	Fourth and fifth nights	Total experiment	First night	All but first night	Total recovery
First REM/NREM period							
N scenes	2	4	9	15	2	4	6
% goggle-world appearance	50.0	50.0	83.3	63.3	0.0	83.3	27.8
Second and third REM/NREM periods							
N scenes	14	39	16	69	10	2	12
% goggle-world appearance	35.7	69.2	54.2	56.5	30.0	0.0	20.0
Fourth and later REM/NREM periods							
N scenes	19	35	19	73	6	2	8
% goggle-world appearance	29.2	32.1	44.4	36.4	25.0	0.0	16.7
Total for night							
N scenes	35	78	44	157	18	8	26
% goggle-world appearance	38.3	50.4	60.6	52.1	18.3	27.8	21.5

TABLE 9.4

Percentage of Complimentary Colored Objects

	Baseline			Experimental Phase				Recovery		
	All but last two nights	Last two nights	Total baseline	First night	Second and third nights	Fourth and fifth nights	Total Experiment	First night	All but first night	Total recovery
First REM/NREM period										
N scenes	3	15	18	3	4	10	17	4	4	8
% complementary objects	28.9	20.9	24.9	13.3	16.7	2.4	10.3	70.6	23.3	54.8
% of baseline total	138.0	99.6	118.9	63.7	79.6	11.5	49.2	337.0	111.5	261.8
Second and third REM/NREM periods										
N scenes	37	43	80	19	39	18	76	18	8	26
% complementary objects	19.3	21.4	20.4	10.8	9.8	17.4	13.1	13.1	15.8	14.0
% of baseline total	92.1	102.4	97.3	51.7	46.9	83.1	62.4	62.8	75.4	67.0
Fourth and later REM/NREM periods										
N scenes	26	47	73	27	44	23	94	15	7	22
% complementary objects	19.5	15.6	17.6	18.7	19.1	12.9	16.6	21.8	13.8	19.1
% of baseline total	93.3	74.6	83.9	89.5	91.4	61.5	79.1	104.2	65.7	91.4
Total for night										
N scenes	66	105	171	49	87	51	187	37	19	56
% complementary objects	22.6	19.3	20.9	14.3	15.2	10.9	13.3	35.2	17.6	29.3
% of baseline total	107.8	92.2	100.0	68.3	72.7	52.0	63.5	168.0	84.2	140.1

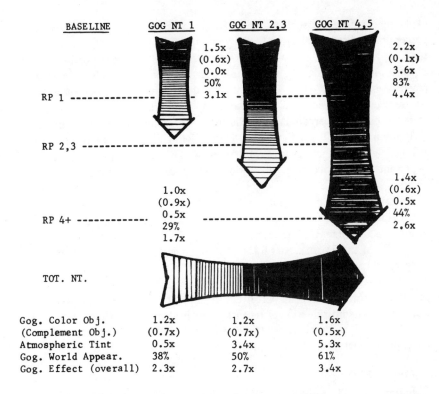

FIG. 9.4.   A summary representation of the general goggle effect in REM dreams as it emerges across nights and by time-of-night (REM-period number) during the red-goggle phase of the experiment. Goggle effect in this illustration is schematically indicated by the length, width, and line frequency in the arrows which represent several data parameters: shifts in goggle (R-O-Y) and complementary (B-BG-G) object colors, atmospheric tint, goggle-world appearance, and goggle effect (overall). (The latter is a rater's wholistic assessment of "goggle effect" on the basis of the subjects' responses to all the data dimensions in the dream-scene questionnaire.) Comparative preliminary values for the selected parameters are presented as vertical vectors for the first REM period (RP 1) and last REM periods (RP 4+) of the first goggle night (GOG NT 1), and RP 1 and RP 4+ of GOG NT 4, 5; and as horizontal vectors for the total night means of GOG NTS 1; 2, 3; and 4, 5.

The goggle effect penetrates into dreams more extensively and in a particular pattern as the goggle phase proceeds. The effect is progressively stronger in the first REM periods from night to night and also tends to invade later REM periods as the goggle phase continues. Though the GOG NT 2, 3 arrow does not adequately reflect it, the effect reaches the last REM periods during this point in the series of goggle-phase nights, and the concentration of the effect merely deepens in the later nights. Numerical values represent proportional increases over comparable values in the baseline phase, thus 2.0x means a doubling of baseline. The baseline value of Gog. World Appear. is judged from several lines of inferences to be about 22%. The small, initial goggle effect in the first REM period of the first night almost disappears by the last REM period, which shows values approximating the baseline figures. Note that in the course of the goggle phase, the amount of complementary object color is reduced tenfold. The greatest penetrance of the goggle effect is in RP 1 of the last goggle nights.

experience before the subjects had even heard about the study. It appears that perceptions experienced prior to the wearing of the goggles may be *recolored* as they are hallucinated in the REM dream. Of course the major portion of goggle objects and effects that are remembered as having a waking reference have been recently experienced. Accordingly, though the dream is composed of raw materials derived from recent waking percepts, evidence is also available that the memory banks of perceptual material may be affected by retrograde processing.

Preliminary analysis of the data from NREM awakenings has not shown as strong a "goggle effect" as in REM dreams. An appreciably stronger goggle effect is present in SO awakening, which does not appear to diminish in the later sleep cycles.

To review our major findings, when chromatic alteration lenses replaced normal vision for a number of days, the dream imagery of REM sleep was rapidly invaded in the first REM periods of each night by the new input, which affected a majority of the dream scenes by the fourth goggle night. In other words, dream imagery did not prove to be impervious to fresh experience. On the contrary, dream imagery reproduced the recently perceived material in abundance and in general the form it had been perceived. In summary, dream content is heavily influenced by the introduction of recently perceived (visual) material, which exerts a quick as well as direct weight (that is, a largely untransformed perceptual loading) upon the visual qualities of the dream.

Control Studies

In designing this study of the effects of perceptual modifications on dreaming, we contemplated the need for a variety of controls. It seemed to us that the first consideration in research of this nature was to be certain that if imagery and content changes are provoked in dreams by visual modifications in waking life, they be attributable to the perceptual shift per se and not to physiological, psychological, or affective influences upon the subjects.

Along these lines, clearly a likely source of indirect contribution to a goggle effect, which might be confounded with a perceptual factor, is a shift in the physiological conditions in which dreaming occurs; a shift, perhaps caused by the induced sensory modifications and the conditions under which they are allowed entry to the CNS. If the obligation to relearn in the service of adaptation to altered environmental conditions results in increases in REM sleep and in its phasic intensity, as suggested by Shapiro (1967) and others, corresponding shifts in dream content would be expected in the direction of more intense imagery. The effect of increases in phasic discharge, as in recovery from REM suppression by drugs, upon the emotional intensity of dreams, has been amply made in recent clinical observations. The implication of this possibility for this study is that our presumed active, independent variable of new perceptual input would not, itself, be the direct cause of the altered imagery of the dream.

Consequently, a study was designed to examine the effects of long-term perceptual alterations in color and illumination on the physiological parameters of sleep (Bowe-Anders, Herman, & Roffwarg, 1974). Subsequent to a period of sleep standardization, three subjects slept four to five baseline nights in the lab immediately followed by four to five goggle nights. The protocol was precisely the same as in the content retrieval experiment, and the subjects were required to continue normal daily routines. However, in this study, no awakenings were carried out and the subjects were allowed to "sleep through." The variables assessed were: total minutes and percentages of REM sleep (REMS) and of NREMS Stages 1, 2, and 3 and 4; latencies to initial Stage 3 and 4 and to REMS, and the intensity of REMS.

Mean values for each subject and for the group during the baseline and experimental phases are represented in Table 9.5. It may be seen that REM percentage remained constant in every subject throughout baseline and experimental conditions. Further, no consistent trends away from baseline values were evidenced in the percentages of NREM Stage 1, or 3 and 4, and in the latency to Stage 3 and 4. Decreases in the percentage of Stage 2 and in the latency to REMS, as well as the increase in REMS intensity in the goggle phase were slight and failed to achieve statistical significance (Friedman two-way analysis of variance). Analyses of the lengths of REMS periods, sleep cycles, and periods of Stage 3 and 4, which are not shown in Table 9.5, uncovered no consistent change between baseline and experimental conditions.

In addition to analysis of variance, we performed a power analysis (Cohen, 1969) on 4 important REM-sleep parameters. This test was performed in order to clarify whether the failure to achieve significant differences between mean values in the baseline and in the goggle phase resulted from the small number of subjects, rather than from the absence of an experimental effect. We found that in order to achieve statistical significance at $< .05$ (assuming that the baseline versus goggle differences for these parameters in the 3 subjects remained constant), 20 subjects would be required for REMS latency, 130 for REMS intensity, 400 for REMS time, and more than 3000 for REMS percentage. These results strongly suggest that significant perceptual readjustments in terms of color and illumination and an associated restriction in peripheral vision, though strongly affecting dream content, do not result in convincing changes in the conventionally measured, physiological parameters of sleep. There is, in these data, neither support for the contention that the goggle effect in dreams results from the increased "pressure" of REM sleep, nor, for that matter, for the reverse.

We have earlier discussed the possibility of contamination of a perceptual effect on dreams from psychological, cognitive (i.e., expectational) and even affective sources. These factors may be summarized under the heading of bias, conceivably operating to affect the subjects' dream telling, even dreams. (See Chapter 3 of this volume for a fuller discussion of bias and dream recall.) It was

TABLE 9.5

Individual and Group Means for Sleep Stage Variables During Baseline and Experimental (Goggle) Phases

		Subject 1		Subject 2		Subject 3		All Subjects	
		Baseline, 5 nights	Experimental, 4 nights	Baseline, 5 nights	Experimental, 3 nights[a]	Baseline, 4 nights	Experimental, 5 nights	Baseline $n = 3$	Experimental $n = 3$
TST (min.)[b]	M	490.5	495.5	475.9	461.5	405.3	419.3	457.2	458.8
	SD	24.7	20.8	46.0	17.3	24.1	6.4	26.3[c]	22.0[c]
REMS (min)	M	115.6	117.8	102.9	97.2	88.0	90.1	102.2	101.7
	SD	12.4	12.5	13.5	10.4	6.7	8.8	8.0[c]	8.3[c]
% REMS	M	23.6	23.8	21.6	21.0	21.8	22.2	22.3	22.3
	SD	2.0	2.2	2.1	1.9	2.5	3.7	0.6[c]	0.8[c]
%NREM 1	M	7.3	6.2	8.0	11.9	8.1	10.8	7.8	9.6
	SD	1.8	1.6	2.5	4.7	1.1	3.0	0.3[c]	1.7[c]
% NREM 2	M	53.8	51.4	57.1	56.4	46.4	39.2	52.4	49.0
	SD	2.2	4.6	2.7	.5	4.4	5.4	3.2[c]	5.1[c]
% NREM 3-4	M	15.3	18.5	13.3	10.7	24.7	29.0	17.8	19.4
	SD	2.1	2.4	3.6	3.1	3.7	7.0	3.5[c]	5.3[c]
REMS latency (min)	M	67.6	66.6	82.4	78.3	65.6	56.3	71.9	67.1
	SD	6.6	6.0	11.6	8.4	4.4	5.1	5.3[c]	6.4[c]
3-4 latency (min)	M	18.5	16.9	24.2	27.4	11.3	8.6	18.0	17.6
	SD	4.7	2.9	4.6	6.9	4.0	2.2	3.7[c]	5.4[c]
REM intensity/ 30-sec epoch	M	1.33	1.36	0.72	1.00	1.42	1.46	1.16	1.27
	SD	.11	.06	.13	.17	.10	.17	0.2[c]	0.1[c]

[a] A portion of the second goggle night of Subject 2 was not recorded because of mechanical difficulties. The mean values for the experimental period are calculated on the basis of Nights 1, 3, 4. [b] TST was the only parameter controlled by the experimental procedure. [c] Standard error of mean in this column, not standard deviation. Reprinted with permission of publisher from: Bowe-Anders, C., Herman, J. H., and Roffwarg, H. P. Effects of goggle-altered color perception on sleep. PERCEPTUAL AND MOTOR SKILLS, 1974, 38, 191-198.

obvious that a need existed for control studies that would help to unravel *perceptual* from (possible) *attentional* contributions to altered color in our nocturnal imagery. Accordingly, we have studied small groups of subjects in a variety of additional goggle experiments which, while not constituting a complete check on sources of artifact, carry some promise of answering certain questions about the two contributions. Each small experiment was designed to account for one or another factor of subject or experimenter expectation.

The control runs were, in part, an attempt to manipulate bias and thereby learn more about its effects on our field of inquiry. In actuality, some of the studies also provided the opportunity for additional investigation of specific parameters of awake perception and their possible counterparts in dream life.

The dark adaptation control.   In this study, which employs the regular red goggle (No. 29 Wratten filters), the subjects were given the orthogonal suggestion that we were "investigating the relationship of dark adaptation in the waking state to dream coloration at night, when the eyes are also normally dark adapted." We recruited subjects for this trial who had no difficulty accepting the rationale offered. The goggle frames were embossed with the phrase "Montefiore X-Ray Dept." The prospective subjects and the laboratory assistant "happened" to walk past the radiology department early in the series of goggle days. The assistant encouraged the subject to come in and look around because the radiologists were also dark adapting. (Dark-adaptation lenses have substantially the same transmission characteristics of No. 29 filters.)

The experimental sequence of nights and awakenings for color content in dreams was exactly the same as in the main study. The perceptual loading of red through No. 29 lenses is equivalent in all respects. However, the assumption is reasonable that some emphasis is taken off *attention to red* because of the substitution of a strong emphasis on dark adaptation.

Provisional analysis of the subject responses show them to be comparable to the results of the main study.

The one-hour and one-day controls.   In the 1-hr experiment, the No. 29 filters were employed, and all the phases of the typical red goggle sequence were run through, with the exception that during the 5-8-day goggle phase, the subjects were instructed to wear the goggles only 1 hr each day. Which hour the goggles were worn was varied from run to run. In some of the 1-hr and 1-day runs, the subjects were told that the goggles contain very strong lenses and that the effect on the retina is considerable.

With respect to the 1-day run, Orne (personal communication, 1974) has pointed out that subjects in a study tend to feel that the maximal experimental effect is slated to occur near the end of the experimental phase, however short or long it is designated to last. In 5-day sensory-deprivation studies, for example, hallucinations tend to appear on the fifth day, but they tend to appear on the second day when the subject knows the protocol terminates on the second day.

Both trials, we feel, provide the same, if not more, attention to and suggestion for a "goggle effect" as in the standard experiment. However, in the 1-hr run, the total perceptual input in each 24-hr period is appreciably less than in the main red-goggle trial. The 1-day run is of interest because the prototype red-goggle study reveals only very minor goggle effects in dreams of the first night. Accordingly, the increase in loading in subject expectation for a goggle effect, owing to the subject's knowledge of the 1-day course and the revealed "strength" of the lenses, accentuates the possibility of a stronger goggle effect in the first (and only) night, based on the attentional factor.

A variation on the 1-hr control was also run by means of which we tried to gain additional insight into the fall of the goggle effect in later REM periods. The question was posed, is the difference in intensity of goggle-related dream material in the early and late REM periods a function of some physiological quality of the later REM periods and dreaming, or simply a function of the recency difference between the early and late REM periods in relation to the time of termination of the red input on the previous evening?

In the run designed to test this question, the subject was awakened after the third REM period and taken for a walk with goggles on around the hospital for 1 hr. After the walk, the subject was returned to bed and the very next REM period was interrupted for a dream interrogation. Whether the intensity of the goggle effect in the collected scenes is more like first or fourth REM periods is the critical issue.

The 1-day runs showed a first-night goggle effect of very small proportions, as in the major experiment; the 1-hr runs have not yet been decoded.

The compensatory color-bias control.   The subjects were put through the same experimental conditions as the standard red-goggle subjects and wore the same lenses. However, at a point just after the baseline or neutral-density filter phase, they were shown the red goggles and invited to put them on. After they wore the goggles for about an hour under bright illumination, the goggles were removed and the subject was requested to peer at an achromatic screen. At the time that the subject experienced the well-known phenomenon of a vivid complementary color (blue-green) afterimage, a "new" lab assistant "aimlessly" mentioned, "We think the same phenomenon occurs in dreaming."

For the compensatory color-bias study, the dream-scene questionnaire was altered so that the interrogator would elicit information about dream coloration against the referent of blue-green imagery rather than as in the regular goggle runs in which the standard is the way the environment looks with the goggles on during the day.

The subject's color experience in dreaming during the goggle phase was gauged alongside of the extent to which the blue-green "suggestion" was taken.

The subject believed the blue-green suggestion strongly, but showed the normal goggle effect. So disturbed at the possibility of "ruining" our study, the subject asked to drop out of the study.

The nonhomogeneous ("dirty") red control.   Subjects were run in the regular red-goggle experimental protocol except that the lenses in their goggles were "dirty," in the radioactive sense. Like the No. 29 filters, the lenses look dark red when held away from the eye (the subjects looked *at* them before the run), and the lenses also confer a strong red tint upon the field of view. However, they "leak" or allow in, wave lengths in lower bands. Accordingly, along with a red background, the subjects saw blue objects in vivid purples and yellow objects in bright orange. The presence of such intense and dramatic object colors is quite unlike the "washed out" effect of the No. 29 Wratten filters on object colors.

Accordingly, because a red tint was cast over all scenery, the subjects approached the nonhomogeneous-red control study with the same red expectation as in the standard study with the No. 29 filters, though the perceptual input was quite distinct in regard to object color. This approach was a further attempt to distinguish an expectational from a visual effect.

These data have not, as yet, been decoded.

Two other control trials that we believed would provide additional information concerning the relationship of perceptual input to dream content are briefly described. The second of the two attempts to provide information about the important differentiation between the *appearance* of color and *wave length* of color.

The black-patch control.   A subject was deprived of all light input during the waking state by means of black opaque lenses placed in the goggle frames. This deprivation of external visual stimulation to the retina and brain (with the exception of dark discharge), we hoped, would serve as a yardstick for the effects of altered color inputs. We must know what will happen to dreams if perceptual input is not only changed, but cut off.

Provisional analysis of the dream data shows a progressive trend to darkly illuminated or blind ("pitch black") dreams.

The "physiological versus the phenomenological" control.   In this experiment, the subjects had to live in special rooms in the laboratory. They were permitted outdoors only when lighting conditions were similar to the lighting allowed to them in the experiment. In the "physiological" study, the subject lived in a brightly illuminated chamber and wore the standard Wratten No. 29 filters. The subject was allowed to travel about outside only under brightly sunlit circumstances. Consequently, indoors or outdoors, the tinted but "washed-out" appearance of the visual environment was maximized. No true reds were seen by the subject, though a copious amount of light in the pure red band constantly impinged upon the retina.

In the "phenomenological" trial the subject wore the same lenses, and lived in a dark room lit only by small and sharply focused sources of light (little Christmas bulbs) and traveled outdoors only at night, when only street and window lights and automobile headlights could be seen against the black surround. These light sources, as well as the little bulbs in the subject's room, were seen all through the study as intense and as "true red." No "washed-out" imagery was experienced by the subject in this condition.

The point should be made that light of exactly the same wave-length character was administered in the two conditions. Only the intensity and phenomenal appearance of the coloration differed. Both conditions were more homogeneous visual experiences than the standard red-goggle trials, which contained both kinds of visual red effects.

The issues in this run are fundamental. The experiment forces an inverse relationship between the amount of red-wave-length energy and the perception of true red. What will the CNS do? Will it take the greater energy load and give a greater red effect of different varieties ("washed-out" *and* true reds) in dreams than in the "phenomenological" run, or will the dreams tend to reflect what was seen in the awake state? Will the dreams be predisposed to "escape"more from one effect than the other?

A preliminary survey of the data reveals a mixed effect, though the dreams, in general, show more of the phenomenal appearance appropriate to the awake condition in each case than the reverse.

Discussion and Amplification of the Data

Our long-term aim is to explore dream formation and sleep physiology relative to perceptual experience. The objective of this particular study was to observe the nature of the color modifications, if any, represented in dreaming when individuals are confronted by an acute, ubiquitous and enduring shift in the coloration of their surroundings. Little in the way of other perceptual changes was provoked by our procedures.

We tried to hold constant our subjects' vantage points as well as their physical and emotional involvements as they confronted their environments, as well as the locales and structural characteristics of the visual environment. An analogous method would change only the phonetics of spoken utterances, leaving unaltered their semantics, quantity, and content.

The chief issue in question was the way the CNS uses (that is, processes) perceptual information into dream imagery. Specifically, following an incessant daily exposure to a filter-rendered reddish-orange world devoid of blues and greens, would subjects' dreams resist, incorporate wholly or partially, modify, or neutralize through generation of opposite coloration, the characteristic effect afforded by viewing through the goggles in the awake state?

All our evidence points to a considerable replay of the awake goggle-effect in the hallucinations of REM sleep. The REM dream, which in baseline dream collection had contained similar and stable levels of red-oranges and blue-greens, in the goggle phase of the experiment exhibited a divergence in the proportion of their representation: a reciprocal increase in the goggle-permitted hues and a decrease in the goggle-screened, or complementary colors.

A sizable increase in the proportion of goggle-permitted colors was observed on the successive goggle nights and the process was least clear on Night 1. Our findings also indicate that the effect was direct — red environment; red dreams. REM dreaming certainly neither avoided the new input, nor showed a tendency for complementary colors to achieve greater representation. The proportion of total coloration assumed by goggle-screened colors in dreams actually declined sharply; in fact, amounting to the most unequivocal feature of the goggle effect. This reduction in goggle-screened colors was overshadowed subjectively by the saliency of the red-orange imagery.

Other Sources of the Effect Not Related to Perceptual Storage?

A separate study (Bowe-Anders et al., 1974) went far towards ruling out the possibility that the experimental wearing of the goggles, by provoking a change in the physiological characteristics of sleep, indirectly induces alterations in the type and intensity of dream imagery. On the contrary, the physiological sleep matrix was so constant across goggle and nongoggle conditions in that study as to constitute further support for our observations as to the stability of the subjects' physical, psychological, and affective states in the experimental period.

Another conceivable source of the goggle effect (that is, the possibility that dark discharge of retinal and higher CNS cells responsible for color discrimination may feed "input" to visual areas during dreaming) also may be eliminated at this point because of the nature of the effect. For in the face of day-long orange-red input to the eyes, and concomitant filtering out of the blue-green spectrum right up to the advent of sleep, one would expect that most spontaneous discharge during sleep would arise only from the ON cells for occluded colors. Virtual quiescence of the depleted orange-red-ON cells for a significant period of time is assured. Only had a goggle effect taken the form of a dreamed increase of the deprived blue-greens, would a dark discharge explanation have to be afforded credence. Since the direction of the data was exactly the reverse of what nocturnal discharge of the blue-green-ON color receptor cells would predict, the activity of these cells may act, if anything, to weaken the red-orange goggle effect that we report in dreaming.

In the absence of final data from our control studies, and the need for other controls and some improvement in procedures, we cannot have complete assurance that the goggle effect in dreams is the result of an alteration in the subjects' perceptual environment, and not referable to subject expectation or suggestion. However, the provisional directions of the control data are strong enough to proceed with considerations of the effect from the perceptual point of view. We must be aware, however, that though the goggle effect in REM dreaming is striking, and likely to represent a valid perceptual influence on nocturnal dreaming, caution should be exercised in generalizing the color-alteration effects to other sensory modalities, and even to other components of visual perception. For example, deviations in auditory experience or gustatory sensation might not gain the access to dreaming that appears to characterize daytime color experience. Careful investigation will be required to determine whether dreams also rapidly reflect changes in other sense data.

With respect to color experience, the question posed by this study, as to whether sense data exert an influence of their own on dream imagery, may be answered strongly in the affirmative. However, it is not at present easy to decide whether goggle-phase dreams merely reflect recent sensory experience, or, in elaborating goggle color, perform adaptational, coping, or "junking" functions. We return to that issue below.

A Deeper Look at the Goggle Effect

Before proceeding further we should fill out our understanding of the recency, and related phenomena characterizing the goggle effect. The term "recency phenomenon" stands for the finding that the REM period dreams, which most predictably displayed goggle imagery and reciprocally reduced baseline levels of complementary colors, were those that were the shortest spaced from the last waking input of each day. This phenomenon continued for as long as the subjects were exposed to the "goggle world." The mosaic of the goggle effect, which is observed with increasing longevity of goggle exposure, may be understood only if the warp of the recency phenomenon is superimposed upon the woof of the progressive whole night deepening of the effect. This latter increase in the penetrance of the whole-night goggle effect was not, as might have been anticipated from the whole phase data, by REM period, localized to the early portion of the night. It was distributed fairly equally to all thirds of the night, the consequence being that the accentuation of goggle effect in the early REM periods was sustained and only lightly augmented during the experimental condition. Accordingly, two vectors — a time-of-night trend (recency phenomenon), and a night-in-phase trend (progressive increase in the whole night effect) — in their intersection throughout the experimental condition, define the goggle effect.

In terms of the parallel to a metabolic study (if information stores can be said to be "metabolized"), the two tendencies of the goggle effect in our perceptual input study amount to:

1. a within-night course, reflecting the highest concentration of a newly introduced constituent shortly after the presleep termination of its infusion, and the progressive diminution in its concentration over time; and

2. a between-night course of heightening nightly curves of concentration, resulting in a serial rise in mean concentration.

The latter finding would indicate that metabolism of the infused constituent does not quite keep pace with the quantity introduced daily. However, the immediate disappearance of the "goggle effect" on the first baseline might indicate that the re-introduction of normal vision rapidly overwhelmes the goggle memory stores.

In regard to the vertical trend, a composite set of measures of goggle effect reveals a falloff from the first to the last REMP of 35%, with the descent in goggle effect more than twice as steep from the middle to the end REM periods as from the first to the middle REM periods. However, the goggle effect in the average last REM periods was still about twice as strong as in baseline (tint- and goggle-world appearance are much stronger in REM Periods 4 and 5 than object color). The horizontal effect, expressed in mean whole-night comparisons, revealed an increase in composite goggle effect of 340%. Of this multiple of 3.4 over baseline goggle values, one-fifth of the change took place in the first goggle night (largely in the first REM period), three-quarters by Night 3, and the remaining one-quarter in Nights 4 and 5.

Some Considerations Concerning Memory and the Recency Phenomenon

What mechanisms might account for this predictable REM-period loading of goggle imagery on the two-dimensional time grid of the goggle phase? Some speculations in terms of memory systems may be warranted. But before presenting them, a difference between types of memory studies should be mentioned.

A study paradigm of awake experiencing relative to sleep reexperiencing in dreaming has a special advantage over studies pertaining to the influence of experience on subsequent mentation phenomena set in the waking state alone. In the latter, the target experience is one of a series of ineluctably continuing experiences; examination for the influence of particular memories upon a current mental behavior must always consider the factor of the intervening and additional experiences. In contrast, in this study of perceptual input in the awake state in reference to dreaming in sleep, an incessant and specific waking input has a sharp termination with the onset of sleep. Its memory may be thought of as isolated from supervening external experiences. The CNS is now in the processing mode of operation rather than in the recipient-plus-processing mode. For purposes of understanding the mechanisms of perceptual "metabolism," the imagery-utilization pattern in sleep of prior perceptual input may be considered only in terms of internal processing. (Of course, this line of argument is enhanced by agreement to neglect two facts pertinent to sleep conditions: (1) that the CNS is never entirely out of the recipient mode in terms of external experience; and (2) that the dreams of one REM period may constitute "perceptual" input for dreams in later REM periods.)

In regard to memory, the data demonstrate that the color information in storage from the most recently experienced environmental settings (the latter held, for purposes of discussion, to be equal in psychological valence) command a high priority for reemergence, that is, hallucinatory reactivation, in the dreams of REM sleep. A phenomenon something like a "last in-first out" system seems to be in operation. It appears that the most recent perceptual experiences tend to blanket earlier stores of perceptual information, at least with respect to their relative availability to the process of dream formation of the physical surround, and particularly in the early REM periods.[5] The later dreams provide relative immunity to the recent input, though as the goggle-phase proceeds, even the terminal REM periods begin, as indicated, to show considerable invasion by the goggle effect.

Two points in the study sequence, the first REM periods of the first goggle day and of the first recovery day, are of particular interest in regard to this phenomenon. In the former, an increase appears in red-orange coloration over baseline values, though not to the degree represented in subsequent leadoff REM periods. Contrariwise, the first recovery-night REM-period dreams display an absence of almost any red-orange coloration, and a more than threefold increase in complementary tones. (Subjects had commented about the beauty and vividness of even the low-saturation blues and greens in their visual sensations on the first day after the goggle phase.) Though the number of total scenes collected from the group in these two REM "locations" is small, the contrast is impressive. What these data point up is the relative ease with which a recent layer of perceptual "silt," however fine, may cover earlier layers, however deep, in terms of their utilization by the earliest REM dreams of the night.

Content Differences and Times of Dreaming

It is likely that the first REM dream more faithfully indicates the color perceptions of the day than any other dream of the night. However, in daily life, this effect goes largely unnoticed because the variety of colors present in most visual situations usually gives the first dream a wide range of selection. In contrast, under the conditions of this study, the change in environmental coloring between the normal and color-altered phases was unmistakeable, and to that degree its coordination with the content of the first dream was striking. Now that this relationship is more apparent, we may wonder at the typical ascription of events of the previous evening, which are found in the first dream of the night, to psychological factors. It should also be emphasized that, although our experimental focus centered on a *change* in perception, the aim of the study is really on the relationship of *perception* to dreaming. The goggle effect, then, is not the consequence of a change in perception, but of perception itself. What the first REM-period data alert us to is that a goggle effect exists every day.

Further correspondences to our "vertical" data have been found in earlier studies about the relationship of contemporaneous material and noncontemporaneous material to time-of-night positioning of REM dreams (Verdone, 1965). Earlier REM periods generally contain remembered experiences and conscious

---

[5]A sharp distinction is not made between memory and storage of experience (information) in this chapter. We would not defend this practice on the grounds of an informed, theoretical position, and would most certainly be willing to accept a delineation.

concerns of the very recent past, frequently including experiences from the wakeful part of the evening. The first dreams of sleep tend to be more reality based and have been found to utilize imagery that is often very little changed from what was recently experienced in the awake state. In contrast, dreaming towards morning appears to be quite liberated from the immediate past. Not only are older memories more frequently located in the later dreams of sleep, but, in addition, these dreams tend to be more abstract, symbolic, and concerned with unconscious themes.

Some Perplexities in Relating Memory Processes to Our Findings

To restate the recency phenomenon in terms of what is known about short-term memory and long-term-memory storage would be convenient. To illustrate, a case could be made for short-term stores being "skimmed off" as perceptual filler for first REM-period dreams, whereas the long-term memories could be said to be deeply "embedded" in information storage, becoming available only in the later hallucinatory eruptions of the night. We have already used the silt .metaphor for recent input; surely the latter REM periods in the ordinal nightly series could be descriptively paralleled to the deeper layers of memory. In this vein, earlier perceived material would "descend" into long-term-memory repositories accessible only to later REM periods, and constitute a more permanent cache. That memories of goggle-phase perception have to become older before the goggle effect reaches the later REM periods, could be supported by the latency of two to three days that exists before an appreciable goggle effect reaches the later REM periods.[6]

Of course, such "explanations" are at best descriptive and merely metaphorical. Our data does indicate that the later REM periods in this study contain somewhat earlier imagery, as we indexed it according to the subjects' recollections concerning age of last exposure, but the time-of-night differences are not great. In fact, we have no good way of truly explaining the mechanisms underlying the attraction of the goggle effect to the early REM periods. An explanation will probably not be forthcoming until considerably more is known about the neurophysiology of information storage and retrieval, as well as of the neurophysiology of imagery transduction.

Problems for the Concept of Long-Term Memory Retrieval in Dreaming

In terms of memory processing, the material derived form SO awakenings provides a fascinating contrast to the REM data. SO "dreams" were obtained

---

[6]Transfer of memories into long-term stores has been found to require only 3-6 hrs (Barondes, 1970). Why, then, would not the experiences of each day find representation in REM Periods 4 and 5 of that night?

from early and late awakenings as were REM dreams, and showed a very substantial transferral of the waking goggle effect into their content. However, in contradistinction to the recency phenomenon evident in the REM goggle effect, SO content maintained its robust goggle effect without reduction all through the night. This difference in memory behavior perhaps points to an important finding: that the memory system subserving SO imagery follows the time course described for the neurochemistry of memory because they both express the operations of an awake system, whereas the memory processes operating in sleep are different.

The possibility is that with respect to color perception, long-term memory and/or retrieval processing, and, therefore, late REM-period retrieval on the first goggle night, does not function very effectively during REM sleep, or in sleep in general. According to this conception, older memories only become available for retrieval in the later REM periods of the night when they have been converted into long-term memories by processes in the awake state. Hence, the latency of a day or two, before the goggle effect shows up in late REM periods. Unfortunately, this speculative formulation runs sharply counter to the data specifically accumulated on assimilation and consolidation of learning during subsequent sleep, which argue persuasively for these processes (see Greenberg & Pearlman, 1974). A conceivable dovetailing of that data and the findings on late REM-period goggle effect in this study, would rely on the contention that long-term memory processing in sleep that is adequate to successful retrieval in sleep, encompasses more complex activities than simple assimilation and consolidation. Surely, obvious inadequacies in long-term processing during dreaming are suggested by the extraordinary evanescence of dream memories.

Also out of step with the putative relationship of short- and long-term memory processes to early- and late-night REM dreams, is the completely unexpected disappearance of the goggle effect in REM Periods 2 and 3 and 4 and 5 in the recovery period. If goggle colors had entered a permanent store available to REM dreams, as suggested by the rising goggle color percentages in the later REM dreams during the goggle phase, they would be expected to be represented in substantial proportions in the later REM periods for at least some period of time after a return to normal viewing. Yet, with the very first day's input of normal colors, goggle tones not only vanished from the first REM period (which can be understood in terms of the recency effect) but also from the subsequent REM periods of the first recovery night. Goggle-color proportions were hardly above baseline levels. The recovery-phase finding then, lends little support to the hypothesis that older perceptual memories are stationed in slow-turnover memory banks, available to later REM dreams after the more quickly circulating, fresher inputs have yielded up to earlier REM activations. Again, however, we must issue the caution that these startling findings may turn out to be truer for memory of color than for form. Color memory is less stable apparently not only in sleep but in the waking state.

Comparison with the SO data may once more be instructive. The SO goggle effect does not fall off very much in the 3-day recovery period. This may again indicate that retrieval processes for any kind of memory are relatively different for REMS and for waking systems. The evidence would appear to argue for a relative dependence of the goggle effect in REMS sleep *at all points in the night* upon the continuation of daily inputs of goggle imagery. This might be so on the basis that either each REM period can avail itself of color memories only from fresh, short-term stores each day, or that latter dreams can express short-term color memories only because they are first manifested and used in early REM periods, and then repeated in the dreams of later REM periods.

The recovery-phase loss of goggle effect in REM dreams forces even such shaky considerations because long-term memories — be they a product of REM processing, awake processing, or both — built up over five days of goggle-phase experience, no longer appear in REM dreams in the proportions that would be expected after such a massive and continuous experience. Or perhaps such information, now locked into long-term and not at all in short-term storage, is only uncovered when evoked by the intermediation of related associations and psychological material.

To put it another way, long-term memory evocation in dreams may work in terms of a slow-discharging system which, unlike short-term memory availability, requires the conjunction of complex psychological accompaniments. Many older themes may compete for expression in the late-sleep dreams, and the ones that emerge may only do so because of the instigation of related, immediate concerns. For this there is considerable evidence from psychological studies. In the recovery period, all the new perceptual material as well as the subjects' orientation, point away from the "goggle" experience. Because, however, the goggle phase did not traumatize the subjects, they did not return to the experience in thought or waking imagery very much, by their own account. In short, it can be contended that the altered imagery, whenever it appeared, was related to short-term memory of the altered color, or to later associative evocations of the long-term memories.

Finally, the metabolic parallel seems to suggest that goggle imagery appears stronger in dreams with each day of the new perceptual influx because the CNS cannot "metabolize" as much input as is daily admitted. Accordingly, the net excess in short-term storage available to REM periods increases. In terms of this explanation, the loss of all but normal quotients of goggle imagery on the first recovery day would result from even one day of cutoff of the altered input, thus permitting almost complete "clearance" of the accumulated excess from the rapid circulation, short-term memory banks. Future studies might attempt to discriminate further whether new input "covers" the previous short-term memories or whether internal metabolism simply "clears" them. In these investigations, after the goggle phase, some subjects would be allowed no new light input during the next day, whereas other subjects would return to normal vision, or to yet another identifiable visual alteration.

Other Ways of Looking at the Rapid Cessation of the Goggle Effect

Though quandaries obviously exist in relating our REM-dream-recall data to memory concepts, we have attempted to create some conceivable explanations along the lines of memory processing. However, the conclusions inspire little in the way of conviction. We are thus prompted to examine other conceptual frameworks into which we may place the data, even though they are at variance with some of our previously stated views.

At least one notion that must be considered is the belief of some workers (Shapiro, 1967; Greenberg & Pearlman, 1974) that REM sleep may be a time of relearning and reprogramming in the CNS in the face of recent perceptual change. It has even been contended that REM sleep parameters will reflect increased REMS activity under such circumstances, though in our studies (Bowe-Anders et al., 1974) we did not show evidence for that position.

Nevertheless, if one takes the position that adaptational functions were at work during the red-goggle study, certain findings seem to make sense, which are otherwise cumbersome to explain. The point here is that the CNS may be demonstrating a goggle effect in its REM hallucinatory productions in an effort to "cope" with and integrate the daytime load. This would be consistent with the finding of a progressively increasing goggle effect that suddenly vanishes when the daytime situation is restored to routine environmental conditions. Such an extraordinarily quick turnabout is difficult to integrate with prevailing memory concepts, but is quite in keeping with the observation that sensory and sensori-motor adaptations, though they develop slowly, rapidly shift back when the environment normalizes.

Similarly, the view that dreaming serves to maintain psychic balance by extruding or "junking" material it cannot deal with, cannot be dismissed because, again, the need for this function would be expected to halt abruptly once the excessive intrusion had been terminated. The data conformed to this expectation.

Why Do We Dream the World As It Is?

To say that *a tendency exists to dream the environment as it is seen,* is to sound perhaps both contentious and obvious: contentious insofar as the statement appears to repudiate the fact of the sometimes fantastic transmutations and transpositions of the real world evident in dream "perception;" obvious in that it is clear that what we experience frequently is reconstituted directly in dreaming.

The reason the statement is made at all is to examine its limits. The fact of the matter is that the goggle effect and particularly the recency phenomenon instruct us about processes that have easily eluded us, owing to the wide range of perceptual inputs that we confront routinely. However, in this study, involving an atypical confinement of color, we had the unusual opportunity to observe that whatever the psychological and situational content of the subjects' dreams, increasingly the dreams displayed the colors in the subjects' very recent perceptual experiences. The subjects could not remember the experiential sources of most of their imagery, which was highly variegated. The settings of our subjects' dreams were very different, and showed a continued accentuation and individual specificity as to the predominant concerns, situations and people in their own lives. These personal themes were not constrained, however, so much as they were accompanied, by the constancy of color perception that the subjects all shared. The goggle effect seemed to exist independently of what was dreamed; it merely colored the content. And, though the goggle imagery was by no means homogeneous in all dreams, it is significant that in a great number of cases the dream scenes were pictorially equivalent, in terms of the shades of color, saturation and illumination, to the monotonous imagery that confronted the subjects while awake.

So legion are the accounts of any and all variety of bizarre appearances and recombinations in dreams, and so convinced are we of enormous individual variation in the creative deployment of perceptual materials to express drives, conflicts and emotions in imagery, that even an elementary knowledge of what may be expected or predicted about the employment of perceptual elements in dreams has been the slave of anecdote. Insufficient awareness has existed that perceptual materials exert their own weight in the representation in dreams; that is, the sense data, in addition to all the other psychological contingencies, have a role to play in dream representation. Individuals may build a variety of emotional and psychological structures in their dreams, but when they mine for the stones to build the structures, they tend to use the color of the stone available in their perceptual quarry.

It is hardly only, highlighting the trivial to point out that dreams make use of what we experience. This is actually a general property of dreaming, as germane to individual variations in dreaming styles and themes as to the use of perceptual materials. Though it is the norm, the fact of simple repetition of experience in dreams has been so disproportionately slighted in comparison to the capabilities for creation and transformation, that it is quite indistinct in our scientific awareness. It is not uncommon for intelligent and informed scientists to ask how color-blind people, or the congenitally deaf, dream. The conclusion is inescapable that dreams are considered so unlimitedly innovative as to allow for the possibility that color-blind individuals, perhaps because of their cognitive awareness of normal coloration, or their emotional desire to dream other than what they see, will somehow transcend their waking sensory restriction.

We must start with, not "discover," the tendency to dream our environments. Small wonder that we dream usually of the countries in which we live, and that the language spoken is our own. In not one of the subjects tested, during the goggle phase in our study did nontransmitted colors sustain their usual proportions, or goggle imagery not increase. Yet, many students of dreaming have entertained serious predictions that the dreams of the goggle phase would be blue-green or unchanged. This indicates that we are not belaboring the obvious.

On the other hand, we must not slight the mutability of the building blocks, and the mind's potential to employ only certain features of them while leaving others out. We have been impressed, with the capacity on the part of the dreaming process for "playfulness" with so-called neutral percepts, when it suits a purpose, just as is often seen with interactional and emotionally meaningful material.

Is the Medium the Message?

In commencing this investigation, we hypothesized that dreamed perceptual elements, carrying the specific, altered coloration we induced, would originate mainly from the red-goggle exposure period. Had this been exclusively so, it would not have required us to question an underlying assumption: that even though the actual origin in waking experience cannot be ascertained for the majority of dreamed elements with goggle-type coloration, the latter have their source in waking experience during the goggle condition.

This assumption must be revised on the basis of the finding of a considerable retrograde coloring effect. Old percepts, seen long before the goggles were worn or even contemplated by the subjects, could appear, not in their natural hues, but in goggle tones. This was not the rule, but was not infrequent. An analysis of these data showed, interestingly, that when a perceptually pregoggle element was dreamed in altered color, it tended to appear in or closer to the first REM period of the night than other pregoggle percepts, dreamed in their original shades.

It is thus possible to conjecture that what was perceived during the goggle phase by the subject was more than a collection of percepts; it was possibly a way of looking at the world, induced by looking through goggles that created the illusion of a differently colored world, without it being actually different in color. The change was in the individual's perceptual apparatus and not truly in the surroundings. If relearning does operate in a new perceptual environment and get repeated in REM sleep, it is conceivable that we dream not only the sense data in the environment, but we dream also the experience of *using* the perceptual modalities at our command at a given time. Accordingly, our retrograde-effect data would suggest that the perceiving process, itself, is dreamed, and that old percepts, as they are hallucinated in dreaming may come under its influence. If subjects were put in a truly red world rather than put behind goggles, the tie of the altered coloration to actual objects might be more absolute; that is, there might be no retrograde effect.

The Roles of Selectivity and Meaning Are Primary to Content

Notwithstanding this unanswered question, the fact remains that the claim that a tendency exists to dream the environment as we see it — underscore *a tendency* — is true. It is meant to emphasize the role of the perceived elements, and, possibly, the current modality of perception, in determining content, so that we may be cautioned from viewing the dream as a tapestry solely under the design of psychological contingencies.

In arguing for some attention to perceptual constancy in relation to dreaming, we must quickly add the necessary qualifications. Current perceptual activity is not a strict governor over what is dreamed. Though some of our subjects wore goggles for eight days, their dreams were never completely without evidence of nontransmitted coloration.

Further, a strict correlation does not exist between what we frequently see and what we dream. How often do we dream of our office desks or kitchen sinks? Selectivity is an important factor in dream life. In quite a few instances in this study, subjects reported dream scenes showing the goggle effect only selectively; for example, the subject's view through a window was affected, but not the room in which the subject stood. Clearly the meaning of objects, places, and people to the dreamer is the strongest determinant of selection for inclusion in dreams. We have argued that when reenactment of objects and people takes place in dreams, the dreamer's recent perceptual experience will, to some degree, influence the modes of appearance.

MANY QUESTIONS REMAIN

We must urge the reader to take comfort in the knowledge of our realization that many features of this study leave questions unanswered. Let us cursorily give mention to just a few, which perhaps can be followed up:

1. Is it possible that a 1-hr goggle exposure just before bedtime each day might have produced our entire effect? What would have been the effect of incomplete, for example, 4-hr-per-day exposures?

2. Is it possible that noncontinuous viewing of the goggle world in association with significant events or emotional upsurge might have given a strong goggle effect in dreams?

3. Is it possible that the higher-than-baseline values of nontransmitted colors on the first goggle day was not due simply to the vividness of blue-green objects and the blue tint seen that day? Could it have been the consequence of novelty? Novelty is one of the strongest magnets for visual attention (even in infants). Should we be alerted that the entire goggle effect may have something to do with novelty, not only with the quantity and way in which things are seen?

4. Our data seemed to show some trend toward a "plateau" in the goggle effect. What would be the effect of longer exposures? Would the effect ever become complete? Might it diminish after the loss of the novelty of the effect?

5. How can we conceptualize the reported effect of subliminal perception in dreaming? It is theorized that subliminal percepts may have a favored route to dream expression because of their "preconscious" character. Have we studied the operations of a different route of entry into the dream?

6. The weight of what we see versus *how* we see it, as indicated, is not clear. Will perceptual memory be different depending on whether it is referable only to the object or whether it is "applied" to the perceptual sense organ?

7. What do these results alert us to in terms of the operations of memory, or perhaps better put, the failure of normal memory processing in REM sleep? The sudden disappearance of an established perceptual inclusion in dream content in the face of only one day of new perceptual input must be checked under circumstances when goggle vision is replaced by the absence of external visual input. We may be at the point of discovering that long-term memories, expressed in dream content, operate on the basis of different laws of retrieval and expression than they do in the waking state. At a time when accumulating evidence indicates that the REM state is a time of synthesis of protein elements in the CNS, the seemingly paradoxical finding confronts us in our data of extraordinary transience of long-term waking memories in dreams, in addition to the already well-known difficulty in dream remembering in the awake state.

8. Is it possible that color constancy is a qualitatively different type of perceptual constancy than some others? Might a different form of visual sensory distortion (one that also did not require a visuomotor alteration), or a change in normal sensory input in another sensory modality, such as a constant odor or low-grade acoustic input, *not* cause the effect on dream content that we observed with color?

9. The expression of the perceptual effect in psychological dream content must be explored to a greater extent in our data. For example, the presence of symbolic material, and primary process transformations of all kinds, will be probed for in the narratives of the goggle dreams; although in preliminary appraisal of the dream content, there was little apparent evidence that continuous exposure to red encouraged an increase in primary process material in the dreams.

As we have pointed out, a considerable incorporation of a purely sensory, perceptual change has been found in the dreams of REM sleep, and at the same time no evidence that the basic phasic-tonic parameters of the REM state were altered. It is exciting to conjecture that a change in perception, which is allied with a systematic and measurable sensory-motor adaptation in the awake state, such as that caused by visual distorting lenses or tilt axis prisms, would evoke not only the expected changes in dream content, but also in the correlated phasic eye-movement pattern of REM sleep. Several studies of this kind are underway in our laboratory under the direction of John Herman, and will be reported at a later date.

As was to be hoped, we have been transported to a new level of inquiry as a result of our preliminary findings. Assuming the general validity of the effect we observed, we are, nevertheless, stimulated to look backwards in reexamination of our method of inducing the change in the perceptual environment, and forward to the necessity of additional experimentation that will help us to further understand the mechansims responsible for our results.

We thought we had constructed an experiment about dreaming that would disentangle the processes of perception from the operations of meaning. Though our hopes have been realized to some extent, we have come upon what many others have observed before — a borderland between the two that will require much more study. Nevertheless, this investigation may provide an improved design for systematic manipulation of experience in waking life in combination with objectified means of observing the effects upon dreaming; a design that may be equal to the task of examining the normative range of interactions of the perceptual and cognitive realms in dream life.

ACKNOWLEDGMENTS

This investigation was supported in part by Research Grant MH-13269, Research Scientist Award MH-18739 (H.P.R.), and Interdepartmental Research Training Grant MH-06418 to Albert Einstein College of Medicine (J.H.), from the National Institute of Mental Health. We would like to thank Stephen Lamstein, Jane Salmon, Regina Wdowiak, Laura Laptook, Michael Fetell and Robert Lupi for their generous assistance in the execution of this investigation.

APPENDIX

DREAM SCENE QUESTIONNAIRE

(1, 2) Code Letters _____

(3, 4, 5) Sheet # _____

(6, 7, 8) Subject Initials _____

    Date _____

(9, 10) Type of Exp. _____

(11, 12) Night # (total) in Experiment ____

(13, 14) Phase of Experiment _____

(15, 16) Night # in Phase _____

(17) Awakening # (total) _____

(18) Stage of this awakening _____

    Clock time of this awakening_____

(19) Awakening # in this stage _____

(20) Period # (see Box III) _____

(21, 22) How long in stage before awakening

    Time gogs removed _____

    Time fell asleep _____

(23, 24, Elapsed time _____
25, 26)

(27, 28, Elapsed TST _____
29)

(30) Scene # _____

    Tape reel letter_____

    Foot # from _____ to _____

    EEG page # _____

"Describe the last scene you saw."
(focus on perceptual material)

RECALL: If no recall at all, skip to #66; if there is recall, but it is not visual in character, skip to #56.

_____

_____

_____

_____

_____

_____

(If there is recall then ask:)

"Are you sure that this experience continued until the moment of awakening? (Ask only once at each awakening) Yes No (If No, skip to #66 and enter 0 for #66).

"As a whole was the scene dimly or brightly lit?" D 0 1 2 3 4 5 B (37)
(score 0 only for visual sense of complete blackness, not simply for absence of visual material; latter is scored −. In either case skip to #56.)

"Were the colors pale and washed out or rich and full?" W 0 1 2 3 4 5 F (38)
(score 0 only for completely achromatic imagery; if subject has a sense of colored imagery but there is no recall of specific coloration, enter −)

WORLD APPEARANCE QUESTION: (ask on goggle and recovery nights only)
"Did this scene appear anything like the world does through the goggles?" Yes No (39)
If Yes: "Explain the similarities and differences." If No: "How was it different?"

_____
_____
_____
_____
_____

OBJECT COLOR QUESTIONS: ask:
1. "What objects did you see?" (up to ten) _____
2. "What was the precise color of the (name object) _____ ?"
3. "How *white* (W), grey, or *black* (B) was the value of this (name object)_____ ?"
4. "Was it a *washed out* (W) or a *full rich* (R) (name color) _____ ?"
5. "Is it possible to see this particular color during the day with the goggles you are wearing now?"

Object	Precise Color Shade	Value W 1 2 3 4 5 B	Saturation W 1 2 3 4 5 R	See with Goggles Yes No D.K.
1.	(37)	(38)	(39)	(40)
2.	(41)	(42)	(43)	(44)
3.	(45)	(46)	(47)	(48)
4.	(49)	(50)	(51)	(52)
5.	(53)	(54)	(55)	(56)
6.	(57)	(58)	(59)	(60)
7.	(61)	(62)	(63)	(64)
8.	(65)	(66)	(67)	(68)
9.	(69)	(70)	(71)	(72)
10.	(73)	(74)	(75)	(76)

(Instructions for 40-45 are on Data Entry Sheet)

"Could you see the light source?" Yes No (46) (if answer is *No*, go to #50)
If Yes − A. "Was it dim or bright?" D 1 2 3 4 5 B (47)
B. "Was there any tint?" Yes No
"What color was the light source tinted?" _____ (48) (if Yes)
C. "Was this a slightly colored (S) (name color) _____ or was it a full rich (R) (name color)_____ S 1 2 3 4 5 R (49)

GENERAL TINT QUESTION:
"Was there any general color tint to this scene?"   Yes   No
if Yes: "What was the color of the tint?"   _____ (50)
          "Was it a slightly colored or a full rich (name color) _____ ?"
                                                          S 1 2 3 4 5 R   (51)

NOTE TO THE INTERROGATOR: If you feel there is a discrepancy among any of the above responses (particularly to the *World Appearance* and *General Tint* questions), clarify here and *change* above responses to most accurately reflect the subject's recall.
COMMENTS: _____
_____
_____
_____
_____

"Was there any *one* object color which was prevalent throughout this scene?"
No   Yes   color: _____ (52) (Note only the *most* prevalent color.)

"Was there anything in this scene whose color was particularly striking?"
No   Yes   object: _____; color: _____ (53)

"Was there anything in the scene which was colored differently than it normally is in the real world?"   No   Yes   object: _____ ; color: _____ (54)
                                                        object : _____ ; color: _____ (55)

"Did you have the feeling that you were wearing the goggles?"   Yes   No   (56)
(ask on goggle, recovery nights, and post-goggle experimental nights only)

"Is the setting of this scene similar to anything actually observed by you?"   Yes   No (57)
If Yes: "How long ago?" _____ (58, 59, 60, 61)
          "Is the scene colored the same or differently as the awake experience?"
                    Same   Diff   (62)

"What emotions did you or anyone else experience in this scene?" _____

If no response, ask: "how did you feel about the (mention a prominent action or object in the scene)?" _____
_____

Enter the two most prominent emotions of *S* (63 & 64) and the most S _____ (63)
prominent emotion of a person in dream other than *S* (65)   S _____ (64)
                                                        Other _____ (65)

	0	1	2	3	4	
	None	Poor	Fair	Good	Excellent	
Recall Rank:	None	Poor	Fair	Good	Excellent	(66)

Did this scene contain a goggle effect in your opinion?

	0	1	2	3	4	
	None	Weak	Mild	Strong	Complete	(67)

State reason: _____
_____
_____

(In #30, number scene being experienced at moment of awakening #1, next earlier #2, next earlier #3, etc.).

DREAM SCENE DATA ENTRY SHEET

Complete in pencil.

FILL IN ALL ENTRIES: wherever a question is inapplicable enter a "—" (dash) next to its number on this sheet; when a series of #'s are skipped, start with a "—," and continue with a vertical line. Always enter letters S̄ and T̄ as shown (with a dash over top).

#		Description	#	Description
1		Specific code letters designated for this experimental run.	40	Enter a two digit # (from 00 to 10) referring to the total # of objects reported for this scene.
2			41	
3		Sheets to be numbered consecutively beginning with 001 and running cumulatively through the experiment. Check last number on previous night and continue.	42	Enter a two digit # (from 00 to 10) which expresses only the # of chromatic objects.
4			43	
5			44	Enter a two digit # (from 00 to 10) which expresses only the # of achromatic objects.
6		Initials for identifying this S for all runs. No other S should have exactly same three letters. Always use three letters. If no middle initial enter a —.	45	
7			46	See the Light Source: Enter 0 for No; 1 for Yes. If answer is No, place — in #'s 47, 48, and 49.
8			47	Brightness of the Light Source: Enter the # circled on the questionnaire.
9		Enter the two numbers given by experiment leader for this run.	48	Tint of the Light Source: Enter 0 for No, or the appropriate code letter from Box IV. (If answer is No, place — in #49.)
10			49	Saturation of the Light Source Tint: Enter the # circled on the questionnaire.
11		Total night number in the exp. beginning with 01; check number on previous night and add 1 for tonight.	50	General Tint: Same instructions as #48. (If answer is No, place — in #51.)
12			51	Saturation of the Tint: Enter the # circled on the questionnaire.
13		Enter Phase of Experiment from Box I. If any question check with experiment leader.		
14				
15		Enter two numbers starting with 01 to designate the total # of nights including tonight spent in lab in this phase.		
16				
17		The total # of awakenings, including this awakening, done so far tonight.		

#	Instructions
18	Enter number from Box II corresponding to EEG stage of this awakening.
19	Total # of awakenings done so far tonight in this EEG stage. (If SOS, total of all types.)
20	Period of this awakening. Enter code # from Box III.
21	Express in minutes beginning with 01 the continuous time of
22	this stage until this arousal.
23	A four digit number beginning with 0001 representing
24	elapsed time in min since gogs were removed today. (On split
25	nights elapsed time is counted from the time the gogs were
26	removed on the previous night.)
27	Enter TST in min until this awakening. Make sure to subtract
28	all awake time. (On split nights, fill in only *after* gogs are
29	worn.)
30	Enter scene # (make sure scenes are numbered according to instructions on back page of questionnaire form).
31 to 35	blank
36	
37	*Illumination of the Scene:* Enter the # circled on questionnaire, or a –.
38	*Saturation of the Scene:* Enter the # circled on questionnaire, or a –.
39	*Goggle World Appearance:* Enter 0 for *No;* 1 for *Yes.*

#	Instructions
52	*Prevalent Color:* Enter 0 for *No* or the appropriate code letter from Box IV.
53	*Striking Color:* Same instructions as #52.
54	*Abnormal Colors:* Enter color code for each of two abn. colors from Box IV. If only one abn. color, enter – in #55; if
55	No abn. colors, enter 0 in 54 and – in 55.
56	*Feeling of Wearing Goggles:* Enter 0 for *No;* 1 for *Yes.*
57	*Observed Dream Setting Before:* Enter 0 for *No;* 1 for *Yes.* (If answer is *No,* place – in #'s 58, 59, 60, 61, 62.)
58	*How Long Ago:* Enter a four digit # in days from 0001 to
59	9999 for how long ago the scene occurred (e.g., 2 years =
60	0730). If period is greater than 9999 enter 999X.
61	
62	*Same or Different Coloration:* Enter 0 for Diff.; 1 for Same.
63	*Emotions of Dreamer:* Choose letters from Box V which correspond best to the two most prominent emotions of the
64	S. If one emotion only, enter – in #64. If no emotions, enter 0 in #63 and – in #64.
65	*Emotions of Another:* Choose letter from Box V code letters for the most prominent emotion of another person in the scene. (If none, enter –.)
66	*Recall Rank:* Enter # circled on questionnaire.
67	Goggle Effect: Enter rank on questionnaire.
68 to 80	blank

347

OBJECT DATA ENTRY COLUMN

Key: swg = see with goggles;
No = 0, Yes = 1, DK = 2

NOTE: In cases when S believes object was colored but color not known, fill in Z under *color*, rank *value* and put a "—" next to *saturation* and *swg*.

1 to 35	repeat entries of 1-35 from opposite side
36	2

OBJECT #1:
37	color (code Box IV)
38	val. (1-5)
39	sat. (1-5)
40	swg

OBJECT #2:
41	color (code Box IV)
42	val. (1-5)
43	sat. (105)
44	swg

OBJECT #3:
45	color (code Box IV)
46	val. (1-5)
47	sat. (1-5)
48	swg

OBJECT #4:
49	color (code Box IV)
50	val. (1-5)
51	sat. (1-5)
52	swg

BOX II
EEG Stage Code

Enter:

1	=	I
2	=	II
3	=	III
4	=	IV
5	=	REM
6	=	SOS, beginning of nt.
7	=	SOS, after REM awakening
8	=	SOS, after NREM awakening

BOX III
Period of Awakening

Period			
0-1st	NREMP	=	1
1st	REMP	=	1
1st-2nd	NREMP	=	2
2nd	REMP	=	2
2nd-3rd	NREMP	=	3
3rd	REMP	=	3
3rd-4th	NREMP	=	4
4th	REMP	=	4
4th-5th	NREMP	=	5
5th	REMP	=	5
5th-6th	NREMP	=	6
6th	REMP	=	6
6th-7th	NREMP	=	7
7th	REMP	=	7

OBJECT #5:

53	color (code Box IV)
54	val. (1-5)
55	sat. (1-5)
56	swg

OBJECT #6:

57	color (code Box IV)
58	val. (1-5)
59	sat. (1-5)
60	swg

OBJECT #7:

61	color (code Box IV)
62	val. (1-5)
63	sat. (1-5)
64	swg

OBJECT #8:

65	color (code Box IV)
66	val. (1-5)
67	sat. (1-5)
68	swg

OBJECT #9:

69	color (code Box IV)
70	val. (1-5)
71	sat. (1-5)
72	swg

OBJECT #10:

73	color (code Box IV)
74	val. (1-5)
75	sat. (1-5)
76	swg
77 to 80	blank

BOX IV
Color Code

Enter	
A	purple
B	blue
C	blue-green
D	green
E	green-yellow
F	yellow
G	orange-yellow
H / I	orange
J	orange-red
K	red
L	violet
M	pink
N	goggle color
P	brown, tan, beige
Q	white
R / S	light grey
T	grey
U	dark grey
V	black
W	metallic silver
X	metallic gold
Y	
Z	don't know

BOX V
Emotion Code

Enter	
A	happiness
B	anger
C	fear
D	envy, jealousy
E	complacency, etc.
F	concern
G	anxiety
H	apprehension
I	shock, surprised
J	affection
K	annoyance
L	doubt
M	depressed
N	confused
P	enjoyable
Q	frustration
R	content
S	ecstatic
T	disappointed
U	detached
V	disgust
W	excitement
X	involved
Y	passion
Z	other

10

The Effects of External Stimuli
Applied Prior to and During Sleep
on Sleep Experience

A. M. Arkin
J. S. Antrobus
City College at the City University of New York

Throughout the long history of the interpretation and study of dreams much observation and discussion have been devoted to the effects of presleep experience on dreams, including the events of the previous day and of sensory stimulation during sleep. The cognitive response of the sleeper to presleep and concurrent sleep sensory stimulation provides us with one of the powerful research tools for the study of how sleep mentation, including dreams, is generated. Since the rules and principles which describe the generation of dreaming belong to more general theories of thought and cognition, presleep experience and sensory stimulation during sleep provide a unique and therefore valuable testing ground for such theories. In the 19th century, sleep-stimulation anecdotes were commonly cited as support for the associationist theory of thinking. For example, the introduction of perfume into a sleeper's room on a hot night was said to be capable of eliciting dreams of tropical romance. Among the secondary benefits of this main research thrust are enlightenment about sensory thresholds, perceptual vigilance, and individual differences during sleep, as well as effects of presleep posthypnotic suggestion as manifested during sleep.

The literature prior to the advent of electrographic technology has been thoroughly reviewed by Freud (1900/1953c) and more recently by Ramsey (1953). Although these reports include many dramatic instances of factors which influence dream content, the observations lack the systematic controls and protections against observer bias that are now required of experimental studies.

The first question asked by contemporary work was whether sleep mentation can be reliably and systematically modified by external stimulation. That is, may we demonstrate such phenomena experimentally? As we shall see, Dement and Wolpert (1958b) and others answered this question with a qualified "yes," that it is possible to observe the phenomenon frequently under laboratory conditions. The second question, in our judgement, is: can we take these observations beyond a set of interesting curiosities and use them to further our understanding about how the dream is constructed? As this review shows, we will be a long time in arriving at an answer.

We will develop the topic as it has been researched during the current electrographic era along the following lines:

1. the effects of stimuli applied *during* sleep on dream content (flashes of light, tones, water sprayed on the skin, tape recording of one's own voice versus that of others, names of persons emotionally close to the sleeper versus indifferent names, and so on);

2. the effects of variables impinging on the subject *prior* to sleep, ranging in time from occurrences during the day (including Freud's "day residue" concept), to events experienced at sleep onset including the hypnagogic phase;

A. studies involving experimental procedures carried out in "normal" wakeful consciousness (specific films, specific drive arousal and frustration, studying, exercise, planned day-time experience, free association at sleep onset, and so on);

B. studies involving presleep hypnosis with posthypnotic suggestions to dream about selected topics or specific content.

EFFECTS OF STIMULI APPLIED DURING SLEEP

Although the studies described under this heading share a common feature — all pertain to the effects of external stimuli applied during sleep on concurrent mentation — they also have many differences: there was considerable variation in the nature of the stimulus, the sleep stage in which it was introduced, and the focus of attention of the investigator. Regarding the latter, some workers were interested in more basic primary and secondary perceptive processes in sleep, whereas others sought to examine higher order cognitive operations. Also some studies were specially designed to assess the effects of external stimuli whereas others only provided incidental observations obtained during the pursuit of other experimental goals. We describe each such category of research separately.

Effects of Sensory Stimulation Introduced During Sleep

The first systematic experimental study of the effects of external stimuli on sleep mentation to utilize electrographic technology was that of Dement and Wolpert (1958b). In an experiment with 12 volunteer subjects, stimuli consisting of either a 1000 Hz tone, a series of light flashes, or a spray of water on the skin were applied during ongoing Stage REM. These stimuli were usually below waking threshold. The subjects were then definitively awakened by a loud bell. The mentation reports elicited following each condition were examined for evidence of: (1) unambiguous *incorporation* of the preawakening stimulus into an ongoing dream; and (2) *modification* of ongoing dream content in some appropriate, recognizable manner other than direct incorporation.

The water-spray stimulus was the most effective by far in producing both types of results. An example of the former outcome was a report in which the subject dreamt of being "squirted" by someone; and of the latter, dreams about sudden rainfalls, or leaking roofs. Following the stimulus of the 1000 Hz tone, a subject reported experiencing the sudden intrusion of a brief roaring sound into the dream. The subject was frightened and thought that either an earthquake was occurring or that a plane had crashed outside of the house in the dream. And after stimulation with light flashes, dream modifications included a sudden fire, a flash of lightning, seeing shooting stars, and a more direct indication of incorporation in which the subject dreamt of the experimenter shining a flashlight into the subject's eyes. Finally, the most frequent incorporations occurring after the sounding of the awakening bell were dream content of the ringing of a telephone or doorbell just as the subject awoke.

The results of 98 tests were available in which the various experimental stimuli, themselves *insufficient* to awaken the subjects, were applied during ongoing Stage REM. 14 of 33 following the water spray (42%), 7 of 30 following light flashes (23%), and 3 of 35 (9%) achieved direct incorporation.

Because of the short latency between stimulation and awakening, those instances in which subjects *were* aroused to full wakefulness by the experimental stimulus, or by the awakening bell provided the best opportunity to evaluate the effectiveness of stimuli in modifying ongoing dream content. Of 15 such occasions following the water spray, 6 (40%) showed such modification; whereas of 204 occasions following the bell, only 20 (10%) revealed similar results. Finally, of 5 instances following the 1000 Hz tone, none of the reports disclosed evidence of dream modification.

Thus the findings of this initial experiment demonstrated that external stimuli, presented during Stage REM could be perceived by the subjects without apparent awakening. Further, they showed that the phenomenon might be similar to waking perception of the stimulus event; or, on the other hand, that such percepts could be transformed in some fashion according to the context of the concurrent mentation of the sleeper.

Is it not interesting and puzzling that this study showed such a relatively small overall proportion of stimulus incorporation (24% of all tests) and experimental modification of dream content (12% of all tests)? Taken at face value, the results suggest that ongoing REM sleep mentation is relatively impervious to intrusions from concomitant external sources. Another partial explanation is that the experimenters judgments of the reports were unduly conservative and literal, thus leading to an underestimate of the magnitude of incorporation of external stimuli and their potential for modification of dream content.

Why the dreamer is more likely to respond to some stimuli, and only on some occasions, is quite relevant to notions of perceptual vigilance during sleep and to models of dream formation. Parametric studies of the effects of stimulus intensity, stimulus modality, and familiarity or history of experience with the stimulus are called for.

Thus, it is not clear why the water spray should have been superior to auditory and visual stimuli in the experimental situation.[1] It is of interest, however, that a parallel clinical situation occurs in enuresis in which dreams about moisture, liquids, and so on are common despite the occurrence of enuretic episodes in NREM rather than REM sleep. The most reasonable explanation is that the sustained stimulation of the urine to the skin affects the content of succeeding REM-sleep dreams in the same manner as did the water spray in the above experimental situation.

Results qualitatively similar to those observed by Dement and Wolpert (1958b) have been reported by others. Thus, using stimuli applied to other types of sensory systems, Baldridge and co-workers (1965, 1966) have published preliminary findings on the effects of thermal stimulation on dreams; incorporations were said to occur in 25% of the occasions. Examples were a dream containing a reference to getting food from a refrigerator following cold skin contact, and another referring to a warm day following a warmth stimulus. In addition, the effects of kinesthetic stimuli (produced by raising and lowering the upper part of a hospital bed) were said to be followed by dreams which were distinguishable from those associated with control nonmovement awakenings. Mentation reports following motion often involved not only specific movement activities but dreams of falling, flying, riding a motor scooter and other indications of increased activity on the part of the dreamer, as well.

Along related lines, incidental observations, made in the course of studies designed for other purposes, indicated that external stimuli, such as tones used to experimentally awaken subjects, are more likely to be incorporated into REM sleep, transformed or misperceived when either the subject's awakening threshold was high or the stimulus was initiated at low intensities and permitted to increase gradually (Goodenough et al., 1965a,b; Rechtschaffen, Hauri, & Zeitlin,

---

[1]More recently, Dement (1972) cited work of his students on the effects of external stimuli on dreams. Unfortunately, the original work is unavailable to us and we can only describe Dement's summary. A number of subjects (total not given) were awakened during REM sleep prior to which tape recordings of stimuli, introduced about 10 sec after REMP onset, had been played at subwaking threshold levels. The stimuli included 12 familiar and evocative sounds such as a rooster crowing, a steam locomotive, a bugle playing reveille, a barking dog, traffic noise and a speech by Martin Luther King, Jr. By contrast to the earlier study (Dement & Wolpert, 1958b), a striking proportion of the sound stimuli influenced dream content: 56%. The locomotive sound was the most effective, and traffic noise the least.

1966). Their findings suggest the importance of stimulus-threshold factors in determining outcomes — a factor not yet systematically investigated.

In the course of designing research in this area, Koulack (1969) properly utilized a technique which would simultaneously ensure cortical registration of the stimulus in all stages of sleep and minimize the production of concurrent arousal bursts of alpha frequencies or body movements. Earlier, Goff et al. (1966) had shown that percutaneous electrical stimulation of the median nerve at the wrist sufficiently intense to elicit a thumb jerk duing wakefulness, is capable of producing cortical responses in all stages of sleep. Accordingly, Koulack (1969) utilized this technique excluding from his main analysis all stimuli associated with EEG alpha frequencies or body movements. Thus, subjects received percutaneous electrical stimulation to the wrist as described, during REM sleep under 5 different conditions, each with awakenings for mentation reports as follows: C_1, no stimulation with awakening 3 min after the first REM; C_2, stimulation at first REM with awakening 30 sec afterward; C_3, stimulation at first REM with awakening after 3 min; C_4, stimulation 3 min after the first REM, with awakening 30 sec later; and C_5, stimulation 3 min after the first REM and awakening delayed for 3 min after stimulus termination. Each wrist was stimulated at least once in each condition and conditions were randomly ordered. Stimuli without awakenings were also applied during NREM sleep. Fifteen awakenings were made for each of 10 adult male subjects, three in each of the conditions, during 4-9 nights each slept in the laboratory. Subjects rated their own dreams on a number of ad hoc rating scales and mood adjective checklist dimensions. Postexperimental interviews were conducted to secure associations to the dreams and additional content. The chief focus of interest was whether the somatosensory electrical stimulus would produce direct and/or indirect stimulus incorporations into the ongoing dream. From both sets of data, direct and indirect dream incorporations were scored by a judge who was unaware of the specific association between the experimental awakening category and the subjects' productions. A second judge, totally unaware of the experimental details, scored edited nocturnal interviews in 7 content areas (such as self-participation or self-activity). In all, 28 subdivisions of such scored material were obtained. Reliability for each judge was evaluated by extent of agreement with the author and was reported as at least 96%. By direct incorporation, Koulack (1969) meant "some sort of direct representation of the stimulus situation in the dream [p. 719]," whereas indirect incorporation referred either to events suggestive to the rater of the stimulus situation or to occasions when subjects were able to connect associatively with the stimulus during the postsleep interview, when such associations related to the more general laboratory or stimulus situation.

The specific hypotheses to be tested were:

1. Stimuli applied during REM sleep in a sequence of six shocks at 2.5-sec intervals would be manifested in mentation reports in both direct and indirect

fashion, as indicated by comparison to reports elicited from nonstimulated conditions in the same subject.

2. Stimuli would enhance self-participation and self-activity in the dream.

3. The greatest dream modification would occur with introduction of stimuli at the beginning of the REM period as opposed to later on.

4. Stimuli presented in NREM sleep would either initiate REM periods or reduce latency to stage REM.

In accordance with Koulack's (1969) prediction, each stimulation condition occasioned significantly more direct and indirect incorporation than occurred with C_1, but contrary to expectations the stimulation conditions did not produce different outcomes among themselves. Maximum indirect incorporation (42%) was attained in C_3, whereas maximum direct incorporation (40%) occurred in C_5. Expectations that stimuli would produce increased presence and activity of oneself in the dreams; that effects would be greatest when stimuli were applied early as opposed to later in the REM period; and that stimuli would initiate or hasten the onset of REMPs were not supported. In addition, direct incorporation was more likely when associated with alpha bursts. Unfortunately, potential gains over other studies in obtaining refined data under improved conditions of stimulus control were not realized because of methodological difficulties. Specifically, Foulkes (1970), in criticizing the work, commented that although the study appeared to demonstrate incorporation of somatosensory stimulation in REM dreams, the lack of control data for stimuli in other modalities made assessment uncertain. Also, a separate control group would have been a useful supplement to using each subject as a self-control (the control baseline having been the number of "incorporations" during the C_1 procedure). Additional problems in evaluating the study included inadequately described dream-scoring categories, inclusion among indirect "incorporations" of any material relating to the general laboratory situation, inadequate Stage REM control awakenings, and a confounding of results of stimulations associated with REM-phasic versus nonphasic differences with early (C_2 and C_3) versus late (C_4 and C_5) conditions.

Children as Subjects in Sensory-Stimulation Experiments in Sleep

Might the maturational level of brain development affect the outcome of external stimuli applied during sleep? One could imagine reasons for predicting either a greater or smaller effect in children than in adults. Relevant information is provided by Foulkes et al. (1969), who sought to determine whether external stimuli were incorporated into children's dreams partly to assess validity of their laboratory dream reports and partly out of the inherent interest residing in the question. After two children between 4½ and 5½ years of age provided two fairly clear-cut but unplanned examples of stimulus effects on dream content, attempts to investigate this possibility more systematically were carried out on four additional children whose age ranged from 4 to 4½ years. On one experimental night each, drops of water, puffs of air, puffs of cotton and an emory board were all lightly applied to the skin of each subject during REM sleep. Only one subject (female) appeared to incorporate a stimulus, and this was on three of the four occasions. The cotton puff was followed by a dream of her sister playing with a cuddly toy lion; the air puff, a dream of a family outing in a boat on a lake, with the wind blowing on her face; the water, a dream that she was with her siblings and spraying a hose. The emory board produced no obvious effect on dream content. In no instance were sleep EEG patterns disrupted and in all cases, stimulation was terminated a few seconds prior to awakening. The results as a whole support the contention that stimulus incorporation is indeed possible in the dreaming child but does not permit meaningful comparisons with results on adults.

Subsequently, Foulkes and Shepherd (1972) performed a more ambitious study. The subject pool consisted of 30 children, 16 of whom were 9-10, and 14 were 3-4 years of age. Awakenings were made after external stimulation on Nights 2 and 9 of a long term study schedule on the content of children's dreams. Mentation reports were obtained from both REM and NREM sleep. The stimuli were a cotton puff dabbed on the face, induced limb movement and a water spray to the skin, each preceding awakening by 5-15 sec.

Fifty-six usable mentation reports were categorized by two independent judges as displaying direct incorporation (related to the subject as a dream character), indirect incorporation (unrelated to the subject), or no incorporation. The incorporation rates were as follows: cotton puff: both judges, 0%; limb movement: Judge 1, 8.5%, Judge 2, 5.6%; water spray: Judge 1, 15.6%, Judge 2, 10.4%. Of Judge 1's six successfully detected-water stimulations, four were categorized as indirect, and two direct; four were in REM and two in NREM sleep. The results were deemed to be generally consistent with those of Dement and Wolpert (1958).

(It should be noted that, in this instance, "direct" versus "indirect" incorporation are used in a somewhat different sense than that of Koulack, (1969) and that of Dement and Wolpert, 1958.)

Effects of Verbal Stimulation

What would happen if, instead of primarily stimulating sensory components of perceptual systems, one chose to observe the effects of verbal stimuli? One might expect in this way to involve more complex cognitive processes. One of the most useful and impressive studies in the entire field of sleep mentation is Berger's (1963) work on experimental modification of dream content by meaningful verbal stimuli. His purpose was to determine whether verbal stimuli would be incorporated or misperceived in some fashion and appear in ongoing dream events, and also whether such occurrences would be related to the emotional significance of the stimulus to the subject. The stimuli were tape recordings of four first names of persons. By suitable objective methods, two were predetermined to possess strong emotional significance for the subject and two were emotionally neutral. The latter were equal to the emotional names in the number of syllables but maximum in phonic contrast.

The experimental plan called for the presentation of a single name 5-10 min after each REM-period onset. On each succeeding occasion, a different name was chosen on a random basis from the set of four specifically selected for each subject. The stimulus was sounded at an intensity sufficient to initially provoke a just discernible change in the EEG without awakening the subject.

Such EEG changes usually consisted of a flattening of the EEG trace, of "humping," of low-voltage, fast activity for 1-2 sec or, only rarely, 1 or 2 sec of alpha rhythm. Four male and four female, "normal" young adults served as subjects.

An approximate total of 10 dreams was obtained from each subject during 4-6 nights of sleep. There were 89 usable reports with approximately equal proportions following emotional and neutral stimulus names. In contrast to the study of Dement and Wolpert (1958b) in which the subjects were aware of the nature of the experiment, not one in Berger's (1963) study seemed to have an awareness of the true aims of the project (as evidenced by their replies to relevant questions put to them, and their expression of genuine surprise upon being informed at the end of the experimental schedule.)

The results were assessed by testing the prediction that both an independent judge and the subjects themselves (for their own dreams) would be able to correctly match each of the four stimulus names with its corresponding mentation report significantly more often than would be expected by chance alone. The assessors were told in advance that "the type of connection to look for is between the dream content and the sound of the name — or any other you may think fit." Both the subjects and the judge did indeed make correct matchings at statistically significant levels (range of $p: \leq .05$ to $\leq .001$) and, furthermore there was a strikingly high level of agreement between them regarding the specific matches. (The subjects had been instructed to state whether their matchings were based either upon a perceived connection between the stimulus names and the reports, or whether they merely made their choice as a guess; the independent judge had been instructed to rate matchings at four levels of confidence, the last level a guess.)

Of the 89 mentation reports used in the assessment, 48 (54%) were scored overall as possessing a "definite connection" to the stimulus name. The manner of the relation varied, however, and appeared to be separable into four different categories, assonance (by far the most frequent), association, direct, and representation. Details are furnished in Table 10.1.

TABLE 10.1

Modes of Relationship between Stimulus Name and Mentation Report

Category	Number of reports	Stimulus name	Features of mentation report illustrative of relationship category
Assonance	31	Robert	Rabbit; was slightly frightened and distorted
		Naomi	An *aim* to *ski*; friend who says *"Oh, show me"*
		Gillian	Came from *Chile* (that is a Chilean); *linen*
		Andrew	La*nd*, cent*ri*fuge, h*and*
Association	6	Maureen	Relevant dream content: being handed back his math book which had been marked in a peculiar manner, similar to the way the English master used to mark books at school.
			Subject's spontaneous associations upon hearing the tape recording of mentation report but still un-apprised of the specific corre-sponding stimulus name: the name of English master had been *More; Maureen* (current girl friend) studied math
Direct	8	Eileen	The subject thought to have shout-ed out the name of current girl-friend, "Eileen" in dream
Representation	3	Leslie	The subject dreamed of an Indian woman with glasses; subject's boyfriend an Indian named Les-lie who occasionally wears glasses
	Total: 48 out of 89 reports		

Berger (1963) indicated his awareness of problematic aspects of the categorizations of his data, stating for example, that

> ... in order to examine the forms in which the stimuli were incorporated into the dream, one must decide which dreams were in fact modified by the stimulus. [For various reasons] there appear to be no adequate criteria by which one can make such judgements and one must rely upon a reasonable, subjective analysis of the dream. The analysis [of the modes of incorporation of the stimuli into the dreams] is there-fore only a tentative one and it must be continually borne in mind that examples quoted may have been arrived at fortuitously [p. 730].

Thus, relationships categorized as assonance were based upon phonic features which the stimulus name and mentation report held in common. Most frequently these resembled the "clang associations" of descriptive psychiatry. More often the dream items repeated single features of the stimulus word-vowels and consonants, either singly or in combination.

Occasions illustrative of the association category arose only during the course of subjects listening to the recordings of their own mentation reports. This provoked spontaneous associations in the the subject which were clearly related to the stimulus name where the mentation report contents themselves had not been previously revealing.

Direct relationships included all instances in which the stimulus was directly incorporated into the dream as an externalized or internalized voice.

Representation was the category reserved for occurrences in which the person bearing the emotional stimulus name appeared either directly in the dream or else "in a disguised or transformed" manner.

In presenting his results, Berger (1963) made the following additional observations and remarks:

1. There were no appreciable differences in the number of correct matchings made for emotional or neutral stimuli or in relation to the sex of the subjects, or between subjects. This result was contrary to one of his hypothesized predictions to the effect that emotional stimuli would be matched more frequently with the proper mentation reports than neutral ones. However, Berger did state that sexual symbols of a Freudian psychoanalytic type tended to appear mainly in association with emotional rather than neutral stimuli.

2. Although the perception of the stimulus name, as manifested by apparent incorporation into dream events, was usually as a single assonant word, such perception frequently occurred as a series of words composed of assonant vowels and consonants. Occasionally, the stimulus word was perceived as a type of auditory "Gestalt" of parts or whole words spoken in succession. For example, "Peter" was thought to have been manifested in the dream as "*t*hree *t*icks" against the name of a firm to whom bills had been paid. On still another occasion, incorporation of the stimulus appeared to be manifested by repetition of one or more letters of the stimulus name in the dream narrative. Thus, "Kenny" was the stimulus to the following dream sequence in which such repetitions occurred: "I was at a *c*oncert . . . some *S*cots *c*haracter was − I think he was mainly a comedian . . . the scen*ery* was some ro*ck* with a *crack* in it." Berger indicated that the manner of incorporation, the relationship betwen the stimulus name and its pattern of appearance in the dream, was consistent with Freud's formulations concerning primary process mentation.

3. Incorporation of the stimulus into the dream events was not associated with the presence of alpha rhythm in the EEG following presentation of the names, nor was there any relation to the frequency of GSR fluctuations. By the

same measures, no differences in arousal were detected in response to neutral versus emotional names. Thus, the likelihood of incorporation bore no relationship to concomitant levels of arousal.

4. Another interesting phenomenon was the high frequency with which subjects spontaneously described the incorporated stimulus as it appeared in the dream events as especially "strange," "odd," "sudden," and "vivid."

Berger's (1963) chief conclusions were that "perception of the external world, be it impaired, does occur during the REM periods associated with dreaming [p. 739]." When the stimulus achieves registration, the sleeper usually does not recognize that it originates in the external world but tends on the contrary to perceive it as if it were part of ongoing sleep-mentation experience. When this occurs, the stimulus, as a rule, appears in a dream with various degrees of transformation. Finally, although Berger stated that perceptual awareness of the stimulus is coincident with its cortical analysis, it is neither generally dependent upon the significance of the stimulus names to the subject, nor upon levels of arousal associated with the stimulus. This latter conclusion is somewhat at variance with implications of an earlier study of Oswald et al. (1960) in which K complexes were more likely to be provoked by sounding the subject's own name, a stimulus of greater emotional significance, as opposed to the names of others. Perhaps the most important difference between the conditions of the two studies is that Berger (1963) tested his subjects during Stage REM whereas Oswald et al. (1960) made their observations during NREM.

Castaldo and Holzman (1967, 1969) performed an interesting variant of Berger's basic approach. A total of 19 subjects participated in the original and a replication study. Five minutes after REM period onsets, sleeping subjects were exposed to tape recordings of isolated words uttered by the subjects recorded at a prior time. All stimuli were made intense enough to produce EEG evidence of registration but not sufficiently intense to awaken the subjects. Shortly afterward they were definitively awakened and mentation reports were obtained following which an interval of free association was elicited. The control condition was a tape recording of another person's voice matched for sex, age, intonation, and the same words played under the same conditions with the same consequent procedure and in counterbalanced order.

Two judges independently rated the mentation reports by means of Likert-type scales which measured aspects of the behavior of dream characters. These aspects included amounts of activity, passivity, helpfulness to others, being helped by others, independence, competence, competitiveness, and assertiveness. The authors stated that the intercorrelations between the scales were quite low, attesting to their statistical independence.

The striking new finding was that reports elicited after recordings of the subject's own voice were judged to be much more likely to contain dream content in which the subject was active, assertive, and independent; whereas in the control condition, hearing another's voice tended to be followed by dreams in which the subject was passive and unassertive. Furthermore, the free association interval following completion of the report was likely to continue into wakefulness whatever active or passive trends had been experimentally initiated while dreaming. In addition, as with Berger's (1963) study, the dreams contained varying degrees and kinds of stimulus incorporation in which repetition of content elements, condensation, and assonance were common forms of response and/or transformation. An example of condensation is provided by a dream containing three references to "pennies," which were in response to the stimulus words "fountain, pen," and after a 1-sec pause, "knee, cap." Another point of agreement with Berger's (1963) study is the demonstration that neutral verbal stimuli are capable of dream incorporation.

Finally, the results indicated quite remarkably that sleeping subjects are better able to discriminate between their own voices and those of others, than while they are awake. This conclusion was drawn on the basis that 89% of the subjects ($N = 20$, combining both the initial experiment and its replication) gave a differential dream incorporation response to the stimuli as compared to only 38% in another group of subjects tested in wakefulness for differential recognition of tape recordings of their own voices versus those of others.

The Effects of External Stimuli on NREM-Mentation: Sensory Stimulation

The first comment in the literature on this point appears in the report of Dement and Wolpert (1958b), mentioning that despite stimulus application during NREM sleep, no dream recall could be elicited following awakenings on any occasion. (The protocol called for 15 stimulations per subject during NREM sleep, 5 times each for the 3 stimulus conditions.) One cannot help but speculate, considering that the study was published in 1958, whether this starkly negative result was partly influenced by the already congealed belief that NREM dreaming was either nonexistent or inconsequential.

Subsequent commentary appears sporadically in the literature as parts of papers devoted to other topics. Thus Rechtschaffen et al. (1963), in the course of a paper on sleep mentation in general, mentioned that two of seven subjects tested showed evidence of incorporating external stimuli into NREM sleep reports. A convincing example was provided in which an experimental tone sounded twice was represented in Stage 2 mentation by a whistling noise repeated on two occasions and interwoven into a dream scene containing dialogue with another dream character. In a subsequent paper on auditory awakening thresholds, Rechtschaffen and Foulkes (1965) commented on the great rarity of incorporations of external stimuli into NREM sleep. Further mention of laboratory observation of incorporation of external stimuli into NREM sleep was made by Foulkes (1966).

Thus, it may be said that no truly systematic study of this problem has been published as yet.

Verbal Stimulation During NREM Sleep

Even though mentation reports were not elicited by Oswald, Taylor and Treisman (1960), their study is worthy of description here because it involves the effects of tape recordings of persons' names within NREM sleep upon K complexes
— an indication of cortical response to external stimulation. Oswald et al.'s
(1960) goal was to test the hypothesis that a sensory stimulus causing arousal
from sleep is preceded by cortical analysis of the personal significance of that
stimulus. The data consisted of electrographic and behavioral responses during
NREM sleep of human sleep-deprived subjects to tape-recorded playbacks of
their own first names versus the names of others throughout the night. Evidence
supporting their hypothesis was derived from the findings that:

1. K complexes occurred significantly more often on stimulation with their
own names versus those of others or their own names played backwards; and this
was observed even in the absence of overt behavioral responses.

2. Polyphasic K-complexes appeared significantly more often after hearing
one's own name played in the forward direction rather than the smaller, less
elaborate K complexes that were more prone to occur following one's own
name played in reverse.

3. Overt awakening responses were significantly more likely after hearing
one's own name than after someone else's.

4. Names played forward were significantly more likely to evoke a GSR than
when played in reverse.

5. It was possible to repeatedly observe persistent lack of response with repetitive playback of the names of others and the sudden sequence of K complexes, GSR, behavioral response, and waking alpha rhythm, beginning as little
as .5 sec. following playback of one's own name. Thus, absence of some electrical response of the brain to repetitive stimulation need not signify cortico-fugal
inhibition of afferent inflow to the cortex, but, rather, failure of response may
indicate that the stimulus, as a *result* of cortical analysis is deemed unimportant.

To bring Oswald et al.'s (1960) contribution up to date, we briefly describe
a recently reported study of McDonald et al. (1975) on the effects of tape recordings of personal names on certain electrographic measures during sleep.
Unfortunately mentation reports were not obtained. Thirteen paid male undergraduate subjects spent 2 nights in the sleep laboratory. Besides the EEG and
EOG, the finger plethysmogram, (FP) and heart rate (HR) were monitored. The
stimuli consisted of tape recordings of 25 monosyllabic male nicknames (Al,
Bill, Jim, Dave, Mike and so on), among which was the subject's own name. This
tape was played a total of 6 times throughout all periods of wakefulness and *all*
stages of sleep such that subjects received their own name stimulus 12 times and
other names 288 times. Interspersed with the names on the tape were brief 500-
Hz tone signals played a total of 156 times. The main relevant results were that

subjects responded differentially in Stage 2 to recordings of their own names, others' names, and the tone stimuli, respectively, in descending order. These effects were manifested in the FP and HR measures, and to a lesser extent by the K-complex response. Similar results were observed in Stage REM for the FP measure, and to a lesser extent in HR. Differential results were not observed in Stage 3-4. The results were deemed consistent with those of Oswald et al. (1960), in that both studies demonstrate information processing during sleep. However, they differ in certain details. First, Oswald's findings pertained only to Stage 2 whereas McDonald et al. (1975) have extended the finding to stage REM, and also showed that FP and HR reflect the stimulus conditions more sensitively than the K-complex indicator. Second, contrary to Oswald et al. (1960) names of others rather than one's own were associated more often with K complexes. To round off this digression on information processing during sleep, we should like to cite the other half of the paper of McDonald et al. (1975). This consisted of an independent study on autonomic concomitants of a wakeful conditioned auditory stimulus presented during sleep. It was found that sleepers were able to retain the wakeful ability to discriminate between the conditioned stimulus and another nonconditioned auditory stimulus. This discrimination was indicated by differential FP, HR, and K-complex responses in Stages 2 and 4; neither K complexes (not normally present in Stage REM), nor differential FP or HR responses occurred in Stage REM, however. In agreement with Williams (1973), who has written an excellent review of information processing during sleep, McDonald et al. (1975) believe that information stored in long-term memory remains most available for processing during sleep in Stage 2, least in Stage 4, and to an intermediate degree in Stage REM particularly if the content is sufficiently meaningful. In addition, stimulus preprocessing and short-term memory storage are demonstrable in all stages of sleep as indicated by the persistence of the FP and HR orienting responses and their potential for habituation throughout.

Not until 1970 was a systematic study performed in the topic area involving the elicitation of NREM as well as REM mentation reports. Using 10 male psychiatric residents as subjects, Castaldo and Shevrin (1970) administered specially designed subwaking threshold stimuli which nevertheless produced convincing EEG signs of stimulus registration. As in 2 earlier experiments by Castaldo and Holzman (1967, 1969), the following stimulus word sequence was employed: "fountain pen," and following the 1-sec pause, "kneecap." This stimulus assembly had been previously shown to produce frequent psychoanalytic-type primary and secondary process associative responses. Typical of the former would be a rebus combination of the "pen" and "knee" part of the stimulus into "penny;" and typical of the latter would be associations conceptually related to the stimuli such as "ink" and "paper" for "fountain pen," and "leg" and "bone" for "kneecap." The authors predicted that following such stimuli, Stage 2 mentation reports would tend to contain conceptual types of responses as opposed to REM reports which would include more rebus-like responses. No effects of the stimuli were discernible after Stage REM awakenings but Stage 2 reports possessed a greater number of words conceptually related to the stimulus word on experimental nights in comparison to the control nights (during which awakenings were carried out without prior auditory stimulation). That is, as expected, Stage 2 was associated with conceptual-type responses to the stimulus. Noteworthy is the lack of REM rebus effects previously observed by Shevrin and Fisher (1967) in response to presleep subliminal stimulation with drawings of a pen and a knee. A further description of presleep stimulus studies is contained in the following section. Castaldo and Shevrin (1970) concluded that their results support the hypothesis of different levels of thought organization associated with REM and NREM sleep.

A more recently published work relevant to REM versus NREM responses is that of Lasaga and Lasaga (1973). Eight young adult females served as subjects in a laboratory study of short-term memory during sleep. Inasmuch as the method involved administration of tape-recorded words, phrases, and numbers to the subjects in all stages of sleep and testing for the efficiency of memory of these stimuli shortly afterward, many opportunities arose to observe incorporation of external events into sleep mentation. Accordingly, many incorporations were reported to occur in Stages 2, 3, and 4, as well as REM. On such occasions, besides instances in which the entire stimulus was correctly perceived and recalled, the experimenters observed incorporations of only part of the stimulus (like "my boy friend" recalled as "friends"), substitutions of another word or words, similar in sound and length to the original stimulus ("your mother" recalled as "you're marvelous"), or else complete distortions of the experimental stimulus. In general, the authors stated that their observations resembled those of Berger (1963).

Although not fitting precisely into our expository categories, a unique experiment of Rechtschaffen and Foulkes (1965) is important to describe. Mentation reports were elicited out of both REM and NREM sleep from subjects whose eyes were kept open artificially throughout the night and before whom visual stimuli were displayed prior to awakenings. A total of seven subjects were studied all of whose eyes had been taped open at the time of retiring. Three of the seven also had a pupillary dilator instilled in amounts sufficient to maintain suitable pupil diameter but insufficient to prevent wakeful identification of ordinary common objects (inasmuch as accommodation was also partially impaired). The visual stimuli included a book, a black X, a moving handkerchief, a coffee pot, and a "do not disturb" sign. The results were that at no time was there evidence of any incorporation into sleep mentation regardless of sleep stage.

It is to be recalled that Dement and Wolpert (1958b) found occasional instances of light flashes influencing dream content, showing that visual sensory stimulation is capable of producing positive effects. It would have been interesting to have used similar stimuli in the Rechtschaffen and Foulkes (1965) study for comparison. It seems on the face of it that perception of light flashes need not involve higher order cognitive resources nor coordinated activity of the oculomotor nuclei in tracking moving patterns. Most of the stimuli used by Rechtschaffen and Foulkes, by contrast, probably would have required the functional availability of higher visual neural circuitry.

In concluding this section, it is safe to say that cognitive responses of some form may occur in both REM and NREM sleep as a result of external stimulation. In addition, such responses when they do occur often involve some transformation of stimulus content or pattern which then seems to "fit in" with ongoing sleep mentation. One must be cautious about accepting the validity of the concept of such stimulus incorporation into dreams. In wakefulness, stimuli are often misperceived and misinterpreted. We do not then say that such stimuli were "incorporated" into our wakeful sequences of consciousness. Many of the reported findings could be explained on whatever bases throw light upon wakeful misperception or misinterpretation, on the sleepers accurately perceiving only a part of a stimulus and elaborating a response to that part only, or upon post-perception transformation or elaboration of sensory elements more accurately registered initially. As yet we have no way of distinguishing between these and other alternatives as well.

It is to be noted that considerable variation exists from study to study as to method, definitions of stimulus "incorporation," and experimental results obtained. What is needed is a group of experiments which will provide us with systematic knowledge of the relationships between stimulus-produced modification of dream content and sensory-stimulus threshold factors, effects of "simple" sensory versus more complex stimuli such as verbal material; individual subject differences in tendencies to have dream modifications; and subjects' tendencies to misperceive and misinterpret similar stimuli during wakefulness; and factors related to specific sleep stages, time into sleep stages, and time of night.

Sleep Mentation as Affected by Conditioning Techniques

Inasmuch as several papers have been published demonstrating the feasibility of eliciting conditioned responses during sleep (both classical and operant types) (Gradess et al., 1971; Granda & Hammack, 1961; McDonald et al., 1975), it is curious that thus far, no reports have appeared describing attempts to condition dream content. Work along these lines is in progress (Antrobus, Arkin & Ellman, 1976; Antrobus, Chapter 18, this volume).

THE EFFECTS OF PRIOR TO SLEEP STIMULUS FACTORS ON SUBSEQUENT SLEEP MENTATION

We will now review a group of studies where the effects of prior to sleep stimuli or the prior to sleep environment on dreaming was investigated. The experimenters test the assumption that dream content will respond to biochemical tissue deficits, drives, or to the arousal of strong emotions. In a sense, this area of investigation includes controlled study of the role of "day-residue material" in dream content. The day residues in dreams refer to dream components which represent an event, experience or thought of the previous day, and it was Freud's belief that in every dream, it is possible to find a connection with an experience of the previous day.

The variety of presleep stimuli has been broad and it seems reasonable to group the studies together, when possible, by similarities in the nature of the stimulus employed. Strictly speaking, the category of the effects of sustained alteration of presleep sensory input on sleep experience belongs here. However, this is the subject of a magnificent experimental study and discussion in Chapter 9 of this volume.

Effects of Biological Drive Frustration on Dream Content

Three reports are available dealing with the effects of frustration of biological drives ordinarily satisfied by oral intake of food or drink. In one study, Dement and Wolpert (1958b) deprived 3 subjects of all fluid for 24 hrs prior to retiring in the laboratory. All subjects were quite thirsty at bedtime. Mentation was sampled from REM sleep on 5 separate nights for each subject yielding a total of 15 mentation reports. The authors concluded, on the basis of their own categorizations, that no content directly portrayed the subject as thirsty or in the act of drinking. Ten dreams were said to be devoid of any direct reference to thirst or drinking whereas 5 were categorized as possibly containing indirect references. An example of the latter was the following mentation report: "While watching tv, I saw a commercial. Two kids were asked what they wanted to drink and one kid started yelling, 'Coca Cola, orange, Pepsi, and everything.'" In actuality, the remaining dreams so categorized were similar in the manner of expression of thirst-related material and the reader might well think that the authors were too stringent in their criteria, possibly resulting in unwarranted exclusion of dreams with material reflecting thirst.

By contrast, Baldridge et al. (1965, 1966) mentioned as preliminary findings the occurrence of dreams with "obsessive reference to food" in some subjects following 24-hr food deprivation. With other subjects under similar experimental conditions, dreams possessing angry content were observed.

Finally, Bokert (1968) performed a more elaborate study to determine the effects of thirst and a related verbal stimulus on dreams. REM sleep reports were obtained under the following conditions from 18 subjects, nurses on night duty, who slept in the laboratory by day:

1. sustained daytime deprivation of food and fluids with ingestion of a salty meal just prior to sleep, to enhance thirst (thirst-alone condition);

2. the same procedure repeated except that in addition, just prior to Stage REM awakenings, the subjects receiving the subwaking-threshold tape-recorded verbal stimulus, "a cool delicious drink of water" (thirst-verbal stimulus condition);

3. a control condition in which the subjects were given a nonsalty meal prior to sleep without prior deprivation of food and fluids.

Each subject experienced all three conditions and hence served as their own controls. The hypotheses to be tested were:

1. Under conditions of thirst alone, dreams would contain a greater amount of thirst-related content than in the control conditions.
2. Under conditions of thirst-verbal stimulus, dreams would contain a greater amount of thirst-related content than both thirst-alone and control conditions.

The REM reports were judged for thirst-related content by three "blind," independent judges (interjudge reliability = .93). Thirst-related content words in mentation reports were those which could be placed in the following categories:

1. words related to thirst sensations (like "thirsty," "parched," "dry," "salty taste");
2. words related to thirst satisfiers:
    a. liquids ("water," "beer," "soda," "fruit juices," "milk," and so on);
    b. foods with high water content ("watermelon," "ice cream," "apples," "tomatoes," and so on);
    c. water in its natural state ("snow," "rain," "ice," "river," "lake," and so on);
3. words related to activities or behavior associated with thirst (for example, all forms of the verb "to drink," "sip," "gulp," "quench," "suck," and so on);
4. words related to places associated with thirst (like "bar," "fountain," "ice-cream parlor," "oasis," "kitchen," and so on);
5. words related to persons associated with thirst (like "bartender," "soda jerk," "waiter" or "waitress," "counterman," and so on);
6. words describing inanimate objects associated with thirst (like "glass," "bottle," "cup," "refrigerator," "straw," and so on).

The results were as follows: in accordance with expectations, the average number of thirst-related words in the mentation reports from either thirst condition exceeded that of the control. Specifically, the average was 2.11 for the thirst-verbal stimulus condition, 1.67 for the thirst-alone condition, and .53 for the control condition ($n = 35$, 41, and 41 dreams, respectively). To control for dream length, the averaged ratings of the three judges were used to obtain the proportion of thirst words in the total verbal output of each dream report. Transforming the data into radians, an analysis of variance was performed which resulted in a significant difference between both thirst conditions and the control ($p < .025$). Interestingly, it was found that the positive effects were observed to a significantly greater degree in the later REM periods of the night rather than the earlier ones — a finding consistent with the progressive increase of the somatic need for water with the passage of time. Additional experimental findings were:

1. The thirst-verbal stimulus condition produced significant variation in subjects' responses. Under this experimental condition:

a. Subjects who appeared to incorporate part of the verbal stimulus into their dreams had a greater amount of additional thirst-related content than subjects who did not incorporate the stimulus. (Incorporation was defined as the appearance in the dream of parts of the verbal stimulus such as "drink," "drinking," "drank," and "water.")

b. Incorporator subjects also had more thirst-related content in the thirst-verbal stimulus condition than in the thirst-alone condition.

2. Dream content was related to aspects of postsleep behavior. Thus, subjects reporting gratifying dreams (containing themes of drinking and/or eating,) actually drank less and rated themselves as less thirsty following sleep than those whose dreams were devoid of such content.

3. The thirst-alone condition was associated with increased REM activity.

Among Bokert's (1968) conclusions were that experimentally intensified somatic needs were capable of modifying dream content accordingly. Furthermore, a key notion related to both Freud's (1900/1953) proposition that dreams represent attempted unconscious wish fulfillments, and some cognitive models of dreaming, which state that the dream may generate a partial solution to a problem, is that the need, state, or problem should be partially reduced by the act of dreaming. Bokert is one of the few workers to directly test this notion, and the implied prediction finds some support in the finding that subjects who gratify their thirst in dream fantasy succeed in reducing their thirst need in postdreaming reality. In addition, the results were deemed consistent with Freud's contention that dreams represent an attempted unconscious wish fulfillment but Bokert also speculated that it was possible for conscious wishes to be so represented independent of reinforcement from repressed unconscious infantile tendencies. Regarding both Freudian and cognitive models, however, one should not lose sight of the limited generality of the findings; effects were detectable solely in a subgroup of subjects.

Finally, Bokert (1968) also asserted that the relatively unimpressive results of Dement and Wolpert (1958b) were due to excessively narrow criteria for thirst-related content which did not allow for a wide range of cognitive representatives of thirst in the dream.

Effects of a Presleep Cognitive-Affective Deficit —
Social Isolation — on Dreaming

In an unusual experiment, testing the effects of a cognitive-affective deficit rather than a physiological one, Wood (1962) worked with five young college graduates who spent five nights in the laboratory. Their second day was spent in solitary confinement. On the average, his subjects showed 60% more REM time but less REM activity in response to this condition. The associated dream content both paralleled and differed from the nature of the presleep wakeful behavior. Just as the day was spent in physical inactivity, the subsequent dreams were also physically inactive; but the physical inactivity tended to involve groups of people standing around talking in a sociable fashion — a contrast to the isolation.

Many procedures, and especially many drugs are capable of suppressing REM sleep; by contrast, only a few drugs are capable of producing increases in REM time percentage (increases which are slight). With the controversial exception of wearing prism lenses which alter optical verticality during wakefulness, and the finding of Rechtschaffen and Verdone (1964) that money incentives are capable of producing slight increases of REM time, the results of Wood (1962) are perhaps unique in reporting an independent variable producing substantial increases. Inasmuch as this outcome preceded publication of the standard scoring manual of Rechtschaffen and Kales (1968), it would therefore be important to either rescore Wood's records or else replicate the experiment.

The Effects of Viewing Films on Subsequent Sleep Mentation

Just as simple sensory stimulation during sleep requires lower order cognitive functioning than complex verbal stimuli, so experimental presleep tissue deficits such as thirst seem to impose a more direct, uncomplicated variable for the mind to deal with than elaborate, thematic-affect-arousing dramatic displays such as films. Might such experimental conditions as the latter be more likely to produce effects on dream content which could serve to enlighten us about dream formation processes? As we shall see, the results once again are mixed.

We, therefore, turn now to a group of seven studies which have in common the employment of a presleep condition of sustained visual stimulation by means of films. Each study compared mentation reports following a bland, neutral film with those following an affect-arousing one, which depending on the study, might provoke anxiety, aggression, or sexual excitement, and correlated the findings in various ways with psychological data. Thus, Foulkes and Rechtschaffen (1964) observed 24 adult subjects who slept in the laboratory for 2 counterbalanced nights following an adaptation night. On experimental nights either a violent or nonviolent film was shown prior to retiring. Five nightly awakenings for mentation reports were made according to the following schedule: 2 NREM, one well prior to the first, and one well after the fourth REM period of the night; and from the early portions of each of the first 3 REM periods.

The results were that the violent film was followed by longer and more imaginative REM sleep reports, and the subjects themselves rated these reports as more vivid, clear, and more emotional than after the nonviolent film. That is, the violent film, far from producing dreams judged to be more violent, aggressive, or unpleasant, was followed by dreams which were exciting and interesting, but without influence over specific drive expression or hedonic tone. This nonspecific increase in intensity of dream experience was observed only in the later stage REM reports and not in either NREM or first-REM-period awakenings. Furthermore, incorporations from either film were rare (5% of 179 reports). Finally, no significant differences were found for either film condition on frequency of stages REM or NREM mentation recall, and on latencies to sleep onset or the first REM period.

A somewhat different result was obtained by Foulkes et al. (1967) in a study on the effects of presleep films on childrens' dreams and sleep. Thirty-two boys were employed as subjects, 16 of whom averaged 7½ years of age and 16, 11¼ years. Prior to sleep they were shown either a film with much aggressive content or one with interesting, albeit rather bland content, in counterbalanced order. One film was a violent western and the other dealt with baseball. Subjects were awakened for REM sleep reports on experimental and control nights, the results of which were categorized on the basis of whether incorporation of the film content into REM sleep mentation had been judged to have occurred. In addition, content analyses, degree of mentation recall, and sleep-cycle parameters were assessed. The results were that 14 of 179 REM sleep reports (8%) were judged to have incorporated elements of the presleep stimulus film. Neither aggressive nor neutral film was more likely to have yielded incorporations. And finally, measures of dream intensity in general and hostile-unpleasant content in particular were *less* following the aggressive film.

Of special interest was the *greater* frequency of "bad" dreams (subjects' own judgments) following the neutral film. In addition, neither film condition typically affected standard parameters of the sleep cycle. Mentation recall was also not significantly affected by the presleep conditions. In effect, then, the likelihood of childrens' incorporation of material from presleep films was close to the 5% observed for adults (Foulkes & Rechtschaffen, 1964), thus finding against the hypothesis that children would possess a greater tendency to employ in a direct, unambiguous manner proximate presleep stimuli in synthesis of their dreams. The decrease in dream vividness and unpleasantness following the aggressive film in children is a finding opposite to that for adults. In explaining this difference, Foulkes et al. (1967) noted that the adults were more emotionally involved in the nonviolent film they had seen (a romantic comedy) than in the violent one, whereas the boys were more attentive to the depictions of hostility. Thus, the combined results suggest that greater interest in the presleep film, regardless of the specific content, is likely to be followed by less vivid dreams. In other words, the observation that less intense and unpleasant dreams followed the better attended, violent film in children was deemed to support the notion that viewing dramas of violence provides emotional catharsis in which aggressive tendencies could be momentarily dissipated and not find expression in the subsequent dreams.

More extensive results with regard to incorporations were apparently obtained by Witkin (1969a) and Witkin and Lewis (1967). Twenty-eight men who worked by night and slept by day underwent the following nonconsecutive five-night experimental schedule: one adaptation night and one night each for seeing films of human birth, human subincision, a neutral film, and receiving psychological suggestions aimed to alter bodily sensations. In some instances, a sixth session was added in which a film was shown of a mother monkey eating her dead infant, following which subjects were required to verbalize their ongoing reverie until they fell asleep (Bertini, 1968). On each night, subjects were awakened for REM sleep-mentation reports. In the following morning, each subject received an extensive inquiry about each mentation report and the entire laboratory experience. Also, each subject received a comprehensive clinical evaluation.

The presleep input was regarded as a source of "tracer elements" whose transformations during subsequent mentation samples could be studied. This voluminous data is still being slowly processed but the authors have volunteered the following impressions which must be regarded as highly tentative:

1. Anxiety arousing films tend to be followed by increases in anxiety ratings of mentation reports.
2. Presleep stimulus material often appeared in dreams in transformed presentations in striking accord with classic Freudian dreamwork mechanisms.
3. Dreams following the neutral film had less obvious sexual symbolism.
4. The laboratory situation, including features of interpersonal relationships, appeared in the dreams.
5. Individual stylistic features in the manner of processing presleep stimuli were discernible.
6. The "tracer elements" reappeared in various guises in the sequential REM periods of the night.
7. There was a higher frequency of "forgotten dreams" on nights following affect arousing stimuli.
8. Dreams following stress films contained features which led to childhood memories (sometimes to one's earliest memory).
9. The sense of conviction as to the relationship between presleep stimuli and their transformed presentation in dreams was maximized by associative material elicited during the following morning.

The authors concluded that presleep stimuli in the laboratory undergo complicated transformational processes, circulate through a network of "cognitive structures" including earliest memories and continue to influence associations in the following morning, all in a cogently discernible manner. One must await publication of the final fully processed results of this study before firm conclusions may be drawn.

From the same laboratory, two subsequent studies appeared, in which specific attempts were made to arouse intense presleep anxiety for the purpose of detecting effects on sleep mentation and electrographic parameters. Thus, Karacan et al. (1966) utilized 16, paid, "normal" college males, who spent 6 nights in the laboratory. After an adaptation and a single baseline night, each subject, prior to retiring, viewed over the next 4 nights, 2 emotionally stressful and 2 neutral films, 1 on each night. Besides the standard EEG, EOG, and EMG recordings, this study was distinctive by virtue of its monitoring REMP erections. The anxiety content of REM reports was assessed by an adaptation of the Nowlis and Nowlis (1956) adjective checklist given to subjects to rate their own sleep experience following each awakening, and also by the Gottschalk et al. (1969) anxiety scale. The results were that no significant differences in anxiety content were observed among film nights; however, dreams high in anxiety content were associated with lack of, or nonsustained erections, without relationship to the nature of the presleep film.

In the second, more recent study, Goodenough et al. (1975) obtained clear-cut positive results on a special subgroup of subjects. The authors reasoned that subjects who were demonstrably more responsive to stress during wakefulness would be more likely to have affect-laden dreams following presleep stress. Specifically, it was hypothesized that with all subjects during REMPs, REM activity, dream affect, respiration rate, and degree of irregularity would be higher on nights following viewing stress films as opposed to nights following viewing neutral films; and that in subjects who showed greater respiratory response to stress films during wakefulness the above effects would be more intense; also, respiratory rate and irregularity were expected to be highly correlated with affect in dream reports.

Accordingly, 28 "normal" male night workers who slept by day were selected as subjects. Each subject slept in the laboratory 5 days each at least 1 week apart. The first session provided for adaptation to the experimental situation and the remaining were used for data collection. During these 4 experimental sessions, 2 stress films (depicting birth and subincision of the penis), and 2 neutral educational travelogues (depicting London and the Western U.S.) were shown to each subject in counterbalanced order.

The data from 366 useful REM-period awakenings (yielding 264 dream reports, a 72% recall rate) consisted of 3 sets of observations:

1. sleep electrographic recordings of the EEG, EOG, EMG, and respiration (thoracic and abdominal components independently measured) (In addition, wakeful measurements of respiration were made during the viewing of the films. This procedure enabled the experimenters to determine and compare the nature of the respiratory responses to the stress films, the neutral films, and the REM sleep experience; and to separate the subjects into a group of wakeful responders and nonresponders.);

2. REM mentation reports elicited 5-10 min after REMP onset (scored by a blind judge for anxiety, hostility-out, hostility-in, and ambiguous hostility on the scales devised by Gottschalk, Winget and Gleser, 1969);

3. mood adjective checklist scores (modified from Nowlis & Nowlis, 1956) obtained in response to a baseline control condition, each film condition and to each REM sleep experience after experimental awakenings.

In comparison to the neutral films, stress films, while being viewed, produced significant wakeful, dysphoric, anxious mood reactions and delayed sleep onset. Viewing stress films likewise resulted in significantly increased dream anxiety and also increased REM-period respiratory irregularity primarily among those subjects, who, in the waking state showed irregular breath patterns in response to stressful film events. In addition, dream affect tended to be related to REM-period respiratory irregularity among those subjects who were wakeful responders to the stress films. This tendency reached statistical significance, however, only on the Gottschalk et al. (1969) hostility measure. The authors concluded that the data supported the hypothesis of congruence between wakefulness and the REM dream regarding the relationship between affect and respiratory irregularity. Thus, laboratory findings partly documented the everyday experience that daytime stress often tends to be followed by emotional dreams.

Arousing a completely different drive state, the effects of presleep sexual stimuli were studied by Cartwright et al. (1969). The experimenters observed 10 young adult students over 5 consecutive nights with the following procedure: reports were collected from all REM periods on 1 initial baseline night without presleep stimulation, and on succeeding nights 2 pornographic films were shown prior to retiring. The records disclosed no evidence of sleep-cycle changes. After the erotic film there was a significant decrease in ability to recall dream content; the number of dream characters per dream was reduced and the number of two-person dreams was increased; also the amount of symbolic representation of the film content was higher than would have been anticipated if the subjects had not been exposed to an erotic movie. This last conclusion was based upon comparison with a similar sample of reports elicited from comparable subjects not seeing a sex film. And finally, the amount of direct incorporation from the laboratory setting was greater than from the movie.

Rather than using an absorbing, attention-arousing presleep visual stimulus, such as a film, Shevrin and Fisher (1967) showed 10 adult females a special subliminal visual stimulus previously demonstrated capable of eliciting primary and/or secondary process-types of cognitive responses. Specifically, drawings of a fountain pen in juxtapositiion to a knee were presented in tachistoscopic fashion. As mentioned above a primary-process type of response would be exemplified by images or words related to the stimuli on the basis of their sounds rather than meanings, and a secondary process type of response on the basis of a conceptual relationship to the stimulus. A typical primary process response is "penny" (pen-knee) and a secondary process response is pencil, ink, bone, or leg, accordingly.

These drawings were flashed before the subjects prior to retiring, and samples of mentation, free imagery, and free association were obtained immediately after the stimulus, and upon awakenings from Stages REM and 2, subsequently. It was hypothesized that REM mentation reports would contain more evidence of primary process thinking, and Stage 2 more evidence of secondary process when each was compared to the other. The hypotheses were supported neither by mentation report nor free imagery analysis, but positive findings were obtained from free associations carried out following all three conditions: presleep and Stages REM and 2; and, furthermore, as predicted, rebus responses were more likely from Stage REM, and conceptual responses more likely from Stage 2. These results are consistent with those of Witkin and Lewis (1967) who also found that free associations elicited on the following morning could be traced to stimuli derived from presleep conditions. Considered together, the observations indicate that perceptual material may be placed into "intermediate-term" memory storage prior to sleep, undergo various transformations and be available for retrieval subsequently under special postsleep conditions; but why primary and secondary process derivatives of the original percepts are detectable in free association only, rather than in mentation reports and free imagery is a puzzle. Certainly in view of Fisher and Paul's (1959) replication of the Pötzl phenomenon, one would have expected clear positive effects in REM mentation reports.

Clues about the status of presleep perceptual material during sleep are provided by an interesting study of DeKoninck and Koulack (1975). Hoping to learn whether dreaming facilitates adaptation to stressful experience, they presented a film featuring body mutilation to a group of subjects before sleep at night and again in the following morning. It was hypothesized that subjects who exhibited a greater mastery of the presleep stress, as manifested by less emotionality following the morning showing of the film, would be those who had more anxiety infused dreams and more dream content related to the film. In order to manipulate the degree of incorporation of film elements and anxiety content of the dreams, a part of the sound track of the film, containing the verbalized self-reproaches of a man guilty of the negligence causing the mutilations, was played during REM sleep. The experimental design provided for separate examination of the effects of the film alone without sound-track stimulation; the effects of the sound track alone without previous viewing of the film; and the effects of combined viewing of the film and sound-track stimulation. This part of the procedure involved 16 "normal" college males. In addition, a separate control group of 8 comparable subjects saw the film twice, each showing being separated by 8 hrs of wakefulness. Wakeful emotionality was scored by means of a modified Nowlis and Nowlis (1956) mood-adjective checklist. Mentation reports were analyzed by two "blind" independent judges using the aggressiveness, friendliness, anger, happiness, sadness, and confusion scales of Hall and Van de Castle (1966). Laboratory-incorporation categories of objects, persons, locations, and situations; film-element incorporations with categories similar to those used for laboratory incorporation; and sound-track incorporations were scored as direct when the subject heard in the dream a voice containing key words uttered in the portion of the sound track played during REM sleep, and as indirect when the subject heard a sound or voice in the dream. In addition, judgments were also made of whether the subject was a dream participant, and also the degree of vividness and bizarreness of the dream.

The results were as follows:

1. The hypothesis that the film would induce stress was supported by comparison of the mood-adjective check-list scores before and after the film. There was a significant increase in anxiety and depression, and a decrease in surgency and social affection.

2. Compared to the baseline, the film with the sound-track stimulus during REM sleep showed a significant increase in the amount of film-element incorporation; whereas the film alone (without the sound-track stimulus) produced no marked difference. This difference in the amount of incorporation occurred mainly in the REM periods of the second half of the night. There was only one instance of a direct incorporation throughout. No effects could be attributed to the sound-track stimulus in sleep alone without previous viewing of the film. In some respects, the augmenting effect of the sound track stimulus resembles that observed by Bokert (1968) for a subgroup of his subjects; that is, for some, the sound stimulus did produce thirst-stimulus incorporation, and with it an increase in thirst-related dream content.

3. Neither film with sound-track stimulation nor the film alone produced increases in the anxiety content of the dream. And this result resembles previous studies showing unimpressive or limited effects of affect-arousing films on dream content.

4. Contrary to expectation, subjects who exhibited more emotionality at the morning presentation of the film tended to be those who had more dream incorporation of film elements. Thus, film incorporation was associated with less, rather than greater, mastery over the experimental stress.

5. The film was followed by a significant increase of sleep-onset latency, averaging 16 min showing that the stress had physiological as well as psychological effects.

In conclusion, the authors viewed the findings in terms of two rival hypotheses both of which assert that dreams serve adaptive functions. One states that we dream about stressful events to acquire mastery over them; the other contends that we dream about events with qualities opposite to those of the reality stress in order to psychologically compensate for them. The authors feel that their experiment does not permit a clear-cut decision as yet.

The Effects of Task Performance on Subsequent Sleep Mentation

The first two categories of presleep-stimulus conditions thus far considered placed the subject in a more or less passive role; that is, the subject had merely to endure drive frustration, perceive stimulus conditions imposed by the experimenter, submit to being wired up, sleep, dream, and report. By contrast, the succeeding group of five studies all required some kind of task performance prior to sleep.

In the first study, Orr et al. (1968) asked seven high-school students to awaken themselves in the laboratory at a preselected time after falling asleep. The target times ranged 250-350 min after sleep onset. Each subject spent five consecutive nights in the laboratory; the first three were control and the last two were experimental nights. Four of the seven subjects were successful in awakening within 16 min of the target time, but the number of subjects was too small to reach statistical significance. At the moment of awakening from these "hits," six Stage REM dreams were available to recall. One contained a reference to a specific time (but other than that time of the specified target); two involved meeting a time commitment; and the others all contained indications of anticipation and apprehension. Such occurrences were not observed on the control no-presleep-task nights of successful subjects; and on none of the nights of the unsuccessful ones. In addition, on experimental nights, the successful subjects had less total sleep and recalled more dreams than on control nights and in comparison to the unsuccessful subjects. The results of the study are at best suggestive but deserve replication with a larger sample and careful mentation-report analysis. It is possible, for instance, that not only may dreams contain more references to time on experimental nights, but other aspects of their organization and content, such as sequential coherence may, also show changes.[2]

In four remaining studies, Baekeland (1971), Baekeland, Resch, and Katz (1968), Hauri (1970) and Cartwright (1974) required their subjects to perform specific behaviors prior to sleep. The presleep activity selected by Baekeland and co-workers in both experiments was 30 min of free association. Over all, they compared the REM sleep reports of 27 experimental subjects to those of 17 controls of whom no presleep task was required. In addition, both subject groups were each further subdivided in accordance with degrees of field dependence versus independence, a cognitive-style index. The free-association interval was divided into thirds and the subjects' subsequently tape-recorded REM mentation reports were divided into nonredundant idea units in accordance with predetermined syntactical rules. Each idea unit in turn was related to the contents of the presleep free-association interval in accordance with a categorization system providing for direct unambiguous incorporation, transformation of free-association elements into the REM reports, and lack of apparent relationship.

[2]That sleep is compatible with cognitive processes subserving awareness of temporal sequencing is indicated by studies of Dement and Kleitman (1957b) who showed that subjects awakened after 5 and 15 min of REM sleep are able to discriminate between correspondingly shorter or longer intervals of dreaming. Congruent results were reported by Koulack (1968) in a study employing subwaking-threshold percutaneous electrical stimuli to the median nerve during REM sleep. Subjects were awakened either 30 sec or 3 min after the stimuli and correct time-category discriminations were demonstrable.

The main findings were that presleep mentation as revealed in the free-association interval was richly represented in REM sleep mentation. The proportion of dream-idea units related to the free-association content ranged from 0.69 in the first REMP to 0.38 in the fourth. In general, the proportion of REM-mentation idea units scored as transformations of free-association elements exceeded the proportion of those scored as incorporations. In addition, cognitive-style factors appeared to play a role. Specifically, the field-independent group had the richest dream content, the greatest number of transformations of presleep free-association items in their dreams, and the greatest tendency to produce such transformations throughout the night. By contrast, the field dependent subjects' dreams were less likely to show transformations beyond the first REMP. Also, elements derived from the first third of the presleep association interval were more discernible in the reports of field-dependent subjects than those derived from the last third. Finally, in comparison to the control subjects, who were not made to carry out presleep tasks, the experimental subjects of whom free association *was* required, recalled more dreams which tended to be higher in references to the experimental situations, degree of unpleasantness, and self-participation. The results were deemed consistent with the idea of a partial causal connection between presleep mentation and REMP reports.

In one of the few studies which examined the effects of presleep conditions on both REM *and* NREM sleep mentation, Hauri (1970) employed 15 adult males as subjects in the following experimental schedule 1 night weekly; 1 adaptation night and 1 night, each in a counterbalanced order, with a 6-hr presleep condition of physical exercise, pleasant relaxation, or challenging mental-task performance. After 3.5 hrs of uninterrupted sleep, subjects were awakened twice each for REM and NREM sleep mentation reports. These were rated by the subjects themselves immediately after rendering each report, and also by independent judges in accordance with a previously standardized procedure. The subjects' own ratings revealed a unique finding: a tendency for Stage REM mentation, to possess less content relating to whatever activity subjects had been involved in prior to sleep. That is, in REM sleep mentation, there was less physical activity after presleep exercise, and less thinking and problem solving after presleep mental effort. The reduction in physical activity was likewise noted in NREM sleep mentation following exercise; but somewhat in contrast, after presleep mental effort, NREM mentation featured a feeling tone of increased tension and greater attempts to influence one's stream of sleep experience. Because of the sparseness of NREM report content, only the Stage REM reports were suitable for the judges' ratings method; and the main significant result of their ratings was that the number of social interactions per character after the mental-effort night was greater than for the other 2 conditions, and that more solitary activity was depicted after presleep exercise and relaxation. In all, only 29 out of 164 mentation reports (17.7%) contained an unambiguous incorporation of some aspect of the experimental situation; and with 1 exception, the presleep experimental activity never "openly intruded into sleep mentation."

Furthermore, a judge, highly sophisticated in dream theory and dream analysis, was unable to distinguish which mentation reports were associated with which presleep condition. Finally, incorporations often seemed concerned with short but psychologically important events of the previous day, whereas longer-lasting events did not appear in sleep mentation in proportion to their wakeful duration alone. Hauri (1970) was impressed by the results of the subjects' own ratings of their REM reports as supporting the notion that dream life is complementary to waking life. He commented on the similarity between his finding and those of Wood (1962), Kramer et al. (1966), and Cartwright et al. (1969). In brief, this model of REM dreaming holds that dream content compensates for whatever characteristics of behavior dominated the presleep condition by depiction of scenes of an opposite or different nature. For example, Wood found that when subjects spent their days in social isolation, their dreams contained greater amounts of socially active and physically passive dream content, such as group conversation, sitting, and "socializing." Similarly, Hauri (1970) found that REM dreams contained less physical activity after exercise and less thinking and problem solving after studying. Of special interest is that this relationship held only for REM dreams, whereas NREM mentation tended to continue in sleep imagination the behaviors prevailing prior to sleep. Thus, after studying, the associated wakeful, tense, emotional atmosphere carried along into the NREM mentation of the night, instead of being "left outside the door" after sleep onset and being succeeded by a type of sleep experience different from that occupying preceding wakefulness.

The last study of the effects of a subject-performed presleep task on subsequent sleep mentation is that of Cartwright (1974a) in which the influence of a conscious wish on REM reports was assessed. She was interested in carrying out an experiment that would also throw light on the meaning and functions of dreams. Thus, she attempted to locate a specific area of psychological tension within each subject, to endow it with saliency by bringing it to the subject's attention and induce a need to resolve the tension just prior to sleep. Regarding these considerations, Cartwright made two general predictions:

1. Dreams following focused awareness of the specific relevant area of tension would tend to possess content elements capable of being related to this tension area.

2. Such dreams would tend to represent a result inversely related to the nature of the resolution as hoped for during wakefulness.

To test these predictions, she employed 17 paid volunteer, college men and women who were self-professed good sleepers. They each slept 2 nights in the laboratory; the first was an adaptation night and the second was for the introduction of the independent variable. During the presleep interval of the latter night, a self- versus ideal-self-trait discrepancy item was identified by an adjective Q-sort technique.

The item with the highest degree of discrepancy between self as actually perceived and self as the subject wished to be was selected as the target presleepstimulus adjective. By means of the same procedure, two control words were selected; a word with a similar degree of self-ideal-self discrepancy but not used as a stimulus adjective and another word without self-ideal-self discrepancy, also not used as a stimulus.

Subjects were then permitted to go to sleep and instructed to verbalize to themselves repeatedly the target-stimulus adjective as they drifted off. Thus, "I wish I were [target word]" e.g. "I wish I could be more *poised. . .*" or more *persevering,* or not so *irritable,* and so on were the kinds of the self-administered presleep stimuli employed. Throughout the night, the subjects were awakened for REM mentation reports, following which they were permitted to resume sleep but were reminded on each such occasion to continue self-administration of the stimulus adjective.

Each REM sleep report was rated separately by a "naive" judge for the presence of each of the selected three adjectives on the basis of the following category system:

1. Adjective describes self.
2. Opposite adjective describes self.
3. Neither adjective nor its opposite describes self.
4. Adjective describes other dream character.
5. Opposite adjective describes other dream character.
6. Neither adjective nor its opposite describes other dream character.

These design features provided the experimenter with an opportunity to discover whether the technique and the instructions to wish for personality change were effective in producing significant incorporation of the trait or its opposite in the dream; whether other personal traits equally characteristic but not brought to the subject's attention were also incorporated into the dream; and whether the manner in which the target trait appeared in the dream represented continuity with waking thought, that is, was consistent with the conscious wish to be different, or whether some other outcome was represented. The results were that 15 of 17 subjects had some evidence of the target word or its opposite being descriptive of the dream characters in 1 or more of their mentation reports ($p < .01$). By contrast, neither of the 2 nontarget words were incorporated to a significant degree. This result indicates, therefore, that the procedure was effective in securing representation in the dreams of items related to the tension area. However, when the instances of incorporation were categorized in accordance with the scheme presented above, only the target words which were the opposite in quality to that wished for reached statistical significance. That is, although the target words tended to be incorporated, few subjects had dreams in which the ideal, wished-for trait was ascribed to the self; rather the opposite held

true — only 2 subjects had instances in their dreams in which their self characters possessed the ideal trait as wished for in wakefulness. The overall results persuaded Cartwright (1970) to conclude that under the experimental conditions
described, dream mentation, though responsive to pre-sleep instructions to attend to specific traits (the wished-for personal quality), revealed differences in
affective values compared to those stated in wakefulness.

The final study reviewed in this section consists of two fascinating related
experiments which are unique because they employed naturalistic stressful presleep stimuli — "sensitivity" group therapy and major surgery (Breger, Hunter,
& Lane, 1971a). Four experimental and 2 control subjects (college students, 3
males and 3 females) participated in the group-therapy project in accordance
with the following schedule: 4 initial laboratory baseline nights for all subjects;
for the experimental subjects, 2 laboratory nights following stressful therapy
sessions during which the subjects and their personal problems were the focus
for group discussion; for the control subjects, 2 laboratory nights, 4 weeks after
the initial baseline. On all laboratory nights, REM sleep-mentation reports were
collected throughout. On all subjects, personality data were derived from a brief
initial interview and the MMPI. In addition, the contents of all group sessions
were tape recorded. All mentation reports were evaluated by means of rating
scales for incorporation of presleep-condition components, for thematic dimensions of the dreams, for cognitive-affective characteristics and by means of a
qualitative psychological analysis. A total of 147 dream reports were collected
from all 6 subjects.

The chief results were that the material aroused during the stressful group
sessions was said to be represented and worked over in the dreams according to
each subject's individual style. The incorporation ratings showed that the central
content of each dream of the experimental subjects was related to the material
discussed in the preceding group session. The manner of both the incorporation
and representation processes tended to be indirect, allusive, symbolic, and
derivative. Dream events often indirectly paralleled wakeful events and blended
with both chronologically older similar anamnestic material. In comparison to
their baseline nights, the control subjects' ratings all changed in the direction of
pleasanter interactions, more adequate and successful roles for both dreamer and
others, and more desirable dream outcomes; whereas for the experimental subjects, the trend was either absence of such change or change in the opposite direction with respect to the same parameters. This differential result was attributed
to the impact of the group-therapy experience.

The surgery study involved five volunteer patients, males and females, all
under the age 65, who were awaiting major surgery; and two control subjects.
Each surgical subject spent four preoperative nights in the laboratory (with a
1 day interval between the last preoperative night and the actual surgery). Post-
operatively, each subject experienced three laboratory nights one to five weeks

afterward. The control subjects underwent a similar nightly schedule but without comparable stress. All subjects were awakened for Stage REM mentation reports throughout. In addition, each subject received an intensive clinical and psychological-test evaluation. Psychological analysis of dream content was said to reveal much incorporated stress—related material both directly and symbolically. Examples were references to repairing mechanical objects or removal of objects from enclosures.

The degree of incorporation was quite marked when the personal meaning of the surgery and individual modes of coping and psychological preparation were taken into account. Of greatest significance regarding the amount of incorporation was the level of preoperative emotional arousal rather than the degree of daily preoccupation with the surgery itself. That is, the dreams, rather than simply reflecting waking experience, seemed to express attempts to deal with unassimilated affect-arousing information. For example, three subjects had actual unexpected stressful experiences with drainage tubes. In each instance, ensuing dreams incorporated and dealt with the incident in a central way. Thus, one such preoperative dream of a male patient exhaustively depicted insertion of tubes into a woman and himself for medical tests, and interwoven with this material were overt descriptions of the subject having sexual relations with her.

In addition to data contained in the case-study material, mentation reports were rated by judges in accordance with 13 scales as follows: degree of incorporation of presleep stimuli (2 scales); thematic dimensions (2 scales: quality of interactions, and the role of the dreamer); formal qualities (6 scales: anxiety, cognitive disturbance, implausibility, involvement, primitivity, and recall); and surgery-related content (3 scales: body imagery, castration, and hostility). The results were said to indicate that the general effects of surgery-related stress was to increase dream anxiety, fragmentation, bizarreness, involvement of dream characters, hostility, concern about the integrity and health of the body for all patients, and worry about specific injury was increased for the males. Some similar elements appeared in the dreams of all patients presumably because of the situation they all had to contend with. Thus, dreams commonly depicted defective objects, references to the acts of cutting, extirpated objects, construction of some innovation or new object, and so on. Such elements were classified as psychological transformations of items of wakeful concern. Also, the individual coping style and psychological meaning of the surgery imparted a characteristic specificity to the dreams of each patient. In general, the same characterological sources for coping strategies manifested in wakefulness appeared in dreams. Fears and conflicts symbolized in dreams rarely occurred without an attempt to resolve or cope with them in some way. A characteristic way in which preoperative stress affected dreams was by repetition of elements and themes. This occurred with nonstress-related components of the preoperative dreams as well as those related to stress and often resulted in constriction of dream content. Also, specific dream symbols or themes were consistently used by certain subjects to represent their central concerns.

Lack of "disguise" was not correlated with increased dream anxiety since few dreams included an actual representation of surgery, whereas some of the most frightening dreams were the most disguised — disguised in the sense that although the subject experienced anxiety in the dream, and in wakefulness as well, the dream content referred to matters other than surgery explicitly. For example, on one preoperative night, a subject dreamed about being threatened by a fellow patient with a gun while they were both involved with cars in a parking lot. In a summary comment, Breger et al. (1971a) stated that "in dreams of all the subjects, the individual fears and conflicts are expressed in altered form. That is, the stress-related stimuli appear to be recoded, symbolized, displaced, or condensed so that their expression is at least one step removed from the primary source of the stress [p. 182]." Furthermore, as in the results with the group-therapy study, stress-related input was said to be integrated with, or assimilated into an organized network of older memories which also appear in the dream content. The authors concluded that their data support the hypothesis that it is affect-related or emotionally arousing information of personal relevance that one tends to dream about. Furthermore, the ensuing transformational processes were deemed consistent with the notion that dreams serve an adaptive function. By means of the transformations and the integration with memories, the psychologically noxious stimuli are believed to be converted into forms which are familiar to the dreamer, and make available psychological resources for coping with the threat.

Aside from criticisms, many of which the authors anticipated and commented upon themselves, the most serious problem with both of these studies stems from the method by which the major analysis of the study was carried out. This portion of the work consisted of dream-by-dream, case-by-case, post hoc studies in which the dream reports of each subject were "analyzed in the context of the presleep experience." The flavor of the analyses may be conveyed by the following excerpt from the case of a male patient about to have surgery for a recurrent peptic ulcer:

> In Dream 5, he must remove the wood-eating moths that could destory or damage trees, symbolizing the ulcerated condition of his stomach. Also: tree trunk = the trunk portion of the body = the trunk of Dream 2 [a storage trunk], all referring to the part of his body to be operated on [Breger et al., 1971, p. 131].

The authors were well aware of the subjectivity in this approach and attempted to check on their analyses by the independent content ratings as described earlier. Although these post hoc analyses are certainly the most interesting part of the study, containing abundant clinically persuasive and dramatic substantiations of the authors' hypotheses, they do not constitute the kind of scientific support that might be provided by independent "blind" analyses of the reports with prior specification of analytic rules and guidelines.

The Experimental and Laboratory Situation as Presleep Conditions Influencing Dreams

This topic certainly deserves review under the general heading of this chapter but all of the relevant work is ably presented and discussed by Cartwright in Chapter 8 of this volume.

Hypnosis and Post-hypnotic Suggestion as a Presleep Condition Affecting Sleep Mentation

In all of the following studies attempts were made to test the traditional view that suitable subjects tend to incorporate and transform material contained in presleep posthypnotic suggestions into their nocturnal dreams. The literature of the pre-electrographic era has been thoroughly reviewed by Tart (1965). In addition a valuable more recent critical review has been contributed by Walker and Johnson (1974).

The first formal work since the advent of modern techniques was carried out by Stoyva (1961). He employed 16 highly hypnotizable subjects, each of whom received presleep suggestions on 6 or more experimental nights, with or without standard hypnotic-induction procedures. Reports were obtained from Stages REM, 2, 3, and 4. Mentation following both presleep conditions contained references to the suggested topics but a larger proportion of hypnotized subjects (44%) reported frequent dreaming on the suggested topic than when they had received suggestion without hypnosis (25%). This effect was manifested in all sleep stages. Stoyva concluded that although hypnotic trance with posthypnotic suggestion was not a requisite for incorporation of presleep suggestions, it increased the probability of such occurrences.

Two subsequent studies were performed by Tart (1964) and Tart and Dick (1970). The first employed 10 highly hypnotizable subjects who received presleep posthypnotic suggestions to dream about a dramatic, anxiety-tinged, threatening narrative in which the subjects were instructed to imagine themselves the central characters. Thirty-eight REM sleep reports were collected after varying intervals of Stage REM had elapsed. Fifty percent of the subjects were judged not to have dreamed at all, in accordance with the posthypnotic suggestion. Those remaining subjects who could fulfill the instructions had dreams which possessed a wide range of evidence of influence, from only a few elements being affected to "almost total control" over the content of the sleep experience. However, the posthypnotic suggestion to dream on a certain topic was deemed to have an inhibiting or suppressing effect on natural dream processes. Tart (1964), therefore, concluded that dreams following posthypnotic suggestions designed to influence natural nocturnal dreaming are best viewed as the outcome of interactions between hypnosis factors and those involved in production of natural Stage REM dreams. In addition, conspicuous by their absence were instances of psychological transformations of hypnotically implanted presleep stimuli which were reported in previous studies (reviewed by Tart, 1965). Finally, it was concluded that equating of dreams occurring in hypnosis and sleep, either spontaneous or in response to specific suggestions is invalid on psychophysiological and psychological grounds.

In the second study, Tart and Dick (1970) employed 13 highly hypnotizable subjects who were given presleep/posthypnotic suggestions to dream in great detail about a presleep narrative they heard prior to retiring. In the course of a 2-night protocol, 2 different stimulus narratives were employed, 1 per night in counterbalanced order. Rather than permit wide variation in the time elapsed since onset of each REM period sampled for mentation (as in the Tart, 1964, study), all subjects were awakened whenever 5-10 min of REM sleep appeared during the night. Tart sought to control his data analysis by having 2 independent judges score every dream report obtained in the study against *both* stimulus narratives without knowing which narrative had been employed on the specific night of the report elicitation. Thus, half the dreams were scored against the wrong stimulus narrative to serve as a control for possible overlapping between spontaneous dream content and presleep narrative. A predetermined scoring system was devised to enable measurement of the degree to which the 2 stimulus narratives affected the dreams following their use on different respective nights. The narratives had been broken down into small specific action-content-like elements and all dreams were examined to assess the extent to which dream reports contained elements relating to both narratives. The total number of possible description items in the narratives averaged 41.5 (40 and 43, respectively, for Narratives 1 and 2).

When a total yield of 78 dream reports were scored against the stimulus narrative actually employed on the associated experimental night, the mean number of narrative elements appearing in the associated dreams ranged from 2.5 to 4 (interjudge reliability coefficient = .98). By contrast, when the same dream reports were scored against the narrative not used on the experimental night concerned, the corresponding mean score ranged from 0.41 to 0.44 ($p < .01$, one-tailed test).

In addition, a more global, thematic analysis of the same narrative-dream-report pairings was carried out, unlike the atomistic, fine-grained initial procedure described above. Two independent judges (reliability coefficient = .85) indicated that specific effects of the narratives were manifested in the dreams of 11 of the 13 subjects. Of the entire pool of dreams, 64.5% possessed thematic qualities clearly related to the associated stimulus narrative, 12.5% had only a tangential relationship, and 21% were apparently unrelated. Eight of the 13 subjects reported at least 1 dream of which the narrative appeared to be the dominant dream content organizer. The authors concluded that although posthypnotic suggestion is a powerful technique for influencing dream content, other nonhypnotic self-training methods described in their discussion are also capable of similar influence.

Barber et al. (1973) criticized Stoyva (1961) for using repeated, authoritative suggestions for his hypnosis group and a permissive manner for his nonhypnosis control group, pointing out that this could have confounded hypnosis factors with the forcefulness in which suggestions were given to either group. In addition, he felt that Tart and Dick (1970), restricting their subject population to highly hypnotizable subjects, imposed upon themselves severe limits as to the generality of their findings. With the design features mentioned above, he hoped to control for these factors, and others. Accordingly, Barber, Walker, and Hahn, Jr. (1973) carried through an elaborate well-controlled study on 77 randomly selected females, half of whom were exposed to a presleep hypnotic induction procedure and half not. In addition, all subjects were given either authoritative, permissive, or no suggestions at all to think and dream about a specific topic: the death of President Kennedy.

In the laboratory, mentation reports were elicited from each REM period and at least once during NREM sleep 45 min after the previous REM-period termination. The results were that presleep suggestions altered the dream content of 25% of the subjects regardless of whether hypnosis had been used. This significantly exceeded the performance of the control subjects receiving no suggestions. Furthermore, the style of the suggestion did play a role after all. That is, presleep suggestions had the greatest effect on dream content of hypnotized subjects when given authoritatively and that of the nonhypnotized when given permissively. Finally, because subjects were randomly selected, it was possible to demonstrate that incorporation of suggested material was not related to the hypnotizability.

Miscellaneous Studies

In Chapter 15 of this volume, the effects of a variety of experimental procedures on sleep utterance are described. However, it is necessary to relate a fascinating study of Evans (1972) and Evans et al. (1969, 1970) which deals with the effect of suggestions administered during REM sleep on sleep behavior. Although elicitation of mentation reports was not part of the procedure, the work has distinct relevance for the topic of mental processes in sleep.

Intrigued by promising exploratory observations, Evans (1972) and Evans et al. (1972) studied the effects of verbal suggestions presented during alpha-free Stage REM on specific subsequent sleep actions. Nineteen male nursing students slept for two nights in the laboratory. Typical examples of the suggestions were "Whenever I say the word 'itch,' your nose will itch until you scratch it;" or "Whenever I say the word 'pillow,' your pillow will feel uncomfortable until you move it." Tests were made of each cue word on at least two different occasions during the same REM period in which the suggestion had been administered (immediate), during all subsequent REM periods of the same night (delayed) and during REM periods of the second night (carry-over). Suggestions were given only once at the first presentation and never repeated throughout (that is, only the cue words were employed on subsequent occasions).

The results were that over the 2 nights, 416 trials were made and 89 correct responses were observed. On the average, 19 subjects responded to a mean of 21% of all cue words (the highest response rate by a subject was 48%). Continuation of REM sleep without alpha was compatible with reception of the cue words as well as execution of appropriate responses shortly afterward. After subjects were awakened in the morning they remembered neither the cue words nor their motor responses.

Perhaps the most striking finding was that these responses could be called forth on subsequent occasions, delayed and carry-over, as well as on a night *five months* after the single initial suggestion was given and without intervening practice. The lack of demonstrable wakeful recall is therefore best characterized as state-dependent amnesia rather than forgetting because the availability of the response was preserved and was demonstrable provided that the initial condition of the suggestion was employed for testing. In addition, there were indirect indications that successful responses might be occasions in which the cue word was incorporated into ongoing dream sequences. Although hypnosis was not used as part of the initial procedure, the best performance was given by subjects who were most highly susceptible to hypnosis as determined at the other times.

DISCUSSION

By now, the reader wll no longer be surprised by comments as to the broad range of variability in reported outcomes in the sleep-research literature. As remarked elsewhere (Chapter 2 of this volume), the arduousness and expense of experiments in this field has often constrained researchers to "make do" with relatively small numbers of subjects. Let us begin therefore by listing the various known sources of variability in experimental results all of which limit the degree to which findings may be generalized:

Individual Differences

Differences in cognitive style, responsiveness, and personality characteristics have been shown to affect the manner and frequency with which external stimuli are incorporated and transformed in sleep mentation (Baekeland 1971; Baekeland, Resch and Katz 1968; Breger, Hunter and Lane 1971a; Goodenough, Witkin, Koulack and Cohen 1975; Witkin 1969a; Witkin and Lewis 1967).

Criteria for Defining the Response

The proportion of occurrences categorized as incorporations or dream modifications according to Dement and Wolpert (1958b) is low compared to that reported by Bokert (1968). This difference is partly attributable to the comparatively strict, conservative criteria employed by the former. Also, some studies utilized subjects to judge their own mentation reports as well as independent judges, and some relied only on judges used in a somewhat inconsistent manner across studies.

Type and Intensity of Stimulus

Dement and Wolpert (1958b) found that water sprayed on the skin during REM sleep, and presleep stimuli, which tended to arouse strong anxiety, were more likely to be incorporated into or modify dream content (Baekeland 1971; Baekeland, Resch and Katz 1968; Breger, Hunter & Lane 1971a; Goodenough, Witkin, Koulack & Cohen 1975; Witkin & Lewis 1967).

Time of Awakening

Some studies awakened subjects for REM sleep reports in a consistent manner within 5-10 min after REM-period onset and others in a comparatively unsystematic manner. Dement and Wolpert (1958b) awakened their subjects 5-20 min and Tart (1964) 6-32 min after REM-period onset. The same variability is true regarding total sleep time and clock time elapsed with respect to mentation report schedules.

Technique of Elicitation of Sleep Mentation and Associated Cognitive Activity

Besides differences in the manner of awakening subjects, it was noted in at least three different investigations that a body of spontaneous associations elicited before (Baekeland, Resch & Katz 1968; Baekland 1971) or after collection of mentation reports (Berger 1963; Shevrin & Fisher, 1967; Witkin & Lewis 1967; Witkin 1969a) enabled judges to discern much more easily, and convincingly, evidence of a relationship between experimental stimuli and sleep mentation. In general, however, apparently successful detections of such relationships were made on the basis of post hoc findings rather than in terms of systematic analysis.

Perhaps one unfortunate characteristic of the experiments testing effects of stimuli applied during sleep has been the general insistence by investigators that only mentation reports following EEG evidence of stimulus registration would be included in the data analyses. This decision has resulted in neglect of opportunities to observe the effects of stimuli which leave the EEG undisturbed. In line with this thought, evidence from several studies demonstrates that it is indeed possible for the sleeper to discriminate between external stimuli in the *absence* of signs of increased activation. (Gradess et al., 1971; Granda & Hammack, 1961; Oswald et al., 1960; Williams, Morlock, Jr., & Morlock, 1966). Perhaps experimental techniques used thus far have mostly permitted us to observe outcomes of forceful intrusion of external stimuli into ongoing sleep mentation within a context of arousal rather than a deft blending or merging of the two without arousal. This remark is supported by Berger's (1963) observation of the high frequency with which mentation seemingly derived from external stimuli seemed to disturb dream continuity, and Koulack's (1969) finding that stimulus incorporation was more likely in association with alpha bursts.

Despite the inconsistencies and misgivings mentioned above, the group of studies as a whole permit us to conclude that incorporation of, and sleep mentation modification by external stimuli (applied prior to, or during sleep), has been demonstrated as a genuine, frequently occurring but by no means inevitable effect. Furthermore, depending upon the factors already cited which promoted variance, the manner of incorporation differed over a wide range. Thus, the most frequent kind of relationship observed between verbal stimuli introduced during sleep and associated sleep mentation was that of assonance. However, direct unambiguous incorporations, although uncommon, were also seen as well as other stimulus transformations involving indirect representations. It is noteworthy that with stimuli applied prior to sleep the reverse was found, with relationships based upon assonance seeming to be relatively infrequent in comparison to indirect representations. At any rate, the overall results lend themselves to the following partial formulation: during sleep, the immediate content of awareness is largely determined by internally produced ongoing stimuli; and, in addition, components of cognitive resources are continuously available for detection and analysis of signals from external sources (Oswald, Taylor & Treisman, 1960). These cognitive components are responsible for three types of decisions following such signal detection and analysis: awakening, ignoring the stimulus, or incorporation and/or modification of sleep mentation in a variety of ways (Dement & Wolpert, 1958b; Berger, 1963). Actually it required no fancy experimentation to tell us this. After all, adults rarely fall out of bed, soldiers, during bombardments, do awaken in response to sudden lulls, sleeping mothers do selectively respond to an infant's cry, and so on. In addition, similar phenomena are observable during wakefulness. The clichéd but valid example involves being lost in a vivid daydream while driving, and preserving adequate cognitive resources for accomplishing both concurrently.

CONCLUSION

Despite the number of carefully executed and sophisticated studies on the experimental manipulation of dream content, the results have told us relatively little about how dreams are constructed. The findings seem rather meager next to the rich elaborate causal links that one may construct post hoc. Knowing the dream, and presleep or sleep stimulus, and knowing something about the cognitive style, personality, and associative patterns of the dreamer, one can frequently make extensive cogent inferences connecting these various sets of items. But post hoc inferences cannot substitute for systematic and predictive studies.

If there is any validity to these post hoc analyses, and our hunch is that there is much that is valid, then we need to do the hard work of spelling out the associative rules that join stimulus to dream response. Until we can articulate these rules, our understanding of the process may remain very rudimentary indeed. In particular, we feel that there is considerable predictive potential in the construction of associative memory networks. There is a variety of association, sorting and clustering techniques which seem potentially useful. Many of them have been extensively developed by psycholinguists and students in the fields of memory and computer simulation of intelligence. For example, the surgical operations performed on Bregar et al.'s (1971a) subjects are concrete examples of the intersection of cutting and fixing procedures. Both cutting and fixing activity appeared in these subjects' dreams but tended to be portrayed in other nonsurgical forms of cutting and fixing. Was a direct, unequivocal depiction of surgery barred from dream experience because it was too threatening or were the situations actually dreamed simply more familar, or derived from "older" memories, and hence more likely to be dreamed about?

The implicit-association model employed thus far is that of classical conditioning, that is, the sound of a bell or sensation of water sprayed on the skin activates memory components of previous pairings of such stimuli with percepts of contiguous events. Yet many of our models of dreaming emphasize goal and motive. Operant-conditioning relationships, in which the stimulus is associated with avoidance, escape, or rewards, seem much more appropriate avenues to the study of effects of external stimuli on dreaming. For example, subjects might be taught, while awake, that pointing to a particular visual stimulus or operating a lever controlling a mental content-bearing visual display will terminate a mildly annoying noise. Or, subjects could be taught to reliably associate photographs depicting ubiquitous cognitive-affective categories with specific, easily recognized sound patterns, receiving small but significant sums of money as reinforcement. Such cognitive-affective categories might include heterosexuality, homosexuality, interpersonal hostility and cruelty, body mutilation, appetizing food, childbirth, death, excretory processes, and depictions of the subjects' earliest childhood memories. Then, after such pairings are well established and maintained by intermittent reinforcement, sleeping subjects would receive the specific sound pattern stimulus, or else the annoying noise stimulus mentioned earlier, and awakened shortly afterward for mentation reports. We might then predict that such stimuli would elicit dreaming of the particular reinforcement-bearing stimulus or common associates thereof. In such a fashion, a large variety of operant-conditioned stimuli could be employed, each representative of major cognitive-affective categories. Eventually, one might be able to construct an experimentally based catalogue of transformational patterns linking external stimulus to dream component. Such a catalogue would doubtless have to be developed with due regard and special provisions for the effects of individual differences, nature of stimulus, stimulus threshold, sleep stage, time of night, and phasic-tonic contexts in association with which the stimulus was applied and from which the subject was awakened. Eventually a catalogue of this type could form the basis of more elaborate systematic studies and hypotheses testing regarding dream formation.

In conclusion, we feel that the size and complexity of human memory has discouraged investigators from the difficult task of developing specific testable models of dream formation. Considerable innovation in both experimental design and data analysis are now in order.

11

The Effects of Drugs
on Sleep Mentation

Arthur M. Arkin
Solomon S. Steiner

City College of The City University of New York

Religious and cultural ceremony worldwide in distribution contains rich anecdotal reference to the effects of drugs on dreams; and popular awareness of such
phenomena is reflected in expressions like "pipe dreams" which relate opium
smoking to blissful, vivid, unrealistic oneiric experience.

By contrast, the scientific literature is sparse — especially if one is determined,
with Aserinsky (1969a), to avoid equating REM sleep time with "dream time."
Although many studies are available that deal with drug effects on Stage REM
parameters (and other sleep stages as well), fewer by far have involved elicitation and analysis of mentation reports. As we have already seen, Stage REM
deprivation does not accomplish total dream deprivation (see Chapters 12 and
13 of this volume). Thus, one is on problematical ground in assuming that drugs
reducing REM sleep time must necessarily reduce dreaming correspondingly and
vice versa.

Despite this caution, one may not overlook reports establishing a positive
correlation between profusion of REMs, and activity content and vividness of
dream experience. (However, see Chapters 6,7, and the Commentary to Chapter
7 of this volume.) For this reason it is appropriate to briefly comment on studies
describing the effects of drugs on electrographic aspects of sleep.

It is difficult to review this literature in a straightforward way, however,
because of several factors (Freemon, 1972), for example:

1. Contradictory results with the same drug have been reported by different
   investigators.
2. Effects of the drug observed over a short interval may be different from
   those seen with long-term administration.

3. Different experimental designs have been employed across studies so that some, for example, have controlled for nonindependence of successive nights and others have not.

4. Some studies have controlled for nightly sleep duration differences and others have not.

5. Some have described effects summed over the entire night, whereas others reported different effects as a result of separate examination of comparable portions of each night.

6. Some drugs have varying effects in small doses.

7. Some studies have employed "normal" paid volunteers and others utilized psychiatric patients.

For the purpose of relating drugs to sleep mentation, however, psychotropic agents may be classified as follows (modified from Freemon, 1972):

1. Drugs which are followed by intense immediate REM sleep rebound in excess of baseline levels on abrupt discontinuation.[1] As stated in Chapter 11 of this volume, such phenomena are usually considered examples of the effects of released accumulations of REM sleep deficit (or "REM pressure"). Among the drugs falling into this category are:

> *sedatives:* barbiturates, glutethimide, methyprylon, ethyl alcohol, diphenhydramine;
>
> *narcotic analgesics:* morphine, heroin;
>
> *sympathomimetic stimulants:* amphetamine, phenmetrazine, diethylpropion, chlorphentermine;
>
> *monoamine oxidase (MAO inhibitors:* phenelzine, tranylcypromine;
>
> *benzodiazepines:* nitrazepam.

(Noteworthy also are the differences in temporal pattern of Stage REM suppression, which may accompany administration of the above drugs. For example, alcohol and barbiturates initially suppress Stage REM but with continual use, the nightly proportion of Stage REM returns toward baseline levels despite their concomitant administration. When these drugs are then abruptly discontinued, however, there is prompt marked rebound in excess of baseline levels from which it is concluded that although Stage REM time levels had previously returned to normal, the drugs used concurrently had held in

---

[1]Oswald (1973) draws attention to differences in REM sleep-rebound responses to different drugs administered for varying durations. For example, the time between drug withdrawal and peak of rebound is said to be approximately related to the time necessary for drug elimination. Thus after withdrawal, peaking of rebound may occur 4 days after fenfluramine, 21 days after a large dose of phenobarbital, 10 days after heroin, and similarly for nitrazepam and large doses of tricyclic antidepressants. It may be noted that what has just been said is partly at variance with the text, (for example, that rebound after fenfluramine is absent, and prompt after barbiturates). The reason for this is that the statements in the text were based upon results of short-term rather than the more recent long-term laboratory follow-ups.

check the compensatory manifestations of the increased REM sleep deficit. This pattern contrasts with that of the MAO inhibitors in which with sufficient phenelzine, for example, Stage REM, after insignificant initial change, may be totally and continuously suppressed for months yielding a huge Stage REM rebound with abrupt discontinuation.)

2. Drugs, which though they significantly suppress Stage REM, tend to be followed by a delayed, and perhaps less intense, REM sleep rebound, or else no significant change above baseline level. Examples of such drugs are:

sedatives: methaqualone (300 mgs or more),[2] meprobamate;
tricyclic antidepressants: imipramine, desimipramine, amitryptiline;
sympathomimetic stimulants: methyl phenidate;
phenothiazines[2]: chlorpromazine (100 mg or more?);
parasympathetic blocking agents: scopolamine, atropine.

3. Sleep producing drugs which do not significantly affect REM during administration, and subsequent to abrupt discontinuation of which, changes in Stage REM are either not detectable, are minimal, or else noticeable in only less than the full complement of Stage REM parameters (such as an increase in REM density alone but without Stage REM rebound).

sedatives: chloral hydrate, methaqualone (lower doses);
benzodiazepines: chlordiazepoxide, diazepam, lorazepam, flurazepam;
sympathomimetic drugs: fenfluramine;
beta-adrenergic blocking agents: propranolol (Dunleavy, MacLean, & Oswald, 1971).

4. Drugs which increase Stage REM:

reserpine;
l-tryptophan;
5-OH-tryptophan;
LSD;
phenothiazines:

(1) chlorpromazine (small doses);
(2) trifluoperazine;
(3) thioridazine;
(4) mesoridazine;

alpha-adrenergic blocking agents: (thymoxamine; Oswald et al., 1975);
anticholinesterase agents: (physostigmine; Sitaram et al., 1976).

5. Drugs which predominantly affect delta sleep:

benzodiazepines: reduction of delta sleep
phenothiazines: chlorpromazine: increase;
amino acids: tryptophan, phenylalanine: increase.

---

[2]In these groups particularly, contradictory results have been reported by different investigators (see Freemon, 1972). Various authorities have suggested that effects are dose related; that is, given in high enough doses, all sedatives will suppress Stage REM.

6. Psychoactive drugs which do not appreciably alter the sleep cycle over all:
   chloral hydrate;
   promethazine;
   lithium (see footnote 2);
   nitrous oxide.

Perhaps the most crucial difference in responses to the two classes of Stage REM suppressant drugs is the factor of the promptness and intensity of Stage REM rebound versus the delayed, less intense rebound (see footnote 1); for, with the former, vivid, anxiety-laden sleep mentation is associated and may become intensified to the point of achieving "breakthroughs" into wakefulness in the form of psychotic deliria following abrupt discontinuation. In addition, it is nevertheless of great interest that REM sleep suppression may occur both with sympathomimetic stimulants, and with sedatives; that sedation may occur without REM sleep suppression, that sedation, as with reserpine, may be accompanied by an increase in REM sleep and that sedation may be accompanied by delta sleep suppression while sparing Stage REM. An additional aspect of such sleep-cycle changes may be corresponding increases of Stages 2 and 3 inasmuch as sleep-onset latency is decreased and total sleep time increased. In certain instances, as with promethazine, there is no alteration of proportions of sleep-cycle stages but a lengthening of each sleep stage accordingly. If the pharmacological action of these various drugs were known in sufficient detail we would be much further along in our understanding of sleep neurochemistry and its contribution to sleep mentation. That different groups of drugs possess different patterns of Stage REM suppression, and tendencies to produce rebound, already indicates that REM sleep suppression per se could not be the sole factor in altering dream content (if indeed such alterations have been firmly established; see below). For example, Fisher et al. (1972) have noted deleterious cognitive changes in a narcoleptic individual on a prolonged phenelzine regimen. Thus, drug-produced alteration of *cognition* may play an essential role in drug-withdrawal vivid dreaming, rather than REM compensation alone.

It is probable, therefore, that different drugs act by different mechanisms to effect similar alterations in the pattern and amount of Stage REM. It is also possible that sleep mentation may be more closely correlated with, and dependent on, the specific mechanisms by which Stage REM is altered rather than with the absolute amount of REM sleep change.

One must also keep in mind that while we are most interested in examining the effects of drugs on sleep mentation, other variables that have been shown to affect sleep mentation have varied across the studies which we comment on below. The type and degree of subject pathology are known to interact with the type and dosage schedule of drugs to alter cognitive processes in the waking state, and it would not be at all surprising if this were shown to be true of sleep states as well. Thus, one must view the effects of drugs on dreams as the outcome of complex interactions between drug-induced neurochemical changes (and the specific mechanisms by which they are brought about) and the endocognitive state and mechanisms of the subjects. It is the end effects of these interactions which finally find expression in sleep mentation.

The remainder of this chapter reviews what little has been published regarding the effects of drugs on sleep mentation and the history of changes in conclusions with new research findings.

THE EFFECTS OF SEDATIVE-HYPNOTIC DRUGS ON SLEEP MENTATION

Exposition of this topic requires description of drug effects on sleep mentation both during administration and following withdrawal, each in relation to individual differences in nature of the drugs, as well as whether the subject population may have been drawn from "normal volunteers" or psychiatric patients. The chief considerations are:

1. Do the drugs concerned have powerful Stage REM-suppressant effects with concurrent build-up of REM-sleep deficit?

2. To what extent are such suppressant effects manifested throughout the entire night rather than lasting for only a shorter interval, permitting a Stage REM rebound in the last third of the night?

That rebound increases in REM sleep may be accompanied by unpleasant dreams and nightmares following barbiturate withdrawal was first noted by Oswald and Priest (1965). Using 2 "normal" volunteers as subjects, 5 initial baseline nights were recorded in the laboratory. Then the subjects received amylobarbitone (400-600 mgs) each night for the ensuing 2 weeks, following which the drug was abruptly discontinued and the subjects observed for an additional 38 days. Sleep was monitored throughout. During the drug phase, there was an initial reduction of Stage REM followed by a gradual return to baseline levels. With abrupt withdrawal, however, there was an intense REM sleep rebound far above baseline amounts, and over this same period, the subjects reported unpleasant dreams and nightmares.

Earlier, it had been demonstrated that under nondrug conditions, the degree of activity and vividness in dreams was associated with REM profusion (Berger & Oswald, 1962). Also, it had been found that subjects while taking presleep barbiturates experienced both a reduction in REM time and REM frequency (Oswald et al., 1963; Baekeland, 1967). And contrariwise, withdrawal of hypnotic drugs accentuated REM profusion (Allen, Kales, & Berger, 1968; Lewis, 1968; Oswald, 1969). These facts, taken together with the finding of vivid, nightmarish dreams during chronic hypnotic-drug withdrawal (Oswald & Priest, 1965), persuaded Carrol, Lewis, and Oswald (1969) to undertake a study in which they made two predictions: (1) that presleep administration of barbiturates would result in tranquil dreams: and (2) that withdrawal of such drugs after administration on consecutive nights would be followed on recovery nights by dream experience exceeding that of baseline or drug nights in richness and vividness (because of the increased Stage REM deficit). To test these hypotheses "three young men" underwent the following experimental procedure:

Night 1: adaptation to laboratory;

Night 2, 3: nonlaboratory, nonexperimental nights;

Nights 4-6: laboratory baseline; placebo administered at time of retiring. Mentation reports were obtained 10 min after onset of the REMPs 2-4 by awakening subjects and inquiring after the content of any mental activity they had been experiencing just before awakening. A standard interview format was used with the Foulkes dream-like-fantasy scale;

Nights 7-9: nonlaboratory nights at home; subjects received bed time placebos;

Night 10: laboratory night repeating the baseline-night procedure, except that subjects were given 200 mgs of sodium amylobarbitone prior to retiring;

Nights 11-16: nonlaboratory nights at home in which subjects took 200 mgs amylobarbitone at bedtime.

Night 17: laboratory night repeating the baseline procedure including the placebo, that is, amylobarbitone withdrawn so that the experimenters could collect mentation reports on a drug-withdrawal night with elevated REM sleep deficit.

Two independent judges rated each mentation report on the Foulkes DF scale, and also as either "active" or "passive" in content. In addition, one of the judges noted whether the reports contained sexual symbolism or content. In all, 27 REM sleep mentation reports were obtained.

The experimenters found significant differences between the DF scores of baseline versus barbiturate conditions (χ^2 = 10.89; $p < 0.01$) and between barbiturate versus drug-withdrawal conditions (χ^2 = 8.01; $p < 0.02$); in each case, the dreams during drug nights were least dream-like. Only three dreams were judged to contain sexual themes and all of them occurred in the withdrawal condition.

In addition, it was found that the probability of obtaining an "active" report was different over all the conditions ($p < 0.05$) and that this difference derived entirely from the differential probability of a "passive" report between placebo and barbiturate conditions ($p < 0.015$). That is, of a total of eight dreams categorized as active, five occurred during the placebo-baseline condition, three during the drug withdrawal condition, and none during the drug condition. Finally, dreams on withdrawal nights did *not* exceed baseline dreams in vividness. The experimenters concluded that barbiturates "alter the dream experience," making it more conceptual and less perceptual, more "thought-like" and less "dream-like.".

Kales et al. (1969a, 1970, 1974) have performed extensive studies on the effects of glutethimide, methyprylon, pentobarbital, chloral hydrate, flurazepam, methaqualone, secobarbital, diphenhydramine, promethazine, diazepam, and chlordiazepoxide on sleep-dream patterns. To begin with, as with Oswald and Priest (1965), Kales and his group were impressed by the spontaneous reports of unpleasant dreams and nightmares by subjects who were experiencing withdrawal from certain sedative-hypnotic drugs under both clinical and laboratory conditions. Thus, both a pentobarbital addict (Kales et al., 1968) and a Tuinal addict (Kales et al. 1969a) during therapeutic drug withdrawal spontaneously described nightmares.

In addition, these investigators carried out systematic laboratory studies of the effects of a number of drugs employing an 8-consecutive-nights protocol with "normal" volunteers. On Nights 1-3 the subjects were given placebos. The first two nights were for adaptation and the third was for baseline data. On Nights 4-6 subjects received the active drug under study, and on Nights 7 and 8, the placebo once more, to examine the effects of drug withdrawal. Among 7 subjects on methyprylon and 5 on glutethimide, 3 subjects made spontaneous reports of unpleasant dreams or nightmares after withdrawal nights, whereas there was no such mention after baseline nights. This observation stimulated Kales et al. (1969b) to conduct an investigation of the effects of these 3 drugs with a 16-consecutive-night protocol in a home, rather than laboratory setting. Chloral hydrate, not a REM sleep suppressant, was compared to glutethimide and methyprylon, both powerful stage REM suppressors. Times of retiring, drug ingestion, and rising times were standardized to allow for 8.5 hr in bed from "lights out" to the waking alarm on the following morning. For each night, immediately after morning awakening, subjects were instructed to write out the total recall of their sleep mentation. The following consecutive nightly schedule was employed:

Nights 1-3: placebo;
Nights 4-6: active drug;
Nights 7-10: placebo (withdrawal);
Nights 11-13: active drug;
Nights 14-16: placebo (withdrawal).

In addition, subjects were required to record their responses to the Clyde mood scale, Nowlis mood adjective check list, and Zuckerman affect adjective check list in order to measure concomitant changes in mood states. Eighteen "normal" adult male volunteers participated, 6 in each study, testing the effects of 500 mg of glutethimide, 300 mg of methyprylon, and 500 mg of chloral hydrate in accordance with the above method. Added to the reports written by the subjects each morning were: (1) the subjects estimate of dream frequency for the night before (irrespective of whether specific content was recalled); (2) the experimenters' ratings of dream frequency based solely upon whether specific content was recalled; (3) the experimenters' ratings of degree of dream detail (minimal, moderate, and maximal detail categories), and; (4) the experimenters' ratings of the unpleasantness of content of only those dreams with dysphoric themes.

The findings were presented in terms of the means of the ratings in each scoring category; unfortunately, a weakness of the study is that neither tests of statistical significance nor coefficients of interrater reliability were provided.

The results for both Stage REM-suppressant drugs were most clear-cut for the first half of the experiment. In comparison to the initial baseline, glutethimide and methyprylon subjects showed decreases throughout in both subjects' and experimenters' estimate of dream-recall frequency, degree of dream detail, and dream unpleasantness; and on the first drug-withdrawal night series, a reversal of this trend was seen such that almost all indices exceeded those of the baseline. The methyprylon subjects provided the sole exception — a trivial one at that — of a slightly lower mean score on the subjects' estimate of their dream-recall frequency. Although this was lower than the initial baseline, it was still higher than the score on the preceding drug nights.

In the second half of the experiment, the results for glutethimide showed the same trend on most of the indices for both of the second drug and withdrawal-night series. However, the methyprylon subjects provided a less-consistent picture. Kales et al., (1969b) explained this on the basis that methyprylon is not as capable as glutethimide in effecting sustained REM sleep suppression.

In summary, with both REM sleep suppressors, a decrease in certain dream-recall categories was noted during drug administration with increases following withdrawal, especially in the degree of recall of dream detail and dream unpleasantness. Comparison data were not presented for chloral hydrate. However, when REM sleep suppressors were withdrawn, dysphoric mood changes (particularly depression) were observed, whereas no significant change was seen with chloral hydrate discontinuance. The authors suggest that the Stage REM rebound, increased dream recall, the unpleasantness, and depression all arise from a common source following REM sleep-suppressant drugs.

In a study on four adult subjects, Oswald et al. (1973) studied the effects of nitrazepam on a variety of human-sleep parameters. Two REM mentation reports were obtained nightly over the following four-week schedule (all administration just prior to retiring): first week, placebo; second week, nitrazepam 10 mg; third week, nitrazepam 20 mg; fourth week, placebo. All reports were scored by means of the DF scale. The results were as follows:

1. *Physiological:* during drug administration both REM profusion and REM time percentage diminished markedly, whereas after drug withdrawal, both measures exceeded baseline levels for as long as two weeks afterward.

2. *Psychological:* during drug administration, dreams were scored as significantly less bizarre, whereas following withdrawal, a striking increase of bizarreness over twice that of the baseline was observed ($p < .001$). This finding was based on 15 dreams elicited during the 1-week baseline phase, 31 dreams during the 2-week drug phase, and 16 dreams during the withdrawal phase.

In the most recent, systematic laboratory study of the influence of sedative-hypnotics on REM sleep mentation, Firth (1974) assessed the effects of amylobarbitone and nitrazepam in comparison to a placebo. His object was to extend and replicate the work of Carroll, Lewis, & Oswald (1969), in the course of which he planned to test the following predictions. During *administration,* both drugs would: (1) reduce the visual aspects of dreaming; (2) produce passive dreams with few activities and social interactions; (3) make REM sleep experience more thought-like and less "real" (Foulkes, Spear & Dymonds, 1966); (4) produce dreams with fewer unpleasant and more happy emotions; (5) reduce eye-movement profusion. In contrast, drug *withdrawal* would result in: (1) very active, unpleasant, visual dreams; (2) increase eye-movement profusion in excess of baseline levels.

Twenty subjects each spent a total of either 7 or 11 nights in the laboratory. They were healthy, paid non-student "normal" volunteers ranging in age from 19 to 26. Each had a total of 3 adaptation nights. Subjects spent 1 week on a placebo (baseline), 1 week on a low-drug dose, 1 week on a high dose, and 1 final week on a placebo (drug withdrawal). Drugs were amylobarbitone (200 and 400 mg), nitrazepam (10 and 20 mg), or placebo. Subjects were assigned randomly, 8 each to amylobarbitone and placebo, and 4 to nitrazepam. The conditions were double blind except for those on nitrazepam, for which it was single blind. Pills were taken nightly before retiring. All subjects were recorded on the first night of each week except the withdrawal week, in which they were recorded on the second withdrawal night. Four subjects in each group were also recorded on the the sixth night of each week. Mentation reports were obtained 7.5 min after onset of the second and fourth REM periods. These reports were analyzed by means of: (1) ratings of the whole report, content analysis, and scores on the psychodynamically oriented scales of Saul et al. (1954) and Whitman (1961); (2) ratings for activity versus passivity, sexiness, anxiety, psychotic thinking, and categorizations as to whether the reports were produced under baseline, drug, or withdrawal conditions; (3) ratings on the DF scale (Foulkes et al., 1966); and (4) content analyses following the system of Hall and Van de Castle (1966). In addition, subjects were required, both at home and in the laboratory, to fill in "visual-analogue scales" to estimate the amount of the previous nights' dreaming, and in some cases, their quality.

Physiological effects. As expected, drug nights for both drugs were characterized by a drastic reduction of REM profusion; and on withdrawal nights, REM activity exceeded that of baseline levels. Figures for statistical significance were given only for baseline versus drug nights ($p < .001$). As indicated below, however, contrary to expectation, REM profusion, as reduced or enhanced by drug action or withdrawal, respectively, was not related to qualities of dreaming. (See Chapters 6 and 7, with Ellman's commentary, for a fuller discussion of relationships between REM profusion and dream-like mentation.)

Effects on dreaming.   Drug-night effects were mostly contrary to predictions. Despite the drastic reduction of REM profusion, dreams were rated just as visually active on drug nights as on baseline nights. None of the psychodynamic scales showed effects, nor did the psychiatrist's ratings for anxiety, sexuality, or psychotic thinking. The experienced sleep-mentation judge was unable to guess better than chance which dreams were collected under baseline or drug conditions. And on the Hall and Van de Castle scales, there were no drug effects on the number of activities, social interactions, and emotions. Several differential drug effects were observed, however. Thus, nitrazepam did reduce the number of bizarre dreams, as reported by Oswald et al. (1973), whereas amylobarbitone was without such effect. And on the Hall and Van de Castle scales, two categories were affected differentially:

1. Nitrazepam reduced the number of dreams with specific looking or watching activity on the part of the dreamer, whereas amylobarbitone was without such effect.

2. Amylobarbitone reduced the number of characters in each dream from a baseline mean of 3.7 to 2.7, whereas nitrazepam was without such effect.

Drug-withdrawal nights, in the main, gave rise to dreams which could not be distinguished by the experienced judge from dreams obtained under baseline or drug conditions. Certain differences were observed across drugs, however. Thus, nitrazepam withdrawal led to an exceptionally large number of bizarre dreams on the Foulkes DF scale, whereas amylobarbitone, surprisingly, was without such effect. On the other hand, amylobarbitone withdrawal led to a mean increase of dream characters to 4.7 per dream whereas nitrazepam withdrawal had no such effect.

Effects on dreams: Subjects' estimates.   Wide individual differences were observed on subjective estimates of dreaming: some reported decreased dreaming while on drugs, others reported increased dreaming on withdrawal, whereas others reported no drug effects at all. One subject reported some quite vivid, aggressively toned dreams while on amylobarbitone; but where results were pooled across subjects, no particular effects were observed. On the first drug withdrawal night, however, which was spent at home, there was a striking rise in the vivid and bizarre quality of dreams as assessed by morning ratings. Further, two subjects spontaneously reported nightmares at home on their first night of withdrawal from 400 mg of amylobarbitone. Thus, for amylobarbitone, the home experience, as reflected by the morning reports of subjects, showed a clear dream-intensification withdrawal effect. This result was disparate from the laboratory finding which showed no such effect, and was possibly due to the laboratory recording occurring on the second withdrawal night, whereas the morning reports displaying these positive effects were those which arose from the first withdrawal night, as mentioned above.

In the course of their discussion, the authors speculated that a possible reason for the difference in results with amylobarbitone withdrawal in the laboratory and at home might involve differences in REM-period length under the two conditions. In the laboratory, REM mentation is experimentally sampled early in the REM period, but at home, the morning recall is derived from REM periods allowed to run their full course. As Foulkes (1966) showed that with increasing REM-period duration, associated dreams become more unpleasant, emotional, anxious, and hostile, it would thus be expected that drug withdrawal dreams at home, which are artifically lengthened by REM-rebound effects, would be more likely to be vivid and nightmarish.

Firth concluded that although the drugs reduced REM activity, they scarcely influenced the visual aspects of dreaming, nor did they affect the activity of dream characters. They do seem capable of producing more "everydayish" dreams, thus indicating that to some extent the qualities of sleep mentation are susceptible to the drug effects. In accord with other studies, drug withdrawal leads to more vivid, bizarre, and dysphoric dreaming although results were manifested in the laboratory only for nitrazepam but not for amylobarbitone; however, such dream intensification and dysphoria was noted for the latter under home conditions.

When one looks at the findings of Oswald and Priest (1965), Carroll et al. (1969), Kales et al. (1969b, 1970, 1974), and Firth (1974), one naturally wonders about the similarities and differences in their results. First, *during drug administration,* Kales et al. (1969b) report a diminution in the frequency and possibly overall amount of dream recall, whereas neither Carroll et al. (1969) nor Firth (1974) specifically describe such effects. In addition, a reduction in dream-like qualities of sleep mentation was found by Kales et al. (1969b) for glutethimide and methyprylon, by Carroll et al. (1969) for amylobarbitone and by Firth (1974) and Oswald et al. (1973) for nitrazepam. However, somewhat differently from Carroll et al. (1969), Firth found that amylobarbitone merely decreased the number of dream characters rather than more drastically affect the dream-like qualities of REM mentation. Also Kales et al. (1969b) and Carroll et al. (1969) reported similarly that glutethimide and methyprylon reduced dream dysphoria, in the former instance, and that amylobarbitone produced tranquil, passive dreams in the latter.

Second, *during drug withdrawal,* more vivid, intense, or nightmarish dreams were observed by Oswald and Priest (1965) and Firth (1974) with amylobarbitone (the latter only while the subjects were at home), by Kales et al. (1969b) for glutethimide and methyprylon and by Oswald et al. (1973) and by Firth (1974) for nitrazepam. By contrast, Carroll et al. (1969) reported no such marked changes with amylobarbitone withdrawal, nor did Firth (1974) (while subjects were in the laboratory).

Thus, the general trend of these studies indicates that with some qualifications, sedative-hypnotic drugs "tone down" or diminish dream intensity and their withdrawal increases it. How may one reconcile the differences in findings? Besides the use of different drugs (barbiturates, nitrazepam, glutethimide and methyprylon), the studies differed with respect to: (1) laboratory REM sleep-awakening mentation reports versus morning recall at home; (2) scales for measurement of dream-like content; (3) statistical procedures in data analysis—Kales et al. (1969b) compared differences in mean values of rating procedures but did not report results of tests of statistical significance or interrater reliability; and (4) size of subject population and organismic factors. Perhaps, only a reevaluation of the effects of a large variety of stage REM-suppressant drugs with uniform methodology and with adequate controls will enable us to answer the questions addressed.

In another paper, Kales et al. (1970) took up two further questions. First, why is it that increased and unpleasant dreaming occurs with some patients and not with others? The authors suggest that "traumatic" hypnotic drug withdrawal is most likely when preceded by a chronically and intensely sustained REM sleep deficit engendered by regular uninterrupted high dosage of long-acting hypnotics. Drug withdrawal in such patients would tend to produce intense REM-sleep rebound and increased dreaming. If severe psychopathology was also present, such dreams would be more likely to be nightmarish or unpleasant. Such an eventuality would be less probable with sporadic use of shorter-acting REM-sleep suppressors which permit discharge of some suppressed REM sleep during the last one or two REM periods of the night.

Second, why do certain patients have nightmares during a drug administration night? Such occurrences are most likely when patients use REM-sleep-suppressant drugs that have a short duration of action. In these cases, Stage REM is suppressed for the first two-thirds of the night and a REM-sleep rebound occurs in the last third producing increased dreaming. Again, should subjects suffer from severe psychopathology, they are more likely to experience nightmares on such occasions.

In a somewhat different study, Hartmann (1968a) had a chance to obtain mentation reports from four acutely psychotic patients who were being treated by prolonged pharmacologically induced sleep (dauerschlaf). The technique involved oral administration of 150 mg of chlorpromazine and 400 mg amobarbital at the onset of the treatment period. Subsequently, for the next 4 days they received 900 mg of chlorpromazine daily and a variable amount of amobarbital (400-1500 mg) in divided doses. All subjects showed some tendency for a Stage REM cycle throughout the 24-hr day. Two subjects possessed a very high total Stage REM time (15-16 hr over the 4 days). In general, dream recall was poor and sparse while under the influence of drugs. The dream content often contained elements reflecting the patient's psychotic state. Two of the three patients who recalled dreams reported unpleasant or anxiety dreams. At least one brief dream was recovered from NREM sleep. It was impossible to estimate the effect of the lack of a normal "day residue" on the dream content. Unfortunately, baseline data were not obtained so that valid estimate of the effects of the drugs on sleep mentation is precluded.

THE GENERAL ASSOCIATION BETWEEN PHARMACOLOGI-CALLY INDUCED INCREASED STAGE REM DEFICIT AND DREAMS CHARACTERIZED BY ANXIETY, UNPLEASANT-NESS, AND UNUSUAL VIVIDNESS

In the section on the effects of sedative-hypnotic drugs, we described the common sequence of the Stage REM-suppressant drug withdrawal after sustained use, followed by REM-sleep rebounds associated with dreams of unusual vividness, unpleasantness, and anxiety, often of nightmarish proportions.

Several authors have commented, that drug induced sudden increased REM-sleep levels regardless of drug class or drug mechanism of action may be associated with similarly intense, dysphoric dreams (Evans et al., 1968; Hartmann, 1970; Kales et al., 1974). Such has indeed been the case under the following circumstances: REM-sleep-rebound states following withdrawal of sustained intake of amphetaming, phenmetrazine, tranycypromine, and alcohol. In addition, administration of reserpine, one of the few substances known to increase Stage REM, has been reported to be associated with increased dreaming and nightmares. Another compound known to increase Stage REM is l-tryptophane, a serotonin precursor. When narcoleptics are given 5 g of this compound prior to bedtime, an inordinate number of Stage REM nightmares with strangled cries were observed (Evans & Oswald, 1966). Also, di-isopropyl fluorophosphate (DFP) is known to increase Stage REM, and clinical intoxication with this drug has likewise been associated with nightmares (Grob et al., 1947). Finally, febrile states are often associated with REM-sleep suppression and Hartmann (1970) speculates that fever nightmares occur during associated REM-sleep-rebound phases.

Both Kales et al. (1970) and Hartmann (1973) have commented that besides elevated REM-sleep deficit, there must be an additional set of factors necessary for the above manifestations. That is, when "normal" subjects are mechanically deprived in the laboratory, their recovery nights characterized by Stage REM rebound, are *not* associated with pronounced nightmarish and unpleasant dreaming. They considered the possibility, therefore, of drug-specific factors and subject differences as playing a role. In addition, mechanical Stage REM deprivation (by awakening subjects at each REM-period onset) engenders fatigue which may be sufficiently intense to outweigh dreaming tendencies.

This purportedly fairly uniform relationship between drug-induced heightened Stage REM deficit and increased dreaming has been hypothesized as providing the basis for delirious states following withdrawal of certain chronically used drugs. For example, clinical syndromes associated with alcoholism have received a great deal of attention along these lines (Feinberg & Evarts, 1969; Greenberg & Pearlman, 1967; Gross et al., 1971). The following typical sequence is suggested: after an initial alcohol-induced Stage REM suppression, with continued intake, REM-sleep levels return to baseline quantities. Concurrently, however, REM-sleep deficit is progressively increased but held in check until a time of future drug withdrawal when a compensating REM-sleep rebound occurs and overwhelms cognitive systems that have been concomitantly impaired by factors associated with drinking. This process produces wakeful hallucinosis and delirium.

With the passage of time, however, this attractive hypothesis has been challenged on a number of grounds. Thus, Laverty (1969) has considered the evidence regarding the effects of alcohol on sleep at the beginning, middle, and end of a bout of heavy drinking. On the basis of his own studies and those already cited, he concludes that the initial REM-sleep-suppressant effect of alcohol is confirmed. With regard to the middle phases, however, he states that the evidence regarding continuation of Stage REM suppression is conflicting. That is, individual differences in the subject populations are marked, and whereas definite sustained suppression does occur, so does adaptation (in that Stage REM time proportions return to normal baseline levels).* Furthermore, during alcohol withdrawal, similar inconsistencies have been found. Thus, in one of his own studies Laverty (1969) noted that only two out of eight subjects, after prolonged drinking bouts, showed Stage REM levels high enough to be described as rebound effects. Laverty (1969) concluded, therefore, that a REM-sleep rebound is not an inevitable or prominent result of the alcohol withdrawal state. Finally, while agreeing that patients in withdrawal delirium do show strikingly high proportions of Stage REM, he doubts that the accompanying hallucinations are a direct result of, or a continuation of, REM sleep increase for the following reasons:

1. Hallucinations may continue during intervals when Stage REM proportions and times are within normal range.
2. Stage REM in delirious states may be misidentified creating scoring errors.
3. Stage REM deficiency as a cause of hallucinatory psychosis is far from established.
4. The CNS disturbances in delirious alcoholics are much more profound and widespread than can be reasonably ascribed primarily to stage REM deprivation and rebound factors.

Along similar lines, Gross et al. (1973) reported that large quantities of alcohol (3.2 g/kg body weight) taken for four to six days markedly suppressed stage REM. However, following withdrawal, significant Stage REM levels in excess of baseline values were not observed.

---

*Such adaptational resumption of baseline REM sleep levels after intense suppression has aslo been noted with chronic amphetamine intake (Feinberg & Evarts, 1969).

Similarly, Wolin and Mello (1973), as a result of a careful study on 14 male chronic alcoholics under controlled conditions, have expressed caution about accepting the hypothesis that drug delirium is merely an intense REM-sleep rebound manifestation. They were interested in the following questions:

1. What are the time relationships between vivid dreams and hallucinations, on the one hand, and alcoholic intoxication and withdrawal, on the other?

2. Do the frequency, intensity, and quality of dream reports and hallucinations show progressive changes from intoxication through withdrawal?

3. Does sustained alcohol use induce cognitive changes that are associated with the onset of hallucinations?

4. To what extent are vivid dream and hallucination intensities correlated with changes in blood alcohol levels during intoxication and with changes in REM activity?

In order to insure opportunities to observe such changes, subjects were selected partly on the basis of a reported prior tendency to experience vivid affect-laden dreams and/or hallucinations during alcoholic intoxication and/or withdrawal.

The overall experimental schedule included a 1-week baseline period, an 11-12 day spontaneous-alcohol-consumption phase and concluded with a minimum of 7 alcohol-abstinence days. The sleep of each subject was electrographically monitored nightly throughout with the exception of an initial 3-night adaptation series. Reports of dreams were obtained by experimenters interviewing subjects each morning with standardized conditions and methods to elicit dream recall of the previous night. Reports of hallucinations were similarly obtained in a standard manner. Cognitive tasks of attention and perceptual organization were likewise administered in a controlled manner in each of the 3 experimental phases. Wolin and Mello (1973) summarized their results as follows:

> The hypothesized continuum of sequential changes that progressed from perceptual alterations to illusions, to vivid dreams, to hallucinations was not confirmed by our observations. Moreover, an alcohol-induced suppression of REM activity followed by REM hyperactivity during alcoholic withdrawal was not consistently observed. Although hallucinations were frequently associated with antecedent REM suppression or insomnia, there are no invariant relationships between hallucinosis and REM activity. Hallucinations were observed during intoxication as well as during alcohol withdrawal. There were no consistent close response relationships between alcohol intake and dreams and hallucinations intensity [p. 296].

In a more recent relevant article available at the time of this writing, Feinberg et al. (1974) have challenged the older literature even more vigorously on the uniformity of REM-sleep rebound following prolonged administration of barbiturates and also the hypothesis that the high level of Stage REM in some patients with delirium tremens represents a rebound phenomenon. In one experiment, three schizophrenic patients and three patients diagnosed as having a personality disorder received placebos for five nights, 200 mg of phenobarbital for four to five nights, followed by placebos (withdrawal phase) for four to five nights. In a second experiment, four medical students had baseline studies for four nights; then 200 mg of secobarbital were administered to one subject for eight nights, and the remaining three received 200 mg of the same drug for one night followed by 100 mg for the succeeding seven nights. All subjects were observed over three consecutive withdrawal nights. The results were that in both studies Stage REM time percentage and REM density were both significantly decreased on drug nights but significant rebounds in excess of baseline levels were not observed on withdrawal nights. Thus, with two different barbiturates, the prevailing expectation of REM-sleep rebound following prior drug-induced suppression was not fulfilled. Furthermore, the authors recommend that consideration be given to whether barbiturate reduction of Stage REM parameters is the consequence of primary inhibition of oculomotor function rather than a sign of a more specific effect on phasic processes in Stage REM. The same idea was thought applicable to some benzodiazepine effects on Stage REM which also may include reduction without rebound.

ADDITIONAL DRUG STUDIES

Imipramine

Whitman et al. (1961) attempted to investigate the effects of imipramine (25 mg), phenobarbital (10 mg), and prochlorperazine (5 mg) on REM sleep mentation. Ten adult "normal" volunteer college students were used as subjects, 5 male and 5 female. Each of the subjects had 1 baseline night and 1 experimental night during which Stage REM mentation was elicited 5 min after REM-period onsets. Each experimental night was preceded by 3 consecutive days, during which the subjects received one of the above drugs 4 times daily. This procedure provided for a total of 10 baseline and 30 experimental nights. The order of each drug series was randomized and administered an a double-blind basis. Seven scales were used by judges (the number of judges was unspecified but interrater reliability = 0.75) to rate the mentation reports on the following content categories: hostility, dependency, anxiety, motility, homosexuality, heterosexuality, and intimacy. A statistically significant result occurred with imipramine administration in that the number of recalled dreams per night decreased and the amount of hostility per word of each dream report increased. In addition, there was a tendency for prochlorperazine to increase the expression of heterosexuality, and phenobarbital that of homosexuality. Finally, nonspecific drug effects manifested themselves with increases in indications of dependency and anxiety and a decrease in intimacy.

It is difficult to draw firm conclusions from this study because of lack of placebo controls and adaptation nights, only one initial baseline night and lack of a postexperimental baseline night.

Kramer et al. (1968) carried out a study on the effects of imipramine on 10 severely depressed, hospitalized patients. On admission to the hospital, each subject was started on 4 imipramine placebo capsules per day, and during the first week slept two nights (Nights 1 and 2) in the laboratory, during which time baseline REM sleep-mentation reports were collected. During the succeeding 3 weeks the patients received the active drug, and the sleep-laboratory procedure (with elicitation of reports) was repeated 1 night per week (Nights 3-5). Comparisons of dream frequency, recall percentage, and content analyses were made between Nights 1 and 5, 2 and 5, and 2 and 3. This design feature permitted comparisons of baseline parameters with those of long-range drug effects over a sustained interval (1-5; & 2-5) as opposed to whatever short-range drug effects were possibly manifested soon after initiating the drug regimen. Two independent judges scored mentation reports on hostility, anxiety, intimacy, heterosexuality, motility, dependency, and homosexuality content categories. Complete results were available for only 7 patients. Contrary to the results of an earlier study (Whitman et al., 1961), on "normal" volunteers, no reduction was observed both in the number of REM periods per night and the frequency of dream recall over all conditions. However, the short-range effects were similar to the earlier study in that significant increases of hostility and anxiety were observed. The long-range effects show an interesting reversal of these results characterized by significantly *decreased* hostility and anxiety, and increases in motility and heterosexuality. To account for their findings, the authors speculated that the imipramine effects in depression occur in two phases: an initial one in which hostility is mobilized, that is shifted from a "bound to a free state," and then discharged by the time the depressed patient is measurably improved. Further, the dream data indicate that when hostile feelings recede in the depressed, tender feelings emerge; and in addition, the motility dimension in dreams mirrors the patients' clinical status. Unfortunately, control studies on a similar depressed population with placebo controls were not carried out. This leaves unanswered the question as to whether the observed changes in dreams were drug effects or simply part of the natural history of the syndrome.

Meprobamate

Whitman, Pierce & Maas (1960) studied the effects of meprobamate on a patient whose clinical diagnosis was not mentioned but was described as possessing pathological character traits and little anxiety. Twenty-six REM sleep reports were collected 5 min after REM-period onset during 8 medication-free nights. The patient then received 400 mg of meprobamate 4 times daily for 7 days, following which REM sleep-mentation reports were collected in the same manner as before,while the medication regimen was continued without interruption. Although the patient was studied over 9 nights (1 day longer than the baseline series) on the drug regimen, only 18 dreams were reported. This reduction in dream recall was consistent with the clinical report of Selling (1955), that meprobamate therapy is associated with decreased dreaming. Three judges scored the report contents on 7-point scales of the following categories: hostility, anxiety, dependency, intimacy, motility, heterosexuality, and homosexuality. Mentation reports elicited under baseline and drug conditions were indistinguishable by both patient and judges on the basis of "gross description." However, the scoring procedure, employing the scales enumerated, yielded significant differences in the direction of greater motility and dependency under the drug condition. These results may not be generalized, however, because only 1 subject was used and because there was no terminal baseline condition following the drug nights for an appropriate control.

A contradictory result to the above was reported by Prigot, Barnes, & Barnard (1957), in a clinical study, to the effect that during meprobamate therapy dream recall was facilitated and furthermore changed in the direction of being more "bizarre," "vivid," "colorful," and "frightening." However, Selling (1954), in the same study mentioned above, claimed that while receiving meprobamate, disturbing dreams were no longer reported by patients.

Benzodiazepines

Chlordiazepoxide

Several clinical investigations have reported that during chlordiazepoxide therapy, a sizable proportion of patients described alterations in dreaming experience. Thus, Toll (1960) mentioned unusually vivid dreaming, and Stanfield (1961) reported nightmares in patient populations. Moore (1962) noted that 16% of 100 patients volunteered excessive dreaming. Maggs and Neville (1964) presented the intriguing observation of 3 cases of recurrent dreams in patients taking this drug.

Finally, Viscott (1968) described, in detail, patients who, while on the drug, experienced extraordinarily vivid, nocturnal, bizarre, affect-laden dreaming often difficult to distinguish from reality, and indeed continuing as intense, prolonged hypnopomic hallucinations, in some instances, after awakening. With one exception, none of those patients were psychotic. The exception was described as a paranoid schizophrenic individual who had no history of prior hallucinations.

Diazepam

Kahn et al. (1970) and Fisher et al. (1973b) have demonstrated that presleep diazepam suppresses or ameliorates Stage 4 night terrors. This effect was attributed to Stage 4 suppression rather than the antianxiety effect of diazepam because thorazine, a drug with antianxiety properties, appeared to exacerbate the night terrors. Some subjects were studied with placebo and dilantin controls, which were without effect.

Monoamine-oxidase inhibitors.   A group of six anxious-depressed patients who provided many reports of dreams on awakening in the morning while drug-free, were unable to recall a single dream during sustained Stage REM suppression brought about by a long-term phenelzine regimen (Wyatt et al., 1971).

Beta-adrenergic blocking agents. Several clinical reports have appeared indicating that beta-adrenergic blocking agents may be implicated in some cases of vivid dreams and nightmares during drug treatment (Atsmon Blum, & Wijsenbeck, 1971; Prichard & Gillam, 1969). In addition, there have been a large number of observations that the same class of drugs may produce hallucinations that are mostly visual and often hypnagogic (Tyrer & Lader, 1973; Atsmon et al., 1971; Gardos et al., 1973; Prichard & Gillam, 1964, 1969; Hinshelwood, 1969; Gillam & Prichard, 1965; Oppelt & Palmer, 1972).

Anticholinesterase Agents

Physostigmine

In a recent study, Sitaram et al. (1976) investigated the outcome of physostigmine administered intravenously to seven sleeping normal adult subjects. The main focus of interest was the effect on REM sleep, and in this connection it was found that .5 mg given during NREM sleep induced the onset of REM sleep, and when administered during REM tended to provoke wakefulness. Doses of 1.0 mg tended to wake subjects regardless of concurrent sleep stage. Compared with a placebo, physostigmine did not alter total REM sleep time, REM density, or any of the NREM sleep stages.

Among subjects who awoke after physostigmine infusion, two reported frightening nightmares. One of these reports came from REM and the other from NREM sleep. A third subject receiving the drug during REM sleep reported "a golden thickness and fluidity throughout my body." Two additional subjects reported dreams when awakened 7 min after REMP onset, each preceded by physostigmine administered during NREM sleep.

In view of the anticholinesterase activity of physostigmine, serving to increase acetylcholine at synapses, the authors conclude that cholinergic mechanisms play a role in the induction of REM sleep and in modulating cortical arousal mechanisms.

In accordance with these contentions, the authors cite work demonstrating the tendency of anticholinergic agents (scopolamine and atropine) to delay REM onset and reduce amounts of REM sleep. In addition, they cite a number of clinical reports of excessive dreaming and nightmares following intake of anticholinesterase drugs.

Tobacco Smoking and Dreams

Baldridge, Whitman, & Ornstein (1967) observed 10 volunteer chronic tabacco-smoking subjects who spent a total of four nights in the laboratory. REM sleep-mentation reports were elicited two nights prior to interrupting smoking and two nights following interruption.

The dreams prior to abstinence were said to "express uncertainity and confusion and a desire to escape." In addition, many reports related to eating.

On the third night following two days of abstinence subjects reported many dreams involved with experience of being restrained or watched. Only a single reference was made to food on this night. On the fourth night (after five days of abstinence), dreams were "generally more serene with some concern about leaving the experiment." No dreams of smoking occurred on any subject night although many reports contained references to the experimental situation. The authors concluded that abstinence from cigarettes was of less direct concern, judging from the mentation reports, than the restraint occasioned by the experiment.

THEORIES OF DRUG EFFECTS ON DREAMS

Not many investigators have formulated a theory of drug effects on dreams. One such attempt (Oswald, 1969b) relates processes involved in neuronal protein synthesis to a variety of findings including the difference in levels of Stage REM rebound levels following deprivation by drugs versus mechanical means. Whether one observes subjects after sustained use of Stage REM-suppressant drugs (like the amphetamines, barbiturates, or tricyclic antidepressants) or even acute overdosage, the height and duration of REM-sleep rebound strikingly exceeds that following deprivation by awakening at each REM-period onset (even though the amounts of deprivation of REM sleep have been "equalized" for both conditions). An additional noteworthy observation is that the peak of the rebound varies under different conditions being considerably delayed with certain drugs. The rate with which this peak is approached seems related to the rate of drug removal, reaching its maximum closely after the final disappearance of the drug from the brain. Oswald (1969b) accordingly hypothesizes that an increase of REM sleep may be a sign of certain types of neuronal repair. Thus, the REM rebound after drug withdrawal is thought indicative of a reshaping of neuronal "machinery," entailing protein synthesis. While not proposing that all kinds of active brain repair are accompanied by REM sleep, he speculates that a REM rebound is likely whenever serotonin or norepinephrine metabolism is involved. In support of his contention, he cites the following:

1. Morphine tolerance increases 5 HT synthesis and its withdrawal leads to increases of REM sleep in excess of baseline levels.
2. Reserpine depletes 5 HT, but at the same time causes increased 5 HT synthesis and amounts of Stage REM.
3. Both l-tryptophan and 5 HTP enhance REM sleep, presumably by increasing 5 HT synthesis.
4. Streptomycin, a protein-synthesis inhibitor, reduces Stage REM.
5. REM sleep is higher in neonates than adults, both in total quantity and proportion of total sleep time. Maturational curves of Stage REM closely approximate the growth and decline of the nervous system.

6. Some cases of human mental retardation have less REM sleep in amount and intensity.

In further support of Oswald (1969b), one can cite the finding of Lester, Chanes, & Condit (1969), that three terminal cancer patients on a diet deficient in tyrosine and phenylalanine experienced a systematic reduction of Stage REM which was reversible with restoration of these amino acids.

More recently, Hartmann (1973) has formulated general theories of the functions of sleep which also take account of drug effects. On the basis of evidence too extensive to be summarized here, he hypothesized a feedback mechanism such that low catecholamine levels produce increases in Stage REM, and Stage REM "in some way restores the catecholamine levels or restores the integrity of catecholaminergic brain systems [Hartmann, 1973, p. 116]," which are important for optimal function in wakefulness. REM-sleep-reducing drugs also deplete brain catecholamines and the REM rebound is seen as the physiological response the goal of which is to restore effective catecholamine functions. In agreement with Oswald (1969b), Hartmann (1973) looks upon Stage REM as an interval of neuronal repair, reorganization, and biochemical synthesis. However, one gains the impression that anabolism and synthesis of macromolecules, such as proteins, are considered by Hartmann to occur especially in NREM (slow-wave) sleep and the products of such biochemical sequences are deemed preparatory, in part, for physiological Stage REM processes.

CONCLUSION

Having read our review of the effects of psychoactive drugs on dream reports, it would be easy to see how one might become discouraged and even conclude that there are no systematic and reliable effects. However, allowing optimism to prevail, the reader might consider that there are a number of important variables and critical methodological differences, all of which are likely to influence studies of the effects of a particular drug on dream reports, and few of which are held constant across experiments with the same drug. The perpetual optimist might consider the effects of drugs on dreams as a vast multidimensional mosaic, with a particular drug being only one dimension of many. The current literature would then be seen as but a few tiles in this vast mosaic. Our goal in these few paragraphs is not to fill in the mosaic but merely to chart its coordinates and leave for future research the task of filling in the individual titles. Perhaps when the mosaic is more complete, we can step back and view the big picture.

First and foremost is the distinction between the chronic (long-term) versus acute effects of drugs on dream reports. For pharmacological, biochemical, and psychological reasons initial effects of a psychoactive agent on dream mentation may be very different from chronic, long-term effects. Therefore, such effects should be considered as a function of the amount of time the subjects have been successively taking the drug. A corollary of this dimension is the effects of withdrawal of a psychoactive drug on dream reports, which in the present literature is sometimes difficult to separate from the effects of the drug itself. This is particularly true if the drug and dose combination are short acting (within an 8-hr night). To belabor the obvious, if the drug in question has cleared from the body in the first 4 hr of an 8-hr night, it is difficult, if not impossible to distinguish the effects of the drug from the effects of withdrawal of the drug on dream reports. This is further confounded by the differences in REM time throughout the night (almost 80% of REM time occurring in the last 3 hr of an 8-hr night of normal sleep).

The drug regimen is another important variable that may influence the outcome of an experiment. An obvious distinction can be made between studies that give single administrations of drugs widely spaced by several days of placebo as compared with studies which administer the drug on consecutive nights. A less obvious distinction exists between drug regimens that, for a variety of reasons are administered four or five times a day or in a fashion which maintains a fairly high and consistent blood level (such as with phenothiazines and butrophenones), and other drug regimens that, while administered on consecutive nights, are given only before retiring. While the patients in both cases may be receiving the drug on consecutive nights, there are marked and prolonged differences in blood level over a 24-hr period for the latter but not the former group.

A sine qua non for pharmacological research, which seems to be absent in the main from the current dream and sleep literature, is the employment of a variety of doses across the same experimental conditions, in the same experiment. It would seem that as difficult as it may be to accomplish, employing more than one dose of a drug in an experiment is an absolute necessity.

Another variable intimately related to both dose of the drug and regimen of drug is the time of night that the drug is active. This is especially so since there are large differences in the amount of time spent in different phases of sleep from one part of the night to another, and phase of sleep is presumed to correlate with dreaming. When interpreting the effects of a particular drug on dreams, it is, therefore, important to keep in mind the time of night that the drug is maximally active. This can be controlled for in a variety of ways among which are: (1) keeping the subject on a regimen that maintains a consistent blood level throughout the night (possibly through the use of spansules); and (2) systematically varying the time of night the drug is active and performing separate analyses on dream reports.

Another critical dimension frequently ignored is the manner in which dream reports are collected. Some studies allow the subjects to sleep through the entire night and rely upon dream reports collected the following morning after the subjects are awakened, while other studies awaken the subjects during REM and other phases of sleep, and collect dream reports at times of awakening throughout the night. While there is no obvious a priori reason to prefer one method over another in all experiments of drugs and dreams, this major difference in methodological approach may account for some of the apparent discrepancies in the existing literature and should certainly be considered as a dimension in future experiments. Lest one think that this is a subtle point, it should be noted that the drug scopolamine, when given in high doses to human subjects, frequently produces bizarre and vivid hallucinations accompanied by disordered thought processes. Yet, once the drug has worn off, the patients are most frequently amnesic for events that transpired under the influence of the drug. One speculates, therefore, as to what we would conclude about the effects of scopolamine on mentation if one relies solely on the reports of the subjects the morning after the drug had been administered the night before.

Another frequent dimension that warrants serious consideration in such studies is the psychological state of the individuals employed as subjects. Obvious distinctions can be made between various categories of psychotic and ostensibly normal subjects. Less obvious distinctions can be made concerning the set and expectancies of subjects as well as the experimenters. Techniques for systematically evaluating such items seem practicable.

Because we feel that it would be presumptuous and impossible to outline the ideal experimental design on the effects of drugs on dream content (as it would be to outline the ideal course of psychotherapy) we have refrained from doing so. We have, however, pointed to a few dimensions and distinctions which we feel are critical in developing our understanding of the effects of drugs on dreams.

Part V

EFFECTS OF REMP DEPRIVATION

12

REM Deprivation: A Review

S. J. Ellman
A. J. Spielman
D. Luck
S. S. Steiner
R. Halperin

City college of the City University of New York
   and
Montefiore Hospital and Medical Center, Albert Einstein College of Medicine

In this chapter we deal primarily with the "psychological" and behavioral effects of deprivation of rapid eye movement (REM) sleep. Our chapter largely overlaps with a recent article by Vogel (1975) which also reviews the behavioral effects of REM deprivation (RD). Since our manuscript was in preparation when Vogel presented his review in 1974, we decided to continue our work, but we must acknowledge our debt to the comprehensive and scholarly effort performed by Dr. Vogel. His review clearly influenced us, although, naturally, he is in no way responsible for the views contained in this work.

In 1960, Dement performed a study in which he asserted that he was dream-depriving subjects. In fact, what he did was awaken people at the beginning of each REM period (REMP) and, using today's terminology, performed the first RD experiment. Dement's (1960a) use of the term "dream deprivation" reflected early views that dreaming, or perhaps all sleep mentation, is confined to REM sleep (Dement & Kleitman, 1957).

However, a variety of developments have led a number of investigators to maintain that not all sleep mentation is confined to the REM period (REMP) and that the biological-behavioral significance of REM sleep might be better conceptualized somewhat apart from the dream experience. The findings of Foulkes (1962) and others (Foulkes, Spear, & Symonds, 1966; Foulkes & Vogel, 1965; Kamiya, 1961), that awakenings from non-REM (NREM) sleep yield mentation reports that are at times quite dreamlike, make it clear that RD is not necessarily dream deprivation. The necessary link between REM sleep and

419

dreaming has also been weakened by both phylogenetic and developmental studies. Almost all mammalian species that have been studied have manifested a type of sleep that can be identified as REM sleep. In addition, numerous studies have shown that infant mammals have much more REM sleep (in both absolute and percentage terms) than adult mammals (Roffwarg, Dement, & Fisher, 1965; Muzio & Dement, 1966). Thus, the discovery that REM sleep occurs in virtually all mammals (Snyder, 1969) and that infants can spend 8-12 hr a day in REM sleep, has led some researchers to hypothesize that the functional significance of REM sleep should not be linked solely or perhaps even primarily, to dreaming. Dement's dream-deprivation experiment then failed to assess, as he had intended, the basic function and significance of dreaming. However, his experiment was a germinal one in the history of sleep research, and few, if any, experiments have had as great an impact on the field.

Although the theme of this book focuses mainly on sleep mentation, we have chosen to include animal studies in this chapter, since, in our view, animal and human RD studies are in many ways inextricably interwoven. After Dement's (1960a) initial RD experiment in humans, he and his collaborators performed extensive RD studies in cats and rats (Cohen & Dement, 1965; Cohen, Mitchell, & Dement, 1968; Cohen, Thomas, Dement, 1970; Dement, 1965; Dement, 1969; Dewson et al., 1967; Ferguson & Dement, 1967, 1968, 1969). On the basis of his animal studies, Dement developed a position that we label a "motivational" hypothesis. Essentially, it is his view that REM sleep is an occasion for the discharge of drive behaviors (Dement, 1969). From this point of view, RD should lead to a higher probability of discharge of drive behaviors in the waking state.

This assumption is compatible with a hydraulic model, and many authors (Sheffield, Roby & Campbell, 1954; Holt, 1976) in other areas have contended that a hydraulic model is not able to explain various behaviors that have been traditionally studied by investigators interested in "learning and motivational" variables. It is beyond the scope of this chapter to attempt to evaluate these arguments, but it is important to report that Dement, to our knowledge, has never presented his hypothesis in a formal manner where he fully spells out the implications of his assumptions[1]. Rather, it has seemed to us that his theoretical position has served as a working hypothesis, and as such has stimulated a good deal of research. Thus, he and his collaborators have looked at the effect of RD on subjects' perceptions on projective tests, on what might generally be termed drive behavior in animals, and on the sleep cycle of schizophrenic patients. Whatever one's view of Dement's hypothesis, to gain a fair representation of his work and the work that he has in part stimulated, it has seemed necessary to us to include animal studies in our review.

[1]We recognize that Dement has published articles in which he has made predictive statements; however he has not, to our knowledge, published a statement of his drive-discharge hypothesis, in which he fully and formally makes a theoretical statement (that is, spells out his postulates and the predictions from these postulates).

Although in our brief historical introduction we have used Dement's work as an illustration, we might just as easily have pointed out that researchers (Dewan, 1969; Greenberg & Pearlman, 1974) who have linked REM sleep with learning and memory variables have used their hypotheses to generate experiments in both humans and animals. At this point in time, the most extensive studies in this area have been in rats and mice.

We will not systematically attempt to evaluate the various theoretical views put forth to explain the behavioral significance of REM sleep, but it is worth noting that these views have rarely been parochial and narrowly focused. Rather, they have often been global (Ephron & Carrington, 1966; Roffwarg et al., 1966), and have attempted to explain elements of psychopathology, mammalian development, drive behavior, learning, memory and so on. Most (if not all) of the theoretical views about REM sleep attempt to explain RD effects, and most of the views that have led to the experiments we review in this chapter have been concerned with data that have been generated from animal and human subjects. We might parenthetically add that this is symptomatic of a good deal of sleep research, but is probably most often the case in the RD literature.

This chapter contains a comprehensive review of the RD literature and, as such, provides background material for Chapter 13 of this volume, in which the effects of RD on sleep mentation are discussed.

In the first section of this chapter we discuss RD in humans, and in the second section, RD in animals. Each section has subdivisions concerned with methodology and with the effects of RD on various behavioral and psychological variables.

THE EFFECTS OF RD IN HUMANS

Sleep-Cycle Changes

In his first RD experiment Dement (1960a) used a "pre-post design" that has frequently been employed in subsequent RD studies. First, the subject is allowed to sleep uninterruptedly for several nights; this baseline (BL) condition provides a standardized sample of the subject's sleep patterns. Following BL nights (five in Dement's study), RD nights are initiated during which the subject is awakened every time upon entering REM sleep. RD nights are followed by recovery (R) nights during which the subject is again allowed to sleep uninterruptedly, as in the BL sequence. In the typical control condition, the subject is awakened during NREM sleep the same number of times as awakened in the RD condition. Thus, in this experiment, the subjects serve as their own control (that is, the same subject goes through both RD and control conditions). Usually, a week or two separates the RD and the control conditions. Since there have been several variations of Dement's original design, we attempt to set down some basic methodological criteria for adequately assessing RD studies.

Two obvious factors in a pre-post design are adequate BL or premeasures, and adequate R, or postmeasures. Various investigators (Agnew, Webb, & Williams,

1966; Dement, Kahn, & Roffwarg, 1965b; Rechtschaffen & Verdone, 1964) have shown that on the first night in a sleep laboratory, subjects show lower REM sleep values in absolute and percentage terms than on subsequent BL nights. Kales et al. (1969) have shown, as have others (Ellman, 1969; Fiss & Ellman, 1973), that only by the third BL night can one obtain stable BL values. Given that this is the case, it is clear that studies which utilize pre-post designs must have at least three BL or adaptation[2] nights to adequately assess the effects of their manipulation on R nights. In addition, the mean of the third and all subsequent BL nights should be used for statistical comparisons.

At least two R nights are needed to assess the effects of RD in studies utilizing four RD nights or less. The need for at least two R nights is particularly important because during RD studies, subjects are frequently deprived of some delta (Stages 3 and 4) sleep (Agnew, Webb, & Williams, 1967; Ellman, 1969). If delta deprivation is great enough, then on the first R night one may see a delta rebound that can displace a potential REM rebound. The REM rebound would then take place on the second R night. As a related point, since BL and R nights are often compared, every attempt should be made to allow subjects approximately the same total sleep time in both conditions. In response to Dement's (1960a) first RD experiment, Barber (1960) has pointed out that control and RD conditions should be counterbalanced. (See Chapter 13 of this volume for a specific example of how counterbalancing can be accomplished.)

As a last general methodological point in human studies, the criteria used for RD can be important. Frequently, a drop in EMG levels (muscle atonia) is an early sign of a REMP, and studies that do not employ EMG measures may allow a subject up to several minutes of REM sleep before an awakening (Kales et al., 1964). Some investigators do not utilize EMG recordings (Cartwright, Monroe, & Palmer, 1967), while others (see Chapter 13 of this volume; Kales et al., 1964) do.

It is quite important to clearly specify the criteria used for RD, particularly in studies reporting negative findings. Moreover, some type of REM-density measure[3] (number of eye movements per unit time) should be calculated for scoring of REM sleep during R nights, since it is possible that high-REM density may

---

[2]Here we are using the terms "baseline" and "adaptation nights" interchangeably, since from a subject's point of view they are identical. On an adaptation night, a subject is treated just as on a BL night, except that no recording is performed. This is a relatively inexpensive way to acclimate subjects to a laboratory. All RD (and sleep) studies should inquire about drug and alcohol habits of subjects. Clearly, for one to two weeks preceding RD and throughout the study, a subject should be drug-free, inasmuch as many drugs influence REM sleep.

[3]REM density is defined as REM-phasic events per unit of REM time. As an example, one may compute the average number of REMs per REM sleep time. Actually, this measure of REM density is usually calculated by computing the number of 2-sec epochs in a REMP that contain one or more REMs. Latency to the first REMP denotes the interval between sleep onset and the first REMP of the night.

substitute for overall REM-time measures of REM rebound. (This point is presented in more detail subsequently in the chapter.)

Dement (1960a) found that for each additional night of RD, more awakenings were required to keep subjects from entering REM sleep. On R nights, they demonstrated elevated amounts of REM sleep (REM rebound), while in the control condition (NREM awakenings), subjects did not display a REM rebound. Thus, they seemed to display a "need" for REM sleep in the sense of attempting to compensate or make up for lost REM sleep. Three other suggestive results have come to be associated with the effects of RD:

1. REM rebound can last for more than one R night (and for as long as four to five R nights).

2. Latency to the first REMP after sleep onset is reduced on the first R night; (REMP latency refers to the time interval between onset of sleep and the first REMP of the night.)

3. During RD, the number of eye movements per REM time (REM density) increases (Dement et al., 1970; Ferguson & Dement, 1968). This can also occur on R nights.

Kales, Hoedemaker, Jacobson, and Lichtenstein (1964) were the first researchers to attempt to replicate Dement's (1960a) findings. Two subjects were REM deprived for 6 nights and showed a large REM rebound during R (REM was elevated 40-70% over BL). Kales et al. (1964) also REM deprived the same subjects for 10 nights and produced an even larger REM rebound. Unfortunately, Kales and co-workers did not specify how many BL nights were employed in the study, nor subject the results to statistical analysis. He reported (as did Dement) that as RD nights progress, the number of awakenings needed to prevent a subject from entering REM increases. This increase is nonmonotonic, although from the first night to the tenth night, mean awakenings increased from 20 to about 40 per night. When Kales et al. (1964) used a NREM awakening control, subjects showed no increase in REM sleep. As in Dement's (1960a) study, conditions were not counterbalanced. Snyder (1963) briefly reported similar results in two subjects, that is, an increased number of awakenings as RD nights progressed, and a REM rebound during R.

Sampson (1965) maintained that Dement's (1960a) findings might be a result of "dream" or REM interruption, as opposed to RD. He proposed to separate these two possibilities by utilizing a method he called "partial sleep deprivation." Sampson allowed subjects to sleep only 2.5 hr per night for five consecutive nights, reasoning that since very little REM (an estimated 10 to 15 min) occurs during the initial 2.5 hr of the night, this procedure would REM deprive subjects without interrupting REMPs. For comparison, the same subjects were REM deprived for five successive nights by awakening them at each REMP onset. Sampson found that both procedures, partial sleep deprivation and dream interruption, produced a REM rebound. While there was no significant difference in

REM rebound, there was a trend in the direction of larger REM rebound following recovery from dream interruption. In addition, dream interruption produced a REM rebound in all six subjects, while partial sleep deprivation produced a REM rebound in only four out of six. Of the two subjects that did not show a REM rebound, one was not adequately assessed during R. The second clearly did not display a REM rebound on any of the three R nights following partial sleep deprivation.

One might argue that a NREM rebound displaced a REM rebound in this subject, since partial sleep deprivation, as its name implies, deprives subjects of both REM and NREM sleep. However, this seems to be an unlikely possibility since, even with total sleep deprivation, one can usually see a REM rebound during the second R night, and this subject showed no effect in three R nights as a result of partial sleep deprivation.

Dement, Greenberg, and Klein (1966) performed two types of studies demonstrating that extended partial RD has a cumulative effect, and that RD effects are reversed only by REM rebound. In the first experiment, after 10 BL nights, 2 subjects were deprived of about 25% of their REM sleep each night for 19 nights. On the first R night, both subjects displayed REM levels that were higher than on any BL night. For one of the two subjects, the effect was small (less than 10 min), and the authors offer as a possible explanation that BL REM levels were spuriously high. From the data they present, there is no reason to assume this, since subjects had 10 BL nights. Moreover, their statistical treatment of the data (simple probability statement) does not allow one to generalize beyond the population of BL nights they sampled. In the second study, after 10 BL nights, two subjects were REM deprived for 5 nights, and then on the 5 subsequent nights, they were allowed REM levels *equal* to those of their BL night. The next 5 nights were "normal" R nights, and both subjects displayed REM rebounds. The conclusion the authors reach is that REM rebound is necessary to dissipate excess REM, or, stated another way, RD effects can be stored over time.

Agnew, Webb, and Williams (1967) performed an interesting study comparing Stage 4 to Stage REM deprivation. Their study is difficult to evaluate because all sleep data is presented in percentages, and there is no way to ascertain whether total sleep time on BL and R nights was held constant. Unless one knows this data, the possibility of artifactually high REM rebound totals is present if total sleep time was greater on R as opposed to BL nights. Obviously, REM rebound could be reported as spuriously low if total sleep time on BL nights is greater than on R nights. Controlling for total sleep time is essential because after the fourth hour of sleep REM percentage[4] increases (Verdone, 1968). Therefore, it is likely that the longer one sleeps, the higher the percentage of REM sleep. Nevertheless, Agnew et al. (1967) reported that selective RD leads to REM rebound, while selective Stage 4 deprivation leads to a Stage 4 rebound. RD

[4]REM percentage is defined as REM time over total sleep time.

produced a selective rebound in that there was no Stage 4 (or any other sleep stage) rebound after RD. On the other hand, even though the authors stated that during Stage 4 deprivation there was virtually no RD (a drop of only 2% per night), on the second and third R nights, subjects displayed elevated REM percentages (REM percentage went from 21 on BL night to 26% on the second and third R night, respectively). This finding may be explained as a partial RD effect. Thus, if a subject displays a percentage loss of 2% per night, then this loss over seven (Stage 4) deprivation nights would be anywhere form 40 to 50 min of REM sleep. This is roughly equivalent to one-half night of RD. This conclusion is a tentative one, since we do not know the absolute values of total sleep time.

Ferguson and Dement (1968) and Dement et al. (1970) have suggested that in RD studies, what is made up is not REMP time per se, but rather phasic events. If this is correct, then it is logically possible to have no elevation in REM time, but a REM rebound in the sense that there are more phasic events per unit time. Although these results are in large part derived from animal studies, and are not replicated, nevertheless it seems to us important in any RD study where rebound is a dependent variable, to report on any measure of phasic activity that is available. Clearly, if phasic events are a crucial element, then the reporting of REM rebound results are not complete without including some measure of phasic activity.

Agnew et al. (1967) report only group data, but in the other four studies[5] we have just reviewed, 20 subjects were administered some type of RD, and 19 of these subjects displayed elevated REM levels on either the first or second R night.[6] In all of the studies, there was an increase from the first to the last deprivation night in the number of awakenings[7] needed to accomplish RD. However, in two studies (Agnew et al., 1967; Kales et al., 1964), total sleep time from BL to R was not mentioned, and in two studies (Dement et al., 1966; Sampson, 1965), there was no NREM awakening control group. Neither of the experiments (Dement, 1960a; Kales et al., 1964) that used the same subjects in both deprivation and control conditions counterbalanced these conditions, although Dement (1960b) has stated that he has counterbalanced conditions and it has no effect on the results obtained. (To our knowledge, he has not published these results.)

[5]Dement and Fisher (1963) report that in studies they conducted, 20 out of 21 subjects displayed REM rebound. We have not included this report because they do not present their data, but only summarized their findings.

[6]One subject in Dement's (1960a) initial dream-deprivation study displayed REM rebound on the second R night. This result can be explained by the fact that this subject reported drinking alcohol before the first R night, and alcohol is a known REM suppressant.

[7]Agnew et al. (1967) used subawakening threshold electric shocks to the foot as their method of sleep stage deprivation, instead of the usual mechanical awakening at each stage onset.

Individual Differences in REM Rebound

Witkin (1970) has stated that the effects of RD have been inconsistent, and that "published reports on REM sleep deprivation in which individual subjects have been included provide striking individual differences in . . .number of awakenings required to maintain REM sleep deprivation and in the extent of subjects' indulgence in REM sleep during recovery [p. 158] . . ." What Witkin calls "striking individual differences" can alternatively be seen as the type of normal error variance encountered in most experiments. The case for individual differences depends on the demonstration that unaccounted-for variance can be explained by an independent variable other than RD. Witkin cites Cartwright et al. (1967) as presenting evidence that differences in response to RD can be accounted for by "psychological" variables. (In addition, Witkin cites the Pivik and Foulkes (1966) study, reviewed in another section of this chapter.) The issue of individual differences in response to RD is a controversial one, and because of this, we review Cartwright's studies in some depth.

In their first study, Cartwright, Monroe, and Palmer (1967) found that REM-deprived subjects on their first R night could be classified as displaying three different response patterns"disruption," "compensation," and "substitution." The disruption pattern is defined as a subject having many Stage 2 intrusions during REMPs, making the sleep record difficult to score by conventional criteria. The compensation pattern is one that Dement and others have typically reported following RD: subjects have an increase in total REM time (REM rebound) and a shortened latency to the first REMP. Cartwright et al. (1967) state that subjects in the substitution group *do not* show a REM rebound following RD. If one elicits mentation reports at REM onset during RD, these subjects also report more dream-like mentation on the Foulkes's (1967) DF scale than do compensator subjects.

In a subsequent study, Cartwright and Ratzel (1972) stated that "the variable which seems likely to be crucial in determining subjects' response to REM deprivation is the degree to which their dream-like activity is restricted to REMPS [p. 277]." In short, substitutors seem to have the ability to have dream-like fantasies that in some way substitute for REM rebound. Cartwright and Ratzel found that subjects who have low onset fantasy (LOF), on the DF scale, for dream reports obtained at REM onset will, as a result of RD, display significantly higher REM rebound, and will have more marked changes in waking behavior than subjects who are high in REM onset fantasy (HOF)[8]. In the language of Cartwright's et al. (1967) previous study, HOFs tend to be substitutors and LOFs tend to be compensators.

Although during the R night the LOFs had a significantly higher percentage of REM sleep than the HOFs (34 versus 24%, respectively), the two groups did

[8]Subjects in this experiment are rated on a Foulkes DF scale; generally, one can say that low scores indicate less dream-like reports than high scores on the scale.

not differ with regard to percentage of REM sleep on the BL night, nor did they differ on the RD nights, on measures such as the number of awakenings needed to accomplish RD, total sleep time, or minutes of REM sleep.

In the data presented, both groups seemed to show some rebound on the R night, as compared to their own BL night; HOFs had about 4% more REM, while LOFs had about 10% more REM. The authors do not state whether the HOF REM rebound is statistically significant (comparing BL and R nights).

On pre-post deprivation test measures, LOFs, as predicted, showed a significant change in the WAIS and on two Rorschach measures (M+ scores and M : sum C scores). Both Rorschach postdeprivation changes were interpreted to mean that the LOF group became more sensitive to internal stimulation. Interestingly, the LOF group showed a 10-point postdeprivation *rise* in IQ score. Most of this rise, according to Cartwright and Ratzel (1972) "could be accounted for by a change in the Picture Arrangement score [p.279] ," (a performance subtest).

In our opinion, Cartwright and collaborators (1967, 1968, 1972) have dealt with fundamental questions that explore the relationship between psychological variables and physiological states. However, there are a number of statistical and methodological questions, any one of which by itself might appear trivial, but when taken together raise some questions about the conclusions one can draw from the present study. The most obvious methodological question arises from the fact that the study employed only one BL night and R night. As noted earlier, to evaluate RD effects, one needs an extended number of BL and R nights. The authors did not use an EMG lead in monitoring their subjects; this may not have had any notable effect on their procedure, but their scoring of necessity differed from the Rechtschaffen-Kales (1968) manual. Moreover, some investigators have reported that the most complete RD in humans is accomplished only with the aid of submental EMG recording.

It is important to note that the authors did not include a measure of REM intensity in their results. These points gain some importance when one takes a close look at some of the data. HOFs on RD nights had an average of 23.2 min of REM, while LOF subjects had an average of 18.4 min of REM. Across 3 RD nights, the mean REM-time difference between groups is 14.4 min. Put in percentage terms (which may be somewhat misleading), the HOF group had 20% more REM time on deprivation nights than did the LOF group. (Although the difference in REM time was not statistically significant, this is in part due to sizable night-to-night variation.) Moreover, in comparing HOF and LOF groups, the HOF group required an average of 10 more awakenings per night (or 30 over 3 nights) to achieve RD ($p = .10$). The fact that the HOFs required more awakenings and had more REM sleep on deprivation nights would seem to indicate at least as great (or perhaps greater) REM "pressure" on deprivation nights, as the LOF group evidenced. It would be interesting to know if the number of awakenings for the HOF group increased as deprivation proceeded, as one would expect in conventional RD experiments.

If we take some of these factors into account, it is possible that the HOFS are not "substitutors," but rather they did not manifest REM rebound in this study because:

1. They had more REM time on deprivation nights.
2. They may have had more intense REMPs on the R night (higher percentage of REMs per unit time).
3. HOF subjects, in addition, may have had somewhat delayed REM rebounds which would not have been seen in this study, since only one R night was allowed.

The authors presented no data about the second point, but it would be crucial to know whether or not REM intensity differed between groups, since Ferguson and Dement (1968) and Dement et al. (1970) have asserted that REM intensity is as important as total REM time in assessing the effects of RD.

Nakazawa et al. (1975) also found that personality variables correlated with subjects' responses to what they called partial RD. For example, introverts tended to show less REM rebound that did extroverts. This study is difficult to interpret because: (1) subjects were allowed only one R night; and (2) the R night was terminated by the subject whenever he awakened spontaneously. It is possible, then, that introverts, who the authors reported are more "neurotic and nervous" than extroverts, also tend to be poorer sleepers. Monroe (1967) has shown that poor sleepers tend to be more neurotic. The lowered REM rebound may simply be a result of introverts' getting up earlier in the morning (resulting in less total sleep time), and therefore displaying less REM rebound. In this type of experiment, the total sleep period for all subjects should be held constant. Prolonged discussion of these results may be premature, since the authors were comparing only ten extrovert with only four introvert subjects.

As a final point in this section, we can say that we share Witkin's (1970) interest in the question of individual differences in response to RD but, in our opinion, there is no firm data for nonpsychotic subjects that has established that there are *systematic* individual differences in response to RD. We can only repeat an earlier statement: One would expect differences in any study; the question is, can these differences in RD studies be explained by a specifiable independent variable? At this point, there is only interesting preliminary data that certainly does not conclusively support Witkin's statements about individual differences in response to RD.

Fantasy and Sleep Mentation

Unfortunately, it seems as if two questions have been joined in evaluating the issue of the effect of RD on psychological variables:

1. Does RD have deleterious effects, that is, can RD trigger or lead to psychosis or "regressive" behavior?
2. Does RD affect psychological variables in the waking state?

Dement (1960a) and Dement and Fisher (1963) initially indicated that 4 or more nights of RD led to tendencies such as anxiety, irritability, and inability to concentrate. They found what they regarded as particularly striking psychotic-like effects in two subjects who were REM deprived 13-15 nights. These two subjects were REM deprived by hand-awakenings and by ancillary administration of amphetamine, a drug that suppresses REM sleep (Rechtschaffen & Maron, 1964). Vogel (1975), Albert (1975), and Dement (1969) have all concluded that these studies were methodologically unsound for the following reasons:

1. NREM control awakenings were often not used.
2. Neither subjects nor experimenters were "blind" with respect to the condition.
3. Most frequently, anecdotal rather than systematic psychometric data was reported.

In addition, the use of a pharmacological agent is a confounding variable.

Although findings of the harmful effects of RD have not been accepted, investigators have been attempting to assess the effects of RD on such variables as fantasy, motor performance, and so on. In two early studies, both Kales et al. (1964) and Sampson (1966) found that RD did not affect performance on tests such as digits forward and backward (Wechsler adult intelligence scale, WAIS) and other types of objective tests.[9] Kales et al. (1964) reported that there were no behavioral changes that could be attributed to RD, while Sampson (1966) reported (in agreement with Dement's (1960a) findings) that REM-deprived subjects developed intense hunger, that is, all subjects reported increased appetite and assorted other types of oral phenomena (increased smoking, desire for special foods, etc.) Subjects also displayed disturbances in their sense of reality or in their "feelings of reality" [p. 316]. Sampson did not report how he quantified the increase of oral phenomena, nor did he run a NREM control condition. Clemes and Dement (1967) studied the effect of six days of RD (six subjects), using mainly unstructured psychological tests, (for example, Holtzman ink blot, TAT-"type" tests, and the Welsh figure preference tests) to evaluate the effects of RD. This study employed a NREM condition and counterbalanced conditions. They found that a number of variables on the Holtzman ink blot and "story (TAT-type) test" were affected by RD. Intensity of need and feeling, as measured by the "story test" and "pathognomic verbalizations" in response to the Holtzman ink blot test showed significant increases, whereas form appropriateness and movement perception in the latter showed decreases following RD. The authors viewed these results as a further confirmation of Dement's (1965) cat experiments (reviewed below) which were reported to show that cats increased "drive" behavior following RD. The interpretation of increases of intensity of need, of

---

[9]Minnesota Multi-Phasic Personality Inventory (MMPI), Nowlis adjective check list, Clyde mood scale, Stroop color work test, word association test, and a complex serial-subtraction test.

feeling and pathognomic verbalization were thought to be signs of increased "drive" to focus subjects on internal as opposed to external events. In a similar way, this changed focus leads to less form appropriateness following RD. Fewer movement responses following RD were seen as "a reduced ability to control" internal perceptions. They quoted Holtzman to the effect that a person needs good "ego control" functions to perceive movement in the ink-blot designs. The contention is that in humans, tests that are not subject to practice effects and tests that are able to measure fantasy production are most likely to detect the effects of RD. The authors caution that their study needs replication because only six subjects participated in the experiment.

At this point in history, one could say that the different test results in the Kales et al. (1964), Sampson (1966), and Clemes and Dement (1967) studies were dependent upon the use of different psychometric measures.

Lerner (1966), in a study that did not utilize polygraphic recordings, concluded that RD enhances the perception of human movement on the Rorschach. From this, she reasoned further that some aspects of REM (or dreaming that takes place during REM) is important in facilitating appropriate body image. Without going further into Lerner's conclusions, from our point of view, her study contained none of the necessary controls that would allow her to make a statement about the effects of RD. Moreover, since she REM deprived subjects with amphetamine, one does not know if her effects are due to RD or are the effects of the drug per se.

Greenberg et al. (1970) found (in four subjects) that RD causes changes in subjects' (three out of four) responses to projective tests "that show a clear pattern for (almost) each subject." The authors' view seems to be that defense mechanisms for three out of four subjects were disrupted by RD. Thus one saw more feelings and wishes in the RD as compared with the BL condition. This conclusion would seem to fit in with "classical Freudian" theory but the authors maintain that their results are better explained by other information processing types of hypotheses. At any rate, this study is difficult to evaluate since there is no quantitative data presented, there are only four subjects in the study and in general the study is presented as a pilot experiment. A related issue was pursued by Greenberg, Pillard & Pearlman (1972) in a study in which they attempted to evaluate the differential adaptability to stress following REM deprivation. Nine subjects were used in that study and the authors concluded that REM deprived subjects displayed less adaptability to stress than NREM control subjects. Cartwright and Ratzel (1972) found that RD enhances only M+ responses, and only for those subjects who displayed a REM rebound (LOFs). Substitutors (HOFs) did not show this enhancement. More importantly, what was considered as responsiveness to inner versus outer stimulation (the M : C ratio) was unchanged in HOFs, but changed significantly in LOFs. In other terms, these subjects became significantly more responsive to internal stimulation. In addition, LOFs' IQ (WAIS) scores became significantly higher, while HOFS' WAIS scores did not significantly change. Since we have previously discussed the methodological problems of this study, it is clear that the Cartwright and Ratzel (1972) findings need to be replicated. However, we think that because these findings correlate changes in REM rebound with changes in waking behaviors (Rorschach and WAIS), these findings deserve more serious consideration than studies that may simply rely on the comparison of two groups, one of which remains unchanged.

Agnew et al. (1967) found that RD (seven nights) caused six subjects "to become less well integrated, less interpersonally effective . . . [and] to show signs of suspicion. [They] seemed introspective and unable to derive support from other people [p. 856]." Their conclusions were based on results derived from the MMPI, Taylor manifest-anxiety scale, Cattell's 16 PF test, and the Pensacola Z scale. They compared Stage 4 and RD conditions and found that psychological changes were unique for each deprivation condition. Agnew et al. (1967) do not present any statistical data on psychological variables.

This study is in contrast to that of Johnson et al. (1974), who found no differences between subjects undergoing REM and Stage 4 deprivation. They used a number of performance tests and, in addition, a mood scale and the primary affect scale, and the Rorschach as scored by the McReynolds Rorschach concept evaluation test (CET). Although Albert (1975) in a RD review presents the Johnson et al. (1974) study as a RD article, it must be pointed out that Johnson et al. administered the Rorschach test after a night of total sleep deprivation following two nights of RD. Clearly, this is a confounding variable if one wants to make statements about RD.

Although the Clemes and Dement (1967), and Cartwright and Ratzel (1972) studies produced seemingly opposite effects on one measure, the authors utilized the same type of concept to explain this result. Thus, Clemes and Dement (1967) find decreased movement responses on the Holtzman, while Cartwright and Ratzel (1972), on a similar test find that RD in some subjects (LOFs) leads to an increased number of movement responses. Both papers explain these changes in terms of subjects' increased focus on internal events. It is, of course, possible that Clemes and Dement's subjects were HOFs and this could account for the discrepancy, except that Cartwright and Ratzel did not find a decrease in M responses in HOFs. However, the Clemes and Dement subjects underwent six days of RD, as compared to three days of RD for Cartwright and Ratzel's subjects. It is possible that there is an interaction between subject type and amount of RD. Regardless of whether this accounts for the differences reported (actually, the Clemes and Dement, 1967, effect was not a strong one), the point should nevertheless be made that if one deems RD to be a physiological-biochemical manipulation, the amount of RD has to be carefully considered. It may be the case, as in many drug studies (Sharpless, 1971), that differing amounts of RD, with some dependent measures, may have opposite effects.

Pivik and Foulkes (1966) were the first to systematically investigate the effect of RD on dream content. They found that RD increased the intensity of

REM mentation reports (as scored on the Foulkes DF scale). In this experiment, REM mentation reports were elicited after the subject had been deprived of REM sleep for 5 RD awakenings. Thus, RD and the mentation awakenings were performed within the same night. Subjects were initially selected on the basis of the MMPI (Bryne repression-sensitization scale). The experimenters chose 20 subjects: 10 "repressers" and 10 "sensitizers". Only the repressers were "significantly" affected by RD, although this may be misleading since:

1. They obtained statistically significant results when both groups were combined.

2. As many sensitizers as repressers (six subjects in each group) showed change in the predicted direction.

3. The DF scale is one which was designed to rate NREM content and, as such, may not be as sensitive to more detailed REM reports (or, in other terms, the scale has a low ceiling for REM reports).

Given this, together with sensitizers having initially higher REM reports, it may be that the DF scale was simply not sensitive to some of the more intense REM mentation reports from sensitizers.

In a second study, termed "A cross-night replication" of the Pivik and Foulkes (1966) study, Foulkes et al. (1968) looked at the effect of RD on REM reports elicited from the night after the RD night. They found that there were no significant differences between mentation reports collected the night after either the NREM-deprivation control or the RD condition. The conditions were counterbalanced and mentation reports were rated blindly. The study, however, suffers from the fact that there was no REM rebound and no shortened latency to the first REMP following RD. Order effects occurred regardless of condition, so that on Night 4, there was always more REM sleep than on any other night.

Their procedure contained neither adaptation nor BL nights, nor an adequate number of R nights. Therefore, there may have been interactions between first-night effects and RD or NREM control effects. Counter-balancing would not control for these interactions, nor could they be taken into account by sophisticated data analysis. Also, subjects were allowed only 6 hr of total sleep time, thus cutting off a period of time where substantial amounts of REM would have occurred. Here, again, the effects of reduced total sleep time interacted with deprivation conditions.

What are the effects of all these possible interactions? At this point, no one really knows, but the authors have concluded that their failure to find significant REM rebound may bring into question the generalizability of RD effects. Moreover, they refer to Cartwright's (1967, 1968) experiments as evidence that RD effects are not as generalizable as one would believe from the past literature. We have discussed the Cartwright and Ratzel (1972) experiment previously (see page 426 of this volume), and we can only suggest that the Foulkes et al. (1968) data are not comparable to any past RD experiments where RD effects have been

found. Because of methodological differences, this experiment makes no interpretable comment on the RD literature and does not adequately assess the effect
of RD on mentation since it is not clear that RD was the major variable being
manipulated.

In our view, the better and/or the more interpretable studies in this area are
the RD experiments that have reported positive results (Agnew et al., 1967;
Clemes & Dement, 1967; Dement, 1960a; Dement & Fisher, 1963; Lerner, 1966;
Pivik & Foulkes, 1966). However, the area is a difficult one to summarize because of two general factors: (1) the small number of subjects that are used in
almost all studies; and (2) that is, that no two studies have utilized the same
methodologies, the same RD procedure, the same number of RD nights, the
same controls, the same dependent variables scored in the same way, and so on.
Moreover, there is now enough suggestive data to indicate that individual differences should clearly be taken into account when looking at the effect of RD
on waking psychological variables.

Schizophrenia

We have already joined Vogel (1975), Albert (1975), and Dement (1969) in stating that no RD study[10] has shown that RD is in any way injurious to one's
mental health. There are, however, several studies that have investigated the
possibility that certain schizophrenics have a unique (or at least rare) reaction to
RD. Two distinct types of results have emerged when investigators have looked
at the effect of RD in a "schizophrenic" population: a "normal" REM rebound,
or no REM rebound. Zarcone et al., (1968, 1969a; Zarcone, 1975), have stated
that actively ill schizophrenics do not display REM rebound, while "inactive"
or schizophrenic patients in remission manifest a larger than normal (control
group) rebound.

Azumi et al. (1967) reported a similar result; they studied only three patients,
and two of the three did not display REM rebound. Gillin et al. (1974), in a
relatively well-controlled study, found that patients who were diagnosed at the
time of the study as not psychotic demonstrated a REM rebound, while actively
ill patients did not. Vogel and Traub (1968c) and de Barros-Ferreira et al. (1973)
report that REM depriving chronic schizophrenic patients produces a REM rebound.

---

[10]In an experiment dealing with the effect of RD on four schizophrenics' responses on
the Rorschach, Zarcone et al. (1974) found that schizophrenics' maladaptive-regression
scores and blatant primary process responses (Level 1) increased. Nonschizophrenic hospitalized patients (a control group of five) did not show increases following RD. However,
they had no NREM awakening control, and therefore one cannot say their results were due
to RD.

These studies have been reviewed extensively, and we may summarize and paraphrase both Vogel (1974) and Gillin and Wyatt (1975) by stating that the results from these experiments (excluding Gillin et al., 1974) are not definitive. The work of Vogel and Traub (1968c), and de Barros-Ferreira et al. (1973) does not comment specifically on the actively ill versus remission issue, since their patients were clearly not actively ill schizophrenics. Vogel and Traub confounded their RD procedure by using amphetamine (a REM suppressant that produces a rapid REM rebound, Rechtschaffen & Maron, 1964). In addition, the patients were continued on psychoactive medication (as was true in the study by Zarcone et al. (1969a), which might affect REM rebound. (In cats, REM rebound is affected by phenothiazines, Cohen et al., 1968; while in normal humans, low doses of phenothiazines do not affect REM rebound, Naiman, Poitrus & Engleman, 1972). The Zarcone et al. (1969a) and Azumi et al. (1967) studies do not present statistical comparisons and utilize few subjects without a control group. Vogel has "analyzed" their data, but the statistical test he used is a low-power non-parametric test. Furthermore, it is not common statistical practice to conclude, as he has, that the hypothesis of Azumi et al. (1967) and Zarcone et al. (1969a) is contradicted because their data do not reach statistical significance. It can only be said that one is not able to reject the null hypothesis. As Gillin and Wyatt (1975) have stated, in the Vogel and Traub (1968a) and de Barros-Fereira et al. (1973) studies, total sleep time increased from BL to R periods.

In a carefully controlled study, Gillin et al. (1974) found that although BL measures of total sleep time and REM sleep did not differ significantly between actively ill and nonpsychotic groups, first R night values of total sleep time and REM sleep did differ significantly. Thus, the nonpsychotic group showed a rise in absolute amounts and percentage of REM sleep on the first R night, while actively ill patients showed a slight nonsignificant decrease in REM time. In this experiment, the major confounding variable is that the nonpsychotic group averaged 53 min more total sleep time on the first R night compared to BL nights, and 71 min more total sleep time on the first R night than did the actively ill group.

This raises at least two possibilities:

1. The actively ill group is simply showing signs of poor sleep and is therefore not able to produce a "classic" REM rebound, and/or the poor sleep of the actively ill group leads to "fragmented" or disrupted REM rebound.

2. The nonpsychotic group is not showing a clear REM rebound, but is showing elevated amounts of REM sleep solely because they had more total sleep time.

One could argue that RD is such a stressful procedure for the actively ill group that the sleep during the first R night is disrupted to some extent. One possibility is that, for actively ill patients, previous RD creates a situation in which one sees effects on the first R night that are analogous to first-night effects in the laboratory in normal subjects (that is, total sleep time and REM time and REM percent are reduced, ostensibly because of some factor, like stress or anxiety). The analogy is that since actively ill patients are easily "disrupted," any strong change in laboratory conditions will bring about something that looks like a first-night effect. If this were the case, then one would expect that REM rebound would occur on a later R night (Gillin et al., 1974, had five R nights), but there were no R nights during which actively ill patients showed statistically significant elevations of REM sleep. There was, however, a small nonsignificant rise in REM time, REM percentage, and total sleep time on the third R night. In addition, "REM latency for the actively ill patients was low on the third night," and in fact, it was significantly lower than for the nonpsychotic ill group, even on the first and second R nights, showed two signs typically associated with increased REM pressure — seemingly large (but nonsignificant) increases in REM density, and shortened REM latency.

There is, then, the alternative possibility that actively ill patients show REM rebound in a fragmented fashion. Using the Gillin et al. (1974) study as an example, it is possible that the rise of REM density and the shortening of REM latency on the first two R nights, coupled with the rise in REM time on the third night, are actually manifestations of REM rebound. This would suggest that, somehow, phasic events (REM density) and amount of REM time might be alternative mechanisms for manifesting REM rebound, and in some way, these mechanisms summate. This type of possibility is a remote one, but gains some slight support if one considers the de Barros-Ferreira et al. (1973) study that maintains that schizophrenics' sleep patterns are difficult to score by conventional criteria, and that there is an intermediate phase (IP) of sleep that contains elements of REM and NREM sleep. [11] It may be that this IP or fragmented phase of sleep is in part yet another vehicle for the manifestation of REM rebound. Thus, perhaps one should attempt to combine REM density measures, REM time measures, and IP sleep measures to obtain a better picture of REM rebound in the actively ill patient. Although we have presented this possible explanation, it is at best a weak alternative, since there is as yet no evidence or way of determining how phasic events summate with amounts of REM, nor is there good evidence for the IP of sleep being a manifestation of REM rebound.

An alternative explanation of the Gillin et al. (1974) results is that neither the actively ill group nor the nonpsychotic control group displayed a REM rebound. This interpretation is based on the fact that the nonpsychotic group had more

[11]Other authors (Cartwright et al., 1967) have maintained that nonpsychotic subjects also show an ambiguous, or IP, phase of sleep, in response to RD.

total sleep time on R nights than the actively ill group. Gillin and co-workers reject this alternative, since both REM time and REM percentage increased significantly on the first R night for the nonpsychotic group. Moreover, an analysis of covariance, in which total sleep time was covaried out, yielded statistically significant differences. The question of an increase in REM percentage is one that has to be evaluated with reference to normative data from subjects age-matched with the patients that participated in the Gillin et al. (1974) study. Verdone (1968) has published such data which shows that by simply allowing subjects to sleep for longer than the 6-7 hr BL sleep in the Gillin et al. (1974) study, REM percentage would be expected to rise approximately 2%. This is true, since there is proportionately more REM sleep in the last two-thirds, as opposed to the first third, of the night. We are thus led to question whether a 5.3% rise is significantly different from a 2% rise in REM sleep.[12] Covariance procedures do not provide a full answer, since covariance methods partial out linear trends, and the amount of REM increase as a function of time increase is not strictly a linear relationship. A simple comparison is available by equating total sleep time of the R and BL nights and comparing REM percentage for this time period.[13] Gillin et al. (1974) performed this type of comparison, and they claim to have found significant differences ($p < .05$ one-tailed t test).

Their use of a one-tailed t-test brings up a more general point, for although Gillin et al. (1974) in their statistical comparisons utilize a variety of conventional multivariate analyses, they frequently compare differences between groups by utilizing a number of one-tail t tests. We would criticize both the use of multiple t tests and the use in this experiment of any one-tail test. As Cohen (1965) has pointed out, it is preferable never to utilize one-tail tests, but if they are utilized, there should be some clear prediction based on indications in a given literature that would warrant the use of one-tail tests. The latter hardly seems appropriate in a controversial area in which two of the four previous experiments have produced contradictory results to the Gillin et al. (1974) findings. Thus, in the analysis where Gillin and co-workers attempt to equate total sleep time between groups, their result does not reach significance ($p = .10$, two-tail t test). In addition, since the use of multiple t tests affects (raises) the p level of the overall experiment, if one were to calculate the experiment-wise p level, a number of their results would no longer be significant. This criticism, however, should not diminish the more sophisticated analyses that Gillin et al. (1974)

---

[12] The control group in the Gillin et al. (1974) study exhibited a 5.3% rise in REM % on R Day 1, as compared to BL. Based on Verdone's (1968) normative data, one would expect the control group's increased TST on R Day 1 to have resulted in a 2% increase in REM.

[13] To illustrate this concretely, one would equate the total sleep time on the first R night with the total sleep time on BL nights (391 min for the control group), and then for this sleep period, compare amounts of REM (REM percentage).

have undertaken, since they have employed analytic techniques that have rarely been utilized in sleep studies.

We may add here parenthetically that we have not discussed a report by Zarcone et al. (1975) that appeared after the Gillin et al. (1974) article. In this article, Zarcone and co-workers presented statistical analysis of data on nine schizophrenic and seven control subjects, and essentially confirmed results from their previous studies. Since we have already commented extensively on the Gillin et al. (1974) report, we will only say here that some of the difficulties we noted in the Gillin et al. (1974) experiment are also present in the Zarcone et al. (1975) report (multiple t tests, the possibility of total sleep time[14] confounding their results, and so on). Their report does contain an important discussion of the conditions under which REM rebound occurs, and a discussion that compares these conditions with RD in "actively ill" schizophrenic subjects. Despite methodological flaws, this is one more report that tends to confirm the Zarcone et al. (1969a) initial findings.

The question of whether actively ill schizophrenics display a REM rebound is part of a larger question of the relationship of REM sleep and schizophrenia, and we have deliberately not pursued questions that would lead to investigations that do not involve RD. In our opinion, Vogel (1975) confuses several issues when he states:

> As I understand it, the hypothesis that lack of REM rebound is a distinctive feature of schizophrenia is based on three poorly supported propositions, viz., a) decreased REM time in acute and actively symptomatic chronic schizophrenics; b) large REM rebounds during the waning phase of depression; and c) abnormally low REM rebound in schizophrenic patients following experiment REMD [p. 755].

It seems to us that the first two points could be false, and if the third is true, the hypothesis still be true. We say "might," because the question would center on whether lack of REM rebound distinguishes actively ill schizophrenics. Thus far, in our opinion, the Gillin et al. (1974) study is the only one that has presented reasonably solid evidence that any independent variable is related to the absence of REM rebound following RD. Their finding of a correlation between field independence and REM rebound is some confirmation of a similar finding by Cartwright et al. (1967) in nonschizophrenic subjects. As Gillin and co-workers have pointed out, their field independence finding was post-hoc and should be interpreted with caution. In a similar way, their investigations, while exemplary, are

_____

[14]Although in the Zarcone et al. (1975) experiment total sleep time was not significantly different between control and schizophrenic groups, the analysis is not adequate since, as we have pointed out, REM percentage is not a strict linear component; therefore, the possibility of interaction terms being significant still exists. In addition, control subjects' first R-night total sleep time was significantly different than their BL total sleep time. This was not true for the actively ill group. This is clearly the more important comparison since REM rebound is determined by the difference in REM percentage between R and BL nights.

by no means definitive for the reasons we attempted to spell out earlier in this section.

RD and Depression

Vogel has been among the main researchers who have consistently pointed out that there is no well-documented evidence that RD is in any way deleterious. In a recent series of investigations Vogel and collaborators (Vogel & Traub 1968a, b, c; Vogel et al. 1975), have maintained that RD is in fact helpful in the treatment of endogenous depression. The study looked at the effect of RD on 34 endogenous and 18 reactive-depressives (as rated by two independent clinicians on a scale derived from Mendels & Cochrane, 1968). Since the effect was limited to endogenous depressives, we can summarize the results by saying that RD was more efficacious than the control condition (NREM awakenings) when clinical improvement was measured by Hamilton (1960) or global scores of depression (Vogel et al., 1975). There was not significant improvement on self-rating depression scales or psychomotor tests (Zung self-rating depression scale, WAIS, and a letter-cancellation test). Vogel et al. (1975) argue that these tests do not correlate with clinical improvement in other studies. While it is true that there were significant differences between RD and control conditions (including subjects who were in the control condition for three weeks and then switched to the RD condition), 16 out of 34 subjects showed no clinical improvement. Of these 16 patients, 4 were transferred to another ward, and for some reason, only 9 subsequently received clinical doses of imipramine hydrochloride (mean of 259 mg per day) over a 4-week period. Of these 9 patients, only 1 improved with imipramine administration, and the authors consider this evidence that patients who do not respond to RD also do not respond to imipramine. In brief, since imipramine is a powerful REM suppressant, the contention is that imipramine works through its REM suppressing action, and if suppressing REM by awakenings does not alleviate depression, then imipramine also should not alleviate depression. A further contention then is that there are two subcategories of endogenous depression, one that responds to REM deprivation and another that is responsive to electroconvulsive treatments (ECT). This is based on Vogel's et al. (1975) finding that ECT did not reduce REM time in depressed patients, and that 6 of 7 patients who did not respond to RD or imipramine (and 1 additional patient who received only RD), did respond to ECT. As a last point Vogel cites the antidepressant-drug literature and maintains that the improvement rate of REM-deprived patients is equal to the improvement rate in most studies that evaluate the efficacy of antidepressants.

The Vogel et al. (1975) study is in many ways a model clinical study in its use of double-blind and crossover techniques, and in its attempt (unlike the RD-schizophrenia studies) to quantify diagnoses and clinical improvement. It seems to us that Vogel and co-workers would agree that while their investigation is a pioneering effort and of great interest, many of their conclusions and internal analyses are post hoc and need replication. Despite this, the study is an important one, for it points to a specification of the mechanisms of at least one type of endogenous depression.

The Effect of RD on Cognitive Functions

A number of workers have attempted to explore the hypothesis that REM sleep is necessary for some aspect of information processing in humans. Two distinct questions have been asked:

1. Is REM sleep a time during which recently learned information is consolidated into long-term memory?

2. Is REM sleep necessary for learning or consolidation of information obtained shortly after the REMP?

Studies investigating the first question employ a paradigm in which training is followed by RD; retention is then assessed. Studies investigating the second question administer training to subjects after RD and then assess learning and retention variables.

Empson and Clarke(1970) presented tape-recorded verbal information to subjects prior to a night of RD- or NREM-control awakenings. Subjects were tested for retention and distortion immediately upon awakening in the morning. RD subjects had lower retention scores and more distortion than NREM controls. The authors note that the study is confounded by total sleep time, since REM-deprived subjects had less sleep and more slow-wave sleep than NREM controls.

Grieser, Greenberg, & Harrison (1972) suggest that RD only affects retention of ego-threatening material. Subjects were selected for high-ego strength, and the task utilized was the Zeigarnik effect. RD subjects had impaired retention compared to NREM controls solely for ego-threatening material. The major problem in this study is the discrepant BL performance between experimental and control subjects.

The study by Lewin and Glaubman (1975) investigated the effects of RD on rote learning (serial memory, clustering memory) and creativity tasks (Guilford's word-fluency test, Guilford's utility test). RD produced a decrement in one of two creativity tasks, and an increment in one of six rote-learning measures. The authors did not control for order effects in that RD and NREM conditions were not counterbalanced.

Ekstrand (1971) tested the hypothesis that spontaneous recovery of a retroactively inhibited response was facilitated through RD (one night). He found no significant results when he compared RD subjects to NREM controls.

Experiments by Allen (1974) and Muzio et al. (1971), using a task learned prior to RD, also yield negative findings. In general, there are no positive findings that lead us to believe that RD affects retention of previously learned tasks.

Chernik (1972), Feldman and Dement (1968), and Feldman (1969) have investigated both the question of whether RD affects recently learned material and whether REM sleep is necessary to consolidate information obtained shortly after the REMP. All three papers reported that RD immediately following a verbal learning task did not impair retention (when RD subjects are compared to NREM-control subjects). In addition, Chernik (1972) found that neither a performance task nor a self-administered mood scale were affected by RD. She stated that her findings did not support Greenberg and Pearlman's (1974) hypothesis that REM sleep was necessary for incompletely learned tasks. (See the animal learning section of this chapter for discussion of Greenberg and Pearlman's hypothesis.) In studies pertaining to the second question, Chernik found that in a verbal learning task acquired immediately after RD, consolidation was unaffected by RD. Feldman and Dement's (1968) findings in similar studies were inconsistent. (It should be noted that Chernik, 1972, did not record and did not control for the interactive effects of administering more than one task to the same subjects.)

At this point in time, there is no replicable data to support the hypothesis that REM sleep is necessary for the retention of information learned immediately following the REMP. We conclude, from the studies cited in this section, that the case for a relationship between RD and human information processing is a weak one. However, since those studies reporting negative findings are not methodologically sound, we do not feel that one should reject the possibility of such a relationship.

The Effect of RD on the Sleep Cycle — Animal Methodology

Although some of the methodological considerations that were raised in the preceding section are relevant to animal RD studies, most experiments that use non-primate species employ methods that differ substantially from human RD studies. There are at least two factors that are related to developing special RD techniques for nonprimate species:

1. Almost all nonprimate species manifest polyphasic, as opposed to diurnal, sleep cycles (this means that if one wants to deprive a rat or cat of all REM sleep, one must monitor the animal 24 hr a day, as opposed to an 8- or 10-hr interval required to REM deprive human subjects.

2. The length of the sleep cycle in most species used in RD studies is substantially shorter than that of humans. It follows that the number of awakenings necessary for RD in the rat or cat is at least 5 to 30 times the number of awakenings necessary for human RD (Morden et al., 1967; Siegel & Gordon, 1965; Steiner & Ellman, 1972b).

These two factors have induced sleep researchers to automate RD. The methods utilized have been: (1) the flower-pot or platform method, in which an animal lives on a stand during the time it is being REM deprived; and (2) techniques which "consolidate" the animal's sleep time by forcing the animal to stay awake at times outside of the selective RD period (Cohen, Thomas, Dement, 1970; Dewson et al., 1967). Frequently, the animal is kept awake by putting it on a treadmill, requiring it to move continuously or suffer some aversive consequence. During time off the treadmill, animals are polygraphically monitored and selectively REM deprived by hand awakenings.

Using the platform method, the animal is placed on an appropriate small platform which is elevated above water. Each time the animal is about to enter REM sleep, it experiences loss of postural muscle tone and falls off the stand and into the water, or loses its balance and simply wakes up trying to remain on the stand. The platform technique entails difficulties that require controls differing from those in human studies. The most obvious factor, and perhaps the most difficult, is that the animal must continuously live on a stand for a prolonged time. A frequently used control for this is a large platform in which the animal is presumably able to obtain REM sleep but has to live in an environment similar to that provided by the small platform.

As Vogel (1975) has pointed out, since the platform method is the one most often used in animal RD studies, it demands close attention. Two questions about the platform method can immediately be asked:

1) Can the small-platform condition selectively deprive the animal of REM sleep?

2. Can the large-platform condition allow the animal significantly more REM sleep than the small-platform condition while remaining an adequate control for the platform environment? Specifically, does the large platform condition control for loss of total sleep time, stress, weight loss, and activity, while allowing the animal to obtain significantly more REM sleep than on the small platform.

To answer the first question (and part of the second), polygraphic recordings must be taken while the animals are on the platforms. Nine studies (Duncan et al., 1968; Fishbein, 1970; Jouvet, Vimont, & Delorme, Mark et al., 1969; Mendelson et al., 1974; Mouret, Pujol, & Kiyuno, 1969; Pujol et al., 1968) report such data: six studies in rats, two in cats, and one study using mice.

In both cat studies, the mouse study, and one rat study (Pujol et al., 1968), no adequate large-platform comparison data is available, and therefore it is difficult to evaluate this technique in these studies. In the only study in which recordings were sampled from mice (Fishbein, 1970), animals were on small platforms (3 cm) for three to five days, while five subjects were placed on large (8 cm) platforms, and recordings were taken for several days. Fishbein did not specify on what day REM time was reduced, nor what time period he was citing in presenting his data.

In four studies[15], rats were the subjects, and in all, after two to three days, animals on small platforms showed significantly less REM sleep than animals on large platforms. However, there was considerable variability among the studies in every sleep measure. For example, Duncan et al. (1968) reported that the five-day mean REM percentage on small platforms was 20% of BL, while large platform REM values were 50% of BL. While Duncan and co-workers presented grouped data (mean of five RD days), Mendelson et al. (1974) compared animals after 24 or 72 hr on the small versus the large platform condition. Mendelson found that after 24 hr of RD, recordings from large and small platforms yielded REM levels that were virtually equal (REM = 9.6%, or 60.2 min of REM on the small platform; REM = 10.5%, or 58.5 min of REM on the large platform). By the fourth 24-hr period (between 72 and 96 hr of RD), animals on the large stand showed REM levels that are virtually equal to BL (REM percentage was somewhat elevated), while subjects on the small stand had significantly lower REM levels when compared to the BL and large-platform subjects (small-platform REM = 8.5%, with 46.6 min of REM time, as compared to large-platform REM = 18.3%, with 105.6 min of REM time). There were no significant differences reported for any group on measures of total sleep time or NREM sleep. Vogel (1975) concluded from this data, that:

> "in studies of rats, using the platform technique for 24 hours or less, dependent variable differences between experimental and control groups cannot be due to REM sleep differences. But in rat studies using this technique for about four days, dependent variable differences . . . could be due to REM sleep deprivation assuming that confounds are controlled" [p. 750]

Vogel's conclusions are reasonable, given the data he is considering, but Mendelson et al. (1974) do not report on a number of factors which Ellman and Steiner (1969a, 1969b) find to be of importance in RD platform studies.[16]

We have found that first, if one is using the platform method, the weight of the animal in relation to the size of the stand is a crucial variable. Furthermore, specifying the weight of the animal at the beginning of the experimental procedure is not satisfactory, since most behavioral experimental procedures from the time of surgery often last 4-10 weeks. During that time, our strain of rats (male albino Sprague-Dawley) can gain 100 to 140 gm. The crucial weighing time is immediately before animals are placed on platforms; subsequent weight

---

[15]To summarize, for one rat study no large-platform polygraphic data is available Pujol, 1968), four studies are reviewed, and the sixth study is the Mark et al. (1969) report, which is not included here because recording was taken only from 10:00 AM to 4:00 PM. We feel that due to the possibility of circadian alterations, this sampling procedure is not adequate.

[16]When we refer to Ellman and Steiner, we are referring to two presentations to an APSS meeting (Ellman & Steiner, 1969a, 1969b), as well as an article by Steiner and Ellman (1972), and more recent unpublished work from our laboratory.

measurements should then be continued throughout. We found that during the first day, four 300 gm rats on stands with a diameter of 7 cm displayed mean REM levels (RD 32 min 5% REM time, versus BL 111 min, 14% REM time) below the 4-day levels of Mendelson et al. (1974). Moreover, there was nothing approaching statistical significance when one compared BL (home cage) versus 7-cm platform condition on either total sleep time or NREM sleep (7-cm platform groups, 82% of BL total sleep time).

Secondly, it seems that the REM reduction observed by Mendelson et al. (1974) during the first 24-hr period, is comparable to a first-night effect in human studies. We found that if one adapts subjects (by placing them on the stand) for 4 days, 10 to 14 days before experimental procedures are performed, then during the first 24-hr experimental period, large-platform subjects' REM levels (95 min) go up to 85% of BL REM levels (111 min). Furthermore, in most rat and cat sleep experiments, lighting conditions during the experiment are carefully specified. Unfortunately, of all the sleep-cycle studies we review, lighting conditions before the experiment have only been specified by Mendelson et al. (1974). This is a possible confounding variable, since Fishman and Roffwarg (1972) have shown that some changes in lighting conditions lead to sleep-cycle changes lasting 2-4 weeks. Standard lighting conditions should be obtained 2-4 weeks before the experiment is begun.

A methodological paper by Mouret et al. (1969) highlights some of the difficulties of the platform technique and will therefore be described in detail. Rats weighing 250-280 gm at the time of operation were placed on either small platforms (4.5-cm diameter) or large platforms (11.5-cm diameter). In the first experiment, animals were recorded continuously during 91 hr on the platforms, and for the following 4.75 hr in their home cages. The animals on small platforms were totally REM deprived, while the animals on large platforms obtained 25% of BL levels of REM sleep. During the 4.75 hr of recovery, both groups exhibited a REM rebound which was markedly smaller in the large platform group. In a second experiment, two groups of animals were again placed on small and large platforms for 91 hr, followed by 4.75 hr of R. In this study, recording cables (for EEG and EMG) were attached only during R. Animals on the small platform had approximately the same amount of REM rebound during R as in the first experiment, while animals on the large platform had no REM rebound. Evidently, animals on the large platform were not REM deprived under these circumstances. Apparently, the burden of the attached recording cables is a necessary condition for RD to be accomplished in rats of this weight on such large platforms. This is a dramatic finding in view of much work where recording is performed only in pilot experiments. It is possible that pilot studies provide markedly different levels of RD, since in the experiment proper versus pilot study, recording cables were not connected to the animals. Furthermore in two reports (Fishbein, 1970; Stern, 1971a), investigators dismiss nonsignificant differences between small- and large-platform groups because they assume that large-platform animals are partially REM deprived. But this may not be the case, if experimental conditions are not the same as pilot conditions. The Mouret et al. (1969) study strongly underscores the absolute necessity for polygraphic recording during all experimental conditions.

The most frequent criticism of the platform technique is that it provides nonspecific stress to the animal, which may be a confounding variable. However, if there is no difference on stress measures or NREM-sleep measures in small- and large-platform conditions, and REM measures do differ, then the differential effect of these conditions on a given dependent variable must be due to differences in REM levels. In rats, three studies reported no differences between animals on large and small platforms on a variety of measures of stress (Ling & Usher, 1969; Morden et al., 1968b; Stern, 1969), whereas a fourth study (Mark et al., 1969) found that animals on small platforms had increased adrenal hypertrophy, as compared to large-platform animals, only on Day 4 of the platform condition. From the fifth to the tenth days, there were no stress differences between animals on the large and small platforms. Therefore, the preponderance of evidence indicates that animals on small and large platforms are stressed to the same extent.[17]

In his review, Vogel (1975) has included total sleep time as a measure of stress. Vogel (1975) concludes that if one compares small platform subjects to baseline subjects, studies that give statistical significance report that total sleep time is significantly reduced in the small platform condition. This is not the case in the Mendelson et al. (1973, 1974) experiment — cited by Vogel (1975) as a superior RD study — that reported no significant differences in total sleep time between any conditions. Moreover, the fact that differences in total sleep time are sometimes found is not surprising, given: (1) the methodological considerations that were raised previously; and (2) that, in our opinion, NREM sleep totals, rather than total sleep levels, is the more useful measure. In any RD experiment, what one attempts to do is to leave NREM sleep intact while eliminating REM sleep. If one is successful in doing this, then obviously there will be less total sleep time. Interestingly, in some experiments (a group in one of our experiments, and in the Mendelson et al., 1974, study) subjects had more NREM sleep in the small-platform condition (in the first 24 hr) than in the large-platform or BL condition.

Although we agree with many of Vogel's (1975) points, we disagree with some. We believe that comparisons between small- and large-platform conditions can yield significant differences after one day:

1. if the appropriate large platform control is used (the appropriate large platform is one that should minimally REM deprive the animal; Plumer et al., 1974,

---

[17]It should be added that animals on both the small and large platforms there were significantly more stressed than nonplatform controls, as shown in experiments (Stern, 1969, Ling, & Usher, 1969; Mark et al., 1969).

have argued that most studies have utilized large platforms that produce contaminating RD in their control animals); and

2. if animals' weights are matched to stand size and an adaptation procedure is used, then sizable REM reductions in the first 24 hr on the small-, but not the large platform conditions can be obtained. (In fact, measures sensitive to REM-sleep changes, such as intracranial self-stimulation measures, can be affected by 22 hr of RD; Steiner & Ellman, 1972a).

Let us now try to summarize the effects of RD on the sleep cycle. Fishbein (1970 see previous comments) showed that mice could be REM deprived differentially, but he did not test for REM rebound. In an unpublished report, he has shown that mice, after one day of RD, will display a statistically significant REM rebound (30-40%) above BL levels. In rats, the experiments that have employed continuous recording and large-platform controls (Mendelson et al., 1974; Mouret et al., 1969; Steiner & Ellman, 1972a) have all demonstrated REM rebound. In an early study, Morden (1967) concluded that RD by hand arousals yielded REM rebounds equivalent to those obtained during deprivation by platform methods (no recording in platform groups). Morden et al. (1967) employed a yoked NREM-awakening control group and a large-platform control group. Steiner and Ellman (1972a) also found that hand awakening and platform RD methods yielded similar results, although the hand awakening condition yielded a (nonsignificant) lower rebound. Siegel and Gordon (1965), using reticular stimulation to REM deprive three cats, found that a combination of 12 hr of reticular stimulation and 12 hr of sleep deprivation (referred to as a brick technique) yielded a large REM rebound (59%). Each subject had a different number of RD days, and there was no recording in what they called their sleep deprivation condition. Foote (1973), in an experiment in which he partially REM deprived cats, showed (over a 16-hr period) a high negative correlation (r ranged from −.022 to −0.86) between amounts of REM recorded in deprivation and R nights. He used a slow-wave sleep-deprivation control, and also controlled for number of arousals.

Dement and his colleagues (Cohen & Dement, 1966; Dement, 1965; Dewson et al., 1967; Ferguson & Dement, 1967) have performed RD studies on cats. In a variety of experiments, they attempted to explore some of the limits of the REM rebound phenomena. In one such experiment, RD continued for 70 days, and it was found that number of awakenings and amount of compensation plateau after 30 days (Dement, 1965). They mentioned that within a given sleep cycle, REM time never reached more than 70% of total sleep time, during R conditions. In most of their cat RD work (Cohen, Duncan, & Dement, 1967; Cohen et al., 1970; Dewson et al., 1967), animals were placed on a treadmill for (typically) 16-hr a day, and off the treadmill for 8 hr. The treadmill ostensibly sleep deprives cats, but no study has reported polygraphic evidence to support this claim. During the 8-hr off the treadmill, RD procedures are performed. This method was designed so that during the 8-hr off-treadmill condition it would comprise a typical RD study, with BL, deprivation, and R periods as well as (at times) a NREM awakening control. The trouble with the entire procedure is that (granting that animals are sleep deprived), it is difficult to assess how the sleep deprivation on the treadmill and RD interact. Also, it is likely that the treadmill does not fully sleep deprive subjects (Ferguson & Dement, 1967; Levitt, 1967). If so, the problem of varying amounts of sleep deprivation coupled with RD is even harder to assess. Despite these issues, it is clear that Dement's (1965) plateau is showing something about the upper limits of REM rebound, and any bio- or neurochemical theory of REM has to explain this data.

Neural Excitability

Many experimental approaches indicate that following RD, central nervous system excitability in the waking state is increased.

In a series of studies, Cohen and collaborators have demonstrated in the rat (Cohen & Dement, 1965) and the cat (Cohen et al., 1967; Cohen et al., 1970), that RD lowers electroconvulsive shock (ECS) thresholds. Owen and Bliss (1970) also found that rats on small stands had decreased seizure thresholds. While they ran a number of control groups, they did not obtain polygraphic recording. Handwerker and Fishbein (1975) found that mice placed on small pedestals have reduced ECS thresholds. No control groups were tested, and no polygraphic data was reported. One contradictory finding has emerged from this line of research. While Cohen and Dement (1968) found that REM depriving mice prolongs the tonic phase of the behavioral convulsion, Handwerker and Fishbein (1975) found that RD shortened the tonic phase.

When all the studies are taken together (including an additional study with mice by Hartmann, Marcus, & Leinoff, 1968), the results are, in the main, consistent and therefore compelling. One can probably conclude that RD lowers ECS thresholds. However, in all of these studies, the lack of polygraphic data does not allow one to comment on how much of a reduction in REM sleep is necessary to produce lowering of ECS thresholds.

In a study of the effects of RD on intracranial self-stimulation[18] (ICSS) in rats, Steiner and Ellman (1972a) found that following RD, ICSS thresholds were lowered and response rates were increased. This study employed two groups of large pedestal controls. Polygraphic sleep recording confirmed that subjects on the small pedestals were deprived of "almost all REM sleep."

---

[18]Sometimes called the Olds phenomenon after Olds (1956), who discovered that rats (and other mammals) find electrical stimulation to certain parts of the brain reinforcing. Put in other terms, animals will work to provide themselves electrical stimulation to some areas of the brain.

In several experiments, RD has been shown to sharpen and intensify neural excitability in sensory systems. In a well-controlled study in the cat, Dewson et al. (1967) demonstrated that RD shortens the refractory period of cortical responses to auditory stimuli. Koppell et al. (1972) studied auditory-evoked potentials during attention tasks, and concluded that following RD, there is greater selective attention when compared to a NREM-awakening control. No measures of waking auditory-evoked potential were obtained in subjects who slept normally. Accordingly, interpretations were confined to the difference between RD and NREM awakening conditions.

Satinoff et al. (1971) REM deprived cats by the platform technique, and measured evoked potentials following brief electrical stimulation. No control groups were run, and no polygraphic sleep data was presented. They conclude that RD does not lead to a general increase in neuronal excitability, but rather to paleocortical excitability and an increase in some type of inhibition which results in sensory filtering.

In summary, various measures of central nervous system excitability are increased following RD. Thresholds of ECS, as well as ICSS, are reduced. Cortical refractory periods are shortened, and selective attention and cortical excitability are enhanced.

Animal Learning and Retention Studies

In evaluating the effect of RD on learning and retention, one must consider: (1) whether appropriate controls are utilized (for example, in animal research, a large-platform control); (2) whether polygraphic recordings were obtained during the experiment and not simply in a pilot study; and (3) whether distinctions are made between learning-retention and performance variables.

As Vogel (1975) has pointed out, in retention tasks in which animals are trained before RD and tested immediately following RD, even if an animal shows a deficit, it may be that some performance variable, as opposed to a retention variable, is being affected (perhaps because of the animal's state and so on). To explore this possibility, one would want to test the animal at some later point. To quote Vogel (1975), "If a performance deficit appeared immediately after REMD but was absent in later testing, then one would have to conclude that REMD impaired performance but not memory of the task [p. 752]." Vogel states that only "Fishbein has used such a control for performance deficit [p. 752]." However, Wolfowitz and Holdstock (1971) and Sagales and Domino (1973) also used this type of control. Although there are several somewhat different variations, the positions in this area that have been spelled out most clearly assert that REM sleep serves as an information-processing state. Thus, Greenberg and Pearlman (1974) see REM sleep as a state that plays an important role in processing what might be labeled as new or unusual information.

While Greenberg and Pearlman hypothesize that REM may be important in both acquisition and retention, Fishbein has stressed the role of REM sleep in retention, and Stern has focused on REM sleep playing a part in the acquisition and retention of any task in the animal's repertoire.

Greenberg and Pearlman (1974) have roughly divided learning situations into ones that are involved in survival value for an organism (REM independent), and other learning situations where the organism is required to assimilate "unusual information" (REM dependent). It is Greenberg and Pearlman's (1974) view that the "assimilation of unusual information requires REM sleep for optimal consolidation [p. 516]." Greenberg and Pearlman regard the distinction they have made as similar to that of Seligman's (1970) distinction between prepared (REM-independent) and unprepared (REM-dependent) learning. (Greenberg and Pearlman's work goes beyond the experiments summarized in this section and they have performed a variety of studies in human as well as animal subjects. One experiment that we have not included in this section is one by Greenberg, Pillard, and Pearlman, 1972, that deals with the effect of RD on stress. In this study they conclude that RD interferes with adaptation to stress.) Pearlman's experiments involving the effect of RD on latent learning[19] and latent extinction[20] are attempts to operationalize and test the REM-independent, REM-dependent distinction. In one experiment in which he looked at the effect of RD on latent learning, Pearlman found that REM-deprived animals did not show an improvement in learning when a reinforcer (food) was introduced into a latent learning situation. On the other hand, control animals (immersed in cold water for 20 min to 1 hr) displayed the normal improvement one would expect in this kind of situation. Such learning was compared to a simpler type of food exploration "learning," in which animals were simply allowed to explore a rectangular box with a niche. He found that RD did not affect this type of "learning." In another study, Pearlman (1973) found that while latent extinction was affected, ordinary extinction was not affected by RD. In addition, he reported that immediate RD affected latent extinction, while RD begun 5 hr after preextinction trials took place did not affect latent extinction. Thus, he concluded that RD affected latent extinction, but not normal extinction, and that latent extinction was affected when RD was administered within a certain time period.

In a study that specifically focused on both the method and timing of RD administration, Pearlman and Greenberg (1973) REM deprived three groups of rats immediately after they had learned a shuttlebox-avoidance task. They REM deprived another group 2 hr after the task. The three groups that were REM deprived immediately after the task were deprived by one of the following tech-

[19]Latent learning refers to learning that has not been manifested in performance. However, performance appears upon introduction of reward contingencies.

[20]Latent extinction refers to extinction without responding. This results from an experience without reinforcement contingencies.

niques: (1) the flower-pot method; or (2) administration of a drug that suppressed REM sleep (5 mg/kg of imipramine or 35 mg/kg of pentobarbital). Another group was simply put back in its home cage after the task. Twenty-four hours after the completion of the task, all animals were tested for retention of the task.

The authors were attempting to show that any method of RD, if applied at the appropriate time, will lead to a learning or retention deficit (in rats, it is apparently within 2 hr of the task being learned). In fact, the groups that received what the authors call immediate RD did show a greater retention deficit than either of the other two groups. All of the Pearlman studies suffer from the fact that polygraphic recordings were not taken; and no platform-control condition was utilized.

The experiment (Pearlman & Greenberg, 1973) in which two different pharmacological agents were used to REM deprive animals, included neither a saline condition (that is, control injections with saline), nor administration of different drug dosages. Both of these procedures are typical controls in pharmacological experiments (Fingl & Woodbury, 1971). In addition, it would have been preferable to have a control condition with a drug that is not a REM-depriving agent. Of course, this is asking for a large number of controls in a given experiment, but unfortunately, if one is using pharmacological agents, then appropriate pharmacological controls are necessary.

Pearlman and Becker (1974), in a study that did employ a saline-control group, found that RD (alternatively 5 mg/kg of imipramine hydrochloride and 4 mg/kg of chlorodiazepoxide hydrochloride) immediately following training, impaired acquisition of a bar-press response. This was true whether training involved the presence of a bar, a visible trained rat who was bar pressing in an adjacent cage, or a visible naive rat in an adjacent cage with no bar. However, the most significant impairment occurred in those subjects trained through observation of a previously trained rat. Also, REM-deprived animals had impaired acquisition of a DRL (differential reinforcement of low rates) 20-sec bar-press response when switched from a continuous-reinforcement response schedule.

In a similar study by the same authors (Pearlman & Becker, 1975), a cooperative-learning task was impaired by immediate RD, as compared to a saline control group. In both experiments, polygraphic recordings were not obtained for experimental animals. In addition, it is difficult in this type of study to differentiate more general drug effects from those related to RD. Moreover, different drug dosages were not employed. This is a crucial control in any drug study.

Stern, on the basis of research that he and Hartmann have conducted (Hartmann & Stern, 1972; Stern, 1971a), has also concluded that RD impairs learning and retention tasks. Stern (1971b) has reported that RD interferes with the acquisition of passive and active avoidance responding and with the acquisition of an appetitive alternation-discrimination task. In these studies, Stern did not find differences between animals on small stands and large stands, but only between small-stand and home-cage animals. Stern's (1971b) contention is that failure to find learning differences following treatment between animals on large and small stands can be interpreted as a failure of 50% vs. 80% RD to produce differential behavioral effects. This may be the case, but the question is circular unless Stern can specify under what RD conditions learning differences can be found. Moreover, it is not necessarily the case, as Plummer et al. (1974) and Mendelson et al. (1974) have shown, that large stand animals have to be deprived of 50% of BL REM sleep values.

Hartmann and Stern (1972) have also performed a RD experiment in which l-dopa (or catecholamine restoration) partially reversed the interfering effects of RD on acquisition and retention. Stern (1971b) has also found that RD does not affect habituation and that this response is not relevant to the question of the effect of RD on learning. In this experiment, Hartmann and Stern did not utilize a large-platform control group, making the experiment difficult to evaluate.

Fishbein, in several studies in mice (Fishbein, 1970, 1971; Fishbein, McGaugh, & Schwarz, 1971; Linden, Bern, & Fishbein, 1975), looked at the effect of RD on retention. Because he and his coworkers employed complicated paradigms, we discuss the design of these experiments with the aid of a schematic diagram. In one experiment (Fishbein, 1971; see Figure 12.1a), animals were first put in a one-trial passive avoidance (PA) situation, and were then immediately placed on RD platforms. Animals were tested for PA retention 1 hr or 1 day after RD. In a study with a similar design (Fishbein et al., 1971; see Figure 12.1b), he again put animals in a PA situation, and then put animals on RD platforms. In this study, at varying points[21] after RD, animals were administered ECS.[22] All animals were then tested for retention 1 day after RD.

In the first experiment (see Figure 12.1a), Fishbein (1971) found that 3 days (but not 1 day) of RD impaired retention 1 hr, but not 24 hr after RD. In the second study (Fishbein et al. 1971 see Figure 12.1b), animals were REM deprived for 48 hr, and when ECS was applied within 3 hr of the RD, retention was impaired. Fishbein et al. (1971) concluded that RD is unique in keeping "the memory trace of a previously learned experience . . . susceptible to disruption (for) several days [p. 82] days." The question as to why ECS must be applied less than 3 hr after RD to disrupt the memory is answered by assuming that, at some time after 60 min and before 3 hr, the memory is converted into a relatively permanent form (long-term storage), and is no longer susceptible to disruption.

[21]ECS was administered 5 min, 30 min, 1 hr, 3 hr, 6 hr, or 12 hr.

[22]ECS is commonly used in memory studies (McGaugh, 1966), and when it is applied at the appropriate time, total or partial amnesia occurs.

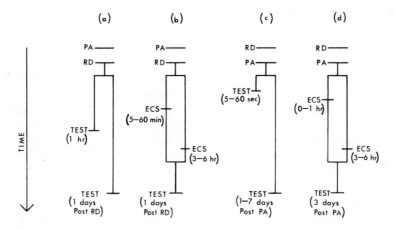

FIG. 12.1.   The diagram is a schematic of the 4 paradigms used by Fishbein et al. (a) Animals were REM deprived after passive avoidance (PA) training. One branch represents animals tested for retention of the PA task 1 hour after REM deprivation (RD), while the other branch represents animals tested 1 day after RD. (b) Animals were REM deprived after PA training and given electro-convulsive shock (ECS) at varying times after RD. Depicted on the left branch are several groups of animals that received ECS 5 to 60 sec after RD. The right branch depicts groups that received ECS from 3 to 6 hours after RD. All groups were tested for retention of the PA task 1 day after the termination of RD. (c) In this design, RD preceded PA training. One branch represents the groups retested for PA retention 5 to 60 sec following PA training. The other branch represents groups retested for PA training 1 to 7 days following PA training. (d) As in Figure 12.1 (c), RD preceded PA training. The left branch represents groups that received ECS 0 to 1 hours following PA training. The right branch represents the groups that received ECS 3 to 6 hours after PA training. All groups were tested for PA retention 3 days following the PA training.

Fishbein (1970), in another experiment, used a different paradigm, in which RD preceded a PA task (see Figure 12.1c), and in which animals were given retention tests at varying times[23] after experience with the task. In this experiment, he found that RD interfered with the retention of the task when retention was tested more than 1 hr after RD, but retention was not affected if the retention test was presented within 1 hr of RD. The paradigm just described was then coupled with ECS (Linden et al., 1975; see Figure 12.1d). ECS was given at varying times[24] after PA training. They found that when ECS is given within 3 hr of RD, long-term memory is impaired. However, when ECS is given more than 3 hr after RD, long-term memory is not impaired. Again, 3 hr appears to be the crucial time, since ECS is not effective when it is given more than 3 hr after RD.

[23]The retention tests were given within 5, 30 sec; 1, 2, 15, 20, 45, 60 min; and then 1, 3, 5, or 7 days after the task.

[24]Immediately; 5, 15, 30, 45 min; 1, 3, 6 hr.

Wolfowitz and Holdstock (1971), in work that was similar to that of Fishbein (1971), reported the same effects in rats.

Sagales and Domino (1973), in looking at the effect of RD in mice on both acquisition and retention, found that RD does not affect acquisition and retention of an active-avoidance task. Their results concerning the effects of RD on retention (eight days after acquisition) are contradictory: in one study, they reported that RD impaired retention, while in a second study, RD did not impair retention. This work is flawed because no recordings were taken to verify whether experimental animals were actually REM deprived, and whether stress control animals were not REM deprived.

Fishbein's (1971), and Wolfowitz and Holdstock's (1971) experiments have the same difficulties that are present in other RD-learning-retention experiments. The appropriate (large-platform) control group was not used, and polygraphic recordings were not taken during the experiments. However, these studies are important because they focus on some other difficulties in conceptualizing the relationship between REM sleep and memory consolidation.

As we understand the REM memory-consolidation hypothesis, new memory traces are kept in labile form until REM sleep occurs. At that point, some process associated with REM facilitates the consolidation of a labile memory trace. Clearly, there can be gradations of this hypothesis. In the strong form, one would maintain that some manifestation of REM sleep is necessary for all long-term memory consolidation. In some weaker form of the hypothesis, one would miaintain that REM sleep is not necessary for, but to some extent facilitates, long-term consolidation.

In terms of this discussion, let us assume that the studies that maintain that RD impairs retention have been well controlled, and that the results are, in fact, due to RD. The question still arises as to whether a memory consolidation hypothesis in the strong form is the only, or even the best, explanation of this data. To point out some of the difficulties, let us briefly review two of Fishbein's experiments. In one experiment (as schematized in Figure 12.1a), Fishbein REM deprived animals after a PA task and then found that retention was impaired when animals were tested shortly after RD, but retention was not impaired when retention tests were performed 24 hr after RD. (The explanation put forth was that RD kept the trace in labile form so that retention was impaired when testing was done shortly after RD. When the animals were allowed REM sleep, the trace was consolidated, and therefore retention was not affected when animals were tested a long time after RD. Compare this experiment with one in which RD preceded the PA task (see Figure 12.1c). In this experiment, short-term memory was not affected, but long-term memory was impaired.[25] Here the

---

[25]We are aware that many authors make finer distinctions about short- and long-term memory consolidation, but we feel that our distinctions are adequate for the purposes of this discussion.

explanation was that RD set up conditions in which a labile trace could not be converted from short- to long-term memory.

In our opinion, from a memory-consolidation standpoint, these two experiments yield contradictory results. Our reasoning is as follows: if RD keeps a memory trace in labile form, then in both experiments the animals are in the same state following RD (see Figure 12.2). Our simple diagram indicates that both experiments should produce animals with labile memory traces at Time A. Since in both experiments animals that are tested a long time after RD are allowed to have REM sleep, what happens to the memory trace should happen uniformly in both experiments, but, in fact, this is not the case. Fishbein (personal communication April, 1976) has indicated to us, that in his (as opposed to Pearlman and Greenberg's 1974), view the strong form of the REM- memory, consolidation hypothesis is not tenable, and some change in the conditions necessary for long-term consolidation must take place, even during RD. Although this is a view that seems to be closer to the data, it is not clear at this point what the testable implications are for this weaker form of the REM memory-consolidation hypothesis. An alternative view that might explain the results of both experiments involves a state-dependent learning effect. In both paradigms, retention deficits depend on the animals being tested in a state that differed from the one during which acquisition took place. Of course, the question still remains whether or not it was RD that influenced even these variables.

The question of why ECS disrupts retention (Fishbein et al. 1971) 0 to 3 hr after RD but not 3 or more hr after RD, is, in our opinion, also not necessarily related to memory-consolidation variables. One might alternatively consider that RD lowers ECS thresholds and that in Fishbein's (1971) experiments, what one

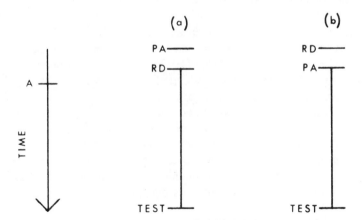

FIG. 12.2.   (a) and (b) refer to the Fishbein et al experiments depicted in Figures 12.1 (a) and 12.1 (c) respectively. In design 2 (a) PA training preceded RD and the PA retention test followed after some specified amount of time. In design 2 (b), RD preceded PA training and the PA retention test follows.

is comparing is a large amount of ECS in the RD condition, as opposed to a smaller amount of ECS in the control condition. Cohen and his collaborators (Cohen & Dement, 1965; Cohen et al., 1967; Cohen et al., 1970) have shown that RD lowers ECS thresholds, and a number of studies have shown that RD increases neural excitability (see previous section of this chapter). Even more importantly, Handwerker and Fishbein (1975) have shown that while RD lowers ECS thresholds, 3 hr later they are back to pre-RD or normal levels. Thus, one can say that in RD-ECS studies, when time of ECS administration has been varied, the effective magnitude of the ECS treatment has also been varied. This is the case, since the stimulus (amount of current) is held constant, while threshold (over time) varies as a function of time from RD. Thus, if one applies ECS immediately after RD, greater neural excitability will result than if one applies the same amount of electricity 3-4 hr after RD. We can conclude that in RD-ECS studies, effective amounts of ECS and time of administration are confounding variables.

The possibility also exists that RD plus ECS will disrupt many tasks that are not well learned or "overlearned." Thus, it might be important to perform a Fishbein-type experiment in which the animal is allowed 3 hr of sleep following PA training and before RD begins. Immediately after RD, the animal would receive ECS and then be given retention trials short and long periods of time after RD. In this experiment, since the animal would be trained 3 hr before RD, one would expect that memory consolidation would take place before RD begins. If in this experiment RD plus ECS affected retention, then the conclusion would be that RD is effective not because it keeps memory traces labile, but primarily because it increases neural excitability and leads to a general disruption of some aspects of the animal's behavior.

Up to this point, we have reviewed studies that only report positive results. There are, however, several reports in the literature that have failed to demonstrate that RD affects either acquisition or retention in animal-learning experiments. For example, Joy and Prinz (1969) utilized a pole-climbing task, and found that neither acquisition nor retention was affected by RD. They did find that when retention tests were given after RD, only then was retention affected. The conclusion the authors draw is that retention following RD is not disrupted when animals are tested under acquisition conditions, but if the retention conditions differ from acquisition conditions, then retention is affected. For the purpose of this review, we say they concluded that RD sets up conditions that induced a type of state-dependent learning. Albert, Cicala, and Siegel (1970) also concluded that REM depriving rats did not affect the acquisition of two different tasks requiring an avoidance response (shuttlebox- and one-way avoidance). They also found that RD did not affect retention of responses in the one-way running-avoidance task. Similarly, Holdstock and Verschoor (1973) found that RD did not affect retention of a learned position response in a T-maze situation. In two related experiments that were reported in very brief fashion,

Miller, Drew, and Schwartz (1971) concluded that RD does not affect retention in a one-trial PA task.

REM Deprivation and Motivation

Although Dement and his co-workers frequently referred to the effect of RD on "motivational" or "drive" states, there have been surprisingly few studies that have systematically tested the effect of RD on behaviors such as eating, drinking, or aggressive and sexual behaviors. Dement (1960a) and Dement and Fisher (1963) initially referred to the effects of RD on human subjects, and we have previously discussed the limitations of these observations. Dement (1965b, 1969) later reported that RD seemed to lead to hyperphagia and hypersexuality in cats. The effect of RD on eating was apparently negligible unless the cats were deprived of food for a period of time before testing. If REM-deprived and -control cats were food deprived, the REM-deprived group ate significantly more than control animals. After RD, it was also reported that 6 out of 12 cats became hypersexual in a manner that was never seen in BL condition or in control animals. (To our knowledge, these observations have never been written up in a full experimental report, so even the mention of these data must be considered anecdotal.)

Two papers using different dependent measures indicated that RD increases aggressive behavior in rats. Morden et al. (1968b) found that RD increases shock-induced fighting, while Sloan (1972) found that RD increases aggression in rats as measured by the Klein-Hall rat aggression scale. Both of these studies had appropriate large-stand control groups, but neither study took polygraphic recordings during experimental procedures. Ferguson and Dement (1969), in a study that REM deprived rats 80-100 hr and then injected them with amphetamine, found that the rats displayed what they termed stereotypic aggressive behavior (in virtually all animals), and "abnormal" sexual behavior (in 9 of 25 animals). Large-stand control animals did not exhibit the same effects. There was no polygraphic recording performed during the experiments. Morden et al. (1968a) also found that RD increased sexual behavior (large-stand control, but no recording).

Although there are a small number of studies, all of them have found that both sexual and aggressive behaviors are facilitated by RD. Unfortunately, none of this work employed polygraphic recordings, but all have used some form of platform control. Steiner and Ellman (1972a) and Cohen et al. (1972) have both looked at the effect of RD on intracranial self-stimulation[26] (ICSS) behavior in

---

[26]ICSS, or self-stimulation, is defined as an animal performing work for an electrical stimulation to the brain. Olds (1956) and many subsequent investigators (see review by German & Bowden, 1974) have mapped a variety of areas in the brain that are self-stimulation sites.

rats. Steiner and Ellman found that RD lowers hypothalamic ICSS thresholds and raises ICSS response rates. They have also shown that nonconvulsive ICSS can reduce REM rebound by 52%. Steiner and Ellman utilized polygraphic recordings and two types of large-platform control (one a yoked large-platform control), and two methods of RD (platform method and hand awakening). As a control for the hand awakening RD method, they employed a NREM awakening control condition. Since Steiner and Ellman (1972a) (and Cohen et al, 1972,) have demonstrated a reciprocal relationship between REM sleep and ICSS, this is additional evidence that in some way RD facilitates motivational states. The result that self-stimulation of a "motivational" area reduces REM rebound has been looked at in a parallel way by Putkonen and Putkonen (1971), who showed that elicitation of hypothalamic rage reactions reduces REM rebound. Although the evidence is sparse at this point, there are no data to contradict the assertion that RD facilitates aggressive, sexual, and ICSS behavior and that ICSS and hypothalamic-elicited rage reactions can substantially reduce REM rebound.

The question of course arises: How can one reconcile evidence linking REM sleep and motivational states with Pearlman and Greenberg's (1974) statements that RD does not affect motivation, or what they have called REM-independent behaviors? Their assertion (which rests on the citation of unpublished data) consists of looking at the effects of RD on rats' bar-press behavior for food. There is little data linking RD and eating, but the Dement (1965) study has stated that in effect, one has to prime the animal or starve it to see the effect of RD on eating behavior. This shouldn't be terribly surprising, since under normal circumstances, there is a rapid ceiling effect in eating behavior. Since Dement (1965b) had already published that normal eating was not affected by RD, Greenberg and Pearlman's (1974) & Pearlman's (1971) similar comments do not come as a surprise. Nevertheless, based on the data from studies looking at sexual, aggressive, and ICSS behavior, what they had called REM-independent behaviors seem not to be REM-independent at all, but rather to be facilitated by REM deprivation.

Dement (1969), in fact, has hypothesized that REM sleep also provides a type of periodic drive discharge; thus, RD should lead to drive facilitation. Ellman and Steiner (1969a, b) have put forth a similar hypothesis, in which they postulate that during REM sleep, at least some elements of the ICSS (or positive reinforcement) neural network are activated. They have further hypothesized that activation of the ICSS network lowers the threshold for a number of "drive" behaviors, or what they have termed stimulus-bound behaviors (SBB).[27] Thus,

---

[27]Stimulus-bound behaviors are those goal-directed behaviors that can be elicited by electrical stimulation to the brain. By goal-directed, we mean that an animal will work to achieve, and can display, a number of alternative motor movements to achieve a given consummatory response. This definition separates stereotypic behaviors from goal-directed behaviors that can be elicited by electrical stimulation.

RD causes a lowering of threshold for the ICSS system, and in turn for SBB sites. This hypothesis attempts to explain why thresholds for sexual, aggressive, eating, and ICSS behaviors are lowered following RD. It also explains why one may see different drive behaviors activated in different animals, since the threshold for any drive behavior can be influenced by at least two internal factors: the threshold at a given site of the specific behavior, and the threshold of the ICSS network. Thus, in a free-moving animal, one may see many drive behaviors or no drive behaviors, activated following RD. However, if one took central-nervous-system measures for eliciting drive or SBB, then all SBB should show a lowering of activation thresholds following RD. In a similar way, priming the animal by starving it would potentiate the effects of RD for a given behavior or behaviors.

The Ellman-Steiner (May 1976) hypothesis may also help explain why RD facilitates some behavior, while impairing the acquisition and/or retention of some tasks. It may be that RD impairs performance by lowering the threshold for a variety of behaviors, thus lowering the probability that the "correct" (from the experimenter's point of view) behavior will be emitted. This might explain why (except in Stern's (1971) studies) behaviors that are not well consolidated are affected by RD, while behaviors that have been more practiced tend not to be affected by RD. In addition, we speculate that the reason why RD is efficacious in alleviating endogenous depression is because RD lowers ICSS and SBB thresholds. In a simplistic way, one can view endogenous depression as a raising of threshold for a variety of drive or SBBs (like sex, aggression, eating, and so on). By REM depriving depressives and lowering ICSS (positive reward) and SBB thresholds, one is increasing the probability of evoking "drive" behaviors (like eating and sex).

It is clear from our review that RD studies share much of the promise and, hopefully temporary, limitations of other areas in sleep research. Despite the methodological difficulties encountered in many RD studies, it seems clear to us that this technique will continue to be of value in helping to understand the many seeming paradoxes uncovered by the discovery of REM sleep.

13

Sleep Mentation as Affected by REMP Deprivation

Arthur M. Arkin
John S. Antrobus
Steven J. Ellman
Jorge Farber

City College of the City University of New York,
    and
Montefiore Hospital & Medical Center

We have seen that REM sleep and dreaming experience of greatest vividness are closely associated in humans and experimental deprivation of REM sleep has produced consistent evidence that a more or less uniform nightly amount of Stage REM is an essential component of normal mammalian homeostasis. Typically, REM-time increases, or tendencies to enter into and persist in REM sleep, occur in roughly direct proportion to the amount of stage REM previously denied the subject (see Chapter 12 of this volume). At the same time, dream-like experience is available or prone to happen, in states of consciousness other than REM sleep, under normal and pathological conditions. Thus NREM sleep, hypnagogic and hypnopompic states, wakeful reveries, waking hypnosis, anesthesias, and hallucinogenic-drug experiences, and the sleep-onset epochs of persons ill with narcolepsy, are well known for their capacities for dream-like experience, often of striking intensity and elaboration.

Confronted by such evidence, one wonders whether increases of REM-sleep deficit, induced by experimental REM deprivation, might result in increases in REM-type mentation in other states of consciousness. For example, inasmuch as dream-like mentation may occur in NREM sleep, is Stage REM deprivation likely to produce intensification of dream-like qualities of NREM mentation? This question is related to another broader problem in psychophysiology: to what extent are specific varieties of phenomenal experience linked to specific constellations of electrographic concomitants? Thus, put in the context of this discussion, we are asking whether the relationship between REM-associated mentation and the REM period, as electrographically defined, is an *obligatory* one; or does the mentation possess some capacity for detachment, such that it may manifest itself in some other state than REM sleep?

In addition, whether Stage REM deprivation is followed by increased NREM dreaming is relevant to an important working assumption widely employed in modern sleep research but which has too long been left untested; that assumption deals with the extent to which REM deprivation equals dream deprivation. As previously described (see Chapter 12 of this volume), prior to the demonstration that dreaming in NREM sleep actually might occur, REM deprivation was indeed equated to dream deprivation by more than one investigator. Thus, if NREM dreaming markedly increased after REM deprivation, REM deprivation might have little or no effect as a dream-depriving operation. That is, the same "amount" of dreaming might occur with REM-deprived subjects as in undisturbed baseline conditions, but merely during NREM sleep instead.

Finally, changes in sleep mentation (both REM and NREM) as a consequence of REM deprivation, might have bearing on another important theme in psychophysiology. Is there a psychological need for dream experience as well as a physiological need for the electrochemical process involved in REM sleep? The hypothesis of a psychological need would predict an enhancement of dream-like characteristics of both NREM and REM mentation under conditions of REM deficit. (Indeed, as mentioned in Chapter 12 of this volume, some previous investigations have reported increases in intensity of REM dreaming following REM deprivation but results have been inconsistent.)

With the above considerations in mind, an experimental program dealing with the effects of REM deprivation on sleep mentation was initiated in 1967. Three large-scale experiments were performed, over a six-year period, each with a different technique and design. The rationale behind the designs are discussed in the introduction to each experiment; but it may be said here that although the hypotheses we sought to test seemed straightforward enough, the exigencies requiring care, and factors requiring control, became extraordinarily complex.

In all three experiments described, we employed as subjects males in attendance at college in the New York City area between the ages of 18 and 26 who were psychologically "normal," without significant organic disease, not active drug users, who were light sleepers (easily aroused) and good dream recallers (spontaneous morning dream recall at home 2-4 times weekly). All subjects were paid volunteers, recruited by placing advertisements on the bulletin boards of placement bureaus at the colleges. In addition, all subjects spent a trial night in the laboratory which provided them with an opportunity to experience the procedure before making their final decision, and enabling us to have a laboratory check on whether they could be sufficiently easily aroused and whether they had a modicum of mentation recall from NREM sleep.

All experiments were performed at the Psychophysiological Laboratory of the City College of New York. Subjects during laboratory studies slept the entire night in a sound-attenuated private room equipped with a bed, a microphone leading to a tape recorder, an intercommunicating device for the convenience of subject and experimenter, a set of electrical leads and a plug box. All electrographic recordings were made with an Offner type R polygraph.

EXPERIMENT 1

Basic Structure of the Experimental Plan

Mentation reports from NREM and REMP sleep were elicited in the laboratory under the following three conditions: initial baseline, REM deprivation, and terminal baseline. Between the retiring and morning rising 8 hr later, the night was divided into approximate thirds. No mentation reports were elicited during the first third. In the last two-thirds of the night, reports were elicited from each third, according to the following plan:

REMP: subjects awakened 5 min after REMP onset;
Stage 2 (REMP-proximate): subjects awakened 5 min after the first spindle occurring since preceding REMP termination;
Stage 2 (REMP-remote): subjects awakened 15 minutes after the first spindle since preceding REMP termination.

Thus a minimum of six reports were elicited each night (two REM and four Stage 2) with a randomized sequence. These design features enabled us to make comparisons of reports under conditions of relatively low- and high-REMP deficit and to observe whether their proximity to stage REM made any difference.

Subjects

Ten subjects were employed in this experiment. They were told that the project was sponsored by the National Institute of Mental Health in an effort to determine the effects of certain commercially used medications (sleeping and "pep" pills), and the effects of disruption of sleep, on all types of mental processes occurring in sleep and upon sleep patterns.

Method of REMP Deprivation and the Experimental Schedule

In devising a REM-deprivation operation, we strove to bring about a significant degree of REMP deficiency without engendering excessive subject fatigue and trauma. We incorporated a suggestion provided by a Dement (1964a) study in which, attempting to maximize REM deprivation, he combined the mechanical awakening-at-each-REMP-onset method with presleep administration of dextroamphetamine (a powerful REMP suppressor; see Chapter 11 of this text). Accordingly, we divided our REMP-deprivation period into two successive stages: an initial REMP-suppressing-drug phase and a following awakening-at-each-REMP-onset phase *without* drugs. The 18-night experimental plan is re-

TABLE 13.1

Sleep Mentation as Affected by REMP Deprivation

Phase	Night	Location	Procedure
Adaptation	1	Laboratory	Bedtime placebo (lactose capsule)
Sleep schedule stabilization	2, 3	Home	Bedtime placebo
Initial baseline	4, 5	Laboratory	Bedtime placebo; mentation reports elicited
REMP deprivation	6, 7, 8	Home	Bedtime amobarbital 200 mg
	9	Home	Bedtime amobarbital 200 mg plus dextro-amphetamine spansule (15 mgs)
	10	Laboratory	No drugs; subject experimentally awakened at each REMP onset
Elevated REMP potential	11, 12	Laboratory	Bedtime placebo; mentation reports obtained
Rest phase	13, 14, 15, 16	Home	Bedtime placebo
Terminal baseline phase	17, 18	Laboratory	Bedtime placebo; mentation reports obtained

presented in Table 13.1. As can be seen, REMP deprivation occurred over a five-consecutive-night series. On Nights 6-8, subjects received 200 mg of amobarbital just prior to retiring. On Night 9, 15 mg of *d*-amphetamine (spansule) was combined with the amobarbital; and on Night 10, REMP deprivation was continued by awakening subjects at each REMP onset alone (omitting presleep drugs.)

It is appropriate at this juncture to state, in anticipation of the discussion section, that our efforts to minimize fatigue were unsuccessful. Contrary to expectations from the literature, one night following presleep administration of *d*-amphetamine, even when antagonized by the hypnogenic effects of amobarbital, resulted in considerable fatigue (as manifested by spontaneous complaint and sleepy behavior when subjects appeared in the laboratory on Night 10.) This fatigue was further compounded by the succeeding night of mechanical REMP deprivation. For this reason, after completing experimental schedules with 10 subjects, we discontinued the above procedure and redesigned our approach (see Experiment 2 below). Despite the small subject population we regarded this phase as a useful exploratory study and carried out the data analysis.

Measurement Procedures

Standard EEG and EOG electrode placements for sleep studies were employed with the exception that the phallo-plethysmograph was substituted for the chin EMG. The reason for this was that we had been experiencing mechanical difficulties with the EMG technique at that time.

Mentation reports were processed in the following manner:

1. The word count of each mentation report was totaled eliminating repeated words and sounds of hesitation ("ah," "um," "er," and so on).

2. Each report was rated by nine independent judges on scales (five to seven steps) based upon the following categories: dreaming, emotionality, action, or movement, reference to the laboratory, number of visual scenes, bizarreness, perceptual vividness, detail of recall, and conceptual thought.

3. Comparisons among all experimental conditions and their interactions were made with a repeated-measures analysis of variance separately for each variable.

Measures of the effectiveness of the REMP-deprivation procedure included: (1) total mean pages of record per night with at least one horizontal REM; (2) mean latency to first REMP of the night (in minutes); and (3) mean REMP time percentage (the absence of the EMG recordings permitted only approximate estimates.) The choice of these measurements was based upon three experimental findings established by others: when REMP deprived subjects are observed on recovery nights, the mean frequency of rapid eye movements and the proportion of total sleep time occupied by REM sleep exceeds that of baseline levels; whereas the time between sleep onset and the first REMP of the night decreases (see Chapter 12 of this volume). By consensus of sleep researchers, these changes are indicators of increased tendencies to enter REM sleep and thus provide a composite index of REM deficit.

Results

Reliabilities of the judges' ratings evaluated separately for each contrast equaled .9.

Most of the variables sharply discriminated between REMP and NREM conditions. Specifically, all but the conceptual and laboratory-reference scales (the latter of which was higher in Stage 2 than Stage REM) were significantly different at the .01 level. Furthermore, the most discriminating scales were action, dreaming, and detail of recall. In addition, the action, dreaming, and emotionality scales also discriminated between REMP-proximate and REMP-remote Stage 2 at the .01 level. Thus, scales were adequately sensitive to the REMP-NREM distinction as well as that between REMP-proximate versus REMP-remote Stage 2 conditions.

Despite the capability of our scales to discriminate between REMP and NREM conditions, *none* yielded a significant interaction of sleep stage with elevated REMP potential as predicted. That is, elevated REMP potential was not associated with increased REMP or Stage 2 dreaming. As a matter of fact, there was a nonsignificant tendency toward *decreases* of the mean ratings on the dreaming and perceptual scales (both $p = .25$) and mean word count of reports ($p = .10$) on nights with elevated REMP deficit.

TABLE 13.2

Measures of the Effectiveness of REMP Deprivation

	Initial baseline		Elevated REMP		Terminal	
	Night 4	Night 5	Night 11	Night 12	Night 17	Night 18
Mean pages with one or more REMS	100	120	186	168	124	160
Mean latency to first REMP (min)	91	94	50	61	90	77
Mean REMP time percentage	22	26	37	33	28	27

Note: See Table 13.1 for experimental schedule.

The measures of the effectiveness of the REMP deprivation can be seen in Table 13.2. These results show that our indices of elevated REMP potential were indeed higher on the REMP recovery nights as expected, particularly on the first night of the pair.

Discussion

It occurred to us that our failure to observe increased dreaming (both REMP and NREM) in response to REMP deprivation might be explained on the basis of four factors.

Fatigue.   As previously described in the procedure section, our efforts to minimize fatigue were not effective. Subjects arrived at the laboratory on REMP recovery nights bearing an expression of tiredness and spontaneously complained of it as well. Fatigue is well known to impair recall of mentation and this factor rather than actually decreased dreaming may have played a role in our negative results.

Impaired motivation.   Our subjects were alert, intelligent, young college persons who were usually intrigued with the novelty and glamor of the first night or two of program, and initially strove to retrieve every wayward, elusive shred of sleep mentation. But this feature quickly lost its luster and they tended to settle for the basic essentials of what was required of them. Thus, progressively diminished motivation may have played a role in suppressing increased amounts of recall on elevated REMP pressure nights.

Disruption of cognitive mechanisms by the experimental procedure.   Presumably, endogenous sources of activation during sleep impinge upon cognitive mechanisms which respond with production or experience of sleep mentation.

It is plausible to assume that such cognitive mechanisms must be intact in order for this to occur just as in the presence of an external patterned stimulus during wakefulness, the lens and pupil of the eye must be capable of proper accommodation and intensity control for adequate perception. Thus, despite the presence of increased REMP, potential dreaming may have been unexpectedly diminished if cognitive mechanisms were disrupted by the experimental procedure and unable to "handle" the increment of activation.

Dissipation of elevated REMP potential.   Although REMP potential was clearly elevated on experimental mentation report collection nights, we may have lost an opportunity to obtain positive results because of untoward REMP deficit "leakage." That is, experimental reports were gathered on nights during which Stage REM was permitted without interference and despite REM deficit in comparison to baseline levels, it was nevertheless insufficient to provide evidence of increased dreaming.

EXPERIMENT 2

In designing the second experiment, we took into account the possible reasons for failure of the first to obtain positive results. Thus, in the interests of minimizing REMP deficit loss, we decided to collect all mentation reports *during* nights of ongoing REMP deprivation rather than on recovery nights. Furthermore, in line with this exigency and because the hypothesis of major interest was that elevated REMP potential produces increased NREM dreaming, we collected reports from Stage 2 only (forestalling even that amount of REMP sleep which would have been permitted had we collected REMP reports as well). Also, in the interests of methodological purity, we avoided adjunctive use of drugs and employed the awakening-at-each REMP-onset technique exclusively, for REMP deprivation. In addition, because we wanted to run a large number of subjects (to maximize chances of identifying even a small effect) we utilized as economical a program as possible for each subject with regard to the number of consecutive nights in the experimental schedule.

We felt that we could accomplish this by comparing Stage 2 mentation reports elicited during three consecutive nights of REMP deprivation with corresponding reports from three consecutive nights of Stage 2-control deprivation; and during the latter, the total number of control awakenings would be made to equal the total required on REMP-deprivation nights. Thus, Stage 2 reports elicited on nights of elevated REMP deficit would be compared to corresponding reports on nights with relatively low-REMP deficit, such nights being otherwise similar with regard to amounts of sleep loss, sleep interruptions, motivation, and fatigue.

To control for order effects, half of our subjects would be run with REMP deprivation first, and Stage 2-control deprivation second; the other half were to be run in reverse order.

Basic Structure of the Experimental Plan

All subjects received a single trial-adaptation night during which a number of awakenings were performed throughout for the purpose of determining whether a modicum of NREM recall was available and also to give the subjects an opportunity to experience the procedure in advance of the actual study (and if they wished, to drop out before beginning the experiment proper).

During the ensuing several days at home and throughout the entire remainder of the experiment, subjects were asked to fill out a sleep log and instructed to stabilize their sleep schedules. They then underwent the following procedure:

> Nights 1-3: REMP deprivation plus elicitation of Stage 2 mentation reports;
> Nights 4-6: rest at home (8 hr uninterrupted sleep each night);
> Nights 7-9: control NREM deprivation plus elicitation of Stage 2 reports.

The first 20 subjects were run in this order and the second 20 were run in reverse with the number of NREM-control-deprivation awakenings on successive nights based upon our experience with the first series. In addition, efforts were made to distribute these control awakenings throughout the night in a pattern similar to that obtained for the initial series. Each laboratory session from the time of "lights out" to final awakening on the following morning was 9 hr.

Method of Deprivation Awakenings

REMP deprivation was accomplished by wakening subjects at each REMP onset by continuous sounding of a loud bell (approximately 80 dB) until the subject switched it off by operation of a hand dynamometer. This switch was adjusted to require intense strength of hand grip sustained for 2 sec in order to break the circuit. Within 5-20 sec, the bell was sounded a second time and its termination managed in the same way.

The rationale for this deprivation procedure was based upon three considerations. First, the sustained, intense, major muscular effort entailed by the highly resistant hand grip switch was expected to be antagonistic to, and incompatible with, the minimal tonic EMG levels characteristic of REM sleep. It was, therefore, expected to be an effective procedure for REM deprivation. Second, the procedure did not involve verbal interchange between the experimenter and the subject, thus reducing a possible source of artifactual "contamination" of subsequent mentation reports. And third, although REM sleep might be effectively interrupted by the procedure, it was hoped that the brevity of each interruption would minimize sleep loss.

NREM deprivation was begun only after the completion of the first REMP and awakening made after typical signs of NREM sleep such as 12-14 Hz spindles, delta-wave sequences, and so on. The technique was otherwise the same as above.

Electrographic Procedures

Standard EEG and EOG electrode placements were used and again, the phallo-plethysmograph was substituted for the EMG.

Schedule of Elicitation of Mentation Reports

A minimum of four Stage 2 mentation reports were obtained in pairs in the middle and final third of each night. The first member of the pair was obtained proximate to the preceding REMP (5 min of continuous Stage 2 after the first spindle appearing after previous REMP termination. These reports were called R-II. The second member was elicited more remote from Stage REM. After completing the R-II report, the subject was permitted to return to sleep; and when the first 5 min of Stage 2, after the first sleep spindle occurred in this context, the subject was awakened again for a mentation report. (These reports were called II-5.)

Automated tape recordings were used throughout to awaken and interrogate the subject. This involved rhythmical repetition of calling the subject's first name; instructing him to "Tell us everything that has been going through your mind;" and inquiring afterward as to whether it had been an image, dream or thought, how vivid and clear recall was and what emotions were associated, respectively.

Indices of Differential REMP Deficit

REMP deficit on REMP-deprivation nights was measured by three separate indicators: (1) the total number of 30-sec epoch pages per night containing at least one horizontal REM; (2) the REMP latency in minutes from sleep onset (first sleep spindle of the night) until first REMP onset; and (3) the total number of awakenings necessary to deprive the subject of as much REMP sleep as possible on the three consecutive nights. The rationale for employment of the frequency of REMs and time latency, from first sleep onset until the first REMP of the night was the same as for Experiment 1. Use of the total number of deprivation awakenings necessary to accomplish REM deprivation was based on the established finding that on successive nights of REM deprivation, the number of awakenings required to forestall REM sleep progressively increases. That is, deprived of REM sleep, the subject "tries harder and harder" to enter the deprived physiological state. This tendency is manifested by ever increasing REMP onsets which in turn occasioned an increasing frequency of deprivation awakenings. Thus, the number of deprivation awakenings on successive nights provides a convenient objective index of REMP deficit (see Chapter 12 of this volume).

Measures of Mentation Qualities

Dream-like mentation was measured in the following manner: 24 reports from each of the 40 subjects were sorted separately by 6 independent judges employing an 8-point Q-sort technique with a forced-normal distribution. The scale emphasized visual imagery, succession of scenes, bizarreness, and a sense that the sleep experience was real. In addition, the total word count of each report was tallied.

Results

Indices of Difference in REMP Deficit on REMP Versus NREM-Control-Deprivation Nights.

Progression in number of awakenings over consecutive nights required for REMP Deprivation. In the forward order (REMP followed by NREM-control deprivation), the mean number of awakening required on the 3 consecutive nights were 37, 53, and 58, respectively.

In the reverse order, the same numbers of awakenings were employed on each corresponding night of the NREM control deprivation series and were distributed as closely as possible, throughout each night in a temporal manner similar to that for the first REMP-deprivation series. This involved some degree of "overshoot" and "undershoot" in the second REMP deprivation series which followed. Untoward dissipation of REMP-onset tendency did not appear to result from this, however, as judged by the decreased latency to the first REMP on REMP-deprivation nights.

Mean number of pages of polygraph record containing at least one horizontal REM. In the forward order, the mean number of pages with one or more horizontal REMS averaged over the 3 consecutive nights was 65.4 for the REMP-deprivation series and 158.4 for the NREM-control nights. Thus, there were 2.4 times more such pages on NREM-control than on REMP-deprivation nights, a marked reduction in REMP phasic events on REMP deprivation nights.

On REMP deprivation nights, the appearance of only one REM on a particular page was both the occasion for including this page in our measure tally and a REMP deprivation awakening. By contrast, on NREM control nights REMs usually occurred in profusion on a particular page and REMP sleep was not interrupted. In either condition, a tally of 1 was entered in the respective total; but it should be obvious that a representative page on a NREM-control night contains many more REM phasic events than on REMP-deprivation nights. That there were 2.4 times more of such *pages* on NREM-control nights, therefore, should be interpreted as indicating a much greater nightly total of REMP phasic events than on REMP-deprivation nights.

As previously mentioned, the number of REMP-deprivation wakenings in the reverse order series (with control-NREM awakenings first) was predetermined on the basis of the mean number of deprivation awakenings on each successive night required for the first 20 subjects who were run in the forward order (that is, with REMP deprivation first). The inevitable result was that with some subjects the number of planned allowed awakenings in the reverse order series fell short of that necessary to eliminate as much REM sleep as had been denied the forward order subjects group. Therefore, an adjustment was required for these subjects in order to use the number of pages with at least one horizontal REM as an index of REM deficit. We reasoned that the most important consideration was a measure of REM deficit prevailing *during* the collection of mentation reports rather than that level occurring after they had been obtained. Thus, on these underestimated nights, instead of the total number of pages per night with at least one horizontal REM, we employed for the comparison the number of such pages preceding the collection of the last pair of mentation reports of the night. Accordingly, in the reverse order, the mean number of pages with at least 1 horizontal REM was 70.4 for REMP and 137.3 for NREM control deprivation nights. Again, a marked reduction of REMP phasic events had been achieved on REM deprivation nights.

Differences in latency to the first REMP. In the forward order, the average latencies in minutes from the first sleep spindle of the night until the onset of the first REMP were 65.3 for the 3 REMP, and 73.6 for the 3 NREM control deprivation nights (difference = 8.3 min).

In the reverse order, corresponding figures were 71.1 for the REMP and 89.3 for the NREM control deprivation nights (difference = 18.2).

Considering all three indices, the results indicate that on REMP-deprivation nights, in either schedule order, the REMP potential was clearly higher than on NREM-control nights.

Comparison of Mean Word Counts of Mentation Reports

Under all conditions, the mean word counts of R-II (elicited proximate to REMPs) was higher than the II-5 reports (elicited remote from REMPs): 130.5 versus 90.7; $p < .01$. On the average, II-5 reports had been obtained 12 min after completion of those from the R-II condition.

Throughout, no order effects were found in mean word counts of reports.

Ratings of Dream-like Mentation

First, the mean rating of *all* NREM reports for *all* nights throughout (R-II and II-5 together) for the first half of the night was 4.35 and 4.55 for the second half. This small increase of the intensity of dream-like mentation in the latter half of the night was significant at the .05 level.

Second, separate analysis of the dream-like ratings for R-II versus II-5 reports revealed that for all nights throughout, R-II reports were more dream-like than II-5 reports. (Mean ratings R-II = 4.73; II-5 = 4.17; $p < .001$.)

In all analyses of dream-like ratings, there were no order effects.

Third, there were *no* significant differences in mean dream-like ratings of reports elicited under REMP deprivation conditions as compared to those elicited during control NREM deprivation.

Discussion

The results point to conclusions similar to those drawn from Experiment 1; that is, REMP deprivation does not result in detectable increases in NREM dreaming. It is possible, however, that an increase in NREM dreaming did indeed occur but was masked by the fatigue and stress associated with the experimental procedure. But an argument against such an interpretation is that although these factors were certainly present, they were not strong enough to obliterate two differential effects previously established by other investigators, namely NREM mentation reports elicited from the second half of the night tend to be more dream-like than those from the first half, and mentation reports elicited shortly after REMP termination tend to possess more words and more dream-like qualities than those elicited more remotely from REMPs (Pivik & Foulkes, 1968; Wolpert & Trosman, 1958; also see Experiment 1, this chapter.) These differential effects were found in our study to persist *despite* the stress of the procedure, and such persistence is evidence that our chosen measures were sufficiently sensitive to small changes. Thus, the results of Experiments 1 and 2 indicate that any possible undetected increase in NREM dreaming in response to REMP deprivation would very likely be an elusive, subtle, and fragile phenomenon in contrast to these previously mentioned stress-resistant effects.

EXPERIMENT 3

Because Experiments 1 and 2 had produced unexpected results that were at variance with some of the work of other investigators (Pivik & Foulkes, 1966) and the expectations of most others, we deemed it essential to perform a new study with more elaborate controls, systematic measurements of all of the known crucial variables, and new refinements—in short, to put our hypotheses, both predictive and retrospective to as critical a test as we could devise with the resources at hand, and at the same time maximize our understanding of possible factors involved.

The main innovations involved using the subject as his own control throughout, as well as counterbalancing the order of the two deprivation conditions;

careful measurement of all variables under three baseline conditions at the beginning, middle, and end of each experimental series; measurement of all variables
on recovery nights as well as deprivation nights; and obtaining REMP and NREM
(including sleep-onset Stage 1 NREM) mentation reports on the same nights
both in association with and remote from phasic events known to occur in these
sleep stages.

Specific Method

Twenty "normal" college men who were light sleepers and good dream recallers were paid subjects. They were run in accordance with the schedule
described below. Each initially acceptable applicant was required to satisfy the
following criterion on a trial laboratory night: report of some clear mentation
with at least one specific item of content in 2 or more of 8 NREM reports elicited throughout the night. Suitable subjects were then asked to stabilize their
sleep cycles for five to seven nights at home, and to keep standardized daily
sleep logs for the remainder of the experiment. Then, they spent three consecutive adaptation nights in the laboratory, the first two of which merely
provided the subjects with an opportunity to get accustomed to the laboratory
bedroom. Thus, electrodes were not attached, no wakeups were performed and
they were permitted to sleep from 11-7 or 12-8. On the third adaptation night,
however, electrodes were attached and six Stage 2 and two Stage REM mentation reports were obtained. After the adaptation series was completed, the experimental schedule proper was carried out as follows[1]:

Nights, 1, 2: initial baseline
Nights 3-5: REMP deprivation
Night 6: recovery

Then, after a rest period at home for three to eight nights, the subject continued in the laboratory as follows:

Nights 7, 8: middle baseline
Nights 9 to 11: NREM control deprivation
Night 12 recovery
Nights 13, 14: terminal baseline

The first 10 subjects were run in the forward order of REMP followed by
NREM control deprivation, the next 10 were in the reverse order. (When the reverse order was employed, the problem arose as to how the experimenter should
determine in advance the number of NREM-control-deprivation awakenings

---

[1]In independent pilot work on four subjects Ellman had obtained initial encouraging
results with this experimental schedule, which he devised.

needed to properly balance the number of REM deprivation awakenings to be carried out in the following half of the schedule. To avoid the minor methodological problem which arose under similar circumstances in Experiment 2, we based our estimate upon the mean number of REM-deprivation awakenings required in the forward order plus a quantity in excess of the mean so as not to "run out" of REM deprivation awakenings subsequently. When it happened that our predetermined number was more than that actually required, we had no choice but to continue the awakenings in Stage 2 until the planned total for the night was exhausted. Although this made for occasional slight excesses in Stage 2 awakenings, it took adequate account of the more urgent exigency of insuring maximal REM deprivation.

Electrographic measurements included the EEG, EOG, and submental EMG with standard electrode placements, monitored throughout each laboratory night.

The Mentation Report Schedule

The schedule was devised so as to enable us to test whether dreaming during sleep onset, Stage 2 or REMP sleep is increased by REMP deprivation. Thus, on each experimental night, the same typical ground plan was employed as follows:

1. A sleep onset mentation report was elicited during the first sequence of rolling-eye movements against a Stage 1 NREM EEG background.

2. As a rule, no additional mentation reports were obtained until 70-90 min of sleep time had elapsed.

3. The remainder of the night was divided into two approximately equal intervals. During each of these, one REMP and three Stage 2 mentation reports were elicited, all in counterbalanced order, yielding a total of nine mentation reports per night (including the sleep onset report).

   a. REMP reports were elicited 2-4 min after REMP onset and equal numbers were obtained in close association with and remote from REM bursts.

   b. Stage 2 mentation reports were elicited at least 15 min after a previous REMP termination and equal numbers obtained in close association with, and remote from, phasic events (phasic EMG suppression and K complexes occurring together or separately).

The technique of mentation-report elicitation involved an initial neutral question as to what had been going through the subjects' minds just prior to awakening and was followed by a standardized interview program to obtain descriptions of the vividness and clarity of the sleep experience, its emotional content, and feeling of reality.

The technique of Stage REM deprivation consisted of awakening subjects at each REMP onset and keeping them awake for at least 2 min by having them do mental arithmetic aloud.

When later on, as the tendency to return immediately to REM sleep became marked, it was necessary to keep subjects awake for as long as 5 min to forestall such REMP resumption.

Processing of Mentation Reports

Four judges, employing an 8-point rating scale (forced-normal distribution) independently sorted 108 reports on each subject. The scale measured dreaming (1 least, and 8 most dream-like). (The issues involved in such measurements are discussed in Chapter 2 of this volume). Throughout, every effort was made to control experimentally or statistically for any effect of time of the night on dreaming.

Scoring of sleep stage parameters was done in accordance with the Manual of Standardized Terminology, Techniques and Scoring System for Sleep Stages of Human Subjects (Rechtschaffen and Kales 1968)

Results

Effectiveness of REMP-Deprivation Procedure (Table 13.3)

Inspection of Table 13.3 reveals drastic reduction of Stage REM on deprivation nights. (For purposes of clarity, the data are tabulated as if stage REM deprivation had been first throughout, that is, with the two counterbalanced orders combined.) Specifically, from baseline Stage REM proportions ranging 20-28%, the range on deprivation nights was reduced to 3-4%.

TABLE 13.3

Total Sleep Time and Sleep Stage Time (Minutes)
by Experimental Nights

Night Sched.	1st B.L.		REMP Dep.			Rec.	Mid B.L.		NREM Dep.			Rec.	Term. B.L.	
	1	2	3	4	5	6	7	8	9	10	11	12	13	14
Tot. Sl.	415	453	331	339	321	470	460	462	378	373	360	462	463	450
TSR	82	103	10	13	13	126	98	103	83	73	77	123	127	108
%SR	20	23	3	4	4	27	22	23	22	20	22	27	28	24
TSN	334	355	321	327	308	345	359	359	295	301	284	339	336	342
%SN	89	79	98	97	96	74	79	78	78	81	79	74	73	76

TABLE 13.4

Mean Ratings for Dream-like Mentation Adjusted for Variations in
Time of Night of Elicitation of Mentation Reports
(Outcome of Analysis of Covariance)

Night Sched.	1st B.L.		REMP Dep.			Rec.	Mid B.L.		NREM Dep.			Rec.	Term. B.L.	
	1	2	3	4	5	6	7	8	9	10	11	12	13	14
Stage														
REM	6.1	5.0	5.7	5.2	5.5	5.5	5.4	5.1	5.7	5.2	5.2	5.1	5.1	4.9
Stage 2 S.O.	4.5	4.2	4.1	3.6	4.1	4.6	4.5	4.5	3.7	4.0	4.0	4.3	4.5	4.3
Stage 1 NREM	4.4	4.3	4.5	4.4	4.7	4.6	4.2	4.4	4.1	4.3	4.2	4.4	4.1	4.2

| ◄——— counterbalanced ———► |

Analysis of Dream-like Qualities of Mentation Reports (Table 13.4)

A grand total of 2504 awakenings were made to obtain mentation reports. Of this number, 557 were from Stage REM (320 REM phasic; 237 REM tonic); 1668 were from Stage 2 (1078 phasic; 590 tonic); and 279 were from Stage 1 NREM.

Since half of the subjects were run in each of the two orders, and each subject went through all conditions, the data was initially treated as a split-plot analysis of variance. Since differences in the two orders were trivial, however, there was no need to take account of the effects of order and its interaction with the other treatment conditions. For the sake of simplicity, we therefore collapsed the two orders and treated the analysis as a randomized block design: Nights 1-14 by time of night (early-late) by class of awakening (1 Stage REM by 2 NREM awakenings) per half of night. Phasic-tonic awakenings were not fully crossed with this classification and were therefore analyzed on a special subset of the total data set. A test (Box 1950) for compound symmetry of the variance-covariance symmetry matrix was carried out on the subject-by-night data matrix; there were no significant violations of the assumptions of compound symmetry. Following adjustment of the means for variation in time of night by analysis of covariance (an overall adjustment was made for the entire night of each subject and not for each condition within each night), the appropriate error terms were computed and a priori comparisons were computed for the hypothesized effects.

Comparison of mean ratings on the three sets of baseline nights revealed the following order effects. Dream-like mentation (Stages 2 and REM together decreased on the second night of each baseline pair ($t = 2.5$; $p < .05$). This effect was strongest for Stage REM ($t = 3.1$; $p < .01$). There was a small but linear decrease in Stage REM dream-like mentation over the three sets of baseline nights (t = 2.95; p ⟨ .01). This effect was not observed in Stage 2 report ratings. Order effects were not detectable for sleep onset Stage 1 NREM reports.

Effects of sleep deprivation (stages REM and 2 together). The most striking effect was reduction in Stage 2 dream-like mentation (t = 5.94; p ⟨ .01). In addition, there was a slight but insignificant increase in Stage REM dreaming (t = 1.26 n.s.). Also, the effects of total sleep reduction over each 3-day deprivation series were not systematic (t for this linear effect = .28). Finally, dream-like qualities of sleep onset Stage 1 mentation remained unchanged throughout.

Effects of stage REM deprivation alone. Comparisons of mean ratings of dream-like mentation on Stage REM- versus Stage 2-deprivation nights revealed *no* significant differences between these two conditions. (t for stages REM and 2 together = −.04; Stage REM alone = .57; for Stage 2 alone = −.10). In addition, neither sleep deprivation per se nor specific sleep-stage deprivation altered phasic-tonic differences (which *were* demonstrable under baseline conditions). Analysis for second order interactions also revealed no significant effects of the experimental variables. And again, REM-sleep deprivation was without detectable effect on mentation associated with sleep onset Stage 1 NREM.

Discussion

Let us review the background to our research. We were impressed by two major considerations:

Empirical Knowledge

Dreaming of the greatest vividness, intensity, and perceptual quality had been deemed to be closely associated with REM sleep, and the degree of activity in dream-event sequences positively correlated with the profusion of REMs (Berger & Oswald, 1962). (But see Chapter 6 of this volume).

Significant amounts of dreaming, though tending to be more conceptual in quality than that associated with Stage REM, occurs in stage 2 sleep; and significant amounts of both perceptual and conceptual dreaming occur during Stage 1 NREM in the course of transitions from wakefulness to sleep.

Normal, mammalian, biological homeostasis requires a more or less uniform nightly amount of REM sleep, which, if curtailed, is followed by progressively more frequent REM-period onsets, and REM time typically undergoes proportionate increases on recovery nights following cessation of experimental REM deprivation.

These facts had raised two questions and much heated debate among researchers in the field. First, does REM deprivation produce corresponding amounts of *dream* deprivation? And second, might there be, in addition to physiological needs for REM sleep, *psychological* needs for vivid dreaming experience? If the latter were true, then dream loss associated with REM deprivation might also result in increased dream-like mentation in physiological states other than REM sleep.

In line with this thought, several incidental observations had suggested that deprivation of REM sleep is capable of producing physiological effects in NREM stages. Thus, REM deprivation had been observed to be followed by:

1. NREM penile erections (whereas in sleep they are normally confined to stage REM; Fisher 1966);
2. brief REM bursts with segments of stage 1 EEG "intruding" into NREM sleep (Sampson, 1965);
3. increases in the frequency of phasic EMG suppression (Dement, 1969) and PGO spiking in NREM sleep (Ferguson & Dement, 1968).

And so, if REM deprivation might result in the manifestation of Stage REM-type physiological events or influences in NREM sleep, why could not REM deprivation also result in increases of REM-type *mentation* in NREM sleep? Consistent with this possibility was the observation that vivid, intense, nightmarish dreaming is associated with recovery nights (and REM rebound) following withdrawal of previously administered REM-suppressant drugs (see Chapter 11 of this volume). That is, during such REM rebound conditions, sleep mentation becomes more intense along with the increased level of physiological activity.

Theoretical Models of Dreaming

An additional stimulus for this research was our wish to test various models of dreaming. By way of example, we briefly comment on predictions made by the classical psychoanalytic, the "motor-output model" of REM period dreaming (Dement, 1967), and certain cognitive models of dream processes Dewan, 1970; Gaarder, 1966; Shapiro, 1967).

Part of the classical psychoanalytic theory of dreaming describes the dream as one way by which partial discharge of instinctual drive tensions may be accomplished. This aspect is referred to, in the literature, by the expression "safety-valve" function of the dream, so-called because levels of drive energy are kept within tolerable limits by permitting quantities to be discharged during sleep in a harmless fashion. This component of the theory implies that dreaming fulfills psychological needs and predicts that if opportunities for REM dreaming are drastically reduced, mentation during NREM sleep would accommodate to the increased drive tension by becoming more dream-like.

The motor-output model of REMP dreaming was formulated by Dement (1967) in an attempt to account for dreaming in all stages of sleep, NREM as well as REM. According to this model, physiological activity in sleep is manifested in a more or less consistent sequence of events which, for descriptive purposes, may be divided conveniently into four phases successively superimposed upon each phase preceding:

1. Basal activity: corresponding to Stage 4 and the quieter intervals of Stages 2 and 3 in later portions of the night. The level of concomitant neural activity is deemed sufficient to support consciousness.

2. Sensory input phase: presumably corresponding to the appearance of PGO spiking (in analogy to experimental observations in the cat), and representing "endogenous stimulation" possessing some of the qualities of activity resulting from sensory stimulation.

3. Peripheral motor inhibition and central activation phase: corresponding to the transition between NREM and REMP sleep. It is characterized by tonic suppression of EMG activity and EEG activation hard on its heels.

4. Central motor output: indicated by the presence of REMs and muscle twitching.

Dream intensity and complexity are at their lowest levels in the basal activity phase and are said to increase as subsequent phases are added until they reach their highest level—the achievement of the "nearly complete psychophysiological integration" represented by the motor output phase. This model predicts that REMP deprivation should result in "more active dreaming or dreams with more activity." (p. 50)

A third group of theorists employ concepts derived from cognitive psychology. Although differing in details, the models of Gaarder, (1966), Shapiro, (1967) and Dewan (1970) share in common the idea that REM sleep is intimately involved with adequately processing information received by the brain during wakefulness. Shapiro and Gaarder both believe that the central nervous system is incapable of completing on-line processing of inputs, with regard to their more remote implications, and simultaneously cope with wakeful adaptational tasks. As Shapiro (1967) put it, "In the absence of sleep, recorded unprocessed data would thus accumulate in sufficient amounts to interfere with the normal activity and decision making of the waking state . . . [p. 73]." Sleep then becomes a requirement for completion of the processing of this residual information without the concomitant burden of dealing with the claims of wakeful life. Dewan, somewhat differently, places major emphasis on REM sleep as an obligatory physiological state uniquely fitted for providing the brain with an opportunity to reprogram itself—an operation necessary for coping with adaptational tasks arising from external and internal sources. In any case, these related theoretical formulations all imply that REM deprivation would seriously impair information processing and central-nervous-system-program maintenance; and presumably this would find reflection in both sleep and wakeful mentation.

With this compelling background, we undertook our research, confident of obtaining positive results in the predicted direction.

We were, therefore, taken by an unexpected surprise when, as described above, the outstanding finding of all three experiments was the lack of demonstrable increases of dreaming in Stages REM, 2 and 1 NREM under conditions of REM deprivation. Furthermore, results were equally negative under conditions which maximally favored positive results, namely, comparing mentation reports elicited in association with, and remote from, both REM and NREM phasic events. In not dissimilar fashion (as set forth in Chapter 14 of this volume) studies of the effects of REM deprivation on wakeful mentation have led to negative, contradictory, unclear or, in any case, quite minimal findings.

Thus, although several physiological states are capable of supporting dream-like mentation, they do not respond to REM deprivation with detectable increases in such mentation. Interestingly, this applied equally to REM sleep mentation as well, inasmuch as no increases in Stage REM dreaming were observed under the experimental condition. And with the same essential outcome with NREM-control deprivation, we conclude that deprivation or disruption of Stages REM and NREM has no specific, typical effect on cognition in the states sampled. Put in another way, mentation-producing processes in three different sleep stages (stages REM, 2, and sleep onset of stage 1 NREM) are relatively independent of any specific factors resulting from REM or NREM sleep deprivation, that is, deprivation or disruption of Stages REM or NREM did not produce characteristic changes in the mentation sampled from Stages REM, 2 or sleep onset Stage 1 NREM.

How do these results compare with those reported by others who have attempted to directly observe the effects of REM deprivation on sleep mentation? In their initial publication Pivik and Foulkes (1966) described an increase in dream-like qualities of mentation reports elicited from the fifth REM period of the night following mechanical deprivation of all preceding REM sleep on the same night. This effect was observed in 12 of 20 subjects. Four showed diminished dream-like qualities and the same number underwent no apparent change. The positive results were yielded chiefly by subjects categorized as repressors, in the Byrne scale (1963) of the MMPI, as opposed to the sensitizers. In a subsequent study, however, Foulkes and Pivik (1968) utilized a cross-night, rather than within-night design, and despite their employing only repressor subjects (to maximize the likelihood of positive findings), dream enhancement was not observed in either REM or NREM sleep following a night of REM deprivation.

Meanwhile, Dement (1967) stated that

> We have taken a brief look at dream recall data obtained from six adult subjects on the first recovery night following either six nights of REM deprivation awakenings or six nights of control arousals. The preliminary analysis suggests that dreams following the former procedure were more active [p. 50].

Unfortunately, no further methodological details were provided in the paper and the study was subsequently discontinued (Dement, personal communication, 1975).

Finally, in comparing Stage REM reports over three consecutive nights of REM deprivation to those elicited under baseline conditions, Cartwright and

Ratzel (1970) failed to observe overall increases of dream-like qualities. However, they did notice that light sleepers intensified their REM-period-onset fantasy more quickly than deep sleepers as deprivation progressed, albeit in no case were values obtained in excess of the baseline. Thus, out of four studies carried out in other laboratories (each of which entailed direct measurement of dream-like qualities of sleep mentation under conditions of REM deprivation) two sets of results were essentially negative, one was indeterminate and one was positive for a subgroup of subjects (repressors) in a within-night design (Pivik and Foulkes, 1966). We return subsequently to issues related to this single positive result.

In thinking about the outcome of our work, several questions have occurred to us:

1. Could subject stress and fatigue have masked positive results?

2. Might individual differences in subjects' propensities to compensate for REM deprivation have been a factor in our not obtaining positive main effects?

3. Is it possible that positive findings were forestalled by ceiling effects attendant upon our choice of good dream-recaller subjects? (That is, increases in dream-like mentation may not have been discernible because of an excessively high initial baseline.)

4. Could positive results have been obtained if NREM mentation reports had been obtained just before REMP onset instead of after REMP termination?

5. Might increases in dream-like mentation have been detected if we had sampled Stages 3 or 4 in addition to those we had selected?

6. Is it possible that increases of dream-like mentation occurred in wakefulness by day instead of during sleep?

Let us now consider these questions in turn.

Stress-fatigue factors. We believe it unlikely that stress and/or fatigue masked differential effects for two reasons. First, our design was constructed in such a fashion that stress-fatigue factors were distributed in a controlled manner, resulting in their being equalized for both REM- and NREM-deprivation conditions; and second, rather subtle, differential previously established correlations between sleep-mentation characteristics and objective indices persisted during the deprivation procedures despite the clearly present stress and fatigue manifestations. Specifically, in Experiment 2, the tendency of Stage 2 mentation to become more dream-like during the latter part as opposed to the early part of the night was preserved; and Stage 2 mentation reports elicited proximate to REM periods remained clearly more dream-like than REM-period-remote reports throughout REM and NREM control deprivation. Furthermore, in Experiment 3, REM mentation elicited in association with REM bursts remained more dream-like than that elicited during REM quiescence throughout all deprivation procedures. (It is to be noted that these findings are in accord with previous reports of other investigators: Pivik & Foulkes, 1968; Wolpert & Trosman, 1958; Molinari & Foulkes, 1969.) We may infer from these findings, therefore, that if cognitive processes were sufficiently intact so as to continue to differentially reflect the above electrographic conditions, they were also capable of differential production and recall of dream-like mentation if such effects were indeed capable of being brought about. In summary, if our measures were sufficiently sensitive to discriminate between mentation elicited from different electrographic conditions, despite stress-fatigue factors, it seems reasonable to expect that they would be sufficiently sensitive to detect increases in dream-like mentation attendant upon REM deprivation if such differences were present in some significant degree.

Individual Difference Factors. With the passage of time, attention of sleep researchers has gradually been drawn to the roles that individual differences might play in producing experimental results, particularly when findings have run counter to previous expectations or have been different among subjects both between and within investigations. Thus, Cartwright et al. (1967; Cartwright & Ratzel, (1972) and Nakazawa et al. (1975) demonstrated individual differences in response to REM deprivation and attempted to relate tendencies toward lack of REM compensation to certain subject personality characteristics. In brief, Cartwright et al. (1967); 1972) reported that normal young adults could be typed as tending to produce three different response patterns to REM deprivation: (1) disruption of the clarity of the electrographic features of the sleep cycle; (2) compensation of previous REM sleep loss manifested by "REM rebound" on the first recovery night (the more or less typical response initially described by Dement (1960); and, (3) substitution in which subjects manifest little or no REM rebound but, in addition, during REM-deprivation nights, recall a greater amount of dream-like mentation from REMP onset awakenings than the compensator subjects. The term substitution was employed to indicate that subjects showing little or no REM compensation are thought able to substitute sleep stages other than REM for the production of dream-like fantasy. Thus, substitutors may heighten dream activity in Stage 2 or at REMP onset and need little or no REM compensation to accomodate for the deprivation of fantasy caused by REM reduction. As a group, substitutor subjects tended to be light sleepers, possess higher baseline-NREM fantasy scores than compensators and be more responsive to internal experience by day (as reflected by Rorshach data).

According to Cartwright's (1967; 1972) formulations, a dream-enhancement effect of REM deprivation may have been discernible in a subgroup of our population if special data analyses had been carried out with due regard for the effects of individual differences between our subjects; and that such positive results were obscured by our not having carried out our data processing beyond assessment of the main effects. That is, Cartwright's position on the effects of REM deprivation is that the "average subject" model (see Chapter 2 of this volume) does not tell the whole story. Much of the association between REM deprivation and dreaming would be revealed in individual differences. Although an

N of 20 is insensitive to anything but large population correlations, we decided to examine our data from the vantage point of Cartwright's (1967; 1972) model.

First, we examined the compensation model by testing whether total REM time on the recovery night following three nights of REM deprivation was negatively correlated with individual differences in dreaming summed over REM onset, NREM, and sleep onset during the three nights of REM deprivation. Squared correlations of .-3, .00, and .12, respectively, between the dreaming variables and total REM time, (TRT) were not sufficiently large to support the assertion that a relationship does exist. Neither is the sample size large enough to support the position that no relationship exists.

It has been our feeling that the variables used by Cartwright to test her model have included variance components which might produce a correlation even if the model were not true. These components should, therefore, be partialled out. Although such partialling is normally done only if the original correlation is significant, we do it here to demonstrate what we consider to be an appropriate form of a test of Cartwright's (1967; 1972) model.

With respect to recovery-night total REM time, the model is really talking about the change in TRT on recovery compared to baseline nights. Accordingly, TRT on baseline nights should be partialled out. Similarly, with respect to dreaming during REM-deprivation and-recovery nights. Cartwright (1967; 1972) is concerned with the change in dreaming relative to dreaming during baseline REM, NREM, and sleep-onset fantasy. Therefore, these variables should also be partialled out; they might be found to differ from one experiment to another and for different aspects of the Cartwright model.

Using the same rationale, we reexamined the Cartwright model using latency to REM onset on the recovery night as the index of the need to engage in fantasy. The model predicts that the less fantasy during REM deprivation, the shorter the REM latency on the subsequent recovery night. The obtained squared correlations of REM onset dreaming, NREM dreaming and sleep-onset dreaming during deprivation nights with REM latency during recovery nights, were only .02, −.08 and .13, respectively. When further corrected for baseline REM latency and baseline dreaming measured during sleep onset, REM and NREM sleep, these correlations were reduced even closer to .0. (Rich, Antrobus, Ellman & Arkin, 1975). We remind the reader that a much larger sample size is required to properly justify the application of these multivariate corrections. Nevertheless, a reasonable test of the model does call for such partialling procedures.

In conclusion, the mixture of negative findings of our work and that of Foulkes, et al. (1968), the positive findings of Pivik and Foulkes (1966), and the indications of the Cartwright et al. (1967; Cartwright & Ratzel, 1972) studies seem best explained with the current information we have by means of the formulations of Antrobus et al. regarding measurement and design in research on sleep mentation reports (see Chapter 3 of this volume). Of special relevance is their demonstration of the futility of using a sample size of less than 20 subjects in order to assess the relationship between sleep stage and mentation report variables. Studies that yielded results inconsistent with ours did not employ more than 16 subjects.

Possible ceiling-effect factors.   Although our subjects were selected for good dream recall, inspection of their baseline-REM and-NREM reports did not suggest any striking higher than average amount of dream-like mentation. Furthermore, the REM reports elicited during the middle and terminal baseline nights of our schedule in Experiment 3 were significantly *less* dream-like than those elicited on the first baseline night. This finding demonstrated flexibility of baseline levels and it is inconsistent with the hypothesis that observation of increases in dream-like mentation were precluded by a baseline that could not be surmounted because it was already at maximal intensity prior to the experiment.

The possibility of increases in NREM dreaming being detectable from pre-REMP NREM instead of post-REMP awakenings.   Setting to one side the technical question of the criteria by which the experimenter might decide that a given NREM epoch was very likely to be followed shortly by a REMP onset, a moment's reflection should make clear that when subjects are awakened frequently throughout the night, the sleep cycle must inevitably be disorganized. That is, under such circumstances pre- and post-REMP may lose any meaning they had under baseline conditions. And, in addition, when REMP onsets occur with progressive frequency, one cannot help but have a large proportion of awakenings within a short time of a prospective REMP. We do not feel, therefore, that our findings could be seriously questioned on these grounds.

The possibility of positive effects being discernible in Stage 3 or 4 mentation reports.   We cannot rule out such a possibility without empirical test. In the interest of avoiding overburdening an already immensely complicated protocol, we did not make provisions for this in our design. Furthermore, we are aware of no experimental finding that would lead one to expect positive results from slow-wave sleep awakenings in the absence of detectable suggestive effects in Stages REM, 2 and sleep onset of Stage 1 NREM.

The possibility of positive effects being discernible in wakeful mentation reports.   This issue is thoroughly reviewed by Hoyt and Singer in Chapter 14 of this volume. We need add nothing further except to say that the evidence does not support the possibility that significant amounts of dream-like mentation appears during wakefulness as a result of REM deprivation.

CONCLUSION

Let us hark back once more to some of our initial questions. What about the question of the need to have a certain amount of dreaming experience? Our results provide no evidence for the existence of such needs. Regardless of whether an unknown proportion of our subjects may have been classifiable as "substitutors" in Cartwright's (1967) terminology, the fact remains that they were all deprived of significant amounts of sleep in which their most vivid dreaming was known to have occurred (during baseline nights) and yet, there was no token of increases or appropriate alteration in dream-like mentation in three different sleep stages on the same nights. Surely, if psychological needs for dream-like fantasy were imperative, there should be some corresponding changes of sleep mentation sampled at other times. So our results speak against this hypothesis. Furthermore, one must conclude that those factors involved in REM sleep which produce manifestations of the need for REM sleep are relatively independent of those factors involved in REM sleep which are involved in dreaming.

Turning now to a related issue: to what extent does REM deprivation "equal" dream deprivation? In contrast to the earlier years of electrographic sleep research it is now generally accepted that dreaming occurs in NREM as well as in REM sleep. Thus, from one point of view, the question is obsolete. However, from another point of view our results indicate that although the sleeper may continue to have dreams during NREM sleep stages, REM deprivation does indeed deprive the subject of REM-sleep-associated dreaming—there is no evidence that the subject makes up for such losses at some other times; so one may conclude REM deprivation equals deprivation of REM-associated dreaming.

Finally, further examination of the results of Experiment 3 discloses that although increases in dream-like fantasy were not detected in any sleep stage in association with REM or NREM deprivation in any of the three experiments, there were differential patterns of change in the qualities of mentation occurring in three different sleep stages over the successive nights of the schedule; and the design of Experiment 3 permitted such tendencies to manifest themselves in the sharpest relief. These patterns are represented in Table 13.5.

First, with regard to order effects, REM mentation showed a significant decrease of dreaming within each set of two baseline nights, and decrease across the three sets of baseline nights as well. In contrast, no statistically significant order effects were observed for Stages 2 and 1 NREM.

TABLE 13.5

Differential Intensities of Dream-like Mentation
in Relation to Sleep Stages and Experimental Schedule

Sleep stage	Experimental Schedule Category		
	Within-baseline-night sets	Across-baseline-nights sets	Sleep-stage deprivation
REM	Significant decrease	Significant decrease	Slight but insignificant increase
Stage 2	Slight but insignificant decrease	No change	Significant decrease
Stage 1 NREM	No change	No change	No change

Second, sleep-stage deprivation (REM or NREM) resulted in a marked decrease in Stage 2 dreaming, a slight but insignificant increase in Stage REM dreaming, and once more, no change in that of Stage 1 NREM.

In summary, three distinct patterns of change were detected in the dreamlike qualities of the three sleep stages in relation to the experimental schedule: (1) Stage REM: order effect decrease within and across baseline sets: Stage 2: decrease during sleep deprivation (REM or NREM); and (3) sleep onset of Stage 1 NREM: no change throughout.

These different response patterns may be a reflection of several factors. For example, subject motivation may be unusually vulnerable during REM sleep awakenings and this might be partly responsible for the precipitous drop in dreaming in REM reports after the first baseline night (see Chapter 2 of this volume). Or it may be possible that, associated with each sleep stage is a somewhat different, more or less independent, organization of psychoneural components subserving cognition, and that the pattern and intensity of activity of each has a determining influence on mentation reports. Similar concepts have been advanced by Wilson and Zung (1966), Routtenberg (1966, 1968), and Freemon (1972).

That is, of the universe of neural-circuit complexes capable of subserving cognition, it is possible that factors associated with each sleep stage tend to selectively recruit more or less specially organized neural-circuitry subsets, and selectively inhibit remaining circuits (which in other stages of the sleep-wakefulness cycle, participate in cognitive processes characteristic of that particular stage). Each such subset would constitute a sleep-stage-associated psychoneural organization capable of cognitive functioning with relative degrees of independence one from the other; and such independence could be manifested in different patterns of cognitive response (in the three sleep stages) to sleep-stage deprivation as described above.

EDITORS' FOREWORD TO CHAPTER 14

It never seems quite possible that the strange fantasy of the night dream and the straight thought of the waking day are created by the same head. The contrast between the two has provoked many theses about what one says and does to the other. We no longer attribute supernatural powers to the dream but we do posit functions that are as extraordinary as the dream is unique. Thus while Fisher's (1965) notion that dreaming helps to avoid insanity had a short life in the research literature, it is sufficiently plausible to enjoy continued acceptance outside. Some physicians in an elite training hospital avoid very early morning surgery and the administration of REM-suppressing tranquilizers in order to minimize risk of psychotic behavior in their patients!

The possibility that one could be deprived of dreaming by eliminating Stage REM sleep made it possible to test experimentally various proposals about the need or function of dreaming. Hoyt and Singer provide us with a systematic review of the experimental literature for and against these notions. In so doing they examing psychoanalytic and cognitive models of dream function.

The latter part of the Chapter turns to an inquiry into which of the various properties of dreaming might have the functions attributed to the whole. They ask whether these properties are unique to REM sleep and unique to dreaming sleep. The inquiry moves on to consider whether some of the so-called functions of dreaming might be handled equally well by daydreaming. At this point they touch bases with Cartwright's model of fantasy and the importance of individual differences in fantasy (see Chapters 12 and 13 of this volume).

Finally, they consider the simple utility of dreaming as a novel distraction from waking stimulation and stress. All in all they not only systematically describe the research on the effects of dreaming on waking experience but suggest alternative ways to formulate the fundamental issues of interest.

J. S. Antrobus

14

Psychological Effects of REM ("Dream") Deprivation upon Waking Mentation

Michael F. Hoyt
University of California, San Francisco

Jerome L. Singer
Yale University

Long before the advent of modern science, man sensed an important link between sleep and dreams and mental well-being. Wie-Po Yang (c. 100-150 A.D.), known as the father of alchemy, advised that if one practiced alchemy falsely, disease would result and "Days and nights will pass without sleep . . . The body will be tired out giving rise to the appearance of insanity. The hundred pulses will stir and boil so violently as to drive away peace of mind and body. "Hippocrates noted the sleep disturbances of many of his patients (Volkan, 1962). Freud (1900/1060), himself a master student of the dream, reminds us of the link between dreams and mental illness observed by many of the great philosophers, recalling, for example, Kant's statement, "The madman is a waking dreamer"; and that of Wundt, "We ourselves, in fact, can experience in dreams almost all the phenomena to be met with in insane asylums." Other early psychiatrists also commented on the similarities between dreaming and madness. Bleuler (1908, cited in Karacan & Williams, 1970), for example, speculated" . . . it may well be possible to show the secondary symptomatology of schizophrenia as wholly identical with that of dreams," and the statements of C. G. Jung (1944), "Let the dreamer walk about and act like one awakened and we have the clinical picture of dementia praecox" and Jackson (1958), "Find out about dreams, and you will find out about insanity", are often quoted. Rosen's (1953) influential psychotherapeutic work continues the view of psychosis as a dream from which one cannot awaken.

Intriguing as these notions are, they were bound to remain at the level of speculation and clinical observation until reliable, objective indicants of dreaming could be identified. The pioneering research of Aserinsky, Dement, Kleitman, and their associates (Aserinsky & Kleitman, 1953, 1955; Dement, 1955; Dement & Kleitman, 1957a; Dement & Wolpert, 1958a; Wolpert & Trosman, 1958) made major contributions toward determining electrographic correlates of vivid nocturnal dreaming. When these early studies were published they seemed to hold promise for bringing to the experimenter for the first time a technique by which subjects could be deprived of dreams, permitting a direct experimental approach to the question, "What are the consequences for waking behavior of not allowing a person to dream?" In order to acquire the clearest picture of the status of current thinking in this area (which is at considerable variance with the simplistic notion that REM sleep and dreaming sleep are coterminal), it is best that we retrace our steps from the nuclear early studies.

The classical biological approach to exploring the function of an organ or system has been extirpation (Dement, 1969). The first "dream deprivation" experiment was conducted by Dement (1960a). After several nights of baseline recording, eight male subjects were REMP deprived for five consecutive nights by being awakened whenever their physiological record indicated they were entering the "emergent Stage 1 EEG-REM period." After this deprivation period, which Dement estimated reduced REMP time about 65-75% of what would have occurred without interference, subjects were allowed five "recovery" nights of undisturbed sleep.

The results of the Dement (1969) study were dramatic:

1. There was a progressive increase in REMP onset "attempts," that is, each night more and more awakenings were necessary to prevent subjects' going into REM sleep.

2. During the recovery phase, there was a marked elevation in REMP time relative to baseline levels.[1]

3. "Psychological disturbances such as anxiety, irritability, and difficulty in concentrating developed during the period of dream deprivation, but these were not catastrophic."

---

[1]This compensation or "rebound" effect has been replicated in numerous studies, including those of Agnew and Webb (1968); Agnew, Webb, and Williams (1967); Azumi and Ewing (1970); Azumi, Takahashi, Takahashi, Maruyama, and Kikuti (1967); Berger and Oswald (1962); Cartwright and Monroe (1968); Cartwright, Monroe, and Palmer (1967); Cartwright and Ratzel (1972); Clemes and Dement (1967); Dement (1965d); Dement and Fisher (1963); Dement and Greenberg (1966); Dement, Greenberg, and Klein (1966); Fisher and Dement (1963); Gulevich, Dement, and Johnson (1966); Johnson, Naitoh, Lubin, and Moses (1972); Kales, Hoedemaker, Jacobson, and Lichtenstein (1964); Rechtschaffen and Maron (1964); Sampson (1965); Snyder (1963); Vogel and Traub (1968c); Vogel, Traub, Ben-Horin, and Meyers (1968); Webb and Agnew (1965); Williams, Hammock, Daly, Dement, and Lubin (1964); Wyatt, Fram, Kupfer, and Snyder (1971); Zarcone, de la Pena, Kopell, and Dement (1970); and Zarcone, Gulevich, Pivik, and Dement (1968). Additional effects of REM deprivation include decrease in latency between sleep onset and beginning of first REM period (Rechtschaffen & Maron, 1964; Sampson, 1965; Vogel & Traub, 1968c and intensification of REM during recovery period (Pivik & Foulkes, 1966).

One subject quit the experiment in a panic, two insisted on stopping their dream-deprivation treatment one night early, at least one subject exhibited serious anxiety and agitation, and five subjects developed marked increases in appetite. None of these physiological or psychological effects were observed during a period of control awakenings (interruptions during non–REM sleep), thus ruling out the possibility that the obtained experimental effects were due to simple sleep loss or irritation/annoyance at repetitive awakenings.

To Dement (1969), these findings suggested:

> It is as though a pressure to dream builds up with the accruing dream deficit during successive dream deprivation nights–a pressure which is first evident in the increasing frequency of attempts to dream, and then, during the recovery period, in a marked increase in total dream time and percentage dream time.... [These results were] tentatively interpreted as indicating that a certain amount of dreaming each night is a necessity .... It is possible that if the dream suppression were carried on long enough a serious disruption of the personality would result.[2]

Subsequent investigations by Kales, Hoedemaker, Jacobson, and Lichtenstein (1964) and by Sampson (1965, 1966) followed up Dement's (1960a) report, each attempting to find systematic evidence of REM-deprivation-induced psychological changes.While both replicated the physiological (REM rebound) effect, neither found any substantial psychological changes to be reflected on the psychometric instruments they employed, although Sampson did report some clinical observations of adverse effects.[3] Clemes and Dement (1976) argued, however, that methodological weaknesses (such as choice of instruments) in the Kales et al. and Sampson studies render them of little value in determining the psychological effects of REM deprivation. To confirm the presence of changes as a function of REM deprivation, Clemes and Dement had six male subjects undergo six consecutive nights each of REM deprivation and six nights of (control) non-REM deprivation. In addition to obtaining the standard rebound effect of

---

[2]The quotation above, equating REM sleep and dreaming, must be regarded as representing an early position of Dement. As more careful inquiry methods have been incorporated into the research on reports following REM and non-REM sleep stage awakenings, the equation of REM sleep and dreaming has come under serious question (Foulkes, 1962). The indications that vivid dreaming could occur also during Stage 1 EEG periods at the onset of sleep without corresponding rapid eye movements had also weakened the link between the dream and the REM cycle (Foulkes 1966; Singer 1966). Further discussion of this issue is presented subsequently in this chapter and in other sections of the book.

[3]Along similar lines, Snyder (1963) very briefly reported that two subjects were "dream deprived" in his laboratory (for an unreported period of time), with the typical physiological effects, but that "It was not possible to demonstrate behavioral or appetite changes in our subjects, but neither were these present in all of Dement's (1960a) subjects." Foulkes, Pivik, Ahrens, and Swanson (1968) also failed to find any deleterious effects, depriving eight subjects of REM for one night (Editors' note: See also Vogel 1974)

increased REM following REM deprivation, Clemes and Dement observed significant changes in responses to projective tasks (Holtzman Inkblot Test and TAT-styled pictures), but not in aesthetic preferences (Welsh Figure Preference Test) or in mood self-reports (Nowlis-Green Mood Checklist). Subjects showed higher intensity of need and feelings and increased pathognomic verbalization on the TAT task; and less form appropriateness and decreased movement with the inkblots which Clemes and Dement (1967) interpreted as "suggestive of reduced ability to control." These findings, seen as indicating heightened drive conditions or depression of certain ego controls under REM deprivation, led Clemes and Dement to recommend projective techniques for clarifying psychological effects of REM deprivation.

Agnew, Webb, and Williams (1967) sought to compare the effects of REM deprivation and Stage 4 deprivation. Their six REM-deprived subjects showed the REM-rebound effect after seven deprivation nights, and the Stage 4 deprivation group ($N = 6$) showed a Stage 4 rebound effect on the first recovery night. No deprivation effects were obtained on performance tasks (such as pursuit-rotor, reaction-time, and paced-addition techniques), but differential psychological effects emerged in a variety of personality assessment instruments: the MMPI, the Pensacola Z scale, the Taylor Manifest Anxiety Scale, and Cattell's PF test. Test-by-test results were unfortunately not reported, but REM-deprived subjects were characterized by Agnew et al. (1967) as having become "less well integrated and less interpersonally effective. They tended to show signs of confusion, suspicion, and withdrawal. These subjects seem anxious, insecure, introspective, and unable to derive support from other people." Whereas Stage REM deprivation was seen as producing a state of higher irritability and lability, Stage 4 resulted in depression and reduced functioning, although no serious psychological or behavioral disruption was reported.[4] Studying 16 experimental and 16 control subjects, Chernik (1972) similarly found no substantial changes, although there was some tendency toward less friendliness, less vigorous activity, and more bewilderment, as assessed by the McNair Mood Scale, following two nights of REM deprivation.

TOTAL AND PARTIAL SLEEP LOSS

REM deprivation can be experimentally accomplished by three basic ways: (1) selective awakening when physiological indicants of REM sleep occur; (2) administration of REM-suppressing drugs (sometimes used in combination with the first method); or (3) total and partial sleep deprivation. Studies of total and

---

[4] A relatively small literature exists concerning the effects of non-REM deprivation. This topic generally falls outside the scope of this Chapter, however, and the interested reader is referred to Johnson (1973) for further discussion.

partial sleep loss can only be of limited value, however, in answering our questions about the consequences of REM deprivation. By nature, they confound REM deprivation with deprivation of other sleep stages, and with problems of general fatigue. Moreover, the results of such studies are not consistent: some, including the first, by Patrick and Gilbert (1896), reported deleterious effects (see Berger & Oswald, 1962; Friedman, Kornfeld, & Bigger, 1973; Luby, Grisell, Frohman, Lees, Cohen, & Gottlieb, 1962; West, Janszen, Lester, & Cornelisoon, 1962), while others report the absence or great reduction of sleep over prolonged periods to be harmless (see Gulevich, Dement, & Johnson, 1966; Jones & Oswald, 1968).

Related lines of research, such as those comparing naturally "long" and "short" sleepers (Hartmann, 1973) and "good" and "poor" sleepers (Monroe, 1967) are also inconclusive with respect to our topic. While such groups may experience different amounts of REM (dream) time, the possible effects of that differential experience are confounded with other potent sources of variance, such as the personality characteristics and life-styles of the subjects.

THE DEVELOPING CONTROVERSY: DOES REM DEPRIVATION PRODUCE MENTAL DISTURBANCE?

By 1963, Dement and Fisher were able to report on 21 cases of REM deprivation. The physiological effects first described by Dement (1960a) had held up, as had the psychological. Of the 11 subjects in the series who had been "dream deprived" 4 or more consecutive nights, "All showed, in one way or another, deteriorating tendencies during the period of dream deprivation which were not apparent during the period of control awakenings. They suffered greater or lesser degrees of anxiety, irritability, inability to concentrate, tiredness, etc. [Dement, 1960a]." Two subjects became somewhat agitated, one showed a marked change in Rorschach responses scored for primary-process manifestations, others showed "evidence of hallucination during photic stimulation at the height of dream deprivation," and six developed ravenous appetites and showed substantial weight gain during REM deprivation.

While these results may seem impressive, Dement and Fisher (1963) approached them conservatively, hoping to conduct "the crucial experiment [which] would be to dream deprive someone for an indefinite number of nights maintaining a reasonable amount of sleep until he either adapted to the procedure or showed some dramatic and unmistakable effect." Such an experiment was begun, with a single subject, but it became more and more difficult to arouse the subject from REM sleep, until, by Night 12 it was almost impossible to awaken him. At that time, during the day the subject had shown only minimal changes, and Dement and Fisher (1963) concluded that "we have not been able to demonstrate that the integrity of the waking personality is dependent on the nightly occurrence of dreaming. All we can say with assurance is that a curtailment of dreaming brings about an increased tendency to dream."

In a subsequent experiment, Dement (1964a) refined his technique in order to increase the completeness and duration of REM deprivation, by using loss of muscle tone as a more sensitive signal of dream onset and by further suppressing REM by presleep administration of dextroamphetamine. Two subjects were REM deprived, one for 15 consecutive nights, the other for 16. One subject showed no real personality change until after the fourteenth night of REM deprivation, and then "loosened up," freely·expressing anger and annoyance, and "wanting to do a variety of things quite impulsively, that normally he would not have considered doing. Among these was the desire to enter a tavern and cheat the waitress out of drinks, as well as a desire to go to a burlesque show." The other subject also showed a dramatic personality change, beginning after the thirteenth night of REM deprivation. Suspiciousness developed, and increased into paranoid ideation, together with a considerable amount of "autistic" material. Dement terminated REM deprivation to protect the subjects, and they returned to normal after the first recovery night.

The experience with these two subjects suggests that REM deprivation does have deleterious psychological effects, but also led Dement (1965d) to re-evaluate his earlier studies:

> "The kind of changes that were seen in the early deprivation experiments were not in evidence in the more recent studies. For example, the last 3 subjects (8, 15, 16 nights of REM deprivation by loss of muscle tone signal) did not become particularly anxious, they did not report any difficulty in concentrating and they did not develop changes in appetite. Since the last three subjects underwent much greater amounts of deprivation, and did not show these effects, it seems likely that the psychological changes observed in earlier studies were an artifact of the experimental procedures and the expectations of the experimenters."[5]

The idea that REM deprivation could be psychologically disruptive was not being dismissed; rather, the quality of the available evidence was being questioned (Dement, 1965c):

> We believe that REM sleep must have some important biological role to play, yet demonstrating this has been remarkably difficult. . . .clear-cut evidence that such deprivation is harmful has not been forthcoming. There have been many hints to this effect, but there have been such difficulties in instituting adequate controls that we have not considered the findings to be conclusive.

This view, however, apparently was not shared by Fisher (1965):

> A considerable amount of controversy has developed as to whether there is a "need" for Stage 1-REM sleep or a "need" for dreaming as a psychological event. It seems to me that such controversy is sterile and leads up a blind alley. There is no doubt that the dream-sleep cycle represents a highly important psychobiological cycle, interference with which can cause serious mental disturbances and, in turn, mental illnesses may be associated with fluctuations in the cycle . . .

[5]The interested reader is referred to Rosenthal and Rosnow (1969) for an extensive discussion of artifacts in behavioral research.

Fisher's theoretical perspective was the psychoanalytic view that dreaming has two basic interrelated functions: (1) the release of tensions via primary-process expression (the "safety-valve" function); and (2) the preservation of sleep by the representation of potentially disturbing wishes as fulfilled. As Freud (1938/1964) put it:

> We shall be taking all our observations into account if we say that every dream is an *attempt* to put aside a disturbance of sleep by means of wish-fulfillment. The dream is thus the guardian of sleep. This attempt can be more or less completely successful; it can also fail—in which case the sleeper wakes up, apparently aroused by the dream itself.

Such a model may be termed "hydraulic," suggesting a system in which

> ... dream deprivation, carried out intensively enough and for a prolonged period of time, might bring about a very large dream deficit, a great intensification of the pressure of instinctual drives toward discharge, eventual eruption of the dream cycle into the waking state and the development of hallucinations, delusions and other psychotic symptoms.(Fisher & Dement, 1963)[6]

Fisher (1965) amplifies this statement, and takes a conclusive position: "The recent work of Hoedemaker et al. [reported by Kales et al., 1964] and Dement [1964a] has demonstrated that such psychotic symptomatology does develop as a result of severe and prolonged dream deprivation."

Dement, who in 1969 again restated his belief that "Experiments involving prolonged REM sleep deprivation have not demonstrated that this procedure is harmful to the organism," was not the only one to disagree with Fisher's (1965) conclusions.[7] Giora (1971), for example, capsulized his views with the statement, "We can sum up, I think, that deprivation (or cessation) of dreaming does not inevitably lead to psychotic breakdown, or to other major disturbances in behavior." Johnson, Naitoh, Lubin, and Moses (1972) similarly observed, "REM deprivation in human subjects does *not* lead to specific psychopathological changes that are common to most subjects." After critically reviewing the research literature, including his own empirical contributions, Vogel (1968) took the position, similar to Dement's, that experimental artifacts could reasonably explain any positive findings that he had obtained: "I do not believe that the

[6]Fisher and Dement (1961, 1963) found a dramatic increase in REM time to occur with the onset of acute psychotic symptomatology. [Editors' note: Dement (1966) later mentioned that "a later re-evaluation suggested that this conclusion was in error and that it (REM time) had actually been reduced. A return to baseline accompanied the remission of the acute phase of the psychosis."] Zarcone, Gulevich, Pivik, and Dement (1968), subsequently also reported evidence of the opposite relationship, that is, a *decrease* in REM time associated with onset of acute psychosis.

[7]In their 1966 demonstration of rebound effects persisting until a delayed recovery period, Dement, Greenberg, and Klein found no psychological or behavioral changes resulting from five consecutive nights of REM deprivation.

studies cited by Fisher—or any other studies for that matter—have " 'demonstrated that hallucinations, delusions, and psychotic symptoms developed as a result of dream deprivation.' " Later, in the same paper, Vogel went on to summarize his view regarding the effects of REM deprivation:

> It may ... be reasonably concluded that REM deprivation does not produce psychological or behavioral disturbances. However, if REM deprivation does produce psychological disruption, it is clear from the studies of both man and animals that at least two weeks of almost complete loss of REM sleep are necessary, that minimal REM sleep protects against development of the presumed harm, and that minimal REM sleep reverses the presumed harm (one recovery night in most). It is doubtful that the necessary conditions for the presumed harm—long and continuous complete REM deprivation—ever occur in the natural state outside the laboratory.[8] This suggests that REM deprivation is not a cause or contributor to clinical illness in man.[9]

REM DEPRIVATION WITH PSYCHOPATHOLOGIC SUBJECTS

Vogel's empirical contributions are particularly interesting because they concern the effects of REM deprivation on already psychologically disturbed subjects. To gain additional information about whether REM deprivation is psychologically harmful or innocuous, and to test Fisher's "spillover model" (Fisher 1965; Fisher & Dement, 1963)—a model which proposes that psychotic symptoms are the intrusion or spillover of increased REM (dreaming) pressure into waking life—Vogel and Traub (1968c) systematically REM deprived five schizophrenics for seven consecutive nights. If Fisher's spillover model is correct, Vogel and Traub reasoned, their subjects would show increased psychotic symptoms during the deprivation period and/or during the early recovery period when REM time is elevated. Their results: subjects showed the standard physiological effects of a progressive increase in the number of required awakenings, with the awakenings becoming increasingly more difficult; a progressive decrease in latency to the first REM period; and REM compensation on recovery nights. Subjects' psychological responses were assessed with an extensive battery of tests (Bender Visual Motor Gestalt Test, Rorschach Inkblot Technique), standardized interviews, and ward-behavior rating schedules (Inpatient Multidimensional Psychotic

[8] At least one exception to this statement can be noted, although it supports Vogel's general argument. Dement (1965d) reported: "We studied a patient who had been taking at least a gram and a half of Tuinal every night for about ten years. This dose was also administered on the recording nights. No REMs were seen during sleep although periods of EEG activation and EMG suppression were present. If no REMs meant no dreaming, then it is likely that the patient had not dreamt for ten years. However, he was in very good shape psychologically."

[9] Some investigators have argued that REM deprivation plays an important role in the "psychosis" that sometimes results from prolonged total sleep deprivation. As we noted earlier, however this research is far from conclusive.

Scale, Psychotic Reaction Profile, Hospital Adjustment Scale). Vogel and Traub reported that there was no intensification of psychotic processes nor any psychological disruption, as indicated by the finding of virtually no changes in all patients on all the assessment instruments employed. In light of their negative findings, Vogel and Traub (1968c) concluded:

> Since our subjects were particularly susceptible to psychological decompensation, and since decompensation did not occur, the present study does not support the hypothesis that REM deprivation is psychologically harmful. The negative psychological findings of this study also do not support the hypothesis that schizophrenic symptoms are precipitated by REM deprivation or are related to marked increases of REM time.

Other studies of REM deprivation involving schizophrenics, however, have not uniformly reported results consistent with those of Vogel and Traub (1968c). For example, Azumi, Takahashi, Takahashi, Maruyama, and Kikuti (1967) deprived four normal and three schizophrenic subjects of REM sleep, generally for five nights, and found a marked depression in the REM rebound of the schizophrenics relative to the normal subjects. Although "no clear-cut psychotic states were induced in either the normal or the schizophrenic group," some minor disturbances did emerge; namely, "normals" complained of feelings of powerlessness and general malaise, although these feelings inexplicably decreased after the third day of REM deprivation, and two of the three schizophrenic subjects began making "non-significant stereotyped body movements." Zarcone, Gulevich, Pivik, and Dement (1968) found schizophrenic patients in remission to show striking REM-rebound effects following two nights of REM deprivation, whereas actively ill schizophrenics showed no REM compensation above baseline levels. Although they did not discuss the psychological effects of REM deprivation on their various groups, Zarcone et al. interpreted their physiological data as suggesting that REM sleep may be implicated in the psychotic process. Koranyi and Lehmann (1960) deprived six chronic schizophrenics of all sleep for 100 hr. This procedure of course confounds REM deprivation with non-REM deprivation and with effects due to general fatigue. Although other specific methodological flaws existed in this study, such as the subjects being continuously able to view one another's reactions, it is interesting to note that all six patients showed severe psychological disruption, five again manifesting the acute psychotic symptoms they had exhibited at the time of their hospital admission, with the sixth patient displaying gross regressive behavioral changes. Finally, in a somewhat different vein, 48 hr of total sleep deprivation (including confounded REM deprivation) has been shown to increase the psychotomimetic effects of LSD on normal subjects (Bliss, Clark, & West, 1959; Safer, 1970).

In the study reported by Vogel, Traub, Ben-Horin, and Meyers (1968), 5 psychotically depressed patients underwent REM deprivation for 7 to 14 nights. Two subjects showed notable clinical *improvement,* 1 minimal improvement, and 2 showed no psychological changes, supporting the prediction that degree of improvement would be directly related to a rapid and steady buildup of REM pressure. While the causes for the psychological gains are somewhat open to question, Vogel et al. emphasized that "it is clear that REM deprivation was not harmful to any of our depressed patients." More recently, Vogel et al. (1974) reported the results of a most impressive study on 49 patients, 33 of whom were ill with an endogenous depressive and 16 with a reactive depressive syndrome. REM deprivation, accomplished mechanically, was beneficial, but only to the endogenous group.

Evidence that REM deprivation might help to alleviate depression was also reported by Wyatt, Fram, Kupfer, and Snyder (1971), who totally suppressed REM sleep (and all indications of dreaming) by the administration of monoamine-oxidase inhibitors (MAOI) to their nonpsychotic anxious-depressed patients. All six subjects' behavior improved markedly when REM sleep was totally absent, although great REM rebounds occurred (up to 250% above normal levels) when the MAOI was discontinued for four of the subjects, with two of the subjects becoming profoundly anxious. Only one subject, who became hypomanic with the postdrug elevation of REM, did not return to his pre-MAOI state. Kramer, Whitman, Baldridge, and Lansky (1965) also report clinical improvement and a reduction of scores on a depression inventory following a 3-week course of im-ipramine, a REM-reducing drug.

DREAMS, KINESTHETIC EXPERIENCE, AND BODY IMAGE

Taking the work of Rorschach and Vold as her point of departure, Lerner (1966, 1967) theorized that ego integrity is dependent on a well-maintained body image, and that "dreams function as reinforcers of body image, and that they do this by providing a relatively unique opportunity for kinesthetic fantasy [1967]." This line of reasoning would suggest, in terms of projective responses to Rorschach cards, that subjects who have been dream deprived would show: (1) more move-ment (M) responses; and (2) a qualitative change in M responses in the direction of body-dissolution imagery. There is an extensive body of literature that links Rorschach human-movement responses to motor inhibition and to imagination (Singer, 1968).

In her test of these hypotheses, Lerner (1966) deprived 20 subjects of REM sleep for 2 nights by bedtime administration of d-amphetamine sulphate and pentobarbital sodium, and tested them with Holtzman inkblots before and after the deprivation. A control group (N = 30) was similarly tested, but without the deprivation treatment. The obtained data supported Lerner's predictions: pre-sumably dream-deprived subjects compensated for their loss by increasing M re-sponses in the Rorschach task; and moreover, "Body-dissolution imagery was rare in non-dream-deprived subjects and frequent in dream-deprived ones, and these differences were highly significant." These results, Lerner argued, support the notion of dream deprivation being a danger to personality integrity, and further suggest that this danger results from disruption of body-image maintenance via fantasized kinesthetic experience, and not from the prevention of drive discharge as one might expect from a Freudian model. Interpretation of these results must be qualified, however, since Lerner did not demonstrate actual REM deprivation but assumed it because of the presumed drug effect.

Consistent with Lerner's (1966) findings, Loveland and Singer (1959) and Palmer (1963) had earlier reported increased Rorschach M responses following a prolonged total sleep deprivation. Clemes and Dement (1967), however, reported a marginally significant ($p < .06$) decrease in their subjects' M responses on the Holtzman Inkblot Test following six consecutive nights of selective REM-sleep deprivation, although they did find REM-deprived subjects to show less form appropriateness with the inkblots and increased pathognomic verbalization on a TAT task. Vogel and Traub (1968c) found no changes in schizophrenics' Rorschach responses following REM deprivation; they do not, however, report scores for separate measures nor do they indicate having specifically examined M responses.

Supporting Clemes and Dement's (1967) statement that ". . . .projective tests appear to hold promise for clarifying psychological effects of selective REM sleep deprivation," several other investigations have reported positive results using projective techniques. Fiss, Klein, and Bokert (1966), for example, found that the TAT stories that subjects made up when interrupted during REM sleep were more "dream-like" (complex, visual, bizarre, emotional, vivid) than were the TAT stories produced upon interruption of non-REM sleep. Extending this line of research, Fiss, Ellman, and Klein (1969) found more dreamlike content in TAT stories told by subjects upon being awakened after completing approximately 75% of a REM sleep period than in stories told upon awakening either at the onset of REM or at the conclusion of a REM period. Moreover, a possible Zeigarnik-like effect was reported: After making up a TAT story, subjects were asked to describe any dreams they had been having before being awakened, and the majority of remembered dreams came after awakenings late in the REM period, that is, interrupted dreams were remembered better than completed ones (Rechtschaffen, Vogel, & Shaikun, 1963, had earlier noted the marked continuity of dream content following repeated REM-sleep interruptions; see also Fiss, Klein, Shollar, & Levine, 1968; Klein, Fiss, Shollar, Dalbeck, Warga, & Gwozdz, 1970.) Finally, Greenberg, Pearlman, Fingar, Kantrowitz, and Kawliche (1970) found three consecutive nights of REM deprivation to result in the overt appearance on projective tests (Rorschach, House-Tree-Person Drawing Test, Holtzman Inkblots) of presumed drive or conflictual material that had previously been well contained (a similar finding had been reported by Fiss et al., 1968), although no consistent effects obtained with respect to conventional variables such as the Rorschach M response.

In light of these equivocal findings, Feldstein (1972) sought to replicate Lerner's (1966) findings by demonstrating a quantitative change in subjects' Rorschach M responses as a result of REM deprivation, while at the same time rectifying some of the methodological problems that rendered earlier studies ambiguous; specifically, Feldstein's was a controlled study using projective-test evaluation, an adequate number of subjects ($N = 19$), and the forced-awakening method, in contrast to drug suppression of REM-sleep—conditions all of which had not been met in any previous study. His findings included the predicted increase in M projections, particularly using Holtzman's scoring system in responses to Holtzman inkblot plates which had been presented to subjects on awakening in the morning after three consecutive nights of REM deprivation. He also found an almost statistically significant increase in pathognomic (somewhat bizarre) verbalization.[10]

Additionally, subjects' field independence or field dependence (see Witkin, Lewis, Hertzman, Machover, Meisser, & Wapner, 1954), an important personality dimension, emerged as an influential determinant of pathognomic verbalization; contrary to prediction, the relatively field-independent group showed the significantly greater increase in pathognomic verbalization. These findings led Feldstein (1972) to conclude cautiously, ". . . it appears that the REM deprivation condition gives rise to a temporary dynamic change in the individual. For some subjects, this means greater attention to an ongoing inner process, while for others, it means retreat from this inner stream."

INDIVIDUAL DIFFERENCES IN RESPONSE TO REM DEPRIVATION

Results such as Feldstein's (1972) point to the importance of considering individual differences in studying the effects of REM deprivation. Beginning with Dement's (1960a) original report, considerable intersubject differences have been repeatedly observed with respect to such variables as amount of time spent

---

[10] Also pertinent here is the finding of Vogel, Giesler, and Barrowclough (1970) that subjects who engaged in physical exercise during periods of REM deprivation showed significantly less REM compensation effects on recovery nights than did control subjects who had not had "substitute" physical activity. It is interesting to speculate if the hyperactive life-styles of naturally "short" sleepers (Hartmann, Backeland, Zwilling, & Hoy, 1971) may in part be substituting for the kinesthetic dream experiences they forego by taking less than the normal amount of REM sleep (Webb & Friel, 1971). The hypothesis is not entirely straightforward, however, since short sleepers curtail both their REM and non-REM sleep. Webb (1969) observes: "I am personally prone to accept the notion that there are differential effects that accrue from differential deprivation. Generally speaking (from personal observation as much as from the data), I would suggest that REM deprivation results in a hyperactive and labile response state, whereas Stage 4 deprivation results in a hypoactive and depressed response state."

in REM sleep, frequency of attempts to enter the REM state, magnitude of the rebound effect, and possible untoward psychological effects.[11] As Witkin (1970) has observed:

> The kind-of-subject factor can be a particularly important contributor to inconsistent results when, as is so often true in monitored sleep research, the number of cases used is small. The importance of individual differences in the effects of REM sleep deprivation lies, however, not so much in their methodological nuisance value as in the route they open to more complete understanding of the function of REM sleep and the consequences of its loss.

Cartwright, Monroe, and Palmer (1967) were able to identify 3 general styles or patterns of adaptation after depriving their 10 subjects of normal REM sleep for 3 consecutive nights. One style, which Cartwright and co-workers called *disruption* was characterized by repeated attempts to enter REM during the deprivation period, but with EEG disruption and no REM rebound during the recovery period; subjects showing this pattern were "poor dreamers," relatively field dependent, and in an earlier study (Cartwright, 1966) had been very disturbed in their reaction to an hallucinogenic drug (piperidyl benzilate). Another response style was called *substitution* by Cartwright et al. (1967) and was characterized by reports of dream-like content upon REM awakenings but with no increase in REM on recovery nights. Subjects in this group, it was suggested, have greater access to their fantasies under all conditions, and could substitute dreaming in other stages for that ordinarily occurring in Stage REM, m;king such compensation unnecessary. Finally, the third style, called *compensation,* was most typical of field-independent persons, and included the standard REM-compensation effect during the recovery period. Subjects in this group were "good dreamers," seemed better able to tolerate REM deprivation, delayed fantasy gratification, and were well controlled during the psychedelic experience induced in the Cartwright (1966) study.

In another study in the same area, Cartwright and Monroe (1968) tested the notion that REM compensation would depend on what type of mental activity was substituted for the interrupted REM sleep during the deprivation period (see Vogel, Giesler, & Barrowclough, 1970). Specifically, their hypothesis, which their data confirmed, was that subjects who were allowed to report their dream mentation upon being awakened from REM sleep would, as a result of having continued access to their fantasies (see Fiss et al, 1966), find it unnecessary to "make up" their lost dream time, and would thus show no REM-rebound effect during the recovery period. And it was also hypothesized that subjects required

---

[11]The work of Foulkes and his collaborators (Foulkes 1966) made clear the fact that vivid dream reports at sleep onset without corresponding REM were obtained from subjects who were more psychologically stable and introspective or imaginative, as measured by questionnaires. The more neurotically inclined patients reported their most vivid dreams during the more intense REM periods much later in the night.

to perform a nonfantasy "filler" task (digit repetition) would be more completely deprived of fantasy mentation; and they did show the REM-compensation effect.

In a follow-up to the Cartwright et al. (1967) and Cartwright and Monroe (1968) studies, Cartwright and Ratzel (1972) explored the idea that the crucial variable in determining subjects' response to REM deprivation is the degree to which their dream-like fantasy is restricted to REM periods. Specifically, Cartwright and Ratzel (1972) predicted that subjects low in REM-onset fantasy (LOF) would show more psychological effects of REM deprivation than would subjects high in REM-onset fantasy (HOF), basing their hypothesis on the idea that:

> HOF subjects are not in any significantly different psychological condition during the waking period following REM deprivation due to their substitution of REM onset fantasy for that usually experienced during the REM time experimentally eliminated. LOF subjects, in contrast, are dream, as well as REM, deprived and so will be in a psychologically different state which will be reflected in a change on their psychollogical test performance."

The hypothesis was empirically supported in a study utilizing 10 subjects in all: following 3 consecutive nights of REM deprivation, LOF subjects showed more postdeprivation changes than HOF subjects. Specifically, LOF subjects showed changes reflecting an increase in accessibility to daytime fantasy: scores improved on the Wechler Adult Intelligence Scale (WAIS), largely accounted for by improvement on the Picture Arrangement subtest; and Rorschach M+ responses increased, and the experience balance shifted toward more introversive responses. Palmer (1963) had reported a similar shift following prolonged total sleep deprivation. Additionally, the increase of REM percentage on recovery nights was significantly greater for LOF subjects than for HOF ones, replicating the substitution-compensation distinction originally made by Cartwright et al. (1967). These findings led Cartwright and Ratzel (1972) to speculatively comment:

> . . . .it appears that subjects who ordinarily do not have much interplay between their internal fantasy and their waking test responses seem to gain something from a little REM loss. Here, the change rather than being in the nature of intrusions of uncontrolled hallucinations which disrupt reality contact, appears to involve a constructive use of fantasy which is integrated with reality responses.*

In a related line of investigation, Pivik and Foulkes (1966) studied the effects of "dream deprivation" on the content of subsequent dreams within a single night. They found that on experimental nights, when the first four REM periods were interrupted, the fifth period was marked by more intense dreams (tending toward the more perceptual, hallucinatory, and bizzare) than was a comparison period on control nights, when sleep interruptions were made during non-REM

---

*Editors' note: Further discussion of the stimulating work of Cartwright and her collaborators may be found in Chapters 12 and 13 of this volume.

periods. This effect was observed for both represser and sensitizer personality types, as determined by scores on Byrne's (Byrne, Barry, & Nelson, 1963) Repression-Sensitization Scale of the MMPI, but was statistically significant only for repressers. As Pivik and Foulkes noted, their dream intensification finding suggested that REM deprivation has immediate experiential, as well as physiological sleep-cycle effects, and points to the repression-sensitization personality dimension as a determining factor of the effects of REM deprivation. These sleep-cycle effects, however, were not observed in a later-attempted cross-night replication (Foulkes, Pivik, Ahrens, & Swanson, 1968), even though *all* subjects in that study were selected to be on the represser end of the continuum.

COGNITIVE-AFFECTIVE INFORMATION-PROCESSING APPROACHES

Various theorists (see Chernik, 1972; Greenberg, 1970) have suggested that REM sleep may play a crucial role in cognitive memory processes. Greenberg and Leiderman (1966), for example, suggested that dreaming transfers perceptions from short- to long-term memory stores, thus clearing the short-term areas for new perceptual input. This is, of course, a somewhat looser use of the concept of short-term memory than prevails in most experimental literature. Similarly, Dewan (1970), casting his theoretical framework in terms of a computer-programming model, has hypothesized that REM sleep involves a preparation for learning and a consolidation of information for long-term memory.

Unfortunately, the data for human subjects are ambiguous. Adelman and Hartmann (1968) deprived subjects of REM sleep by administration of appropriate suppressant drugs and found a decrement in short-term memory for nonsense syllables learned on the morning following deprivation. Studying 18 subjects, Feldman and Dement (1968) reported a long-term memory decrement for a serial anticipation task learned after one night of REM deprivation; but in a follow-up experiment, Feldman (cited in Chernik, 1972) was unable to replicate the effect following two nights of REM deprivation. Empson and Clarke's (1970) subjects listened to a tape-recorded list of nouns, 5 sentences, and a prose passage just before going to sleep; 10 subjects were REM deprived, 10 not; upon awakening, the REM-deprived group recalled less of all 3 types of material, especially the prose passage. In their study of 4 subjects, however, Greenberg et al. (1970) found 3 consecutive nights of REM deprivation to have no significant effects on the learning of paired word associates, and Chernik (1972), in a carefully controlled experiment, found 2 nights of REM deprivation to produce no significant differences between 16 experimental and 16 control subjects "on post-deprivation recall of paired-associate adjectives learned prior to deprivation or on the post-deprivation serial learning of trigrams." In light of the negative paired-associate results of the Greenberg et al. (1970) study, Greenberg (1970) concluded, somewhat hastily perhaps, "Thus it seems that dreaming is not involved in purely cognitive memory," but did suggest that dreaming may play an important role in what he calls "emotionally meaningful learning" and the psychological integration of emotional events.

The idea of dreaming serving as an arena for the "working over" of emotional material is not new. Freud (1920/1960), for example, interpreted the repetitive nightmares seen in war neuroses as unsuccessful attempts by the ego to master traumatic material. Similar theoretical positions, stressing the adaptive, coping functions of dreams, have been elaborated by numerous writers (see Greenberg, Pearlman, & Gampel, 1972). Laboratory evidence that stressful stimuli are incorporated into dreams has been reported by Witkin and Lewis (1965) and Collins, Davison, and Breger (1967), using emotionally-charged films as stimuli; by Whitman, Pierce, Maas, and Baldridge (1962), who found the experimental situation frequently appearing in their subjects' dreams; by Breger, Hunter, and Lane (1971a), who found surgical and group therapy patients' dreams to involve aspects of their stressful experiences; and by Greenberg, Pearlman, and Gampel (1972), who demonstrated a clear relationship between the psychological state of war-neurotic patients and the physiological (REM) concomitants of dreaming.

To experimentally test the hypothesis that dreams serve an ego-adaptive function, Greenberg, Pillard, and Pearlman (1972) had their subjects view twice an anxiety-provoking film of a medical autopsy, with a night of monitored sleep between viewings. Five subjects were allowed undisturbed sleep, nine were REM deprived, and six others awakened from non-REM sleep the same number of times a paired REM-deprivation subject was awakened. The Greenberg et al. (1972) data indicated that "for those who showed a significant anxiety response to the first viewing, the dream deprived group showed significantly less adaptation to the second viewing than the other two groups," results which the authors interpreted as supporting the hypothesis that dreaming aids adaptation to anxiety-provoking stimuli. Greenberg, Pillard, and Pearlman (1972) suggested:

> The person's initial defensive reaction (to a stressful situation) is usually of an emergency or generalized type (such as global denial or repression.) Then, during the dream experience . . . . the individual's characteristic defenses for that particular set of emotions and memories are used to deal with the current threat. If the stress is reexperienced, he now has available his characteristic (for him most efficient) means of dealing with the threat. Thus, re-exposure to the stress should not produce the initial degree of anxiety.[12]

[12]There are schools of psychotherapy (see Singer, 1971, 1974a) that have patients engage in intensive, more-or-less guided daydreaming, believing the fantasy experience to be, in and of itself, beneficial. Similarly in a preliminary report, Cartwright (1970) has described solutions to TAT-based problems reached after a night of sleep with dreaming as "more active, reasonable, and more ego integrated" than solutions reached after equal periods of normal wakefulness.

REM DEPRIVATION AND/OR DREAM DEPRIVATION?

Of what is one deprived in REM deprivation? Many researchers in the area have, on the basis of the correlation between REM and dream reports upon awakening, used the terms *REM sleep* and *dreaming* interchangeably, assuming that deprivation of the former is deprivation of the latter. But is this equation justified? The evidence suggests it is not.

First of all, there is the simple fact that the correlation between REM and dream reports is not unitary: REM sometimes occur without concomitant dreaming, and equally important, dream mentation sometimes occurs during non-REM sleep (Foulkes, 1962; Kales, Hoedemaker, Jacobson, Kales, Paulson, & Wilson, 1967; Rechtschaffen, Verdone, & Wheaton, 1963), and can even extend into the waking period (Fiss et al., 1966).* And then there is the suggestion (Cartwright & Monroe, 1968; Vogel et al., 1970) that other forms of activity can apparently substitute for interrupted REM sleep, obviating need for subsequent REM compensation. Additionally, evidence is now emerging (Globus, 1966; Kripke, 1972; Kripke & Sonnenschein, 1973; Othmer, Hayden, & Segelbaum, 1969) that REM cycles are not restricted to sleep, but rather, that the approximately 90-min REM cycle continues throughout wakefulness. Finally, as several writers (e.g., Giora, 1971; Klinger, 1971; Kubie, 1962; Singer, 1966) have pointed out, mental activity is varying but incessant, continuously flowing in what Kubie (1962) calls "the preconscious stream." With other avenues for fantasy available (such as artistic activity, daydreaming, play, television), the concept of successful, prolonged "dream" deprivation seems dubious. As the evidence we have reviewed demonstrates, fantasy expression is phenomenologically mercurial: if temporarily blocked in one channel, the "preconscious stream" seems to shift its "flow" into another outlet. This interference with a habitual mode of expression may be temporarily somewhat disturbing to the economy of the personality, but generally does not eventuate in serious disruption owing to the plasticity of the system, that is, alternative modes are soon found.*

However, as Giora (1971) puts it, "one *is* deprived of something, if not of dreams, in REM deprivation." Some theorists (eg., Kleitman, 1963, 1970; Snyder, 1963) have viewed dreaming as a mere epiphemonenon or habitual, functionless accompaniment of the physiological processes associated with REM sleep. Other writers (see Johnson, 1973; Snyder, 1967) have also assigned the subjective, psychological experience of dreaming a minor role, instead emphasizing hypothetical cognitive mechanisms underlying the REM state. Dement (1965c,

---

*Editors' note: Strictly speaking, it was not dream mentation itself that Fiss and co-workers found to extend into the waking period but rather the increased likelihood of elaborating dream-like protocols in response to TAT cards following REMP awakenings.

1969) has focused attention on the biochemical aspects of REM sleep.[13] But whatever the final conclusion, it seems REM must play some important role:

> The REM phenomenon is so ubiquitous, so complex, and so well represented in terms of brain areas allocated to its structures and mechanisms that it is not likely to have evolved solely as a caprice of nature. We must therefore assume that it does have a vital role to play—a role which we will eventually be able to describe with precision and profit [Dement, 1969].

SOME THEORETICAL APPROACHES AND IMPLICATIONS

An effort to address the question of REM function called for by Dement has recently been presented by Hartmann (1973). Indeed it is perhaps the most intriguing theoretical approach yet proposed to integrate REM sleep, dream content, and daytime mentation. The details of his position need not be elaborated on in this chapter; but, essentially, they emphasize quite different functions for NREM and REM sleep cycles. Using S sleep to denote NREM and D sleep to denote REM, Hartmann proposes that S sleep has a general physiological restorative function essential for normal bodily processes, while D sleep has a more specialized role in relation to the "reprogramming" of complex unfinished businesses of the day, stresses, and the strain of maintaining alertness and focussed attention. Hartmann proposes that a critical balance of the catecholamines is necessary for optimal information processing and organized thought which characterizes the waking state. To a certain extent the complexity of daily information processing depletes the catecholamine balance, and requires its restoration during sleep. Support for the general position is detailed at some length in Hartmann's book. The special qualities of night dream, particularly as manifested during D sleep, reflect the absence of the "flexible focused attention," organized environmental patterning, and a "feedback-modulated internal guidance system." Hartmann (1973) writes, "It is exactly these subtle feedback guidance systems, especially characteristic of mammalian waking brain function, which I have suggested wear out somewhat during tiredness and may be completely shunted out for repairs during D-sleep."

In effect, Hartmann's proposal is that while the dream itself in its content may have no special significance in producing any physiological change, it

---

[13]Fisher (1965) dismisses the idea of considering the function of REM sleep solely in terms of underlying somatic and physiochemical processes without attention to the concomitant psychic events of dreaming: "Dement's idea that the function of REM sleep is to clear the nervous system of some endogenous metabolite is not more informative than some equivalent statement that the function of thought is to clear the nervous system of the acetylcholine used up in the transmission of nervous impulses involved in psychic activity."

may represent a kind of "window" into the underlying physiochemical processes. During D sleep, in effect then, new connections are being formed, especially with respect to those cortical areas served by the ascending catecholamine pathways. These new associative links are presumably between various unfinished elements from daytime experience and older "pathways." Hartmann points out that the concept of the Freudian wish is not critical here. Since childhood memories are of course a part of the great substrate of memory schema, they are likely to be organized around drives or wishes. A high percentage of linkages between the "day residue" and such wish-related materials is therefore evident when examining dream reports.

A key portion of Hartmann's argument, particularly with respect to the way in which the dream may provide a clue about the nature of the processes underlying D sleep, is his presentation of a series of functions, such as subtle emotionality, indications of fatigue, highly focused and distractible attention, reduction in logical thought, and the lack of "continuing sense of self." All seem to be characteristic of dreaming thought. Hartmann (1973) writes:

> ... those functions ... which occur in waking but *not* in dreaming, are functions of the cortex under the influence of catecholaminergic neuronal systems; those I see as being repaired during sleep and perhaps 'shunted out' for purposes of repair and reworking; thus the dream can show us the functioning of the brain when the catecholamine influence is removed.

Admittedly, Hartmann's position is speculative, but it allows us an entry point to raise a question about much of the literature on the presumed influence of REM sleep deprivation on daytime mentation. There is presently a tremendous imbalance in the emphasis of the dream-research literature on the nature of thought during sleep in relation to the complexity of the daytime thought processes. Very few of the investigators have sought to examine the complexity and richness of ongoing waking cognitive activity. The tendency, as a matter of fact, is to write as if the normal stream of consciousness and sequence of mental processes of the waking adult or child is characterized by a kind of logic and orderliness and freedom from wishfulness, speculation, and fantasy. Yet extensive research carried out by Singer (1966, 1974b) and various collaborators (Antrobus, Singer, Goldstein, & Fortgang, 1970) suggests that daytime mentation is more or less continuous and full of imagery, illogical leaps, and wishful or frightening sequences of fantasy and anticipation. Content analyses suggest that night dreams often contain fairly complex secondary process thinking, and daytime thought trends in structure and content are comparable to night dream contents (Starker, 1974).

A study that also raises some question about the emphasis on night-dream cycles and points the way toward an entire new direction for research has been that by Kripke and Sonnenschein (1973). The evidence reported by those authors of a 90-min daily cycle during a 10-hr waking period with daydreaming, characterized by vivid fantasies, minimal rapid eye movement, and elevated alpha rhythms recurring regularly raises the possibility that what is seen at night during sleep is only a small fraction of the complex cognitive processing underway.

Although the extensive work on daydreaming and the stream of thought has not as yet emphasized the cyclical patterning observed by Kripke and Sonnenschein, much of this research also makes clear the extent to which there is indeed considerable variability and fluctuation in the levels of cognitive activity produced. Subjects seated in darkened rooms with the task of detecting signals which require highly focused attention in order to produce accurate responses (if questioned every 15 sec) report a very high frequency of fantasy-like thoughts. These are predominantly visual images. They include a range of content from fairly logical through somewhat bizarre or unusual fantasies (Singer, 1974b; 1975; Antrobus, Singer, Goldstein, & Fortgang, 1970) Add to this evidence the indications, by now well established, that a considerable amount of thought activity occurs even in non-REM sleep and indeed that it is difficult frequently to discriminate these contents (Van de Castle, 1971).

We are left with the possibility that the differences in mentation between day and night may not be as readily attributable to fundamental physiological processes as Hartmann (1973) and others would suggest. As a matter of fact, Hartmann's theory of catecholamine restoration is not incompatible with the view that much daytime thought is made up of brief fantasies, images, and slightly bizarre turns of logic. Abstract, logical, and highly concentrated mentation is generally accepted as more demanding and can be carried on only briefly. Head's (1926) concept of central vigilance, so fragile and so susceptible to fatigue or brain damage, comes to mind. Perhaps catecholaminergic restoration is going on much more of the time than just during nocturnal D sleep.

A possibility that also might be considered is that the act of shutting one's eyes or in general relaxing, which of course characterizes sleep, drastically reduces the information-processing load on the sensory system. If we can make the assumption that the brain is actively processing material in its long-term storage system more or less continuously, and that such processing activity is, in effect, the very way in which the brain stores material (rather than simply putting it in a *place* as one might characterize computer storage), then reducing the *external* information load might increase the degree of awareness of this other *internal* source of stimulation. It is easy enough to produce material that bears all of the characteristics of dreamlike thought by having subjects relax with eyes open or shut on a couch or an easy chair and engaging in one of the kinds of "imagery trips" employed in the European mental imagery methods (Singer, 1974b). There are also indications that if we are engaging in daydreaming or elaborate fantasies, whether involuntarily or upon demand, we find it necessary to fix our eyes or to gaze upon some blank wall in order to reduce the elaborate visual content that characterizes extended searches of the long-term memory system (Antrobus, Antrobus, & Singer, 1964, Singer & Antrobus, 1965, Singer, Greenberg, & Antrobus, 1971).

In addition to these studies of ongoing mentation, there is ample evidence from large-scale data collection through questionnaires and interviews to the effect that most normal adults reported considerable amounts of daydreaming and related cognitive activity during the day (Singer & Antrobus, 1963; Singer & Antrobus, 1972). Indeed, factor-analytic studies, using various forms of the Imaginal Processes Inventory developed by Singer and Antrobus, (1972) have yielded replicable factors on a variety of young adult samples, suggesting at least three major patterns of ongoing thought: guilt-negatively toned emotional daydreaming, anxious-distractible daydreaming, and positive vivid styles of daydreaming. Starker (1974) has recently presented evidence that night-dream logs of subjects who represent extremes on each of these daydreaming patterns are characterized by comparable content preoccupations. Extensive research by Giambra (1975) on the pattern of daydreaming associated with the aging process from late adolescence through the 70s has also replicated the basic factors described above and has found differential reductions in the three factors with increasing age. His data suggest that positive-vivid daydreaming shows relatively little decline over the life span compared with the more negatively toned daydream patterns.

It seems a reasonable possibility, therefore, that the nature of human thought is continuous with certain fluctuation in the degree of "logicality" or formal organizational characterizing such thought, depending probably to a great extent on a combination of information-processing load, task demand, social role demand, and cognitive style or intellectual capacity of the individual. The so-called fanciful nature of many kinds of daydreams need not necessarily be viewed as indications of regression or primitive thought. They may probably be regarded as alternative approaches to problem solution and anticipatory planning which may have useful functions in their own right. In this sense, the so-called "regression in the service of the ego" (Kris, 1952) that is frequently reported in the case of creative individuals may simply represent a more flexible and differentiated facet of human thought capacity that may be appropriate for certain types of problem solutions in both the sciences and the arts. Indeed, there are indications that persons who are capable of extensive and elaborate waking thought, such as artists and scientists, may also produce more complicated and interesting nightdream material. The much-cited instance of Kekulé discovering the carbon ring in his dream must be regarded in the light of his already being an established and imaginative investigator who probably spent a good deal of waking time thinking about the same problem.

We ought not overlook the great role that individual differences might play in the effects of REM deprivation on daytime thought. What can we make of the findings of Cartwright and her collaborators (e.g., 1967, 1972), of Feldstein (1972), or the differences observed by Hartmann (1973) between long and short sleepers? Unfortunately, without comparable measures in these studies it is hard to make definitive statements about the specific patterns of individual differences. There are suggestions that persons more attuned to or accepting of daytime fantasy (which might include Cartwright and Ratzel's [1972] high-REM-onset dreamers) are less needful of the "biochemical" support of REM sleep. Foulkes (1966) had found greater psychological-mindedness and inner-living characteristic of persons who produced more sleep-onset dreams. We need studies that take into account more fully the daytime mentation patterns of persons who are later subjected to interruptions in REM sleep. Hartmann's (1973) "long sleepers," who are characterized as more given to worry and dysphoric moods but who also seem more creative and nonconformist than his "short sleepers," might be tested for daydreaming behavior on the Singer-Antrobus (1972) Imaginal Processes Inventory and then studied by a Kripke-Sonnenschein interruption method throughout the days prior to several nights of REM deprivation. Such a study might help us tie down the presumed continuity between daytime mentation and the function of REM sleep by indicating whether certain patterns of daydreaming and night-sleeping tendencies were linked to differential patterns of resolution of unfinished business by daytime-fantasy activity as against nighttime REM-dream patterns.

The presumed differences in logic and organization between waking and sleeping mentation may be regarded at the cognitive level, first, as a consequence of the change in complexity of ongoing processing of externally derived material; and second, as a function of the nature of attributions assigned to sleep by the individual in a social context. (See Jones, Kanouse, Kelley, Nisbett, Valins, & Weiner [1971] for a discussion of attribution theory.) Social psychology has recently examined much more extensively the ways in which people assign causes to behavior. There is reason to believe that group pressures, for example, may play as much a role in our method of describing emotions as in any distinctive character that emotions may have purely on a physiological basis. That such social attribution processes do indeed play an important part in relieving insomnia has been reasonably well demonstrated (Davison, Tsujimoto, & Glaros, 1973; Storms & Nisbett, 1970). In effect, the various reasons we give ourselves for going to sleep and for what we expect during sleep may play a key role, not only in how quickly we get to sleep or how well we sleep, but in the kinds of thought content in general we are likely to experience during the night and what we are likely to reminisce and rehearse and, therefore, remember as dreams upon awakening in the morning.

This somewhat extended discussion should lead the reader to be more cautious in making assumptions about presumed daytime consequences of various nocturnal-sleep-cycle-deprivation states. Indeed, we would probably be well advised to concentrate more extensively on a significant analysis of first, the topography or possible cyclical pattern of ongoing daytime reverie; and second, various conditions that demand different levels of cognitive functioning and their potential effects upon sleep. The position taken here, then, is that much thinking involves sets of expectations and anticipations, as well as evaluations of ongoing events. These form the stream of consciousness. Behavior such as ease or difficulty of falling asleep would then depend in part on the relationship to the setting of expectations and the interpretation of sleep assigned by the individual. Certainly it is clear that no matter how fatigued an individual may be, the knowledge that some major event of great importance awaits upon awakening in the morning may lead to extreme difficulty in actually falling asleep, as the unfinished content and anticipation of this event runs round and round in the individual's head while he or she prepares for sleep.

It seems unlikely that sleep alone or, specifically, REM sleep, provides any sufficient restorative function or problem solution for the day's unfinished activities. Most studies of dream content reveal a predominance of negative or problematic material, although admittedly, without quite the degree of emotional edge that one finds in daytime worries. It is possible to regard going to sleep as providing a change of style that reduces the complexity and tension which characterizes much unfinished business in one's daily life. It therefore leads at least to a temporary diversion from the previous day's aroused affects of anger or distress. By distracting ourselves from the high level of the day's tension, we can awaken in the morning in a better mood. Indeed, to the extent that dream content does by its nature involve the intermingling of jumbled elements of previous experience with material from the remote past and hence involves a certain amount of novelty, our mood may be one of interest and curiosity, which, as we awake in familiar surroundings, turns to a mild experience of pleasure or joy (Tomkins, 1962, 1963). These notions are, of course, also speculative, but again they point out the possibility that we need to review the emphasis in studies of night dreaming to take into account the broader patterns of ongoing cognitive and emotional functioning of the individual and the social context which may play a role in determining one's orientation towards sleep and one's expectations about dreams and related cognitive activity during sleep. The well-demonstrated physiological changes characterized by interruptions in the regular cycle of Stage 1-REM sleep are certainly worth studying. The assumption that these processes are specific to certain cognitive and imaginative psychological functions is far from demonstrated. The time seems ripe to study more extensively daytime cycles, cognitive styles, and daydreaming patterns; and then to observe their impact on patterns of day and night physiological cycles.

One approach might be to examine careful ratings of thought content obtained from daytime mentation reports at different points of the Kripke-Sonnenschein (1973) 90-min cycle and to compare them with differences between REM- and non-REM- or deprived- and nondeprived-REM-state reports of mentation. If there is a fundamental physiological process involved in generating nighttime REM mentation (as a function, for example, of catecholaminergic restoration or a similar theory) than one should find gross differences in ratings of the logical structure or organizational characteristics of daytime and nocturnal reports. REM deprivation might lead to more clear-cut alterations of daytime mentation, somewhat along the line reported by Feldstein (1972) using Rorschach measures of pathological responses. At least the possibility of testing a set of fairly specific hypotheses including some alternative deductions critical to theory exists if we can begin to take more seriously the possible continuity of day and nighttime mental activity and include our waking stream of consciousness (Singer, 1974b) with its complex meanderings as part of our effort to understand the dream process.

Part **VI**

CLINICAL PHENOMENA IN RELATION TO SLEEP MENTATION

15

Sleeptalking

Arthur M. Arkin
City College of the City University of New York

In this chapter I am concerned chiefly with the scientific literature on somniloquy which has come to my attention or has been published since my first review (Arkin, 1966). Readers interested in details of the descriptive psychiatry of sleep talking, and in the history of related scientific psychoanalytic and philosophic commentary are referred to this earlier paper.

Sleeptalking (somniloquy) is defined as the utterance of speech or other psychologically meaningful sound in association with sleep, without simultaneous subjective critical awareness of the event.

How Common is Sleeptalking?

It is generally agreed that sleep speech is more frequent than is appreciated, largely because potential observers are usually asleep when episodes take place (Arkin, 1966; Arkin et al., 1970a), and the sleep talkers themselves tend to have no memory of the event. The most recent known attempt to estimate the incidence of somniloquy was made by Gahagan (1936), who asked 228 male and 331 female college students to fill out an extensive 23-item questionnaire pertaining to such sleep characteristics as dreams, recurrent dreams, sleepwalking, sleeptalking, and the like. Of this group, 65 and 57% of the females and males, respectively, reported a history of sleep talking (combined percentage 61%). Of those so reporting, 176 (51% of erstwhile sleeptalkers) stated that sleeptalking had persisted until the time of the survey. Gahagan believed that the elusiveness of the phenomenon makes any figure, based on self-report, lower than the real incidence. For this reason Gahagan (1936) concluded that a "history of sleeptalking should be considered normative, i.e. modal [p. 234]."

In our own laboratory investigations (Arkin et al. 1970a), it was usually an easy matter to obtain experimental subjects volunteering a current sleep-talking history. Our pool of paid subjects consisted of 17 females and 26 males. Two were high-school students, 1 was a medical technician, and 1 was a professional subject in the teaching of medical hypnosis, and the remaining 39 were college students or recent graduates. With a few exceptions, our subjects volunteered in response to advertisements for sleeptalkers, posted at the placement bureaus of several colleges in New York City.

Baseline records of undisturbed nights' sleep were recorded with 13 subjects. This yielded a total of 206 speeches uttered during 53 such nights (mean = 3.9 speeches per night). Ten subjects spoke 1 or more words at least once, one merely moaned, groaned and emitted other types of sounds and the remainder failed to vocalize in any significant manner.

In an independent study, MacNeilage (1971) found that of 5 subjects who volunteered a history of sleep-talking 4 somniloquized at least once in 6 nights, and uttered a total of 28 speeches and 54 nonlinguistic vocalizations in the same period.

Are Specific Organismic Factors Associated with Sleep-Talking Propensities?

More than 70 paid adult volunteer subjects who alleged that they had spoken in their sleep at some time in their lives were interviewed. It was our impression that sleep talking per se was not associated with any specific psychiatric syndrome. The symptom occurred in a wide range of personalities, namely people with borderline schizophrenia, psychoneuroses, and character neuroses of various types, overt homosexuality and, those with insignificant or no easily detectable psychopathology. Sleeptalking is apparently so widespread that it was difficult to locate individuals in a college population who have *never* been told by someone, at least once in their lives, that they had talked in their sleep. Comparison of the sleep talkers with a nonsleeptalking control group from the same college populations (by means of a life-history questionnaire and interview) revealed no psychodynamic or genetic patterns typical of sleeptalkers in contrast to the non-sleeptalkers. This conclusion finds considerable support from an independent study of Bone et al. (1973), in which 27 males and 39 female sleeptalking college students were compared to 12 male and 19 female non-sleeptalkers by means of a test of 16 Personality Factors. Differences were revealed for only two factors: female sleeptalkers scored higher on radicalism ($t = 2.95; p = .01$); and male sleeptalkers scored lower on superego strength ($t = 2.08; p = .05$). These results seem more or less consistent with our earlier conclusion that sleeptalkers do not differ from nonsleeptalkers in any gross, striking manner; and that the two groups are more similar than different (Arkin 1966). However, Mac-Neilage et al. (1971, 1972, 1973) found a significant association on questionnaire responses between subjects' estimates of their sleeptalking propensities and their estimates of their dream recall. That is, while subjects with high recall of dreams may or may not sleep-talk, subjects who recall few dreams are much less likely to be sleep-talkers (MacNeilage, 1971, p. 100).

Finally, several investigators have reported that subjects with somnambulism and night terrors also tend to talk in their sleep. (Fisher et al. 1973a; Gastaut & Broughton, 1965; Kahn et al., 1973; Kales & Jacobson, 1967).

Thus, the future possibility of finding subtle psychological differences between sleep talkers and "silent sleepers" cannot be excluded.

Do Available Laboratory Studies Throw Any Light on the Issue of Specific Physiological Factors?

MacNeilage (1971) selected 5 subjects who were good dream recallers and who had claimed that they talked in their sleep at least occasionally. In the laboratory, over a period of 6 nights, 3 subjects talked in their sleep on 27 occasions, 1 talked only once and 1 not at all over the same period. (The latter 2 were grouped as nonsleeptalkers). The speech musculature of the sleeptalkers displayed much more frequent and intense occasions of electromyographic activity through the night (although only a small proportion of such occurrences was associated with actual vocalization).

Considering the information available from all known studies, the importance of physiologic factors is strongly indicated by the striking individual differences among subjects, with respect to quantity of sleep speech, the sleep stages with which the somniloquy tends to be associated, and the content and degree of linguistic correctness of the speeches. The details of these differences become apparent as we proceed. However, samples are too small and the variability of the phenomena too large to permit definitive statements to be made as to degrees of association between possible specific organismic factors and the above parameters.

What Are the Electrographic Concomitants of Somniloquy?

In general, the electrographic characteristics of most sleep speech occurrences are consistent with those criteria described for "movement arousal" episodes (regardless of sleep stage) by Rechtschaffen and Kales (1968; Arkin et al., 1970c; Cohen et al., 1965; Gastaut & Broughton, 1965; Kamiya, 1961; MacNeilage 1971; Rechtschaffen et al, 1962; Szabo & Waitsuk, 1971; Tani et al., 1966). This does not make the two identical, however. For example, the question is still unanswered as to why some such movement arousals are accompanied by vocalization and others not. Also, there is great variability in electrographic concomitants of sleep-speech episodes both within and across subjects. Because of this variability, meaningful quantitive comparison is difficult and most commentary in the literature (with a few minor exceptions (Cohen et al., 1965;

TABLE 15.1

Somniloquy in Association with Sleep Stages

Study	Number of subjects	Total number of episodes	Percentage by sleep stage (rounded off)	
			NREM	REM
Kamiya (1961)	Not specified	98	88	12
Szabo et al. (1971)	10	Not specified	100	0
Gastaut and Broughton (1965)	Not specified	Not specified	92 By sleep stages 1 = 33 2 = 33 3 = 17 4 = 9	8
Rechtschaffen et al. (1962)[a]	28	84	92 1 = 0 2 = 63 3-4 = 29	8
Rechtschaffen et al. (1967)[a]	28	28	86 1 = 0 2 = 43 3-4 = 43	14
Tani et al. (1966)	3	8	0	100
MacNeilage (1971)	4	28	82 1 = 11 2 = 68 3 = 3	18
Arkin et al. (1970a)[b]	10	206	52 1 = 4 2 = 19 3 = 13 4 = 16	48
Arkin et al. (1970a)[b]	9	105	81 1 = 1 2 = 27 3 = 26 4 = 27	19

[a]Because of the possibility that the distribution of sleep speech episodes among the various sleep stages was biased by data from a minority of the subjects, Rechtschaffen et al. (1962) recalculated their results on the "basis of one incident selected at random from each subject. This calculation reduced the number of incidents to 28, of which 4 (14%) were in REM periods, 12 (43%) were in Stage 2, and 12 (43%) were in Stages 3 and 4 [p. 420]."

In attempting to arrive at a comparable value of the central tendencies of the data from our own subjects (Arkin et al. 1970a), we determined the average percentage (*across* subjects) of sleep speech episodes in each sleep stage (not tabulated). The results were as follows: NREM Stage 1, .9%; Stage 2, 21.5%; Stage 3, 21.5%; and Stage 4, 28.5%; total NREM

MacNeilage 1971; Tani et al., 1966;) describes what seem typical on the basis of inspection of large numbers of records rather than precise measurements.

What Are the Relationships Between Somniloquy Episodes and the Various Stages of Sleep During Which They Are Prone To Occur?

There is general agreement that most sleeptalking occurs in association with stage NREM sleep although a definite, albeit smaller, proportion of episodes occur in association with stage REM.

Furthermore, I wish to emphasize again that among our own subjects, individual differences were marked, that is, some were loquacious, others somewhat reticent; some spoke entirely in association with NREM sleep, others both in association with NREM and stage REM (our most prolific sleeptalker spoke predominantly in association with stage REM.) Rechtschaffen et al. (1962) also noted that stage REM episodes occurred with subjects who also produced NREM incidents. The results of reports in literature are presented in Table 15-1.

The data of Tani et al. (1966), and our own (Arkin et al., 1970a) in the table are the results from baseline nights of undisturbed sleep. The experimental conditions for the entire populations of the other studies were heterogeneous, including baseline nights, nights with experimental awakenings and possibly other types of unspecified manipulations.

In summary, about 80% or more of sleep-utterance episodes are associated with NREM sleep and 20% or less with stage REM.

Does Somniloquy Tend to Occur at Certain Times of the Night and/or in Association with Specific Portions of the Sleep Cycle?

Rechtschaffen et al. (1962) concluded that "the chance sleep-talking would occur during any one particular hour of sleep was about as great as the chance that it would occur during any other hour [p. 421]," and that "NREM" sleep-

---

72.3%; Stage REM, 27.7%. Omitting the exceptionally prolific Stage REM sleeptalker mentioned above yielded NREM Stage 1, 0.1%; Stage 2, 22.5%; Stage 3, 23.9%; and Stage 4, 31.4%; total NREM, 77.9%; Stage REM, 22.1%.

[b]The first entry with 10 subjects contains an unrepresentative high percentage of Stage REM-associated sleep speech. This "disproportion" is the result of our most voluble sleeptalker who contributed 101 speeches to our total sample of sleep speeches collected under conditions of baseline undistrubed sleep. The subject spoke mostly in association with Stage REM and uttered 79 of our 99 Stage REM speeches. The second entry with 9 subjects omits the contribution of this unusual subject and the results more closely resemble those of the other studies.

talking never initiated REM periods p. 421]." In attempting to evaluate our observations (Arkin et al., 1970a) with regard to the same question, the entire
nightly sleep period and each REM period and NREM period of the night were
each divided into tenths and the occurrences of all sleep speech in each such
time interval were tabulated for each baseline record for all subjects on whom
baseline sleep was recorded. This procedure failed to disclose any well-marked
tendencies and these results were, therefore, consistent with those of Rechtschaffen et al., (1962). There was a suggestion, however, of slight increases in frequency during the second 10th and the eighth 10th of the entire sleep period
and also the last 10th of each NREM and REM period. Moreover, we observed
16 instances of sleep speech and 12 additional nonspeech vocalizations in NREM
sleep just preceding stage REM sleep, many of them occurring at or immediately
before REM sleep onset. Thus, although one cannot say that NREM speech
"initiated" the REM sleep in any causal sense, it is clear that the above temporal
sequence is observable.

The lack of any tendency of sleep-speech episodes to cluster in some specific
portion of the night provides an interesting contrast with "night terrors" which
do indeed tend to occur more frequently during the first two hours of sleep
(Fisher et al., 1973a). Thus, two syndromes both characterized by sleep-associated utterances nevertheless display different temporal patterning.

What is the Degree of Concordance between the Contents of Sleep Speech and the Mentation Recalled by the Subject Upon Being Awakened Immediately after the Utterance? And How Is This Related to the Sleep Stage and Time of Night in Association with Which the Utterance Occurred?

Kamiya (1961) reported that a comparison of sleep-speech content and mentation elicited upon waking the subject afterward failed to disclose any obvious
relationship. The data, however, were too meager to support definite conclusions.

Rechtschaffen et al., (1962), in a more extensive work, mentioned that of
two awakenings following stage REM-associated speech, the content of one mentation report bore an unambiguous relationship to the sleep speech (classified
as first-order concordance below). In addition, 9 of 12 (75%) awakenings following stage NREM-associated speech resulted in the recall of at least some cognitive content which the subject believed had occurred just prior to the awakening.
In 7 of these 9 NREM awakenings (58.3%), a relationship between the content
of the mentation report and the sleep speech could be inferred (presumably
classifiable as either first or second order concordance below). The remaining 2
sleep speech-mentation report pairs (16.7%) seemed devoid of concordance.

In their study of episodic phenomena during sleep, Gastaut and Broughton
(1965) agreed with Rechtschaffen et al., (1962) that the content of several of
their observed REM sleep speeches "related to dreaming." By contrast, however,

Gastaut and Broughton (1965) associated NREM speeches with a "lack of re-called dreaming," and concluded that the speeches "are not exteriorized symptoms of true oneiric activity [p. 208]." Furthermore, they expressed a belief that NREM sleep speech is "liberated from low level continuous mental life during sleep" or else stems from "simple perceptual confusion during abrupt awakening [Gastaut & Broughton, 1965, p. 208]."

Neither Kamiya (1961) nor Gastaut and Broughton (1965) mentioned the number of sleep-speech-mentation report pairs on which they based their conclusions.

Arkin et al. (1967, 1970b) have published their findings based on 166 sleep speech-mentation report pairs uttered by 28 paid chronic sleeptalking subjects in the laboratory. The content of each sleep speech was compared to its associated wakeful mentation report with regard to similarities and differences in *manifest* content alone. Each such associated pair was scored as showing:

1. *first-order concordance* when they possessed in common one or more words, phrases, or other clearly identifying feature, e.g. REM-sleep speech, ". . . telling her how I can tell . . . that really likes;" associated mentation report, "I was thinking how I can tell philosopher better than the other—how much more I liked them," and so on;

2. *second-order concordance* when they possessed in common some specific feature of mental content or subject matter but did not share identical words, phrases, and so on, e.g. Stage 3 sleep speech, "No good as a dry dock;" associated mentation report, "This . . . one passage where it says . . . the hull of a ship, single mast, single boom for a cutway sail," and so on;

3. *third-order concordance* when the only element of concordance between the sleep speech and mentation report was the latter's containing a reference to someone (usually the subject) vocalizing. Thus a post-utterance mentation report describing someone as "talking," "saying," "asking," and so on was scored separately as third-order concordance if recall of an event involved vocalization without additional specific commonalities, that is, if criteria for second- or first-order concordances were not fulfilled;

4. *no discernible concordance* when concordance was not discernible on the basis of the manifest content of both speech and report, despite mentation having been recalled, and criteria for third-order concordance were not fulfilled.

5. *no mentation recalled.*

The most relevant results are presented in Table 15.2.

For the population examined in Table 15.2 one may conclude (disregarding Stage 1 NREM pairs because of their small number) the following:

1. Sleep utterance-mentation-report concordance tends to be greatest for Stage REM, least for Stage 3-4 and intermediate for Stage 2.

2. Recall of mentation after sleep utterance is most likely after Stage REM, least for Stage 3-4 and intermediate for Stage 2.

TABLE 15.2

Sleep Utterance: Mentation Report-Pair
Concordance in Relation to Sleep Stage

Sleep Stage	Total number of utterances	Order of concordance[a]				None discerned	No recall
		First	Second	Third	Combined		
REM	24	8 (33.3)	5 (20.8)	6 (25.0)	19 (79.2)	4 (16.7)	1 (4.2)
2	85	15 (17.6)	7 (8.2)	17 (20.0)	39 (45.8)	28 (32.9)	18 (21.2)
3-4	52	5 (9.6)	4 (7.7)	2 (3.8)	11 (21.1)	21 (40.4)	20 (38.5)
1 NREM	5	3 (60.0)	1 (20.0)	0.0	4 (80.0)	0.0	1 (20.0)

[a]Percentage of total utterances in parentheses.

3. No discernible concordance between sleep utterance and recalled mentation is most likely with Stage 3-4, least with Stage REM and intermediate with Stage 2.

Comparison with the results reported by Rechtschaffen et al. (1962) shows that in our data a somewhat smaller proportion of concordance and a higher proportion of no recall were found in NREM pairs. It should be noted, however, that only 12 NREM awakenings were performed by them and the differences could be related to differences in size of sample. Their findings on REM sleep speech are consistent with ours but their data contained only 2 stage REM pairs. The REM sleep-speech findings reported by Gastaut and Broughton (1965) are likewise consistent with ours, but they did not mention the number of speech-report pairs in their paper.

With regard to the speech associated with night terrors arising in association with Stage 4, Gastaut and Broughton (1965) were impressed by the nearly complete tendency for amnesia during full wakefulness for the mental content associated with the episode. However, some instances were described which might be included in our categories of first and second order concordance, but no differential proportions were mentioned. By contrast, our data contain a sizeable number of instances of recall as well as concordance. This may be explained on the basis that our sample contained many instances of Stage 4-associated sleep speeches which were bland in quality and apparently not infused with anxiety—a type of nocturnal episode which is quite different from a night terror. This indicates the importance of stressing once more that sleep speech is not a unitary phenomenon but rather one in which important subject differences exist as well as differences within the same subject from one sleep speech to the next, depending on a number of factors. This view is further borne out by a recent study of Fisher et al. (1974), presenting contrasting findings to those of Gastaut and

Broughton (1965). In their study with 11 subjects, 58% of night-terror arousals were followed by recall of mentation described as occurring prior to full achievement of subjective wakefulness, after termination of the attack. In addition, many striking instances of first- and second-order concordance were observed between "night-terror speech" and the following mentation report. In conformity with our own results, such concordance was more likely in episodes with milder levels of arousal. (Arkin et al., 1970b, 1972).

Finally, MacNeilage (1971) observed only one instance of a direct relationship (first-order concordance) between a sleep speech and a mentation report in a population of 16 pairs. This speech was associated with Stage "Alpha," considered by MacNeilage to be a "transitional" phase between sleep and wakefulness. In addition, she found that 44% of mentation reports following sleep speech to contain verbal content (third-order concordance?), most of her sample occurring in association with Stage 2.

What Are the Characteristics of the Sleep Utterances Themselves?

It is not possible to give a brief description of sleep utterances because they possess almost as much variability as those of wakefulness (Arkin, 1967). Although the majority of sleep speeches contain at least a few words, some consist of only one, such as "good," "no," "okay," "yes'," or Mm-*hm,"* others are of paragraph length, occasionally in excess of one hundred words. Most speeches last a few seconds or less, but longer ones may continue for a minute or more. The range of clarity extends fron unintelligible mumbles to crystal-clear words. The belief is widespread that most sleep speech is indistinct. We have been repeatedly surprised, however, by utterances which, unclear when heard over the intercom, turned out to contain some clear *sotto voce* or whispered speech on the tape recording. Often, speeches contain silent pauses, in which case the context suggests sleep dialogues with hallucinated partners, sometimes resembling one side of a telephone conversation. Another frequent occurrence is sudden interruption of a speech in the middle, followed by sustained silence or an apparently meaningless mumbled petering out. The hearer is left with a feeling that a thought has been fragmented or left incomplete.

Of major interest are the structural features of sleep speech. Evaluation of these aspects were perforce based upon fragments of varying completeness. When associated with REM sleep, they were somewhat more likely to be correct in syntax, inflection and word structure. Almost all cases of marked abnormality were associated with NREM sleep and could be arranged on a continuum from no or mild disturbance to sheer gibberish, in which clang associations and recurrent utterances were prominent with occasional "neologisms." The latter especially occurred in association with Stage 3-4 in the first half of the night, and often had an explosive quality with rapid emission of words. It is particularly the sleep speeches with degrees of disorganization which bear striking resemblances to aphasic utterances and, in a sense, may provide a physiological model of aphasia (Arkin and Brown, 1971).

Turning to the content of sleep speech, one is struck first by the *rarity* of secrets. This provides a contrast to widely held popular belief and frequent use of sleep talking in literature as a technical means by which the "real truth" comes to light. (Witness Othello's convinced response to Iago's account of the alleged sleep talking of Cassio.) From a moral point of view, however, most of the somniloquy observed in the laboratory is prosaic and would not ruffle the strictest censor. In our entire population, only five or six speeches uttered by four males and one female contained references to what might flout conventional sensibilities. One made an oblique reference to male homosexuality. The other five utilized crude slang expressions for the female genitial, sexual intercourse, and feces. But the majority of intelligible, clear utterances sound like fragments of overheard, unremarkable daily conversations. References to gossip, school matters, newspapers, entertainment, art, science, the experimental situation itself, food, philosophical discussion, and the like were all common.

Another item of interest is the affective qualities of somniloquy. Not infrequently, sleep speeches involve tense, anxious and dramatic fragments. Doubtless many of these are examples of a variety of NREM night terrors and REM nightmares (Fisher et al., 1973a). The most common affect, however, is one of conversational blandness appropriate in quality to the content of the speech but of somewhat diminished intensity. But the range is broad. Subjects chuckled, laughed, sang, whimpered, sounded petulant, sulky, childish, irritable, sarcastic, displayed intense anger with shouting, anxiety of all degrees, sobbing with both fear and remorse, and finally an inchoate, nonspecific high-intensity affect accompanying the discharge of the outburst-like vocalizations mentioned above with clang associations and recurrent utterances.

Finally, another group of sleeptalking phenomena resemble words and sounds one utters in solitude while awake. Exclamatory words, phrases, sounds of surprise, curiosity, pleasure, agreement, and so on are common. In addition, one encounters utterances resembling wakeful vocal self-priming or stimulation as if someone were following a recipe or other stepwise task, and wondering aloud what to do next.

Are Techniques Available by Which Sleep Talking May Be
Experimentally Influenced?

Following the introduction of modern electrographic technique, I became intrigued by the possibility of gaining control over sleeptalking with the object of obtaining first hand, "hot off the griddle," reports of ongoing sleep mentation (much as a television commentator gives an on-the-spot account of an event.) I hoped in this fashion to get a report of a dream in progress influenced as little as possible by interference from cognitive factors operating during retrospective recall after awakening.

The basic feature of the technique in the first attempt consisted in hypnotizing sleeptalkers prior to retiring for the night and giving them posthypnotic suggestions that they would sleep and dream normally in the laboratory, just as they do at home, but that the occurrence of a natural dream would be a posthypnotic signal for them to talk in their sleep and describe the dream as it was going on without awakening. In addition attempts were made to increase the amount of sleeptalking by giving posthypnotic suggestions to talk in their sleep more than before. The subjects were then aroused out of the hypnotic trance to normal wakefulness, whereupon they were permitted to go to sleep. Needless to say, results fell short of the ideal goal specified in the post-hypnotic suggestion. Out of eight subjects, a striking result was obtained with one, a less striking but convincing result was obtained in a second, an equivocal result in a third, and either no effect or a diminution of sleeptalking in the remainder, to the point of total suppression (Arkin et al., 1966b). With our best subject we obtained the results demonstrated in Table 15.3.

The mean frequency of sleep speech over 9 first baseline nights was .8 per night (total speeches = 7) all of which occurred in the first half of the night, all of which were associated with NREM sleep, and 71% of which were more than 15 min from the nearest REM period. By contrast, the mean frequency of sleep speech over 23 nights employing posthypnotic suggestion was 10.0 per night (total speeches = 230). Of this latter total, 27% occurred in the first half of the night, and 73% in the second; also, 35% were associated with stage REM, and an additional 4% occurred at either REMP onset or termination. Of the remaining 61% uttered in association with NREM sleep, 64% occurred less than 15 min from the nearest REMP. The mean frequency of sleep speech over the 6 terminal baseline nights was 7.8 (total speeches = 47). Of this latter total, 79% occurred in the first half of the night and only 10.6% over the entire night were in association with stage REM; and of the 89.4% occurring in association with NREM sleep, 57.4% were more, and 42.6% less, than 15 min from the nearest REMP.

Thus, all procedures utilizing posthypnotic suggestion resulted in a marked increase in mean total number of speeches per night, a shift in location of the bulk of speeches from the first to the second half of the night, initiation of speeches during REM sleep, and an increase of NREM speeches closely associated with the nearest REM period. Tart (Personal Communication, 1974) has independently demonstrated the effectiveness of this technique for the experimental production of sleeptalking.

In addition, a certain number of awakenings following sleep utterances were performed on 9 experimental nights separate from the above. After 8 REM-associated speech awakenings, recalled mentation displayed first order concordance in 87.5% of the cases; and after 35 NREM associated speeches, wakeful

TABLE 15.3

Results of Posthypnotically Stimulated Sleeptalking with Our Best Subject

Experimental condition and number of nights	Mean episodes per night	Percentage first half night	Percentage during REM sleep	Percentage NREM sleep	Percentage NREM more than 15 min from nearest REM period	Percentage NREM less than 15 min from nearest REM period
First baseline, 9	0.8 (N = 7)	100.0	.0	100.0	71.4	18.6
All posthypnotic hypnotic suggestion, 23	10.0 (N = 230)	27.0	39	61.0	36.0	64.0
Terminal baseline, 6	7.8 (N = 47)	79.0	10.6	89.4	57.4	42.6

mentation reports displayed 20% first order concordance. The quality of speech, number of words and emotion resembled that of many of our spontaneous sleep-talkers not subjected to the hypnosis technique. However, the proportions of first order concordance were sonewhat higher with the posthypnotic subject than with the spontaneous sleeptalkers not subjected to the hypnosis technique: stage REM 87.5; versus 33.3% respectively; NREM 20 versus 13.6% respectively.

In another experimental study, a significant increase in sleeptalking was observed during recovery nights following two prior consecutive nights in which subjects took a dextroamphetamine spansule (15 mg) and pentobarbital (100 mg) prior to sleep (Arkin et al. 1968). Although at that time our result was attributed to the increased "REM pressure" usually following presleep ingestion of this drug combination, it is now known that other stages of sleep are also affected by this procedure. Whatever the underlying mechanism, it is, nonetheless, an instance of experimental stimulation of somniloquy.

Aarons (1970) has reported preliminary findings on attempts to condition sleep vocalization by escape-avoidance techniques. Using three paid male students (ages 22-23) who were apparently in good mental and physical health and without a history of sleeptalking or other sleep disturbance, the EEG, EOG (electro-oculogram), submental EMG, respiration, and voice were monitored for a total of three control-adaptation and eight experimental nights. The basic strategy was that of shaping and developing operant responses of avoidance behavior. The termination of various combinations of noxious light and sound stimuli applied during sleep was first made contingent upon *any* vocalization and by gradual steps changed to requiring increasing overt verbalization as the desired operant response. The goal was the elicitation of speech of sufficient duration, intensity, and clarity to be easily comprehensible without awakening the subject. For a number of reasons, the procedure was not strictly uniform. In general, most of the experimental nights were carried out without informing the subjects of the desired goal, but in the latter part of the series, they were explicitly told that the purpose of the experiment was to produce sleeptalking and that if they spoke, the unpleasant stimuli would cease. No subject vocalized during the control night whereas all vocalized during experimental nights, in a large variety of ways. Thus, groans and unintelligible mumbling, clearly enunciated coherent words, phrases, and sentences were all observed. In addition, there was a similarly broad spectrum of affective tone and content both related and unrelated to the experimental situation. One subject increased in responsiveness over three nights and another decreased over four. Total responses per session were obtained over a range of 28-100% of the stimulation trials with 57% transient awakenings. Responses, in weighted percentage for response sample size accompanied by alterations of the EEG but without alpha evidence for awakening, were distributed by sleep stage as follows: Stage 1 NREM, 62% (N = 10); Stage 2, 88% (N = 40); Stage 3, 70% (N = 27); Stage 4, 96% (N = 22); Stage

REM, 40% (N = 10). Aarons regards his study as possessing numerous limitations, however, and is cautious about making generalizations. More experimentation is necessary to assess the extent to which the reported conditioned sleep speeches resemble spontaneous somniloquy observed in "natural" sleeptalkers as to content, electrographic correlates, and concordance with mentation reports elicited immediately afterward. Moreover, the effects of aversive techniques in training subjects to talk in their sleep may have powerful biasing influences over each of these parameters.

Still more recently, Bertini and Pontalti (1971) claimed to be able to train nonsleeptalkers to "free associate" in response to white noise during wakefulness. After this response was well established, the subjects were exposed to the same white-noise stimulus in the laboratory during REM sleep and were said to free associate in response without awakening. On the other hand, Hauri (1972) attempted to replicate this work and failed to produce sleeptalking during Stage REM. Subjects often reported that they "heard the white noise in their dreams, but when they realized that they were now supposed to talk, they 'lost' their dream experience [Hauri, 1972, p. 61]. Hauri did report, however, that spontaneous, sleeptalking increased during the experiment, especially in Stages 2 and 3.

Finally, in the course of our own work, it was observed that frequent awakening of subjects and requiring them to perform verbal tasks aloud (giving mentation reports or performance of mental arithmetic aloud) resulted in the appearance of spontaneous sleep speech in two separate populations of nonsleeptalker subjects who were selected only on the basis of being light sleepers and good dream recallers (for another project) (Arkin et al. 1970a & b; Farber et al., 1973). It is of interest that such sleeptalking experimentally produced in nonsleeptalkers, occurs most frequently in Stage 2 sleep. (They also occurred often in Stages 3-4 and Stage REM). Electrographically, phenomenologically, and content-wise, the episodes were undistinguishable from those of chronic sleep talkers. In addition, it was observed that frequent awakening of chronic sleeptalkers for mentation reports resulted in increases of sleep speech (Arkin et al., 1973).

Is it Possible for an Experimenter to Engage in Conversation with a Sleeptalker without Awakening the Subject?

The old clinical and scientific literature contains many accounts of "conversations" between somniloquists and a wakeful companion for which the sleeptalker either has complete or partial amnesia (Arkin, 1966). Knowing of my interest in sleeptalking, at least six intelligent conscientious couples in recent years have volunteered that they can regularly engage their respective partners in prolonged sleep conversation with the sleeptalker experiencing complete lack of recall in the morning. Attempts to observe this phenomenon in the laboratory have met with partial success (Arkin et al., 1966a). The reason for this qualified comment is that thus far, the dialogues recorded do not seem as sustained as those described in the anecdotal reports of the above reliable persons. It is possible that the laboratory, its equipment, and an experimenter who is not an intimate of the subject may have an inhibiting effect.

There are two techniques which may be useful: the "answering method," and the "provocation method." Using the former, the experimenter waits patiently for the sleeping subject to talk and attempts to answer audibly in the same spirit, intensity, and on the same topic as if conversing empathically with a wakeful partner. In so doing, the experimenter should strive to "feel his way" into the experiential world of the subject at the instant and respond accordingly for as many interchanges as possible. With the latter technique, the experimenter softly speaks to the at-the-moment "silent" sleeper using the subject's or another's name, word, or topic which the experimenter knows is of interest to the subject. When the sleeptalking is thus initiated, the experimenter continues with the answering method.

In general, during the actual vocalization, the accompanying electrographic background, when readable, is that of Stage 1 NREM.

Rather Than Being a Valid Reflection of Sleep Mentation, Is It Possible That Sleeptalking Merely Indicates the Mental Content of the Movement-Arousal Episode (As Defined by Standard Criteria) and Is Essentially Unrelated To Sleep Mentation As Such?

The results of studies in several different laboratories have a bearing on this question.

First, with regard to Stage REM-associated sleeptalking, the high proportion of concordance between sleep-speech content and the usual relatively elaborate REM sleep-mentation reports described as dreams by the subject, provides convincing evidence that REM-associated sleep speech arises out of and reflects previous ongoing REM sleep mentation. On the other hand, the same conclusion with regard to NREM-associated utterances cannot be drawn so easily. This caution is required by the lack of well-established electrographic correlates of NREM sleep mentation in contrast to those of Stage REM. That is, in the latter instance, electrographic signs of Stage REM permit a reasonably valid inference that dream-like mentation was in progress immediately prior to the actual onset of the sleep utterance and continuous with it, whereas this would not be the case with NREM sleep.

An effort was made by us (Arkin et al., 1972) to approach this problem by comparing NREM mentation reports elicited immediately after NREM-associated sleep utterance to reports elicited during NREM "silent sleep." We sought to evaluate the following hypothesis: many NREM associated utterances are the outgrowths of previous streams of *ongoing* NREM mentation which, from time to time, find expression in overt vocalization of the subject.

Evidence that this could indeed occur would be important because we would then possess a spontaneous subject-emitted, objective indicator of the presence and content of some NREM mentation. Support for this hypothesis would require the following three findings:

1. An analysis of the general content of mentation reports elicited immediately after NREM-associated utterances would reveal no significant differences from reports elicited from NREM "silent" sleep, that is, sleep without proximate sleep vocalization.

2. There would be no significant differences in the total word counts of the mentation reports elicited from these two conditions; and also no significant difference in proportion of reports categorized by judges as lacking in content altogether.

3. By contrast, on awakening the subject after NREM sleep utterance, the frequency with which the subject recalls an imagined occurrence in which the sleeper was vocalizing would be *greater* than after an interval of NREM silent sleep. Examples of such occurrences would be those in which the subject reports, "I was (or we were) talking, discussing, teaching, arguing, conversing, and so on" in an imagined incident prior to being awakened.

We obtained our data from the first 23 of the 28 subjects utilized in our study of the degree of concordance between the content of sleep speech and the associated wakeful mentation (Arkin et al., 1970b). Only their NREM reports were employed and from this pool, we set up pairs each consisting of one report associated with sleep utterance and one associated with silent sleep. Both members of a given pair came from the same subject, from the same night and were also chosen to minimize the difference in time elapsed between the two reports. This procedure yielded a total of 74 pairs of reports for initial data processing. (Of the 23 subjects, 4 yielded 1 report pair each; 7, 2 each; 4, 3 each; 3, 4 each; 4, 6 each; and 1, 8 pairs).

Content analysis and total word counts were made on the entire population of report pairs. The content analytic categories included visual content, action, number of characters, self-representation, bizarreness-incongruity, interpersonal action, emotion, references to the laboratory-experimental situation, references to work and/or school, mentation absent or unscorable, subject vocalizing, and other verbal categories. Eight of the 11 reliability coefficients for 2 dependent judges ranged from .70 to .89. The coefficients for the remaining 3 categories (emotion, bizarreness, and visual content) were below acceptable levels, but were deemed spuriously low largely because of the low frequency and the low overall amount of variability of these items in the entire report population, (Arkin, 1973b). No significant differences were found between the mean total-word counts, frequency of mentation recall, the content analysis categories in the 2 groups of reports with *one* clear exception: reports after sleep utterance were much more likely to contain an indication of the subject vocalizing in an imaginary sleep experience (33.8% after sleep utterance versus 12.2% from silent sleep). An additional 6.7% of both groups of mentation reports contained references to other verbal categories (such as "others vocalizing," anticipated vocalization," and so on. This brought the total proportion of reports containing references to verbal content to 40.5% after sleep speech and 18.9% from silent sleep, a difference of 21.6%. It was therefore concluded that many NREM-associated sleep utterances arise out of ongoing streams of NREM mentation and provide valid indices of NREM mental content because the 2 types of reports were indistinguishable with the sole exception as described. These results are closely consistent with those subsequently reported by MacNeilage (1971). Her findings were that the proportions of reports judged as reflecting dreams, coherent dreams, containing visual content and finally physical activity were uniformly but only slightly higher after sleep utterance than after silent sleep (mean difference, 5.5%; range, 1.5-7.7%). This difference is presumed to be statistically insignificant inasmuch as levels were not reported. By contrast, the percentage of reports elicited after sleeptalking categorized as possessing verbal content was 43.8 as opposed to 23.1 for the controls, a difference of 20.7%. The figures from the two laboratories were, therefore, in close agreement.

Finally, Fisher et al. (1974), in a study of night terrors (which feature speech and vocalization), report that on several occasions, awakened subjects described mentation prior to the spontaneous terrifying arousal which possessed content out of which the night terror seemed to develop, for example, one subject remembered political discussions preceding a night terror of falling off a cliff in a baby carriage. These observations accord with out conclusion that many NREM sleep speeches are outgrowths of previous ongoing streams of NREM mentation.

A Conceptual Scheme for the Formulation of Sleep Utterance and Related Phenomena

Preparatory discussion of two considerations are necessary to make my exposition clear. First, in what senses may we say that when a subject somniloquizes, he is in fact "talking in his sleep;" and second, how shall we view the concept of psychic dissociation which, as mentioned in my previous papers (Arkin, 1967, 1974b), seems useful in accounting for sleep utterance.

At the outset it is necessary to note that a universally accepted, unambiguous definition of sleep has not yet been formulated. Although, polygraphic parameters, particularly those derived from the combined use of the EEG, submental EMG, and EOG, have been used by sleep researchers for providing the most pragmatic criteria yet available, there are, nevertheless exceptions and transitional states not conveniently subsumed under them. For our purposes, it will suffice to cite two recent authoritative views. Thus, Dement and Mittler (1973) indicate that the cardinal feature of wakefulness is the efficiency of discriminatory reactivity to the environment or perceptual "environmental engagement". They ask us to imagine an individual whose eyes are taped open and who is required to make a motor response to light flashes whenever they are presented. At some point, the individual fails to respond. The moment of sleep onset is taken by the authors as coinciding with this moment of "perceptual disengagement" as betokened by the response failure—and such response failure may occur in the presence of a wakeful EEG. They continue by remarking upon their existing uncertainty concerning the precise temporal relationships between loss of discriminatory reactivity and the usually accepted EEG signs of sleep.

Likewise, Johnson (1970) evaluates the evidence for unique correspondence between electrographic signs and mentally defined states. Reviewing the then present state of the art in electrographic assessment of sleep and states of awareness as described by a mentation report, actually, he considered the state of consciousness to possess priority over electrographic measures and further, that the assessment of the state of consciousness was a prerequisite to interpretation of the EEG.

Earlier in this chapter, it was established that the typical episode of somniloquy occurs within the electrographic context of a movement arousal episode. Rechtschaffen and Kales (1968) classify such events in a pragmatic somewhat arbitrary manner. If their duration exceeds half of the duration of the epoch simultaneously obscuring the EEG and EOG tracings, they are categorized as (MT) muscle tension. In such cases, they are counted neither as unambiguous sleep nor wakefulness because of currently insufficient knowledge of their behavioral correlates. If, on the other hand, half of the epoch or less is occupied by a movement-arousal incident, its sleep-stage classification depends upon the electrographic characteristics of the readable remainder of the record. The category "movement arousal," therefore, is not necessarily considered incompatible with ongoing sleep but is recommended to the experimenter as a herald of some impending change in whatever sleep state had obtained before its occurrence.

Moreover, in many instances observed in our laboratory the EEG was artifact-free at the exact moment of utterance and fulfilled the criteria of unambiguous sleep. Similar findings have been reported by others during episodes of somnambulism; that is, coordinated motor activity was maintained in the presence of electroencephalographically unambiguous slow-wave sleep (Broughton, 1973; Jacobson & Kales, 1967; Kales & Jacobson 1967).

The relevant point to be gleaned from these previous comments is that despite certain electrographic signs of increased arousal, a subject may nevertheless be, or remain, *psychologically* asleep, especially if such occurrences are immediately preceded and rapidly followed by unambiguous electrographic correlates of sleep. This latter sequence actually describes the electrographic structure of a typical sleep-utterance episode. In other words, psychological and electrographic sleep may often be slightly out of phase. Further support for this suggestion arises from the demonstration that when subjects are awakened, there is a time lag in the full recovery of wakeful critical reactivity even though typical electrographic signs of wakefulness prevail. Experimental results of others reviewed by

Tebbs (1972) demonstrate that postawakening performance decrements may range from 25 to 360% below full wakeful levels, and that although the rate of recovery is most rapid during the few minutes following the awakening, complete recovery may require as long as 25 min. Findings consistent with these have been reported by Feltin and Broughton (1966) and Scott (1969). In addition, Broughton (1968) has demonstrated the carry-over of NREM sleep components of the occipital visual evoked potential, or increased latencies and decreased amplitudes of later components into immediately following wakefulness.

The second relevant area to be discussed is that of psychic dissociation. In a recent paper, Hilgard (1973) published a neo-dissociationist theory which accounts nicely for somniloquy. Its basic assumption is that unity in personal cognition is precarious and unstable. Self-perception and conception of self as agent, maintained largely through continuity of memory, is a function of the "executive ego." The latter normally has ascendancy over a hierarchy of cognitive subsystems themselves mutually autonomous and concurrently interactive in varying degree. Each subsystem, which may operate outside of awareness, has an input and output system with feedback enabling it to seek or avoid input and enhance or inhibit output. These formulations provide a conceptual scaffolding for the following phenomena observable in connection with sleep utterances:

1. They express input from endogenous sources, that is, vocalization appears to arise spontaneously requiring no external stimuli.

2. They often accompany and/or reflect the content and the subject's imagined participation within streams of mentation associated with sleep. This is demonstrated by variable degrees of concordance with recalled mentation elicited during immediately subsequent wakefulness.

3. The content of the sleep speech may be ample and yet bear no discernible relationship to the equally ample content of the immediately following mentation report. This suggests the possibility of multiple dissociated concurrent streams of mentation.

4. There is a lack of simultaneous critical awareness of external reality at the moment of the occurrence. That is, when accompanied by sleep consciousness the subject treats the sleep-imagined experience associated with the sleep utterance as if it were real. Furthermore, when receiving a threshold arousal stimulus, the subject describes experiences and behaves in accordance with customarily expected characteristics of one who has been asleep and has just been awakened.

5. There is a strong tendency for amnesia which is more marked for mentation accompanying NREM than REM sleep utterances.

6. Lack of associated recalled mentation is often total, that is, the subject may deny recall of any preawakening experience whatsoever. Inasmuch as this outcome is usual when sleep utterances possess marked degrees of linguistic disorganization, the possibility exists that such speech emissions may occur in the absence of awareness.

7. The psycholinguistic integrity of the emitted speech tends to possess broadly varying degrees of disturbance, often resembling ictal automatism or types of aphasia (Serafetinides 1966). Thus, we might express somniloquy in terms of Hilgard's (1973) theory as follows: during slumber, the sleep executive ego acquires ascendancy over its wakeful counterpart. Its related subordinate semiautonomous cognitive systems include those mediating imagery, covert utterance, overt utterance, moral codes, and memory which in turn is subdivided into echoic, short-term and long-term components. Accordingly, our definition of somniloquy may now be reformulated as follows: *somniloquy is the output of the overt-utterance system during psychological sleep (v.s.) occurring in varying degrees of dissociation from the memory and imagery subsystems along a continuum from minimal to apparently complete dissociations, while, at the same time, with little or no dissociation from individual moral-code subsystems.*

This last item indicates that sleep speech, no matter how dissociated from other cognitive structures, has, nevertheless, little autonomy from moral-code subsystems judging from the rarity of exposure of secrets under conditions which would seem to actually facilitate revealing them. This provides an interesting sidelight upon the tenacity of moral-code systems in their role of modulation of psychological outputs.

16

Night Terrors and Anxiety Dreams

Edwin Kahn
Charles Fisher
Adele Edwards
Queensborough Community College
  and
Mount Sinai Medical Center

A distinction has been made between the night terror which occurs with very rare exception out of Stages 3 and 4 sleep, and the more common anxiety dream or nightmare which arises from REM sleep.[1] The night terror is usually an event of the early part of the night when most Stage 4 is present, while the nightmare can take place in any REM period. Also the night terror is physiologically much more intense than the REM nightmare (heart rates have almost tripled for the night terror while in the REM anxiety dream the greatest heart rate acceleration at our laboratory was from 76 to 92 beats per min). The lesser intensity of the REM anxiety dream may be at least partially explained by the fact that during REM the physiological activation provides a buffer which prevents extreme terror. Finally, night terrors occur in an arousal state (arousal out of Stages 3 and 4 sleep) while anxiety dreams occur during sleep, in the midst of an ongoing REM period and terminate on arousal.

The following is a summary of our laboratory's findings on night terrors, detailed accounts of which have been reported elsewhere (Fisher, et al., 1970, 1973a, 1974b; Kahn et al., 1972, 1973).

The severe Stage 4 night terror consists of perhaps the greatest heart rate acceleration possible in man (in a typical severe arousal heart rate accelerated

---

[1] In their original publication (Fisher et al. 1970), the authors described an exceptional form of frightening arousal occurring in association with Stage 2 sleep. The concomitant anxiety tended to be more severe than REM anxiety dreams but much less than that related to Stage 4 night terrors. Prior to awakening, similar to the latter, there was no change in heart or respiratory rate but after awakening, only moderate increases were observed. One such Stage 2 episode was described as an occurrence of moaning followed by spontaneous awakening with a report of content about receiving a severed human leg as a Christmas gift.

from 64 bpm to 152 bpm within 15 to 30 sec) with screams of enormous intensity, cursing, motility, increases in respiratory rate and especially amplitude, and a sharp increase in skin conductance. The episode is of brief duration, heart rate decelerating 45 to 90 sec after the moment of onset, and returning to normal baseline levels within 2 to 4 min. Most subjects characteristically fell asleep shortly after an episode, and in several with multiple terrors it was not unusual for another one to occur 15 to 30 min later when they were back in Stage 4. There seemed to be a sex difference in incidence; although considerably more women responded to our newspaper ad soliciting nightmare sufferers, 10 of the 12 night-terror subjects were men.

Although arising out of Stage 4 (approximately two-thirds of the night terrors occurred during the first NREM period when most Stage 4 occurs) the episode actually takes place as part of an arousal response, characterized by a waking EEG pattern (see Broughton, 1968, below). When the night terror occurred in the first NREM period, the mean time from sleep onset to the first night terror was 44.5 min showing how early in the night these episodes will occur.

One consistent finding was that the intensity of the night terror was correlated with the amount of Stage 4 preceding the attack, that is, the more Stage 4 the more severe the episode. Thus, for *each* of the three subjects with the most frequent arousals, amount of preceding Stage 4 correlated significantly with the heart-rate change at arousal and this relationship was further confirmed for the other subjects with fewer arousals. It was speculated that with increased duration of Stage 4 sleep becomes "deeper," and with deepening sleep there is an increasing potential for loss of ego control, eventuating in the uninhibited release of terrifying repressed impulses.

Since night terrors occurred out of Stage 4 it was hypothesized that a way to curtail them would be to administer a drug that suppressed Stage 4. Kales et al. (1970) reported that diazepam had such an effect, therefore it was tried. In four of six subjects it was found that 5-20 mg of diazepam taken at bedtime suppressed night terrors which returned when the subject was taken off drug or given placebo. In the remaining two subjects, diazepam reduced night terrors, however, the reduction persisted during the off-drug period. One subject differed in that night terrors occurred during each NREM period, so that toward morning when Stages 3 and 4 were absent, night terrors occurred out of Stage 2. Diazepam suppressed this subject's Stage 2 as well as Stage 4 night terrors, indicating that the drug could exert its effect independent of sleep stage.

In other findings, night terrors were elicited in two of three subjects when buzzers were sounded in slow-wave sleep. The buzzer-elicited night terrors were, on the average, of the same severity as those arising spontaneously. Clinical EEGs performed on three of the subjects with the most frequent night terrors (in two it was recorded just preceding and during severe night terrors) indicated no pathology in the tracing. Sleep heart rates for night-terror subjects were in the normal range and were significantly lower than for subjects who had

REM nightmares   or anxiety dreams, the latter showing elevated sleep heart rates.

The night terror is one of three major Stage 4 sleep disorders, the others being somnambulism and enuresis. Broughton (1968) and Gastaut and Broughton (1965) formulated some unifying ideas about these three disorders by considering them disorders of arousal. The authors noted that each of these disorders occurred during arousal from delta sleep, associated with alpha EEG, body movement, mental confusion, and disorientation, relative nonreactivity to external stimuli, and amnesia for the episode. They also took the position that because of amnesia it is virtually impossible to demonstrate that preceding NREM content is the trigger of night-terror attacks. Any content could be determined by the physiological changes occurring during arousal, for example, respiratory changes giving rise to feelings of suffocating and choking, increases in heart rate giving rise to fear of death, this formulation being a restatement of the old James-Lange theory. Broughton and Gastaut (1965) further speculated that thoughts may be rationalizations of the autonomic components of the attack or that during the postarousal period a return of waking conflict occurs through a clouded sensorium. Therefore, in Broughton and Gastaut's view it is unlikely that the night terror is triggered by ongoing NREM mentation.

In our investigation of night terrors it was observed that distinct content was often reported following these episodes. To help resolve the question of whether or not the night terror can be initiated by ongoing NREM mentation a thorough review of our night-terror arousal interviews was made to determine the frequency and nature of the reported content.

THE EXPERIMENT

Method

Twelve adult Stage 4-night-terror subjects (10 males and 2 females) were studied for a total of over 250 nights. A night terror was defined as a NREM arousal when heart rate reached a level of 108 bpm or more during any 15-sec postarousal interval.* By this definition we have observed over 275 night terrors at the laboratory. About half of the night terrors came from Subject 1, who was studied during 98 nights.

*Editors' note: In the papers referred to earlier in which the authors provide more extensive detail than is possible here, a separate category of "milder arousals" was described which was defined by heart rates of less than 108 bpm. The associated findings in this group, especially regarding the nature of recalled mentation, presented some important differences in comparison with those of the more severe night terrors. For example, the content resembled many of the sleep speeches recorded by Arkin and co-worker (see Chapter 15 of this volume) uttered by subjects defining themselves as chronic sleeptalkers rather than night-terror sufferers.

The subjects slept undisturbed while EEG, eye movement, heart rates, and respiratory rates were recorded. When a spontaneous awakening occurred, subjects were interviewed by the experimenter for content through a two-way intercom. A tape recorder was operated through the night to record all arousals and interviews.

Half of the subjects on some nights were studied on diazepam and other drugs in attempts to suppress night terrors. Drug as well as baseline nights were combined in this study so that a greater number of night terrors could be sampled. There was minimal effect of drug on amount of recall and content.

Abstracts of the arousal interviews were prepared which eliminated irrelevant detail. Each arousal was then labeled as recall, vague recall, or no recall by two judges working independently of each other.

Further details of method and subjects can be found in our earlier report (Fisher et al., 1974).

Results

Table 16.1 presents the number and percentage of instances of recall, vague recall, and no recall for all spontaneous night-terror arousals in eight subjects who had at least three night-terror episodes. Of the four remaining subjects with fewer arousals, two had 100% recall for two and one night terrors, respectively, and the other two subjects had no recall whatsoever for the same number of night terrors. Recall for night-terror arousals was 58% (65% when including vague recall), calculated by the mean of subject percentages.

TABLE 16.1

Number and Percentage Recall, Vague Recall, and No Recall
of Night Terrors (heart rate > 108 bpm)

		Number			Percentage		
Subject	Number of nights	Recall	Vague recall	No recall	Recall	Vague recall	No recall
1	92	112	13	38	69	8	23
2	32	5	6	10	24	28	48
3	31	12	2	11	48	8	44
4	48	6	1	0	86	14	0
5	9	0	0	33	0	0	100
6	13	3	0	0	100	0	0
7	4	2	0	1	67	0	33
12	16	12	0	5	71	0	29
					58[a]	7[a]	35[a]

[a]Percentage means.

Some of the most severe night terrors involved being crushed or struck by some sudden force, things closing in or being entrapped in a small area, being left alone or abandoned, and choking on or swallowing something, such as electrode wires. In Subjects 1 and 2 there was a tendency to better recall the most severe night terrors. It seemed that these two subjects were more fully aroused by the more severe terror and thus were more alert and better able to report detailed content, whereas in milder arousals the subjects were groggy, confused and unmotivated, and recall was impaired.

To illustrate more clearly the content associated with night-terror episodes, examples are given of six of the subjects' night-terror reports.

Subject 1 the most extensively studied subject, had repetitive and frequent night terrors of choking on something, such as the electrodes, tapes, and so on, and also had several very severe night terrors of being trapped in a small space. After one of the severest night terrors observed at the laboratory (heart rate went from 56 to 164 bpm within 1 min the subject gave the following report:

> *Somebody said . . . somebody . . . oh shit . . . somebody said something,* I don't even remember what this person said. All of a sudden I felt on all sides of me like, uh, metal, or stone doors. In other words I was someplace, probably in a basement, and like on every side of me was, except one, which I could sort of see maybe a window, every side was like stone or something, stopped up, almost like when I was in a tomb. *And so I started . . . uh, screaming.* I didn't realize that there was still a . . . an opening of some kind.

The screaming probably coincides with the onset of the arousal reaction. Note the brief content of someone speaking *before* the terrifying imagery appeared and the subject's statement that the content caused the screaming. Other night terrors of this subject who, it is to be noted was violently opposed to the United States policy of involvement in Vietnam, were swallowing and choking on an American flag (occurring at the height of the protest movement), choking on something that had been cut and severed, perhaps belonging to the experimenter, "I swallowed the whole thing," The subject also recalled being squeezed between a bus and wall.

After one of the night terrors where heart rate went from 60 to 120 bpm, subject 1 reported "One of the people here asked to have the light on . . . So I said it was okay. There was a hard time finding it. It was very dark. I thought they wanted to . . . And that's where I got panicky . . . I don't know what it was that really frightened me, the boxes themselves in front of me . . ." Although the content is not especially clear, from the above report it seems that some unavailable thought associated with ongoing NREM content ("And that's where I got panicky") instigated the episode.

Much of Subject 1's report content was repetitive and brief like the choking on wires and being entangled in electrodes, the repetitiveness giving the impression of postarousal elaborations of the intense autonomic responses. However, as noted in the illustrations above, other contents were distinct and specific and seem to rule out postarousal elaborations.

Subject 4, in a disturbing arousal that did not, by the heart-rate criterion, reach night-terror intensity (heart rate went from 48 to 92 bpm) reported the feeling of a snake in bed. He screamed to his girl friend, who he imagined was lying beside him, "Lights! I got a snake or something here!! Get the lights on, please, Can you get the lights on? *Can you get the fucking lights on,* goddamnit! Are you awake?"

After the episode subject 4 reported:

> I felt like I was going to have a nightmare . . . I had sensations there was something on the bed like a snake . . . it was damned low and moving up towards me, moving up the bed . . . The potential fear . . . might be the most interesting thing, namely, you build up a certain panic about *not being able to turn the lights on;* that seems to be one of the most important goals in a situation like that. Otherwise I thought I was with Mary Liz because I was actually talking to her, telling her to turn on the lights.

It would appear that the mental content of the snake, or something, in the bed triggered this episode.

In other night-terror arousals this Subject 4 often felt that he was being threatened or victimized by the sleep laboratory or others. In one very severe arousal, in which he ripped off the electrodes, he reported he was on a car trip requiring a reservation or tickets, such as to the Rose Bowl. He was with his sister and brother-in-law and suddenly felt as if someone was going to do something to him, like hit him over the head, shoot him, or humiliate him in some way. He wanted to get out of the situation and rip off the electrodes. This subject, who was sophisticated about the distinction between Stage 4 and REM sleep, then asked, "Was it a Stage 4 night terror . . . cause there was a lot of dream content there?"

Subject 2 had excellent recall for very severe arousals. In one the subject believed he had rolled over into the "wrong slot" and was about to be stepped on by the experimenter who was coming into the room (heart rate went from 80 to 160 bpm). The subject screamed during this episode:

> AOH! AAH!—HEY HEY, WATCH—WATCH—WATCH—WATCH—WATCH—Watch!! What's with me? Hold it . . . Hold it . . . Hold it . . . It wasn't me now! IT's NOT ME ANYMORE!! Oh, shit, you are *stepping on me now,* Dummy!! Hey, I switched . . . I'm here now. I'm here now. I'm in the middle position now. There you go. Okay?

After the night terror, and the heart rate returned to normal, the subject gave the following description of the arousal:

> In the room, you know, and, like someone was going to step on me . . . It was like—just like—It was a mixup like, you were doing—You weren't doing me harm purposely, you know what I mean? You follow me? . . . Well, someone was coming in. I didn't know who was coming to fix something up here and, I was like in the wrong slot. And you didn't realize I was in this wrong spot and *you were stepping on—you were stepping on me,* or something like this, and then I'm trying to tell you like I'm here. I'm over here. I'm over here, or something like this, I don't know. But it was violent there for a couple of seconds, yes. It was. Because I had a burst of energy . . .

In another of Subject 2's night terrors the room was shrinking and coming down on the subject, and in a third the subject experienced being left alone by someone on a rowboat in the middle of nowhere on a rough ocean, the other person disappearing in the distance. The latter was so severe that the subject ripped the electrodes off and we have no record of the heart-rate acceleration.

Subject 6 had two very severe arousals, ripping off the electrodes and later recalling vivid and detailed content. In one, the hull of a ship came down on and caught the subject beneath it, not crushed but trapped. In the other, the subject fell off a cliff while sitting in an English baby carriage on an endless fall, feeling helpless and shocked. Preceding the fall there was a political discussion with a neighbor whose radical political beliefs the subject strongly disagreed with. It also turned out that this neighbor owned an English stroller resembling the one the subject was trapped in during the night terror. The subject reported, "Falling, calling for help, and then waking up occurred at that very second."

Subject 3 reported in about half of the arousals strong physiological sensations, such as heart pounding and difficulty breathing. Although Subject 3's recall was, in general, poor, several "dream-like" contents were reported, like warriors or soldiers on horseback rattling their swords, while the leader talked to the group and the horses were about to charge. In one night terror in which heart rate went from 50 to 128 bpm, the subject screamed, "Help! Hey! Help! Hey get! It's near my throat! Things choking me! Something is stuck in my throat!" During the postarousal interview the subject reported, *"Something is choking in my throat ... It is choking in my throat, whatever the fuck is in there ... I just want to know why, I'd like to know what the hell is in my throat. It just woke me up that's all!"* The subjects last statement may be taken as evidence that content initiated the arousal.

Subject 12 often reported "dream-like imagery, for example, in one night terror, Martha Raye, at age 20 was helping the experimenter put electrodes on the subject, who wanted to tell them that the stuff on the head was too tightly fit. Suddenly no one was there and the subject awoke frightened. Subject 12's most fearful arousal, during which the electrodes were ripped off, was that a shelf in the room was closing in. The theme of a threatening person in the room appeared quite frequently in this subject's night terrors.

Discussion

The results reported indicate that recall of content associated with spontaneous arousal from night terrors is much better than has been reported by Broughton (1968). The degree of recall, a mean of 58%, is similar to the 70.0 and 61.5% recall at nonspontaneous awakenings from Stages 3-4 sleep in normal young adults reported by Foulkes (1962) and Arkin, et al. (1970 a & b), respectively.

An important problem, of difficult resolution, is the temporal relationships of the content recalled from Stage 4 night terrors; that is, does the psychic content refer to events that took place during the prearousal period of Stages 3-4 sleep just prior to the sudden onset of the night terror; or the postarousal period lasting not more than 1 to 2 min and characterized by marked autonomic activation, sleeptalking, and other utterances such as cries, screams and cursing, and return of motility. Recalled content may refer to one or both periods in a given instance.

Broughton (1970) believed that any content retrieved from night terrors is probably postarousal, either an elaboration of the intense autonomic changes that occur or a return to waking conflict. In our study, during the postarousal period some content may have been elaborated, as Broughton emphasized, like fears of dying associated with pounding of the heart (Subjects 1 and 3), or of choking in response to respiratory difficulty (Subject 1). Elaborated content may also occur in response to environmental circumstances, like Subject 1's frequent report of being left alone or abandoned. Most often, it is impossible to decide whether such content (dying, choking, or being abandoned) represented pre- or postarousal events.

However, a considerable amount of the content reported by our subjects was extremely vivid and so clearly described that it is difficult to imagine that it was postarousal mentation. Furthermore, in several instances, the subjects reported that it was because of the content that they became panicky, aroused, and began screaming (like Subject 1's report of being in a tomb, Subject 1 in the dark, and Subject 3 choking on something). Now that the existence of NREM mentation has been firmly established, there is little reason to doubt that such prearousal NREM content could initiate night-terror episodes.

Arkin et al. (1970a, 1972) have extensively studied mentation reports following NREM-sleeptalking episodes. They believe that the sleep speech often reflects the content of NREM sleep mentation, since content reports immediately after NREM sleep speech and NREM silent sleep show no differences except that there are more references in the former to the subject's talking. They also demonstrated concordance between sleep speech and recalled mentation, which, according to their argument, suggests that this recalled mentation frequently reflects ongoing NREM mentation. We have illustrated several instances of concordance between sleep speech and reported mentation during night-terror episodes (Fisher et al., 1974) However, we doubt in the situation of night terror or sleeptalking episodes, whether this constitutes proof of prearousal content as Arkin seems to contend, since the concordance could simply reflect mentation during the screaming and/or speech episodes which take place during arousal periods and not NREM sleep.

In two of three subjects, night terrors have been induced by sounding a buzzer during slow-wave, Stages 3-4 sleep (Fisher et al., 1970). One other subject reported that night terrors while in the army were set off by someone slamming the barracks door, or by other noise. These night terrors, induced by external stimuli, are perhaps the best evidence for mental activity playing no role in precipitating the episodes (Broughton, 1970). It might be postulated that in predisposed individuals, terrors can be "set off" by either of two types of stimulation:

(1) endogenous, in the form of mental activity occurring in NREM sleep; and (2) exogenous, in the form of a loud noise or other external stimulation.

One subject, subject 5, had no recall from 33 arousals classified as night terrorrs. It is interesting that Subject 5 was the only subject of three (Subjects 1, 3, and 5) in whom it was impossible to induce night terrors with a buzzer. In fact, the subject could not be aroused from Stages 3-4 sleep even with an extremely loud buzzer. This finding supports Zimmerman's (1970) hypothesis that NREM recall is related to amount of cerebral activation, that is, Subject 5, as evidenced by the high-arousal threshold, was a very deep sleeper (much less cerebral activation) with an NREM recall of zero.

A frequent very frightening content was that the room was closing in or shrinking; for three subjects the room was closing in, a fourth imagined being enclosed by the hull of the ship and a fifth reported a shelf in the room getting closer. This may be typical of night terrors at home or especially stimulated by the experimental situation, because the sleep room was quite small, located in the basement, with no outdoor view.

In four of six subjects with the most reported content, aspects of the sleep laboratory occurred in over 50% of the reports. Therefore, this has not been a study of night-terror content in general, but in a particular situation, that is, a laboratory. Nevertheless, there was very considerable overlap between content noted in the laboratory and that reported to have occurred at home before the investigation or during nonlaboratory nights during its course. Thus, Subject 1, whose most frequently reported content at the laboratory was choking on the wires or electrodes, reported that night terror content at home also involved choking, but not on wires. At home the subject would choke on or swallow such things as nails, a shirt, part of the subject's own throat, an itemized list for a tax return, and so on. His wife reported that he sometimes spit when he awakened as if he had swallowed something and wanted to get rid of it. This shows for Subject 1 that although the laboratory influenced the details of the content, the underlying theme may not have been different from what it was at home.

The REM nightmares show a gradual acceleration of heart and respiratory rates during sleep immediately prior to spontaneous arousals (Fisher et al., 1970; Kahn et al., 1972), however, the acceleration is not nearly as great as for the Stage 4 night terror. For example, in one of the most severe REM nightmares observed at the laboratory, heart rate went from 76 to 92 bpm and respiration from 18 to 30 breaths per min in the several minutes of REM sleep preceding spontaneous arousal. The Stage 4 night terror has *never* manifested *any* physiological change just prior to the sudden onset of the episode. This finding suggests that in the Stage 4 night terror the frightening content does not build up gradually as in the REM anxiety dream, rather it occurs suddenly, immediately igniting the arousal reaction. There may be ongoing neutral NREM thoughts which then touch upon an intense conflict area of the subject, producing simultaneously a terrifying image or thought and the intense arousal reaction, as in the example of Subject 6's night terror about the English stroller.

Of the three classical characteristics of nightmares discussed by Jones (1911, 1959) and others, intense dread, paralysis, and oppression on the chest, only the first, intense dread, has been found in this study to be a consistent characteristic of night terrors.

None of the night-terror content involved fear of paralysis. Liddon (1967) noted that during REM sleep there is a loss of muscle tone, and that this lack of tone may be related to the traditional report of paralysis in the nightmare. He further noted that some of the symptoms of narcolepsy are sleep paralysis, hypnagogic hallucinations, and sleep-onset REM periods (see Rechtschaffen & Dement, 1970) and speculated that those persons experiencing frightening dreams of paralysis, who had been described in the literature as victims of the nightmare, actually suffered from narcolepsy. It is of interest that in our studies the one content report of paralysis associated with considerable fear came from a sleep-onset REM period from Subject 3, who consistently had sleep-onset REM periods but none of the other symptoms of narcolepsy.

SUMMARY

In their studies on Stage 4 night terrors, Broughton and Gastaut took the position that ongoing NREM mentation did *not* trigger these episodes. In this study we made a careful review of our night terror data and found content recalled from 58% of 272 night-terror arousals in 8 subjects. A distinction was made between "prearousal" and "postarousal" mental content. In many instances it is difficult or impossible to determine whether the reported content refers to one or both of these periods. Some content was brief and repetitive and may have been postarousal elaboration of the intense autonomic response, but much was vivid, unusual, and sometimes detailed, more likely originating in the prearousal period. Also, in several instances the subject reported that the frightening content caused him to scream and ignited the episode.

ACKNOWLEDGMENTS

This research was supported by United States Public Health Service Grant MH03267.

The topic of this chapter is fascinating, dealing, as it does, with a dramatic, mysterious, awesome phenomenon known to the ancients and throughout non-Western cultures as well. Not only does it possess obvious clinical importance, but electrographicly controlled study of night terrors and nightmares has much to teach us about the basic psychophysiology of sleep mentation; and the foregoing chapter provides excellent coverage of the issues relevant to sleep mentation.

An aspect of this area of research which has claimed the attention of both Fisher, Kahn et al (1974), and Gastaut and Broughton (1965, is the issue of whether mentation exists prior to the onset of the arousal episode, and whether it is related to the succeeding events of the night-terror episode proper.

The question is: which comes first? Does ongoing mentation play a role in triggering the night-terror arousal episode?; or does the latter emerge from a "physiological vacuum" following which emergence the intense automatic arousal becomes the primary instigator of the concomitant terrifying mentation? If the latter were true, then the occasions and content of night-terror episodes would provide no psychological information about prior sleep mentation, but rather, reflect primarily the arousal episode proper.

Because this consideration possesses the greatest relevance to work in sleep mentation generally, my comments, necessarily brief because of space limitations are confined to this issue alone.

Our problem will be much simplified if we agree at the outset that, much like the situation with common sleeptalking, (an intersecting aberration) night terrors are not a unitary phenomenon but, rather, a final common path of differing configurations of factors. Thus, individual differences across subjects and between one episode to the next within subjects must account for a significant portion of the variance. This is consistent with the impressive variability observed regarding recall and qualities of associated mentation, frequency and times of occurrence, responsiveness to diazepam, intensity of associated physiological changes and clinical course.

From the work described, the following types of night-terror termination outcomes seem to be useful considerations for the problem at hand. With return of full wakefulness and efficient communicative contact with the experimenter, the subject:

1. recalls no mentation whatsoever;
2. recalls mentation which bears no discernible relation to the content of utterances emitted during the night terror arousal;

3. recalls mentation which is clearly concordant with the content of the utterances and in addition, the earliest item of such recalled sequences is something clearly terrifying;

4. recalls mentation clearly concordant with the utterances but with the difference that the earliest item is clearly of a nonterrifying quality and *precedes* in the subject's recall, the point of onset of fearful mental content and anguished vocalizations.

Fisher, Kahn et al. (1974) suggest that the last sequence described (no. 4) indicates an example in which prior ongoing sleep mentation is succeeded by the night-terror arousal proper with its concomitant anxiety-infused content. In this case, it seems reasonable to hypothesize that prior nonanxiety-laden sleep mentation was associatively related to repressed conflictual material reflecting psychic traumata, stirred up the latter, and thus led to the night-terror arousal.

With outcome no. 3, however, there is no recall of prior nonanxious type sleep mentation. It seems to the experimenter as though the subject is asleep one instant and in the very next, plunges precipitously into the night-terror-arousal episode which is neither sleep nor wakefulness but rather a special state of consciousness. Such an interpretation of the data in this type of outcome finds strong support in the reports of Gastaut and Broughton (1965) and Kahn, Fisher *et al.* (Chapter 16 this volume) that the "Stage 4 night terror has never manifested *any* physiological change just prior to the sudden onset of the episode."

That is, the reported lack of any prearousal-episode physiological change seems consistent with the hypothesis that the episode was not preceded by sleep mentation possessing potentialities for increasing arousal levels. If, on the contrary, there had been some sort of electrographic change prior to the marked increase in EMG levels or EEG activation associated with the episode proper, then one might reasonably infer the possibility of prearousal mentation capable of triggering or leading to the night terror.

At this point some questions arise. One of the key electrographic indicators of arousal was heart-rate change. Was the method of evaluating heart rate change the most appropriate to the task at hand? For this purpose, Fisher, Kahn, et al. (1973) calculated the mean heart rate for the 2.5 min interval before night-terror-arousal onset, and Gastaut and Broughton (1965) likewise relied upon mean heart-rate determinations over an unspecified time interval. Is it not possible that changes occurring during the few seconds immediately preceding the onset of the arousal were undetected because they were overshadowed and "canceled out" by fluctuations in the much larger tally of heart beats recorded from the bulk of the total measurement interval? That such a possibility must be taken seriously is shown by the work of Townsend et al. (1975). They studied heart-rate changes preceding body movements and in a "pseudomovement" control condition during sleep in 5 "normal" adult males. Instead of determining mean heart-rate levels, over relatively large epochs, Townsend et al. (1975)

based their findings on a "beat-by-beat heart rate analysis for 20 pre-body movement onset beats through 10 beats following the onset of movement. Group beat-by-beat heart rate averages for spontaneous movements in Stage 2 and REM sleep were calculated using the average response for each subject [p. 218]." They found that spontaneous movements in the observed sleep stages were preceded by significant heart-rate increases beginning approximately 8 sec (beats 20 through, 15) before the onset of the movement. The results were interpreted as supporting an hypothesis that the heart-rate acceleration before spontaneous movements in sleep may be triggered by internal arousal stimuli which, like movements, have sleep-stage-specific rates of occurrence.

Guilleminault and Brusset (1973) provide an additional set of observations that demonstrate the possibility of detectable physiological changes prior to night-terror-arousal episodes. A single subject, (a young male schizophrenic who developed night terrors after hospitalization) was studied for 14 nights distributed in three groups of 4 or 5 nights over a period of 80 days. The clinical picture was very similar to the severe episodes described by Fisher, Kahn *et al.* (1975) and by Gastaut and Broughton (1965). Arousals from Stages 4 and 2 were *always* preceded by somatic changes 30 to 60 sec prior to the behavioral arousal proper. The heart rate would change from 80 to 100 or 120 bpm; respiratory rate and patterns likewise underwent changes, and occasional body movements and vocalizations occurred. *Only* after these changes were EEG modifications observed (consisting of a pattern similar to wakefulness) and behaviorally, the patient seemed to be in the throes of a night-terror arousal proper. (Author's italics).

A third observation that physiological changes may occur shortly prior to the actual night-terror-arousal onset, is provided by a polygraphic record reproduced in a paper by Gastaut and Broughton (1965). The first sign of electrographic change in a stage 3 sleep epoch was a series of K complexes followed very soon by a unidirectional eye movement. In the 1-sec interval after the onset of the first change, the heart rate rose from 56 to 63 bpm. It was not until about 4 sec after the initial change that EMG levels increased and produced EEG artifacts. By this time, the heart rate had risen to 72 bpm. If we count the instant of EMG increase as signaling the point of onset of the arousal episode proper, then a heart-rate increase of 16 bpm occurred over the 4-5 sec interval prior to the beginning of the arousal depicted in the figure. Might it not have been that this prelude was accompanied by mentation leading into the anxiety-infused experience of the night terror proper?

Finally, on a number of occasions, (but unfortunately not routinely), heart rate was monitored on several of our sleeptalker subjects and a tendency toward increased heart rate was observed, particularly in the 5 heartbeats preceding increased EMG levels and EEG artifact or alpha indicating arousal. We have too few subjects and observations, however, to enable us to assert that this is a general trend.

In summary, evidence exists from more than one laboratory, that if heart rate is determined on a beat-by-beat basis just prior to arousal episodes (rather than calculation of the mean heart rate over a relatively long preceding interval), detection of prearousal cardio-acceleration is possible. Thus, the prearousal state is not necessarily a "physiological vacuum." If this hypothesis could be validated, it would suggest that a group of night-terror-arousal subjects might experience nonretrievable mentation prior to the arousal episode proper—mentation in association with which the heart beats faster. This would in no way vitiate in principle a category of episodes in which the arousal does indeed emerge abruptly from a prior state without detectable physiological perturbation and devoid of associated mentation.

A. M. ARKIN

AUTHOR'S REBUTTAL TO EDITOR'S COMMENTS
ON CHAPTER 16

Arkin argues very cogently that evidence exists from three laboratories in which night terrors have been investigated, that if heart rate is determined on a beat-by-beat basis just prior to arousal episodes, rather than by calculation of the mean heart rate over a relatively long preceding interval, as was done by Fisher, et al. (1973, 1974), detection of prearousal cardio-acceleration is possible. During our extensive work with night terrors we were much preoccupied with the problem discussed by Arkin. Although it is true that in our heart-rate calculations we utilized mean heart-rate figures, varying .5-2.5 min, we paid special attention to and closely examined the heart rates in the few seconds immediately preceding the physiological and behavioral indicators of the arousal reaction. We were never able to demonstrate any acceleration during these brief intervals. We had occasion to examine at least several hundred prearousal heart and respiratory rates. We paid just as careful attention to respiratory rate and amplitude. In many instances we calculated, in millimeters, peak-to-peak distance between respirations and again were unable to demonstrate respiratory acceleration. Good examples of this cardio-respiratory stability can be seen in Figures 1 and 2 (Fisher et al., 1973) and Figure 2 (Fisher et al., 1974) In these figures it is to be noted that the best indicator of the onset of the night terror is a break in the respiratory rhythm.

The three observations cited by Arkin in the literature as supporting his point of view do not seem very convincing. The investigation by Townsend et al. (1975) dealt with normal body movements arising spontaneously out of Stages 2 and REM sleep, not Stage 4. Such normal body movements may be triggered by internal arousal stimuli qualitatively different from the gross or somnambulistic body movements characteristic of the night terror arousal reaction.

It is difficult to interpret the observations reported by Guilleminault and Brusset (1973). They dealt with a single atypical subject, a young male schizophrenic, who showed a marked sleep disturbance characterized by paucity of Stage 1 REM and a marked excess of Stage 4, and who was, during the period of study, on a variety of tranquilizing and hypnotic drugs.

Although Gastaut and Broughton (1965) were the first to describe the arousal reaction in relation to the night terror, their description of it differed from ours in one important respect, in that they located the period of screaming and other vocalization at the end of the night-terror episode rather than at its very beginning, as we found to be universally the case. It is our impression that the particular episode that they chose as an illustration (Figures 10a and 10b of the Gastaut & Broughton, 1965 experiment) also appears somewhat ambiguous and atypical.

First, the EEG appears to be quite low voltage and devoid of slow waves characteristic of Stage 3 or 4. Second, the onset of the arousal appears to be atypically gradual. We would, however, locate it immediately following the last heartbeat at the rate of 56 bpm. the indicators of arousal being the eye movement, a slight irregularity of the respiration at that point, and what appears to be the onset of alpha simultaneously.

Although it would fit in with my preconceived notions and prejudices that a group of night-terror-arousal subjects, as Arkin suggests, might experience non-retrievable mentation in association with which the heart beats faster, I do not find the evidence he marshaled in favor of this contention very persuasive and find myself rather uncomfortably stuck with the concept of the prearousal state as a "physiological vacuum."

Charles Fisher

Part VII

IMPLICATIONS AND
NEW DIRECTIONS

17

Contemporary Sleep Research and Clinical Practice

Arthur M. Arkin

City College of the City Univeristy of New York

The history of modern theory of dream formation and interpretation begins with the Traumdeutung of Freud (1900/1953c), a monumental work, which treats in depth a heroic list of subjects. Among the topics dealt with are theories of psychic structure and function, psychosexual development, psychological processes involved in dream production, psychological and biological "purposes" and principles and manifested or reflected in dreams, and specifications for a technique and theory of dream interpretation. As time passed, clinicians and theoreticians (including Freud himself) made further contributions and emendations to his original formulations, and some propounded rival theories of varying scope and cogency. For historical purposes, it is important to realize that this evolution occurred on the basis of continuing clinical experience, rather than laboratory research.

With the advent of the electrographic era in sleep investigations, a number of workers have attempted to evaluate or modify classical clinical theories, as well as make comparisons between them, all in the light of these new findings.[1] Since it is impossible in a short space to review this literature adequately, I shall limit myself to selected comments regarding, what appear to me, the most germane topics, and then sketch out those aspects of the new knowledge which have been useful in my own clinical practice.

[1]The chief contributions along these lines are those of Altschuler (1966), Anders (1974, Breger (1967, 1969) Breger *et al.* (1971b), Dallett (1973), Fisher (1965), Foulkes (1964, 1966), Foulkes et al. (1973), Foulkes and Vogel (1974), Greenberg and Pearlman (1974), Hawkins (1966), Holt (1967), Whitman (1974), Whitman et al. (1970), and Zetzel (1970). In addition, several collections of relevant articles and commentary are to be found in Dement (1964a), Fisher and Breger (1969), Hartmann (1970), Holt (1967), Kramer et al. (1969), Madow and Snow (1970). Of special interest is Jones' (1970a) comprehensive review of clinical dream theory, with suggested reformulations in the light of laboratory findings. This should be read in conjunction with Umbarger's (1974) critique.

The most fruitful point of departure, I imagine, is the issue of the process of dream formation; and in this regard, the chief considerations are the contributions made by physiological, and by psychological factors, respectively. A basic assumption of the prevailing clinical psychological theories of dreaming (despite their marked diversity) has been that dreaming occurs in a nonpredictable, erratic manner—and then only as a result of a complex interaction of suitable psychological variables. (Some clinical theories merely imply this assumption, whereas others, such as the classical Freudian psychoanalytic theory, provide specific details regarding the interaction of these psychological prerequisites of dreaming.) However, the new laboratory findings demonstrate a certain rhythmicity to vivid dreaming experience, which tends to occur in association with electrographically defined stages and events of the sleep cycle (especially, REM sleep) and the time of night as well, (see Chapters 1 and 6 of this volume). In light of this fact, the assumption of aperiodic, and exclusively *psychologically caused* dreaming must be challenged. The need for revision is made all the more compelling by the demonstration of the higher diurnal proportion of REM sleep in premature babies, neonates, and small children in comparison to older humans, as well as the ubiquity of REM sleep in most mammals. That is, these findings establish even more forcefully that physiological processes have primacy over psychological processes, and that occasions for dreaming are subject to regularly recurring physiological factors. By contrast, classical Freudian dream-instigation theory specified that dreaming occurs as a final outcome of a psychological process necessarily driven by the activated or disinhibited psychic energy investing a repressed wish; that is, no repressed wish, no dream. The laboratory findings, however, indicate that biological rhythmic factors are the main initiators of dreaming occasions.

But it is one thing to state that the primary instigators and constraints of dreaming are factors derived from biological rhythms and another to deny that psychological factors may be crucial determinants of the content of sleep mentation, the sequence of its events, and the efficiency of dream recall on awakening. This statement is consistent with a recent view of mind as an emergent property of cerebral activity which once evolved acquires casual efficacy in its own right and becomes manifested in the course of interaction with physiological processes. For example, Sperry's (1969, 1970) modified Concept of Consciousness contends that

> conscious phenomena as direct emergent properties of cerebral activity do interact with and causally determine the brain process . . . also that the neurophysiology controls the mental effects, and the mental properties in turn control the neurophysiology . . . and that the conscious phenomena are in a position of higher command, as it were, located at the top of the organizational hierarchy [p. 534].

Sperry adroitly defends his conceptualizations against a charge that his approach is basically dualistic in the traditional philosophical sense. But to discuss this further here would be an excessive digression, and the reader is referred to Sperry's fascinating papers.

In examining the common procedures of using dreams in clinical practice, one notes that despite marked differences in conceptualizations regarding dreams and dreaming, all known influential clinical approaches operate with two basic assumptions: that dreams, like poetry, possess components of "*non-o*bvious *m*eaning" (*NOM* components); and that when a patient relates a dream in the therapeutic session it provides the therapist with important opportunities for formulation and appropriate utilization of interpretations as a means of furthering therapeutic progress. Indeed, the purpose of a theory of dream interpretation is to describe a systematic approach to decoding NOM components so that "they can be inserted into the chain of intelligible waking mental acts." (Freud, 1900/ 1953c). The therapist may employ his interpretations in a variety of ways. For example, suppose a patient is troubled with anxiety, shyness, and feelings of inability to feel himself genuinely masculine. He has a dream in which he depicts himself as being trampled by a horse. The patients' life history and the current contexts of his life suggests to the therapist that being trampled by a horse is an NOM component derived from the patient's unconscious feminine wishes. If the patient is a poor candidate for insight therapy, the therapist may respond to his interpretation of the NOM component by recommending that the patient undertake a muscle-building program in an effort to counteract his conscious feelings of inadequacy; or if the patient has been progressing well in insight therapy, the therapist may make comments designed to prepare the patient to hear and integrate at some future time specific information regarding his unconscious feminine strivings; or, again, if the patient has given "signs of readiness" and has adequately worked through material used in defenses, the therapist may choose to explicitly utter forthwith, information describing the patient's unconscious feminine strivings. In any case, the interpretive process involves an implicit or explicit decoding or transformation of NOM components into easily understood verbal expressions, that is, "obvious meaning components." Put more precisely, to the extent that the NOM components of psychically derived outputs can be expressed in accordance with the rules of simple and complex well-formed formulae of propositional calculus, such components will achieve corresponding degrees of clarity. One might well ask why bother with dream interpretation at all in clinical practice? Clearly the answer is that decoded NOM components provide important essential clues for the therapist regarding the difficulties of the patient, not easily obtainable in any other way. (For a recent vigorous exposition and defense of this viewpoint, see Greenson, 1970.)

Returning now to the Traumdeutung, one must again take into account that Freud attempted to set forth therein much more than a theory and technique of dream interpretation in the narrow sense; and this consideration provides the basis for an important distinction. One could usefully describe the specific theory of the technique of decoding NOM components as the set of *nuclear* concepts in a theory of dream interpretation; and to describe all other related thought regarding the "function" of dreams, or assertions concerning basic, omnipresent structure of dreams, as *peripheral* and unessential to the validity of the former.

Examples of such peripheral features are those considering dreams as preservers of sleep, psychic "safety valves," or as strictly differentiable into manifest and latent content domains. Similarly classifiable as peripheral concepts would be certain non-Freudian ideas such as considering dreaming as *necessarily* providing occasions for solving problems, planning for the future or compensating for intrapsychic dysharmony.

NOM-components might include transparent or transformed derivatives of such phenomena as memories from the recent and remote past (as far back as infancy), affects of all types, unmastered acute and chronic stress of situations, life goals, philosophic and religious matters, and psychological conflict (both conscious and unconscious). The domain of NOM components encompasses classical Freudian latent content and the sphere of hermeneutics (Ricoeur, 1970), as subsets of a still broader category. Actually, that which is included in the category of meaningfulness is so complex as to defy concise description. For example, Odgen and Richards (1945) discuss no less than 16 different usages of the meaning of "meaning." For example, the "meaning" of an expression may pertain to aspects of denotation, connotation, intentions, implication, emotion, prognostication, emphasis, memories, associations, encoding, and other related considerations. (See Appendix 17.2 for their complete list.)

For the most part, these various aspects of "meaning" seem capable of description and inclusion within the cognitive-affective information-processing models formulated by such theorists as Lindsay and Norman (1972), Anderson (1975), and Mandler (1975). *For the purpose of my exposition, "meaning" is to be understood in its broadest possible sense to include conscious and unconscious meanings of all verbal and non-verbal forms of expression of the psyche as they might be differentially represented throughout the stages of psychological development.*[2]

It is therefore, invalid and simplistic to seek *the* underlying meaning of a dream. Langer's (1957) comment should make this clear:

> The fact that very few of our words are purely technical, and few of our images purely utilitarian, gives our lives a background of closely woven multiple meanings against which all conscious experiences and interpretations are measured. Every object that emerges into the focus of attention has meaning beyond the 'fact' in which it figures. It serves by turns, and sometimes even at once, for insight and theory and behavior, in nondiscursive knowledge and discursive reason, in wishful fancy, or as a sign eliciting conditioned reflex action." (p. 285)

Working clinically with dream material most often entails delineation and elucidation of psychological transformational processes in a large variety of contexts. Such transformations may progress equally in two directions: from the primitive, regressed or concrete, to the more mature, organized and verbal; or proceed along the opposite pathway. Thus, a wide-eyed baby climbing up a

[2]Further treatment of this subject may be found in Church (1961), Peterfreund and Schwartz (1971) Peterfreund & Franceschini (1973), Hospers (1967), Schafer (1970, Cherry (1966), Schimek (1975), Lindsay and Norman (1972), Palumbo (1973), Rubinstein (1974), Horowitz (1972).

pole in a dream may be, in part, a transformation of an actual awe-arousing percept of an erect penis on the evening before the dream; and it may also be a way of transforming an item of self-characterization—considering oneself to be a naive baby. The former is an illustration of the transformation of a wakeful percept (which stimulated intense affect) into a remote, disguised and emotionally toned-down concrete representation; the latter is an example of the use of the same concrete image to represent a comparatively abstract idea, that of inappropriate naivete. One finds numerous examples of such transformations in Freud's writings on dreams, in Sharpe's (1949) *Dream Analysis* and in Bonime's (1962) *The Clinical Use of Dreams.*

A recent treatment of this theme may be found in the work of Jones (1970a, c) who recommends that the term transformation be substituted whenever we come across the terms disguise, distortion, or censorship in dream literature. It is in accounting for this area that Freudian theory excels; and laboratory experience has repeatedly provided abundant *in vivo* examples of the specific mechanisms of dream work that Freud described. Furthermore, experimental data bear out Freud's clinically important contentions of the ubiquitousness of psychic temporal and formal regression as features of sleep mentation (Baekeland et al (1968); Berger, (1963); Breger et al. (1971b); Fisher and Paul, (1959); Pötzl et al. (1962); Shervin and Fisher (1967); Witkin cited in Kramer (1969).

Do results of laboratory study affect the clinician's assertion that dreams possess NOM components? A broad spectrum of personal opinion prevails among sleep researchers who, at one extreme, are skeptical about the validity of the concept of the meaningfulness of dreams. Thus, Kleitman (1963) seems content to see little more in dreams than the outcome of "crude" or "inefficient" cerebral-cortical activity. At the other end of the spectrum, many investigators are convinced that dreams do indeed possess NOM components which are capable of being decoded—a belief in which I share.[3]

Despite numerous competing approaches to dream interpretation, it is fair to say that the most elaborate influential, and provocative has been that of Freud. Certainly the bulk of criticism stemming from both clinical and laboratory sources has been directed at his theories. It is curious, therefore, that with few exceptions, the focus of scientific evaluation has been *early* Freudian theory. And what is generally ignored are many of the theory's complexities, Freud's qualifying comments made during the course of later revisions, and certainly the implications for dream theory of the newer post-Freudian developments in psychoanalytic thought.

I should, therefore, like to collate and discuss a series of propositions which are intended to provide a modern framework for the clinical use of dreams.

---

[3]Lewis (1968); Foulkes (1964, 1966); Foulkes and Vogel (1974); Kramer et al. (1975); Greenberg and Pearlman (1973); Whitman (1974; and Fisher (1965). The difficulties of validating such interpretations are at least not *more* formidable than those involved in validating most other clinical hypotheses (Eagle (1973); Rubinstein (1973); Sherwood (1969, 1973); Shope (1973).

Drawing upon the corpus of Freudian thought and its continued evolution in the hands of his followers, it is also consistent with the new laboratory studies of dreams. The basic scheme consists of a set of psychological components which interact with biological and sociocultural factors. As such, it is capable of accommodating dream-forming influences derived not only from classical Freudian considerations but from factors upon which attention has been focused by other clinical theorists. Such factors include attempts to solve problems and to cope with adaptational demands, as well as dream forming influences which are reflections of existential predicaments, and those which bear the imprints and effects of sociocultural factors. It is my freely admitted bias that the many valuable contributions of non- and neo-Freudians to the practice of dream interpretation can be easily and harmoniously incorporated into such a *contemporary* Freudian scheme, but the reverse is not feasible.

The Elaboration of Mentation Is An Autonomous Ego Function

[Hartmann, 1939]

This proposition contends that the production and maintenance of the stream of mental events is an outgrowth of developmental-constitutional-neuropsychological factors which, in ongoing interaction with the external *milieu,* result in differentiated, flexibly organized cognitive processes and structures. Inherent in this statement is the idea that the ego is biologically endowed with a certain degree of independence from influences arising from the id and from external reality, and is thus capable of functioning "on its own" (Rapaport, 1967). Thus, studies of mentation reports under a variety of experimental conditions, obtained during all stages of sleep and wakefulness, attest to the existence of ongoing endogenously produced mentation. Such mentation is detectable from all stages of sleep (Foulkes, 1966) and is virtually impossible to suppress for sustained intervals during wakefulness (Singer, 1974).

Characteristics of Ongoing Mentation, Both Qualitative and Quantitative, Are Correlated with Concomitant Stages of Sleep and Sustained Wakefulness, Each as Modified By The Basic Rest-Activity Cycle (BRAC)

That characteristics of mentation are associated with stages of the sleep cycle has been amply documented in Chapter 6 of this volume. Variation in wakeful mentation as a function of the BRAC is perhaps less striking, but research in this area has only recently begun and various studies (Foulkes, 1966; Foulkes and Fleisher, 1975; Friedman and Fisher, 1967; Globus, 1970; Hartmann, 1968b; Kleitman, 1970b; Lavie & Kripke, 1975) already point to reliable correlations. The essential implication, however, is that quite independently of motivational-affective factors, cognition is subject to crucial constraints and influences arising from neuropsychological factors inherent in particular states of consciousness. For example, one of the cognitive resources of wakeful, vigilant consciousness is the optional capability to impose and monitor an overall, logical integration and coherence on prolonged intervals of mentation, and to maintain sustained critical reactivity to afferent impulses. This option is much less available or else not usually recruited in states of reverie, sleep, and sleep-onset consciousness. In these latter states of diminished vigilance, mentation is more fluid and fragmentary, less organized in a logical, sequential, coherent manner, and proceeds in patterns well described as the "primary mental process" (Freud, 1900/1953c). The looseness of logical relationship between one item of low-vigilance mentation and its successors presumably confers upon sleep mentation a vulnerability to influence by momentary perturbations arising from fluctuating psychological factors, and shifts in patterns of endogenous activation. Such vulnerability may become manifested in the relatively chaotic qualities of sleep mentation.

It is of interest to suggest that just as the incoherent features of schizophrenic mentation can be explained by an immediacy hypothesis (Salzinger, 1971), so might be similar characteristics of sleep consciousness. According to Salzinger's (1971) formulation, schizophrenics' behavior " ... is more often controlled by stimuli which are immediate in their spatial and temporal environment than is that of normals [p. 601]." Among such controlling stimuli are those comprised of the subjects' immediately prior responses or emitted signals. Salzinger (1971) goes on to state that " ... unless an individual is able to respond to relatively remote response-produced stimuli (his prior verbal behavior) his speech would only make sense for short segments [p. 604]." Presumably, the same principles of immediacy could play a role in governing the pattern of ongoing sleep mentation and thus partly explain its diminished coherence and intelligibility. That is, each item of mentation would have prepotent influence over its immediate successor, rather than the latter being responsive to a remote mentation item occurring much earlier. The entire mentation sequence viewed in the large would then tend to lack coherence and often to seem chaotic. Thus, Salzinger's principle of immediacy describes a factor involved in those primary process characteristics of sleep mentation to which Freud (1900/1953c) applied the term "formal regression" wherein primitive methods of expression and representation are substituted for the usual ones.

Subject to Constraints and Influences Originating From Neuropsychological Variables Peculiar to Different States of Consciousness, the Specific Content and the Event Sequence of Ongoing Mentation Are Governed by Four Sets of Factors

The Principle of Multiple Function (Waelder, 1936)
Current Adaptational Tendencies and Requirements (Hartmann, 1939)
Epigenetic Phase Factors (Erikson, 1954; 1963)
Determinants of Modes of Thought Representation (Horowitz, 1972)

During the course of a psychotherapeutic session in which more or less free verbal expression is encouraged, one observes a succession of verbal and nonverbal behavioral sequences. One is apt to be bewildered unless some system is available for ordering this material. Organizing principles are needed which are sufficiently broad so that no significant area of human life is slighted or overlooked. One must be able to understand the behavioral sequences as being simultaneously determined by a host of psychological factors which in turn have been constrained, molded and partly derived from biological and sociological variables. Foremost among the psychological factors are conscious and unconscious components of instinctual urges, ethics, cognition, executive and mediating functions, psycholinguistics, interpersonal and intrafamilial relationships, and adaptational and coping mechanisms, all in the context of the specific developmental history of the individual. And this realm of the psychological is interwoven with and derived from biological factors (such as biological rhythms, physiological mechanisms, and our animal heritage), and from sociological influences (such as cultural and subcultural, racial, socioeconomic, class, political, interfamilial, and population-density factors.)

The concept of the ongoing psyche existing independently, but also in interactive and derivation relation to biological and sociological factors is set forth in a clinically useful manner by selective, combined formulations of Freud (1900/1953), Waelder (1936), Hartmann (1939), and Erikson (1954, 1963) as cited above, and formally presented within Rapaport's (1960) attempt at systematizing psychoanalytic theory.

First, the principle of multiple function states that all behavior (including mentation) is elaborated by the ego, during the course of which it fulfills, by means of varying combinations of active and passive coping processes, the simultaneous requirements of the id, superego, adaptation to reality, and attempts to achieve belated mastery over previous traumata (Waelder, 1936). Thus, each behavioral phenomenon is a product of synthetic ego activity in which suitable compromises are arranged between these various psychic agencies and thus, no single factor may be invoked as a sole cause. (To those who are put off by psychoanalytic terminology, similar basic ideas were expressed by Aristotle when he noted that man is unique among animals because he is able to formulate plans and rules which take into simultaneous account his needs for pleasure, virtue and prosperity; Ross, 1964).

Second, in his radical development of the psychoanalytic theory of adaptation, Hartmann (1939) formulated the concepts of primary autonomous ego apparatuses and their development out of innate elements present at birth. Such apparatuses subserve perception, memory, anticipation, motility, and threshold functions for each. They arise independently of the id and, in Rapaport's paraphrasing (1967), they provide the "primary guarantees" of the organism's fitting in with (adaptedness to) its neonatal environment. As development proceeds, apparatuses of secondary autonomy, originating either from instinctual modes and vicissitudes, or from defensive structures formed during conflict solution, undergo a "change of function" and serve as additional resources for adaptation. In contrast to primary autonomous apparatuses which are "innate," secondary autonomous apparatuses arise from "experience." The essential point here is that both sets of autonomous ego apparatuses ordinarily function in a relatively conflict-free manner in subserving the needs of adaptation to the psychosocial environment and play critical roles in fashioning parameters of mentation.

Third, Erikson's (1954a, 1963) important conceptualizations involve an epigenetic scheme of ego evolution which:

> ... encompasses the kind and sequence of certain universal psychosocial crises which are defined, on the one hand, by potentialities and limitations of developmental stages (physical, psychosexual, ego) and, on the other, by the universal punctuation of human life by successive and systematic 'life tasks' within social and cultural institutions [1954a, p. 155].

And during the therapeutic session, by means of these three organizing perspectives, one may discern in the patient's stream of mentation, dominant and subordinate themes within multidimensional and multicontextual networks. Each of these themes, in turn, has a past history, a future orientation, patterns of transition, a "depth," and a "surface." They may also be seen from a different vantage point as simultaneous self-disclosures and motivated concealments, as ways of seeking after diverse gratifications and shielding one's vulnerabilities, as types of adaptation to interpersonal situations, and other forms of psychological existence.

Fourth, it is fruitful to view the patient's mental content as outputs of a thought-representation system which functions in accordance with combinations of three modes of thought representation: enaction, imagery, and lexical expression (Horowitz, 1972, 1975). Minor, abbreviated trial actions involving anticipatory or concurrent tensing of various muscle groups may carry out or reflect thinking by enactive representation of stored psychomotor information. Examples of complex enactions are gestures, facial expressions, and bodily postures.

Imagery expresses information by mentation with sensory qualities embodying visual, auditory, tactile, olfactory-gustatory, kinesthetic, and other similar components. Examples of complex imagery formations are provided by introjects, visual symbols, fantasies, body images, and interpersonal role relationships.

Lexical modes of thought representation are the outcome of epigenetic development from earlier modes of enactive and image representation. Lexical representation involves the use of words to express thoughts, and in its quintessential form is carried out without action (no subvocal speech) and imagery (no auditory, visual, or kinesthetic accompaniments). But lexical representation does not replace enactive and image thinking, which themselves undergo continued epigenetic development and persist throughout life.

Under normal conditions, the three modes of thought representation interact, blend and merge in the course of mentation-sequence production.

Of cardinal importance is the principle that information represented in one mode is capable of free and effortless translation into the other representational modes. Actually, information becomes fully processed and assimilated to the extent that is has acquired cross-modal translation. For example, Horowitz (1972) describes an incident during a therapeutic session in which a patient's awareness of her own facial grimace led to a visual memory image of her mother's face disfigured by injury, and then to its lexical expression including conceptualizations of her pathological identification with this feature of her mother—a factor in the patient's self-perception as ugly.

An additional feature of Horowitz's model is the assumption of regulatory processes at the boundaries of the three subsystems responsible for representation in the three modes. These processes control entries and exits of information from one subsystem to another. Furthermore, besides external inputs, the representational system is generally activated by internally derived inputs of information from conscious and unconscious sources. These input sources may govern the representational system in parallel or reciprocal fashion in varying mixtures. That is, the stream of mentation may show influences of both external and internal stimuli under moderate levels of activation during routine wakefulness. In the presence of high influxes from the surround, however, external rather than internal stimuli gain ascendancy in the representational system (a bomb blast would overide an erotic fantasy); and with low-level external influx or inhibition of stimuli from the surround, internal usually take precedence over external sources of information (absorption in a reverie or dream tends to supplant traffic noise).

A variety of dynamic and cognitive physiological factors influence the functioning of the boundary control systems leading to fluctuations in momentary and sustained patterns of thought representation in the three modes. For example, visual could predominate over lexical representation or vice versa in accordance with defensive requirements. The defense of isolation could involve inhibition of cross-modal translation—a warded-off idea or affect that acquired representation mostly as an image at the expense of lexical translation would be reduced in conceptual meanings and implications with consequent diminution of emotional response; or lexical intellectualization of the therapist's interpretations could bleach imagery of its affective charge. Distortion and displacement could be the outcome of mistranslations between subsystems. In another context, if a memory were initially encoded solely in the image and enactive systems, it might not be capable of conscious expression in the lexical mode.

The qualities of dreaming experience could result in part from shifts in the proportions of factors governing thought representation in the three modes. During sleep, the enactive and lexical systems undergo physiological attenuation and at the same time, particularly in REM sleep, there is relative intensification of internal sources of information. Such conditions approximate those Horowitz (1975) describes as favoring hallucinatory experience in wakefulness. These include relative reduction of external input with no relative decrease, or even relative increase, of the receptivity of the representational system, augmentation of internal input due to arousal of ideas and affects derived from drive states, and degrees of disinhibition of internal inputs. Under these circumstances, the representational system tends to function predominantly in the image mode which, unencumbered by influx or constraints from the real surround, and the rules of the lexical system, produce dreams.

From the point of view of Horowitz's (1972) model, psychoanalytic

working through a given set of ideas and emotions would include crosstranslation of information between modes without censorship or distortion. When crosstranslation is possible, then there can be full establishment of all appropriate association connections. The resultant multifaceted representation is probably essential for some types of change in cognitive structures [p. 816] . . .

I should like to emphasize that my employment of metapsychoanalytic theoretical concepts for the purposes of this chapter is not to be construed as insistence on their ultimate scientific validity. I am well aware of the mounting controversy which is leading many outstanding psychoanalytic theoreticians to question whether continued adherence to Freudian meta-psychological formulations, even if refurbished and updated, is likely to be useful in the future (e. g. Rubinstein, 1967, 1975; Klein, 1969; Palumbo, 1973; Peterfreund & Schwartz, 1971). The main point is that to adequately account for the characteristics of mentation sequences in all states of consciousness, a set of perspectives possessed of sufficient dimensional scope and interactive components is required. The problems, after all, are most complicated. It seems injudicious to strive zealously for theoretical parsimony if the result is conceptual poverty. In addition, whether an organizing scheme is formulated in Freudian metapsychological terms is immaterial as long as it contains theoretical provisions for whatever valid empirical considerations are subsumed under the psychoanalytic dynamic, economic, structural, genetic, adaptive, and topographic points of view (Rapaport, 1960).

Turning now to sleep mentation proper, it seems appropriate to assume that just as *wakeful* behavior sequences (including the stream of mentation) are completely determined by psychological factors as previously indicated, so do psychological variables determine *sleep* mentation—and to assume also that such determination occurs within constraints set up by the rhythmic biological and physiological factors which are reflected in the sleep cycle. As an analogy, one might imagine a group of children at school whose behavior is controlled to some degree by the school schedule with its concomitant rules and regulations. That is, the periodicity and structure of the school schedule is analogized to that of the sleep cycle. Under normal conditions, the behavior of the children would stand in rough correspondence to sleep mentation, such that the relative quiet and motionless of recumbent rest periods correspond to no—or minimal—content sleep mentation reports; the sustained intervals of organized verbal and conceptual activity involved in instruction, study and discussion correspond to modal NREM reports; and the periods of free play correspond to modal REM reports. During free play, the children would not be totally without external constraints but would nevertheless utilize such ludic materials as crayons, dolls, toys, masks, their own bodies, and so on, for enactment of unique, highly varied, loosely organized, often chaotic behavior sequences. The latter would reflect such influences as the children's instinctual urges, moral values, unconscious fantasies and memories, future strivings, sociocultural background, expectancies, cognitive skills, and inborn proclivities. Similar analogies could easily be imagined for persons of any age and in the midst of any epigenetic phase. In Horowitz's (1972) terms one might view NREM sleep as an occasion which permits varying mixtures of both lexical and image modes of thought representation, with lexical often overshadowing image expression; whereas in REM sleep, the opposite situation prevails—image modes of representation have the ascendancy over lexical forms.

To repeat: Whatever specific psychological variables might be considered as determinants of wakeful behavioral sequences could likewise codetermine sleepmentation events along with neuropsychological factors inherent in sleep states of consciousness (such as diminished critical reactivity and "regressive" alterations of cognition). Thus, there seems to be no reason to assume incompatability between biological components of the sleep cycle, the determining influence of psychological factors in fashioning dreams, and dreams being the vehicles of NOM components. As such, decoded dream reports may yield information capable of elucidating problems in clinical psychiatric diagnosis, psychodynamic and psychogenetic formulations, transference and countertransference situations, planning treatment, evaluating its momentary status, assessing the readiness for specific interpretations and, finally, therapy termination (Whitman et al., 1970).

With regard to the specific techniques of clinical dream analysis and interpretation, I have found, along with so many other clinicians, that the most useful are those described by Freud (1900, 1953c), Sharpe (1949), and Erikson (1954a). Each of these authors approaches dream interpretation by considering the patient's associations to elements of the dream report, total behavior during the session, recent events in the patient's life, all within the context of life history, personality structure, repertoire of mental transformational processes, and public and private symbolism. In my opinion, the new sleep research contains nothing to contravene these nuclear features (see above) of their respective approaches.

Such a format for analysis and interpretation of dreams seems entirely compatible with recent cognitive-psychological and information processing formulations. (Anderson 1975; Lindsay & Norman 1972; Mandler, 1975). Taken as a group, such models utilize components subserving:

1. reception of inputs;
2. subjective interpretation of such inputs;
3. processing of inputs by a complicated system of memory networks, including memory networks, the structure and content of which are accessible to free-association procedures;

4. psychological transformational processes operating at each stage of information processing;

5. encoding, production, and monitoring of outputs.

In addition, these models contain provisions for articulation with psychological factors related to motivation, affect, and adaptation. Actually, the outline of dream analysis presented by Erikson (1954a) in his excellent paper sets forth the principles of modern psychoanalytic interpretation in the senses indicated earlier in the chapter. (This outline is included as Appendix 17.1 at the end of the chapter.)

Patients, in the Course of Psychological Adaptation to the Therapeutic Situation, May Alter Many Characteristic, Sustained Cognitive, Motivational and Attention-Deployment Patterns, Leading to Changes in the Quantity and Quality of Dream Recall, as Well as Instigation or Intensification of Psychic "Censorship" in Specific Transferential and Counter-transferential Contexts

In attempting to relate the new sleep-research findings to the clinical use of dreams, it is essential to keep in mind the nature of the data upon which various investigators have based their conclusions—conclusions as to the psychological characteristics of "good" versus "poor" dream recallers, and vivid NREM dreamers; also conclusions concerning the qualities of REM mentation in subjects belonging to various nosological groups, or whether REM reports may be judged as representing attempted fulfillment of unconscious wishes.

First, and foremost, with rare exceptions the subjects were *not* involved in the research study as a direct means of obtaining relief from personal distress. Rather, they participated in varying degrees out of financial need, intellectual or career interest, and emotionally compliant predispositions to requests of scientific researchers.

Second, the time period of involvement was for a more or less comparatively brief interval, the duration of which was specified in advance. The usual conditions were such that the subjects were likely to perceive the study situation as short-lived, and as noninstrumental in securing amelioration of suffering or bringing about personality change. These conditions are consistent with the expectation that after completion of the study, they would return psychologically to the *status quo ante.*

In summary, clinical conditions, in which the primary goals of the undertaking are therapeutic in nature, contain crucial exigencies not present under research conditions in which the ostensible primary goal is the increase of scientific knowledge. This is far from saying that research findings are inapplicable, but rather that they may not be applied to clinical settings piecemeal and without consideration for the altered circumstances inherent in clinical contexts.

The initiation of a psychotherapeutic relationship entails more than "establishing rapport," carrying out therapists' instructions, and permitting transference phenomena to emerge; it also requires the patient to carry out a process of psychological adaptation to this unique situation. For example, the expression of hitherto unverbalized emotionally charged material in the therapeutic setting inevitably results in shifts in previously existing equilibria which functioned in more or less stable fashion. Added to this are the effects of the therapist's various interventions, including not only interpretations, but factors arising from the necessary practical arrangements (session schedule, fees, and cancellation policies). As transferential tendencies and defenses are mobilized and interact with whatever therapist behaviors are manifested, processes involved in the formation of dreams and associated NOM components are likely to be significantly influenced.

Accordingly, although Freud probably overestimated the role of intrapsychic censorship in the dream formation of people not absorbed in therapy or self-examination, clinical literature is replete with convincing illustrative examples of the operation of censorship mechanisms during psychoanalytic treatment (Luborsky, 1967). To what extent censorship, disguise, and indirect expression, are active during dreaming in "everyday life" is an imponderable question, but the hypothesis of its activity during mentation in clinical contexts makes intelligible many otherwise puzzling or unnoticed events. This assertion is borne out by at least three studies in which patients in psychotherapy or psychoanalysis had their dreams concomitantly monitored in the laboratory (Breger et al., 1971b; Greenberg & Pearlman, 1973; Whitman et al., 1963). Furthermore, it is common clinical experience that patients who claim that they never, or rarely, recall dreams often become "good dream recallers" as therapy proceeds. It is, therefore, of great interest that controlled studies of dream recall demonstrate that it is indeed possible for many "normal" individuals to significantly increase their rate of dream recall, even if their recall is poor prior to the onset of the study. (Cory et al., 1975; Domhoff & Gerson, 1967; Meier et al., 1968).

A final study supporting the contention that long term psychological patterns related to dreaming are subject to alteration by the therapy situation has been reported by Cartwright et al. (1975). A group of self-referred patients seeking psychotherapy was considered unlikely to remain in long-term treatment because the patients had impaired access to their internal lives and also suffered from poor ability to discuss their inner experience. A subgroup of these patients received training in the laboratory in recalling and discussing their REMP dreams. This resulted in improved dream recall and a diminished dropout rate in comparison to three different control groups.

In summary, much evidence is available indicating the validity of the assertion that long-standing psychological patterns involved in dreaming are subject to change in clinical contexts, and that the evaluation of such change provides additional opportunities for psychological interpretation.

Afterthoughts

The foregoing discussion of problems of dream interpretation has not done full justice to the relevance of the new sleep research for clinical practice. It has been shown that a heterogenous group of sleep-related syndromes need not arise primarily out of psychological conflict (although psychological factors may subsequently play crucial determining roles). For example, enuretic episodes need not be concurrent with dreaming; they are usually not associated with REM sleep, and dreams with urine-related content recalled in the following morning may have resulted from stimulus incorporation of the sensation of moisture on the skin derived from previous bed-wetting in the same night (Gastaut & Broughton, 1965). Similarly, disorders such as narcolepsy, somnambulism, night terrors, cluster migraine, nocturnal asthma, bruxism, paroxysmal head banging, and certain other syndromes involving excessive, disrupted or insufficient sleep, while being strongly influenced by psychological factors, usually require some biochemical-physiological components in the formulation of their essential etiological backgrounds (Williams et al., 1974). Limitations of space, however, precluded further comment.

ACKNOWLEDGMENTS

I wish to thank Irving Paul (Department of Psychology, CUNY) and Alfred Lilienfeld (Department of Psychiatry, New York University Medical School) for their helpful critical suggestions.

APPENDIX 1

Erikson's (1954a) Outline of Clinical Dream Analysis with slight modifications

   A. Features and configurations of the sleep mentation report (manifest dream).
1. Psycholinguistic – general quality, spoken words, word play.
2. Sensory – general quality, variety, range and intensity and specific sensory foci
3. Spatial – quality of extension and dominant vectors
4. Temporal – general quality of succession and time perspective
5. Somatic – general quality of body feeling, body zones and organ modes
6. Interpersonal – general social grouping, changing social vectors. "object relations" and points of identification
7. Affective – general quality of affective atmosphere, inventory and range of affects, and points of affective change.
9. Summary and correlation of configurational trends

   B. Links between manifest and latent-dream material: (Erikson took pains to add the following important ideas in this context – "On closer inspection, then, the radical differentiation between a manifest and a latent dream, while necessary as a means of localizing what is 'most latent,' diffuses in a complicated continuum of more manifest and more latent items which are sometimes to be found by a radical disposal of the manifest configuration, sometimes by a careful scrutiny of it") (Erikson (1954a - p. 154).

1. Associations;
2. Symbols

C. Analysis of latent dream material:
   1. Inputs occurring during sleep
   2. Delayed inputs (day residue)
   3. Acute life conflicts
   4. Dominant transference conflict
   5. Repetitive conflicts
   6. Associated basic childhood conflict
   7. Common denominators: "wishes," drives, needs, methods of defense, denial, and distortion.

D. Reconstruction

   1. Life cycle
      a. present phase
      b. corresponding infantile phase
      c. defect, accident, or affliction
      d. psychosexual fixation
      e. psychosexual arrest.

   2. Social process: collective identity
      a. ideal prototypes
      b. evil prototypes
      c. opportunities and barriers

   3. Ego identity and lifespan
      a. mechanisms of defense
      b. mechanisms of integration

Using the above outline in an ingenious, complex and subtle manner, Erikson deepened and enlarged upon Freud's (1900/1953c) analysis of his own historic "Irma" dream – the first dream in history subjected to psychoanalytic interpretation. The details can only be appreciated by a close reading of the paper.

APPENDIX 2

The various Senses of the term "Meaning" (as modified and condensed from Ogden and Richards (1945)

Meaning may be:
1. that which is signified by a term or event
2. that which is denoted by a term
3. that which is connoted by a term, word or person-produced event
4. the place of any item in a conceptual system or context
5. the practical consequences of an item or event
   a. in our future experience
   b. with regard to theoretical implications or entailments of statements.
6. an activity projected into an object
7. the goals of volitions and intentions as manifested in real action and/or in fantasy
8. emotion aroused by any input
9. that which is related to a sign by a chosen relation
10. the mnemic effects of any input including complex groups of associations.
11. that to which the user, producer or interpreter of symbols and/or products of the imagination
    a. actually refers or expresses
    b. ought to be referring or expressing
    c. believes oneself to be referring or expressing
12. conceptualizations involving
    a. intrinsic properties
    b. essences
13. unique unanalysable relationships between items

Certainly, this catalogue of the meanings of "meaning" is neither exhaustive nor the only useful approach to the subject. The related literature is awesomely voluminous.

18

Dreaming for Cognition

John S. Antrobus

City College of the City University of New York

The study of dreaming and related sleep mentation has been largely untouched by the renaissance of cognitive psychology over the past quarter century. Theories about how dreams are formed, their meaning, and function have been dominated by the psychoanalytic point of view described by Freud (1900/1953c) at the turn of the century in terms of the scientific and mechanical concepts available at that time. Regardless of the theoretical merits of the psychoanalytic position, it can benefit from the rapid developments of cognitive psychology only to the extent that it relinquishes its private language and constructs for the more "interdisciplinary" language of information-processing models. The study of sleep mentation can, in turn, I think, make a contribution to cognitive psychology, to the study of concept formation, abstraction, retrieval from sensory specific memory, and more. I believe that this contribution will be realized only when the raw data of the sleep-mentation reports have been translated into the elementary working units of information-processing and related models. In this chapter I suggest how such a tssk might begin.

There is good reason to expect that the examination of dreaming and sleep mentation might contribute significantly to cognitive psychology. In the first place, any comprehensive model to thought and imagery must be able to account for how sleep mentation is produced. Secondly, the distinctions between waking and sleeping mentation and, indeed, among sleep mentation of different sleep states provides a naturally occurring method for isolating different qualities of thought and imagery that is simply not available in the waking state.

The meager contribution of the study of dreaming to cognitive psychology thus far may be attributed to, in my opinion, the inability of anyone to achieve even a modest predictive control over the content, the objects, and events of the mentation report. One cannot cut strong models on soft data! I suggest some possible experimental techniques for, hopefully, improving this situation. A vital issue in cognitive psychology at this time concerns the nature of concepts and categories in semantic memory. This issue turns, in part, around the question of whether a category is defined in relation to specific best instances of a category (dog = my black Labrador) or in terms of a list of abstract features which represent all of the attributes of the category (Collins & Loftus, 1975; Quillian, 1968; Rommetveit, 1968; Rosch, 1975; Rumelhart, Lindsay & Norman, 1972). It seems to me that this issue is related to assumptions underlying the art of what for millennia has been known as the interpretation of dreams, or the "meaning" of the dream.

DREAMS, SYMBOLS, CONCEPTS, AND FEATURES

I used "interpretation" and "meaning" in the most general sense of an object or event symbolizing, representing, or standing for another object or event. Let us symbolize the features or attributes of two persons, objects, or events as two sets of features, A and B, where the intersection, A B, represents their common features. Since features vary in terms of their ability to define membership in a category, Event A should represent Event B as a function of the number of the features which A and B share in common, AB. These common features also define the common class membership of Events A and B. Thus, a cigar and a pen might represent one another in that they are both members of a class whose features are cylindrical, hand held, and functional for humans. Similarly, blood moving through a vein may be represented by a train moving along a track to the extent that they are both instances of a class of moving things whose paths are defined by continuous parallel boundaries. The members of these pairs are so dissimilar, their common features so few, that the members of each pair are not readily recognized as instances of the same concept. When such a category is employed in the waking state, the category instance is generally identified as a metaphor by the use of "as" or "like." With respect to dreaming we are faced with the option either that the symbols are figments of the interpreter's imagination or that most dream thought and imagery is of this remote symbolic, metaphoric character. If the latter is true, then the study of sleep mentation may be able to offer something unique to the study of category membership and concept formation. Let us look at a specific example: the presurgery situation of a logger and a portion of one of his dreams described by Breger, Hunter, and Lane (1971a). The logger is awaiting an "aneuryectomy [an operation in which a damaged portion of a blood vessel is removed] to clear the vascular blockage in his leg." A portion of his dream is:

> We was working on a train . . . a work train . . . this Oregon crew had to come over on account of some washout or something . . . So we saw them come down to that last station and do some switching. We figured . . . also they came across the bridge up there someplace and hooked over onto our railroad. We was . . . looking at this other

engine and . . . we lined the switch, it seemed like our switch . . . it was a funny thing. They had to come off this private (rail)road onto ours and them switches weren't a standard switch. We had to dig some rocks out of the ground . . . and throw this switch over. And I was doing that, I was helping . . . I can't tell you what a switch is, instead of them just being flapped over and locked down to the padlock they was flapped over, the ends of two pipes together and there was a piece of this crooked zigzag piece of iron that was run first in one pipe and then the other so you couldn't lift the one out . . . and we was digging them things out of them pipes so we could throw the switch for them guys so they wouldn't have to stop . . . they hadn't used that switch it seemed like for years and naturally the sand and dust had blowed into these pipes and it was all rusty. It took quite a while . . .
[Breger, et al., 1971a, 118-119].

There is a double representation in this report of some features of the impending surgery. The veins are similar to the railway track and also to the pipes of the switch. Blood moving through the veins is similar to the train moving on the track and to the piece of iron running through the pipes. Vascular obstruction is represented by the train stopped because of the jammed switch and the piece of iron stuck by rust and sand in the pipes of the switch. At a higher point in each hierarchy, surgery is represented by fixing the switch to let the train through, and digging the pipe liner.

Let us assume that many of the elements of the dream exist in long-term memory prior to the dream but that this particular construction or combination of the elements is novel. Since this dream did not previously exist in memory, it could not have been searched for in long-term memory as one searches for a word to symbolize an event or even as one searches for a familiar visual symbol, a saying or a well-known parable to stand for a complex event. Construction of the dream events seem more similar to the creation of an original metaphoric parable or fable.

The merit of metaphor is its ability to describe complex relations among elements effectively and efficiently. "Sour grapes" communicates a set of relations that cannot otherwise be accurately described in a single word or phrase. But improved efficiency of communication is hardly a plausible reason for the use of metaphor in the dream. If a picture is worth a thousand words, then the primarily visual dream should be an efficient medium for the direct transmission of information without metaphor. If the patient is concerned about the impending aneuryectomy, then an explicit dream of the surgery would obviously contain more information about the surgery than the metaphor of a blocked railroad switch.

Is the thought of surgery too aversive for the dream? Although there is no empirical evidence one way or the other on this matter, my subjective opinion is that the metaphoric quality of dreams seems to be present regardless of the affective quality of the event presumably symbolized. The high incidence of nightmares gives little credence to the notion that dreams avoid painful affects. Freud's (1900/1953c) proposal that most dreams involve disguise for even more noxious impulses does not stand alone outside of his elaborate theory of mental process.

There are alternate possibilities though little empirical evidence to choose among them. Let us consider the possibility that the dream is produced from features preserved from the original event in the waking state. The loss of almost any of the original features of the waking event and substitution with alternate features yields an event which satisfies the definition of a metaphor (see Skinner, 1957). The question of interest then becomes, "Is the loss of features random or due to systematic cognitive operations which occur between the waking event and the dream?" My personal impression, again, is that the loss of features is not random. Those dreams, which appear to be symbolic or metaphoric extensions of previous waking experiences, are likely to share organization and relational characteristics, actions and values but not visual features, despite the fact that the sensory mode of the dream is predominantly visual. It is not the number of features shared in the waking situation and dream but rather the complexity of the organization within which the elements are related to one another. I am impressed by the conceptual sophistication of a system that can create the compound metaphors of the stopped train and jammed switch out of a vascular blockage. One would be hard pressed to do as well when fully awake.

Considered from the viewpoint of the concept acquisition, it is difficult to imagine how the logger's dream could be created from his surgery situation unless that original concept were first described and stored somewhere in terms of its component features and their relation to one another. If the similarity of the dream to surgery is other than happenstance, the vein, track, and pipe are members of the same category by reason of their common features of parallel boundaries (see Figure 18.1); just as blood, train, and iron bar share the features of substance moving within parallel boundaries. Similarly, the more complexly organized events, surgically removing obstruction in vein, turning the switch to let the engine through, and clearing sand and rust to operate the switch, may be regarded as instances of a single, but more complex category. Because the common ground shared by these specific instances is so remote from the instances themselves, the only plausible way to account for their membership in the same category is by reason of their common features.

The criteria for describing the relationship between waking experience and sleep-mentation reports in terms of their common features and relations might include:

1. all features common to persons, objects, relationships, and actions of both waking- and sleeping-report sets;

2. the features organized according to relations and actions common to the waking and sleeping sets;

3. when common features are redundant, retaining only the most specific, particular features in preference to more abstract features (to facilitate efficient description). (Thus, *cylindrical* might describe the most specific feature shared by *vein* and *pipe*, but it is too specific as a common feature of *vein* and *railroad*

track. In the latter case, the more abstract features, or elements, of *long-contains substance-directs moving substance-boundary* might be more appropriate.)

The use of words to describe visual features introduces an arbitrary element into the process. Considerable work would be required to achieve high interjudge reliability of descriptions such as those in Figure 18.1. But high reliability of judgments in such a loosely controlled experimental situation is not essential to an experimental test of the assumptions upon which descriptions such as those in Figure 18.1 are based. And it is the validity of these assumptions rather than the validity of the description of the relation between an individual's waking-sleep experience which is of prime interest here. Now that the judgment process has been briefly described, let us look at the underlying assumptions relevant to cognitive psychology.

We assume that the waking event is stored in memory in a form that is more abstract than the waking verbal description of the experience. It is an empirical question as to just how abstract the form of storage is. The abstract elements may be visual features of objects and actions but may include qualitative and affective qualities such as intention or fear. These features and characteristics need not be stored at the single address of the specific waking experience. Thus, the entire concept described in Figure 18.1a might be stored at or crossreferenced with, and later recalled from such addresses as blood, fix, and clean.

The evidence at hand gives us little basis for determining whether the organization of features (for example, see Figure 19.1a) provided the initiating condition for constructing the dream, or whether the logging fantasy came first and some element of the logging scene was responsible for the retrieval of the abstract organization of features from long-term memory. Certainly, the undesirable state of the patient's aneurysm and forthcoming aneuryectomy constitute sufficient cause for either to initiate the dream. But if the aneurysm were the major trigger for the dream we might expect the dream to include specific visual elements of the patient's symptoms and proposed surgery. Let us suppose, however, that the concept Figure 18.1a has an independent status in memory, and that the abstract features of *blocked* or *fix* are as adequate a trigger for the generation of thought and imagery as are aneurysm and aneuryctomy. If *blockage, obstruction, repair,* and *fix* have a longer history of frequent usage in the context of logging, then one might expect the features of Figure 18.1a to be applied to a logging context as in Figures 18.1b and 18.1c.

My own reading of sleep-mentation reports suggests that the most marked similarity between the sleep report and the pressing personal concerns, conflicts, or desires of the waking state occurs at the point of an abstract organization, such as that described in Figure 18.1a rather than at the level of specific persons, objects, and the contents of the sleep report. Although the content occasionally includes specific elements from the previous day, it more commonly consists of persons and objects stored in memory years before. To the extent that the primary motivation for the dream is associated with a personal concern or

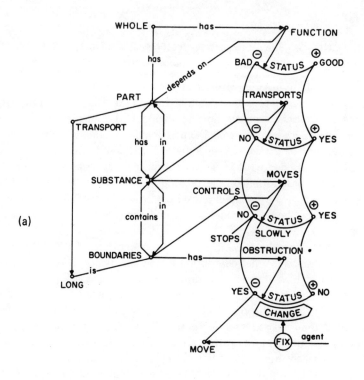

(a)

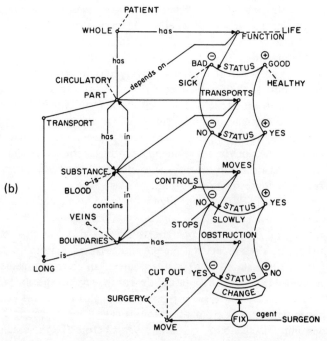

(b)

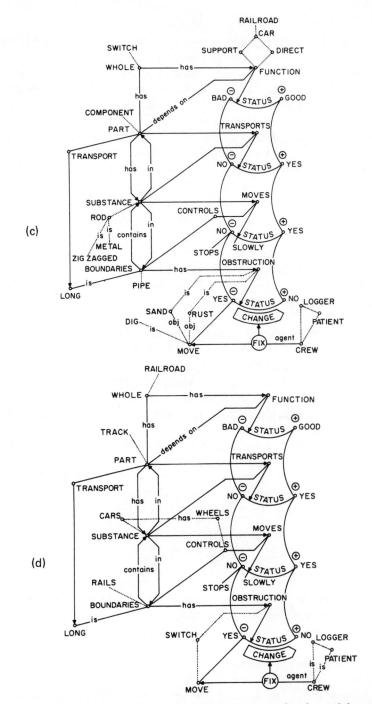

FIG. 18.1. Organization of elements in waking pre-surgery situation and dream of logger, described by Breger, Lane and Hunter (1971a): (a) Abstract elements; (b) Abstract elements— with surgery situation; (c) Abstract elements—with first portion of dream; (d) Abstract elements—with second portion of dream.

conflict aroused during the previous day, or is continuous over a period of preceding days and weeks, this motivation appears more likely to be stored in the abstract form I have described. If this is indeed the case, this abstract organization might be considered the "active" unit for the retrieval of events in memory which have the required features. However, since many characteristics of a dream appear to be invented rather than recalled, we must consider the possibility that the construction of the dream procedes jointly or alternately both with the retrieval of objects and events which satisfy multiple feature criteria and with the construction of novel events, again, according to the criteria of abstract features.

EXPERIMENTAL STRATEGY

Speculation beyond this point is idle without independent experimental manipulation of the abstract organization and the specific concrete content. An experimental technique currently being evaluated in our laboratory might be helpful. Waking subjects are trained, in an avoidance procedure, to discriminate specific classes of visual stimuli. Each stimulus class is associated with a specific combination of tones which are later presented during sleep. Preliminary evidence suggests that subjects dream of events that have many of the same features as the originally conditioned visual stimulus, yet the specific persons and objects in the dream may be quite different than the conditioned stimuli. For example, a female subject dreamed of cutting a pie with a kitchen knife, in response to a tone previously associated with the unconditioned stimulus of a man cutting the bark of a tree with a cane knife.

If research along these lines continues to support the notion that the criteria for dream imagery are visual features, rather than specific persons and objects, the next step should be the determination of the upper limit of the specificity or particularity of these feature criteria and the complexity of their organization.

BIZARRENESS AND INDEPENDENT-FEATURE GENERATORS

So far, we have considered the potential contribution to cognitive psychology only of the relation between waking and dreaming experience. Let us now look at the relations among elements within the sleep-mentation report. It is those relationships that we call "bizarre" for their improbable occurrence in waking experience that have the greatest potential for suggesting characteristics of cognitive processes that are not apparent to us from the study of waking behavior. That elements are produced which stand in improbably relationship to one another suggests a "failure" to coordinate the processes that produce the elements.

This presumed failure implies, of course, that the elements or events in question may be produced independently of each other. I suggest that we study sleep-mentation reports systematically from the context of current models of independent memory systems and modality-specific information processes to see if any new illumination can be thrown on the questions now being investigated.

An important issue in perception and memory concerns the relative independence of abstract and sensory modality-specific systems of meaning (Brewer, 1974). Sleep mentation reports contain many instances where detailed information in one sensory modality is unrelated or even contradictory to the dreamer's description of the purpose, function or meaning of the reported event. Subjects may report a contradiction between the visual identity and the "real" identity of a dream character, "... my ... younger brother and he was a little girl—it seemed natural in the dream ... (Breger, Hunter & Lane, 1971a, p. 55). In this case, incompatible characteristics are sustained by visual features on the one hand and abstract in the sense of nonsensory features, on the other. Is this dream produced by two semiindependent generators? If so, which one is leading the way? What kind of information is passed from one generator to the other?

In many reports the dreamer or actor, observer or interpreter seems to respond to improbable events as though one part of the system doesn't understand why the other, usually the visual system, does what it does, as demonstrated by a report collected in our laboratory: "... my mother was touching the finger-nails of my niece and I noticed that one of them was flatter than the others. And my niece said, 'Yes'. And I laughed at that and after we were talking why that was that ... we thought that probably she hit herself and that was the reason."

The overall impression produced by such reports is that the left cortical hem-ishpere is standing helplessly by, watching the right hemisphere do its thing—often badly—and making plausible explanations when possible. Ehrlichman and An-trobus (1974), Bakan (1975) and Cohen (1975) have argued elsewhere that the simpler visual functions of the right hemisphere dominate the subjective experience of REM sleep. The improbable combination of *brother* seen as *girl* in the above cited dream implies a lack of coordination between visual features and the more abstract meaning of brother, which is consistent with a drop in communication between hemispheres during REM sleep.

Although the majority of the bizarre relations in dreams seem to be visual, it is also true that visual imagery predominates in nearly all REM mentation and dream reports. Systematic classification of the sensory and abstract characteristics of mentation reports is needed to clarify these suggested associations.

Inferences about auditory imagery and speech during sleep are often mis-leading. The majority of references to speech are "about" what some character was talking about rather than quotations of what was actually said. It seems to me that if the sleeper can impose the meaning *my brother* on the visual image *little girl,* then the sleeper can also impose the meaning of a conversation upon a dream in which no auditory imagery is actually produced. Although quotes appropriate to the visual context of the dream are occasionally reported, quotations that are emphasized as verbatim often consist of neologisms: "Califar, Califar," and so on or "Avercrombie, [spelled out] I kept repeating it to myself," and isolation phrases that the sleeper has been repeating endlessly: "In the Calex bibliography you have to. In the Calex . . . [and so on]." Unlike the situation with bizarre visual imagery, the sleeper offers no meaningful interpretation of the bizarre speech. These neologisms are similar to those often observed in response to external stimulation by meaningful speech during sleep (see Chapter 10 of this volume). These repetitive reports suggest that acoustic processes are occasionally dominant but tend to be independent of the visual and more general-meaning features. Such repetitions are reminiscent of repetitive tunes and phrases that, even when one is awake, occasionally run through one's head untouched by the rest of one's experience.

This apparent independence of speech and meaning raises my skepticism about whether reported conversations during sleep have ever known acoustic features or any analogue thereof. The issue should be pursued, both for the sake of understanding the production of dreaming and for knowledge of how sensory systems are coordinated with meaning. As a first step we must determine whether phrases such as, "they were talking about . . ." may be emitted when the subject is still able to recall specific words and phrases of the dream. Robert Schnee, in our laboratory, is attempting to find out whether instructions to report all specific words spoken within the dream will produce words that are otherwise lost because the subject finds it more convenient to report a summary of the meaning or gist of a conversation. Jenkins (1974) and Bransford and Franks (1971) have shown that specific words and phrases are rapidly lost as a subject automatically transforms sentences into more abstract form. Perhaps during sleep this transformation occurs for speech but not visual imagery, thereby accounting for the predominance of visual imagery in REM reports. Unfortunately, little is known about the similarity of this feature-extraction and abstraction process in speech compared to visual memory. Furthermore, no systematic work has been done on the abstraction of longer narratives or on narratives of combined visual and verbal material. The Bransford and Franks (1971) experiments deal with single sentences. Research on these issues on either side of the sleeping-waking boundary would enhance knowledge on the other side.

The portrayal in dreams of private internal events, such as emotional or affective responses, is worthy of special comment. The use of verbal metaphors, such as "elated," "depressed," "high," and "cool" to describe emotional states, has nowhere been better described than in Skinner's (1959) paper, "The Operational Analysis of Psychological Terms." The notion that the verbal metaphor shares some critical features with the emotional event runs into trouble because the metaphoric event is a public event or action, whereas the emotional event is private and we have no language to describe it directly. Skinner proposes that a metaphor such as "depressed" works because some of the private internal responses to being physically pressed or pushed down are similar to some of the private internal events we call "feeling depressed." The shared features (characteristics of internal responses) are not in the public, verbal, or visual event but a subset of hypothetical private events.

In my opinion, a similar set of assumptions is required to account for a visual dream that is a metaphor for a private affective event or emotional state. To illustrate, I describe a dream that appears to be a visual metaphor for an emotional state, but in which the visual metaphor is quite similar to another well-established metaphor in the language. Since this particular subject has, indeed, described feelings in terms of that metaphor one might wonder whether the visual dream is directly representing the feelings, or perhaps, simply representing the visual features of the metaphor.

A subject in Breger, Hunter & Lane's (1971a) group-therapy study has just been turned against by three peers in a session of penetrating verbal crossfire. At the end of the session, the subject says, "I feel like everything's dropped out underneath me . . . (and now I don't) give a hang about anything." The subject reported after the awakening, "I was in a swimming pool . . . all the water dripped out . . . I was swimming along . . . then there was nothing left . . . Everything dropped out right underneath me . . . I could feel myself falling [p. 47]." We are given: Element 1, a verbal report of Element 2, an imagined visual event which, in turn, is a "literal" representation of Element 3, a verbal phrase *dropped out* recently emitted in the waking state, which verbal phrase is a metaphor describing State 4, spatial movement, which can be encoded Element 5, visually by a third party observer but also has State 6, private interoceptive features for the hanging, falling, dropping, or let-down party.

Skinner would suggest, I think, that some of the State 6, private, interoceptive responses to being let down or dropping in physical space are similar to State 7, some of the interoceptive responses to the social rejection which Breger's subject is experiencing. And not all of the features of State 7 are represented in State 6. Since the internal response cannot be observed by the social community it cannot be directly labeled. The metaphoric name is the closest publicly namable event available that permits the private response to be communicated verbally to another party. Following Skinner's (1959) analysis, and viewing the dream as a private event, the initial stimulus for the dream would be State 7, those interoceptive responses to the social rejection of the previous day which are similar to State 6 above. This analysis would seem particularly plausible if the dreamer were creating the visual metaphor from scratch, going through the sequence of States $(7 \cap 6) - (2)$ omitting State 3.

When metaphors such as *depressed, the bottom dropped out,* or *let down* become highly overlearned from fequent usage, one would expect that their usage in the sense above as a description of State 7, does not involve moving through the entire stimulus-response chain of States $(7 \cap 6)$ to State 2 omitting Stage 3. This suggests to me that the visual dream State 2, might be triggered directly, or at least influenced by the verbal stimulus, State 3, without any influence of the private stimulus State 7.

These informal observations must now be developed into formal methods of analyzing sleep-mentation reports. Such analysis must systematically describe the kind and frequency of improbable relationships in terms of features and more abstract characteristics. This analysis should indicate whether the improbable relations are randomly distributed with respect to type or whether they are organized in any pattern. If the latter is true, is the organization consistent with any particular relationship among semi-independent feature generators responsible for the production of visual imagery, speech, and meaning? If a particular organization is implied, does it also suggest a hierarchy as such that sleep mentation is initiated or controlled by one part of the system and passively observed by another? For example, is the dream initiated by a general abstract subsystem, or by a (visual) modality-specific subsystem in which meanings are encoded by features that, in turn, are decoded by an internal observer system, and so on? Or are the visual persons and objects of the dream initially produced without regard to meaning; the dream then procedes as other units of the cognitive system respond to what was originally a meaningless image? An even looser possibility is that communication among all units or subsystems is poorer than during wakefulness, varies systematically with sleep stage and perhaps hemispheric dominance, as well as other factors on which we have no handle. For example, if some reports have only visual imagery and some are only speech, we might conclude that encoding in the two modalities can be quite independent. If the two, in turn, are associated with different sleep stages and the sleep stages are associated with differences in EEG activity in visual and speech centers, we may join the sleep model to biological and general cognitive models. Visual dreams vary greatly in the sense of participation of the dreamers. Some are viewed as scenes in a movie or television program; in others, the dreamer is a full participant. For dreams somewhere in between, the dreamer may be frustrated at the inability to physically (visually) carry out one's intentions. Some have attributed these dreams to inhibition of the motor system and, therefore, absence of proprioceptive feedback, caused by phasic locus coeruleus activity in REM sleep. If so, such dreams should be more frequent during phasic events. Arkin and I propose that dreams of motor disturbance may be associated with increased activity of the vestibular nuclei during REM sleep. This possibility could be tested by caloric stimulation of the middle ear. Yet another possibility is that variation in participation, as against simply observing, are due to fluctuations in interhemispheric communication at the level of the corpus collosum, or simply fluctuation in EEG power within the left hemisphere.

Systematic analyses of mentation reports is an approrpiate first step narrowing these options that experimental studies can follow. In the meanwhile, it is not too unreasonable to hope that the unusual characteristics of sleep mentation will reveal, if through a glass darkly, properties of the cognitive system not readily observed in the study of waking processes.

References

Adair, J. G., & Epstein, J. Verbal cues in the mediation of experimenter bias. Paper presented at the meeting of the Midwestern Psychological Association, Chicago, May, 1967.

Aarons, L. Evoked sleep-talking. *Perceptual and Motor Skills,* 1976, *31,* 27-40.

Adelman, S., & Hartmann, E. Psychological effects of amitriptyline-induced dream deprivation. Paper presented at the meeting of the Association for the Psychophysiological Study of Sleep, Denver, 1968.

Adler, A. On the interpretation of dreams. *International Journal of Individual Psychology,* 1936, *2,* 3-16.

Adler, A. *What life should mean to you.* New York: Capricorn, 1958.

Agnew, H. W., & Webb, W. B., Jr. The displacement of stage 4 and REM sleep within a full night of sleep. *Psychophysiology,* 1968, *5,* 142-148.

Agnew, H. W., Webb, W. B. Jr., & Williams, R. L. The first night effect: An EEG study of sleep. *Psychophysiology,* 1966, *2,* 263-266.

Agnew, H. W., Webb, W. B., Jr., & Williams, R. L. Comparison of stage four and REM sleep deprivation. *Perceptual and Motor Skills,* 1967, *24,* 851-858.

Albert, I. B. REM sleep deprivation. *Biological Psychiatry,* 1975, *10,* 341-351.

Albert, I., Cicala, G. A., & Siegel, J. The behavioral effects of REM sleep deprivation in rats. *Psychophysiology,* 1970, *6,* 550-560.

Alexander, L. Dreams in Paris. In R. Flores (Ed.), *The psychoanalytic reader.* Vol. 1. New York: International Universities Press, 1948.

Allen, S. REM sleep and memory. *Proceedings of the Second European Congress on Sleep Research,* Rome, Italy, 1974.

Allen, C., Kales, A., & Berger, R. J. An analysis of the effect of glutethimide on REM density. *Psychonomic Science,* 1968, *12,* 329-330.

Altschuler, K. Z. Comment on recent sleep research related to psychoanalytic theory. *Archives of General Psychiatry,* 1966, *15,* 235-239.

Altschuler, K. Z., Barad, M., & Goldfarb, A. I. A Survey of dreams in the aged, Part II. *Archives of General Psychiatry,* 1963, *8,* 33-37.

Amadeo, M., & Gomez, E. Eye movements, attention and dreaming in subjects with life-long blindness. *Canadian Psychiatric Association Journal,* 1966, *11,* 501-507.

Anders, T. F. An overview of recent sleep and dream research. In L. Goldberger & Rosen (Eds.). *Psychoanalysis and contemporary science,* Vol. 3. New York: International Universities Press, 1974.

Anderson, B. F. *Cognitive psychology: The study of knowing, learning and thinking.* New York: Academic Press, 1975.

Antrobus, J. S., Antrobus, J. S., & Fisher, C. Discrimination of dreaming and non-dreaming sleep. *Archives of General Psychiatry,* 1965, *12,* 395-401.

Antrobus, J. S., Antrobus, J. S., & Singer, J. L. Eye movements accompanying daydreaming, visual imagery, and thought suppression. *Journal of Abnormal and Social Psychology,* 1964, *69,* 244-252.

Antrobus, J. S., Arkin, A. M., & Ellman, S. J. Dreaming, operant control, and meaning structure. National Institute of Mental Health Grant Proposal, September, 1976.

Antrobus, J. S., Arkin, A. M., & Toth, M. F. The effects of REM period deprivation on sleep mentation. *Psychophysiology,* 1970, *7,* 332. (Abstract)

Antrobus, J. S., Arkin, A. M., & Toth, M. The effects of REMP deprivation on sleep mentation. *Sleep Research,* 1972, *1,* 156.

Antrobus, J. S., Dement, W., & Fisher, C. Patterns of dreaming and dream recall: An EEG study. *Journal of Abnormal and Social Psychology,* 1964, *69,* 341-344.

Antrobus, J. S., Ezrachi, O., & Arkin, A. M. K-complexes and dreaming in Stage 2 sleep. Unpublished manuscript, 1973.

Antrobus, J. S., Pass, R., Luck, D., Sanders, K., Ellman, S., & Arkin, A. M. Discrimination of REM/NREM reports. *Sleep Research,* 1974, *3,* 102. (Abstract)

Antrobus, J. S., Rich, K., Pass, R., Nelson, W. T., & Sanders, K. Multiple linear regression of mentation reports on REM/NREM sleep. *Sleep Research,* 1973, *2,* 104.

Antrobus, J. S., Schnee, R. K., Offer, V., & Silverman, S. A psycholinguistic scoring manual for mentation reports. Unpublished test, ETS test collection, Educational Testing Service, Princeton, New Jersey.

Antrobus, J. S., Singer, J. L., Goldstein, S., & Fortgang, M. Mind-wandering and cognitive structure. *Transactions of the New York Academy of Science,* 1970, *32,* 242-252.

Arkin, A. M. Sleep talking: A review. *Journal of Nervous and Mental Disease,* 1966, *143,* 101-122.

Arkin, A. M. The degree of concordance between sleep-talking and mentation recalled in wakefulness. Paper presented at the meeting of the Association for the Psychophysiological Study of Sleep, Santa Monica, April, 1967. *Psychophysiology,* 1968, *4,* 396. (Abstract)

Arkin, A. M. Qualitative observations on sleep utterance in the laboratory. In The Atti del Simposio Internazionale sulla psicolifisiologica del sonno e del sogno. Proceedings of an International Symposium, Rome, 1967. Bertini, M. (Ed.) Milan: Editrice Vita e Pensiero Milan, 1970.

Arkin, A. M. Review of MacNeilage, P. F. & MacNeilage, L. A., Central processes controlling speech production during sleeping and waking. *Sleep Research,* 1974, *3,* 331-333. (a)

Arkin, A. M. Somniloquy as the output of dissociated cognitive subsystems. Paper presented at the meeting of the Association for the Psychophysiological Study of Sleep, Jackson Hole, May, 1974. (b)

Arkin, A. M., & Antrobus, J. S. Sleep mentation as affected by REMP deprivation. Progress report to National Institute of Mental Health, MH 13866-03. 1970.

Arkin, A. M., Antrobus, J. S., Toth, M. F., & Baker, J. The effects of chemically induced REMP deprivation on sleep vocalization and NREM mentation — An initial exploration. Paper presented at the meeting of the Association for the Psychophysiological Study of Sleep, Denver, March, 1968. *Psychophysiology,* 1968, *5,* 217. (Abstract)

Arkin, A. M., Antrobus, J. S., Toth, M. F., Baker, J., & Jackler, F. A comparison of the content of mentation reports elicited after non-rapid eye movement (NREM) associated sleep utterance and NREM "silent" sleep. *Journal of Nervous and Mental Disease,* 1972, *155*(6), 427–435.

Arkin, A. M., & Brown, J. W. Resemblances between NREM associated sleep speech, drowsy speech, and aphasic and schizophrenic speech. Paper presented at the Association for the Psychophysiological Study of Sleep, First International Congress, Bruges, June, 1971. *Psychophysiology*, 1972, *9*, 140. (Abstract)

Arkin, A. M., Farber, J., Antrobus, J. S., Ellman, S. J., & Nelson, W. T. The effects of repeated sleep interruption and elicited verbalization on sleep speech frequency of chronic sleep talkers: Preliminary observations. *Sleep Research*, 1973, *2*, 105.

Arkin, A. M., Hastey, J. M., & Reiser, M. F. Dialogue between sleeptalkers and the experimenter. Paper presented at the meeting of the Association for the Psychophysiological Study of Sleep, Gainesville, March, 1966.(a)

Arkin, A. M., Hastey, J. M., & Reiser, M. F. Post-hypnotically stimulated sleep-talking. *Journal of Nervous and Mental Disease*, ·1966, *142*, 293-309. (b)

Arkin, A. M., Sanders, K. I., Ellman, S. J., Antrobus, J. S., Farber, J., & Nelson, W. T., Jr. The rarity of pain sensation in sleep mentation reports. Paper presented at the meeting of the Association for the Psychophysiological Study of Sleep, Edinburgh. May, 1975.

Arkin, A. M., Toth, M., Baker, J., & Hastey, J. M. The frequency of sleep-talking in the laboratory among chronic sleep-talkers and good dream recallers. *Journal of Nervous and Mental Disease*, 1970, *151*, 369-374. (a)

Arkin, A. M., Toth, M. F., Baker, J., & Hastey, J. M. The degree of concordance between the content of sleep talking and mentation recalled in wakefulness. *Journal of Nervous and Mental Disease*, 1970, *151*, 375-393. (b)

Arkin, A. M., Toth, M. F., & Ezrachi, O. Electrographic aspects of sleep-talking. Paper presented at the meeting of the Association for the Psychophysiological Study of Sleep, Santa Fe, March, 1970. *Psychophysiology*, 1970, *7*, 354. (Abstract)

Arlow, J. A., & Brenner, C. *Psychoanalytic concepts and the structural theory*. New York: International Universities Press, 1964.

Arseni, C., & Petrovici, I. N. Epilepsy in temproal lobe tumors. *European Neurology*, 1971, *5*, 201-214.

Asahina, K. Paradoxical phase and reverse paradoxical phase in human subjects. *Journal of the Physiology Society of Japan*, 1962, *24*, 443-450.

Aserinsky, E. Brain wave pattern during the rapid eye movement period of sleep. *The Physiologist*, 1965, *8*, 104, (a) (Abstract)

Aserinsky, E Periodic respiratory pattern occurring in conjunction with eye movements during sleep. *Science*, 1965, *150*, 763-766. (b)

Aserinsky, E. Physiological activity associated with segments of the rapid eye movement period. In S. S. Kety, E. V. Evarts, & H. L. Williams (Eds.), *Sleep and altered states of consciousness*. Baltimore: Williams & Wilkins, 1967.

Aserinsky, E. Drugs and dreams: A synthesis in drugs and dreams. *Experimental Medicine and Surgery*, 1969, *27*, 237-244. (a)

Aserinsky, E. The maximal capacity for sleep: Rapid eye movement density as an index of sleep satiety. *Biological Psychiatry*, 1969, *1*, 147-159. (b)

Aserinsky, E. Rapid eye movement density and pattern in the sleep of normal young adults. *Psychophysiology*, 1971, *8*, 361-375.

Aserinsky, E., & Kleitman, N. Regularly occurring periods of eye motility and concomitant phenomena during sleep. *Science*, 1953, *118*, 273-274.

Aserinsky, E., & Kleitman, N. Two types of ocular motility occurring during sleep. *Journal of Applied Physiology*, 1955, *8*, 1-10.

Atkinson, R. C., & Shiffrin, R. M. Human memory: A proposed system and its control processes. In K. W. Spence and J. T. Spence (Eds.), *The psychology of learning and motivation: Advances in research and theory*, Vol. 2. New York: Academic Press, 1968.

Atsmon, A., Blum, I., Wijsenbeek, H., Maoz, B., Steiner, M., & Ziegelman, G. The short-term effects of adrenergic-blocking agents in a small group of psychotic patients. *Psychiatria, Neurologia, Neurochirurgia*, 1971, *74*, 251-258.

Austin, M. D. Dream recall and the bias of intellectual ability. *Nature,* 1971, *231,* 59-60.

Azumi, K., & Ewing, J. A. The effects of REM deprivation on GSR during sleep. Paper presented at the meeting of the Association for the Psychophysiological Study of Sleep, Santa Fe, New Mexico, 1970. *Psychophysiology,* 1970, *7,* 301. (Abstract)

Azumi, K., Takahashi, S., Takahashi, K., Maruyama, N., & Kikuti, S. The effects of dream deprivation on chronic schizophrenics and normal adults: A comparative study. *Folia Psychiatrica et Neurologica Japonica,* 1967, *21,* 205-225.

Baekeland, F. Pentobarbital and dextroamphetamine sulphate: Effects of the sleep cycle in man. *Psychopharmacologia,* 1967, *11,* 388-396.

Baekeland, F. Correlates of home dream recall: Reported home sleep characteristics and home dream recall. *Comprehensive Psychiatry,* 1969, *10,* 482-491.

Baekeland, F. Correlates of home dream recall: 1. Rem sleep in the laboratory as a predictor of home dream recall. *Journal of Nervous and Mental Disease,* 1970, *150,* 209-214.

Baekeland, F. Effects of pre-sleep procedures and cognitive style on dream content. *Perceptual and Motor Skills,* 1971, *32,* 63-69.

Baekeland, F., & Lasky, R. The morning recall of rapid eye movement period reports given earlier in the night. *Journal of Nervous and Mental Disease,* 1968, *147,* 570-579.

Baekeland, F., Resch, R., & Katz, D. D. Pre-sleep mentation and dream reports. *Archives of General Psychiatry,* 1968, *19,* 300-311.

Bakan, P. Dreaming, REM sleep, and the right hemisphere. Paper presented at the meeting of the Association for the Psychophysiological Study of Sleep, Edinburgh, May, 1975.

Baldridge, B. J. Physical concomitants of dreaming and the effect of stimulation on dreams. *Ohio State Medical Journal,* 1966, *62,* 1271-1279.

Baldridge, B. J. Review of Hauri, P. & Van de Castle, R. L., Psychophysiological parallels in dreams. *Sleep Research,* 1974, *3,* 312-314.

Baldridge, B. J., Whitman, R. M., & Kramer, M. A comparison of variability of some physiological functions during dreaming while telling the dream and during dream playback. Paper presented at the Association for the Psychophysiological Study of Sleep, Chicago, 1962.

Baldridge, B. J., Whitman, R. M., Kramer, M., Ornstein, P. H., & Lansky, L. The effect of external physical stimuli on dream content. Paper presented at the meeting of the Association for the Psychophysiological Study of Sleep, Washington, 1965.

Baldridge, B. J., Whitman, R. M., & Ornstein, P. H. Smoking and dreams. Paper presented at the meeting of the Association for the Psychophysiological Study of Sleep, Santa Monica, California, 1967.

Barad, M., Altschuler, K. Z., & Goldfarb, A. I. A survey of dreams in aged persons. *Archives of General Psychiatry,* 1961, *4,* 419-424.

Barber, B. Factors underlying individual differences in rate of dream reporting. *Psychophysiology,* 1969, *6,* 247-248. (Abstract)

Barber, T. X. Letter to the editor, *Science,* 1960, *132,* 1417-1418.

Barber, T. X., Calverley, D. S., Forgione, A. M., Peaker, J. D., Chaves, J. F., & Bowen, B. Five attempts to replicate the experimenter bias effect. *Journal of Consulting and Clinical Psychology,* 1969, *33,* 1-6.

Barber, T. X., Walker, P. C., & Hahn, K. W., Jr. Effects of hypnotic induction and suggestions on nocturnal dreaming and thinking. *Journal of Abnormal Psychology,* 1973, *82,* 414-427.

Barrett, T. R., & Ekstrand, B. R. Effects of sleep on memory: III. Controlling for time-of-day effects. *Journal of Experimental Psychology,* 1972, *96,* 321-327.

Barondes, S. H. Multiple steps in the biology of memory. In: F. O. Smith (Ed.), *The neurosciences:Second Study program.* New York: Rockefeller University Press, 1970.

Barros-Ferreira, M. de, Goldsteinas, L., & Lairy, G. C. REM sleep deprivation in chronic schizophrenics: Effects on the dynamics of fast sleep. *Electroencephalography and Clinical Neurophysiology,* 1973, *34,* 561-569.

Baust, W., & Bohnert, B. The regulation of heart rate during sleep. *Experimental Brain Research*, 1969, *7*, 169-180.

Baust, W., & Engel, R. Correlations between heart rate, respiration and dream content. *Pflugers Archives*, 1970, *319*, 139.

Beck, A. T., & Hurvich, M. S. Psychological correlates of depression. I. Frequency of "masochistic" dream content in a private practice sample. *Psychosomatic Medicine*, 1959, *21*, 50-55.

Beck, A. T., & Ward, C. H. Dreams of depressed patients. *Archives of General Psychiatry*, 1961, *5*, 462-467.

Belvedere, E., & Foulkes, D. Telepathy and dreams: A failure to replicate. Paper presented at the meeting of the Association for the Psychophysiological Study of Sleep, Bruges, Belgium, June, 1971.

Benedek, T., & Rubenstein, B. B. The correlations between ovarian activity and psychodynamic processes: I. The ovulative phase and II. The menstrual phase. *Psychosomatic Medicine*, 1939, *1*, 245-270; 446-485.

Berger, R. J. Tonus of extrinsic laryngcal muscles during sleep and dreaming. *Science*, 1969, *134*, 840.

Berger, R. J. Experimental modification of dream content by meaningful verbal stimuli. *British Journal of Psychiatry*, 1963, *109*, 722-740.

Berger, R. J. Physiological characteristics of sleep. In A. Kales (Ed.) *Sleep: Physiology and pathology*. Philadelphia: Lippincott, 1969.

Berger, R. J., Olley, P., & Oswald, I. The EEG, eye movements, and dreams of the blind. *Quarterly Journal of Experimental Psychology*, 1962, *14*, 183-186.

Berger, R. J., & Oswald, I. Effects of sleep deprivation on behavior, subsequent sleep, and dreaming. *Journal of Mental Science*, 1962, *108*, 457–465. (a)

Berger, R. J., & Oswald, I. Eye movements during active and passive dreams. *Science*, 1962, *137*, 601. (b)

Berger, R. J., & Walker, J. M. Oculomotor coordination following REM and non-REM sleep periods. *Journal of Experimental Psychology*, 1972, *94*, 216-234.

Berlucchi, G. Callosal activity in unrestrained, unanesthetized cats. *Archives of Italian Biology*, 1964, *103*, 623-624.

Berlucchi, G. Electroencephalographic studies in "split-brain" cats. *Electroencephalography and Clinical Neurophysiology*, 1966, *20*, 348-356.

Bertini, M. Procesi de transformazione simbolica nel periodo del dormiveglia e nel sogno (studio sperimentale). Estratta dalla Rivista IKON-Milano, Suppl. al N. 65-66, Aprile-Settembre, 1968.

Bertini, M., & Pontalti, C. Clinical perspectives of a new technique in dream research. Paper presented at the meeting of the Association for the Psychophysiological Study of Sleep, Bruges, 1971.

Bizzi, E., & Brooks, O. Functional connections between pontine rceticular formation and lateral geniculate nucleus during deep sleep. *Archives Italiennes de Biologie*, 1963, *101*, 648-666.

Blank, H. R. Dreams of the blind. *Psychoanalytic Quarterly*, 1958, *27*, 158-174.

Bleuler, E. *Dementia Praecox*, 1908. Cited by R. L. Williams, The relationship of sleep disturbances to psychopathology. *International Psychiatric Clinics*, 1970, *7*, 93-111.

Bliss, E. L., Clark, L. D., & West, C. D. Studies of sleep deprivation-relationship to schizophrenia. *Archives of Neurology and Psychiatry*, 1959, *81*, 348-359.

Blum, G. A. *Model of the mind*. New York: Wiley, 1961.

Bogen, J. E. The other side of the brain II: An appositional mind. *Bulletin of the Los Angeles Neurological Society*, 1969, *34*, 135-162.

Bokert, E. The effects of thirst and a related verbal stimulus on dream reports. *Dissertation Abstracts*, 1968, *28*, 4753B.

Bone, R. N. Extraversion, neuroticism, and dream recall. *Psychological Reports*, 1968, *23*, 922.

Bone, R. N., & Corlett, F. Brief report: Frequency of dream recall, creativity, and a control for anxiety, *Psychological Reports, 1968, 22*, 1355-1356.

Bone, R. W., Hopkins, O. C., Buttermore, G., Jr., Belcher, M. M., McIntyre, C. I., Calef, R. S., & Cowling, L. N. Sixteen personality correlates of sleep-talkers. Paper presented at the meeting of the Association for the Psychophysiological Study of Sleep, San Diego, May, 1973.

Bone, R. N., Nelson, A. E., & McAllister, D. S. Dream recall and repression-sensitization. *Psychological Reports, 1970, 27,* 766.

Bone, R. N., Thomas, T. A., & Kinsolving, D. L Relationship of rod-and-frame scores to dream recall. *Psychological Reports, 1972, 30,* 58.

Bonime, W. *The clinical use of dreams.* New York: Basic Books, 1962.

Bosinelli, M., Cicogna, P., & Molinari, S. The tonic phasic model and the feeling of self-participation in different stages of sleep. Unpublished manuscript, 1973, Institite of Psychology of the Medical Faculty of the University of Bologna, Italy.

Bosinelli, M., Molinari, S., Bagnaresi, G., & Salzarulo, P. Caratteristiche dell attitiva psico-fisiologica durante il sonno. Un contributo alle techniche di valutazion. *Rivista Sperimentale di Freiatria, 1968, 92,* 128-150.

Boss, M. *The analysis of dreams.* New York: Philosophical Library, 1958.

Bowe-Anders, C., Herman, J. H., & Roffwarg, H. P. Effects of goggle-altered color perception on sleep. *Perceptual and Motor Skills, 1974, 38,* 191-198.

Box, G. E. P. Problems in analysis of growth and wear curves. *Biometrics, 1950, 6,* 362-389.

Bradley, C., & Meddis, R. Arousal threshold in dreaming sleep. *Physiological Psychology, 1974, 2,* 109-110.

Bransford, J. D., & Franks, J. J. The abstraction of linguistic ideas. *Cognitive Psychology, 1971, 2,* 331-350.

Breger, L. Function of dreams. *Journal of Abnormal Psychology, 1967, 72,* 1-28.

Breger, L. Children's dreams and personality development. In J. Fisher & L. Breger (Eds.) *The meaning of dreams: Recent insights from the laboratory.* California Mental Health Research Symposium, No. 3, 1969.

Breger, L. Dream function: An information processing model. In L. Berger (Ed.), *Clinical-cognitive psychology – models and integrations.* Englewood Cliffs, N.J.: Prentice-Hall, Inc., 1969.

Breger, L., Hunter, I., & Lane, R. W. The effects of stress on dreams. *Psychological Issues, 1971, 7* (3, Monograph 27). (a)

Breger, L., Hunter, I., & Lane, R. *The effect of stress on dreams.* New York: International Universities Press, 1971. (b)

Brewer, W. F. The problem of meaning and the interrelations of the higher mental process. In W. B. Weiner & D. S. Palermo (Eds.), *Cognition and Symbolic processes.* Hillsdale, N.J.: Erlbaum, 1974.

Brooks, O. C. Localization of the lateral geniculate nucleus monophasic waves associated with paradoxical sleep in the cat. *Electroencephalography and Clinical Neurophysiology, 1967, 23,* 123-133.

Brooks, O. C. Waves associated with eye movement in the awake and sleeping cat. *Electroencephalography and Clinical Neurophysiology, 1968, 24,* 532-541.

Broughton, R. Sleep disorders: Disorders of arousal? *Science, 1968, 159,* 1070-1078.

Broughton, R. Confusional sleep disorders: Inter-relationship with memory consolidation and retrieval in sleep. In T. J. Boag, & D. Campbell (Eds.), *A triune concept of brain and behavior.* Toronto: University of Toronto Press, 1973.

Broughton, R. J., Poire, R., & Tassinari, C. A. The electrodermogram (Tarchanoff effect) during sleep. *Electroencephalography and Clinical Neurophysiology, 1965, 18,* 691-708.

Burch, N. Data processing of psychophysiological recordings. In L. D. Proctor & W. R. Adey (Eds.), *Symposium on the analysis of central nervous system and cardiovascular data using computer methods.* Washington, D. C.: National Aeronautics and Space Administration, 1965.

Byrne, D., Barry, J., & Nelson, D. Relation of the revised Repression-Sensitization scale to measures of self-description. *Psychological Reports,* 1963, *13,* 323-334.

Calkins, M. W. Statistics of dreams. *American Journal of Psychology,* 1893, *5,* 311-343.

Campbell, D. T., & Fiske, D. W. Convergent and discriminant validation by the multi-trait multimethod matrix. *Psychological Bulletin,* 1959, *56,* 82-105.

Carrington, P. Dreams and schizophrenia. *Archives of General Psychiatry,* 1972, *26,* 343-350.

Carroll, D., Lewis, S. A., & Oswald, I. Effect of barbiturates on dream content. *Nature,* 1969, *223,* 865-866.

Cartwright, R. D. Dream and drug-induced fantasy behavior. A comparative study. *Archives of General Psychiatry,* 1966, *15,* 7-15.

Cartwright, R. D. Dreams as compared to other forms of fantasy. In M. Kramer, R. M. Whitman, B. J. Baldridge, & P. H. Ornstein (Eds.), *Dream psychology and the new biology of dreaming.* Springfield, Ill.: Charles C. Thomas, 1969.

Cartwright, R. D. The effect of dream opportunity on daytime problem resolution: A preliminary report of a pilot study. Paper presented at the meeting of the Association for the Psychophysiological Study of Sleep, Santa Fe, New Mexico, 1970. *Psychophysiology,* 1970, *7,* 332. (Abstract)

Cartwright, R. D. Sleep fantasy in normal and schizophrenic persons. *Journal of Abnormal Psychology,* 1972, *80,* 275-279.

Cartwright, R. D. The influence of a conscious wish on dreams: A methodological study of dream meaning and function. *Journal of Abnormal Psychology,* 1974, *83,* 387-393. (a)

Cartwright, R. D. Problem solving: Waking and dreaming. *Journal of Abnormal Psychology,* 1974, *83,* 451-455. (b)

Cartwright, R. D., Bernick, N., Borowitz, G., & Kling, A. Effect of an erotic movie on the sleep and dreams of young men. *Archives of General Psychiatry,* 1969, *20,* 263-271.

Cartwright, R., & Monroe, L. Relation of dreaming and REM sleep: The effects of REM deprivation under two different conditions. *Journal of Personality and Social Psychology,* 1968, *10,* 69-74.

Cartwright, R. D., Monroe, L. J., & Palmer, C. Individual differences in response to REM deprivation. *Archives of General Psychiatry,* 1967, *16,* 297-303.

Cartwright, R. D., & Ratzel, R. Light and deep sleeper differences: Fantasy scores from REM, stage 2 and REM deprivation awakenings. Paper presented at the meeting of the Association for the Psychophysiological Study of Sleep, Santa Fe, New Mexico, 1970.

Cartwright, R. D., & Ratzel, R. W. Effects of dream loss on waking behaviors. *Archives of General Psychiatry,* 1972, *27,* 277-280.

Cartwright, R. D., Weiner, L., & Wicklund, J. Effects of lab training in dream recall on psychotherapy behavior. Paper presented at the meeting of the Association for the Psychophysiological Study of Sleep, Edinburgh, 1975.

Castaldo, V., & Holzman, P. The effect of hearing one's voice on sleep mentation. *Journal of Nervous and Mental Disease,* 1967, *144,* 2-13.

Castaldo, V., & Holzman, P. The effects of hearing one's own voice on dreaming content: A replication. *Journal of Nervous and Mental Disease,* 1969, *148,* 74-82.

Castaldo, V., & Shevrin, H. Different effect of auditory stimulus as a function of rapid eye movement and non-rapid eye movement sleep. *Journal of Nervous and Mental Disease,* 1970, *150,* 195-200.

Chernik, D. A. Effect of REM sleep deprivation on learning and recall by humans. *Perceptual and Motor Skills,* 1972, *34,* 283-294.

Cherry, C. *On human communication.* (2nd ed.) Cambridge, Mass.: M.I.T. Press, 1966.

Church, J. *Language and the discovery of reality.* New York: Vintage Books, 1961.

Clausen, J. Family structure, socialization and personality. In L. W. Hoffman & M. C. Hoffman (Eds.), *Review of child development research,* Vol. 2 New York: Russell Sage Foundation, 1966.

Clemes, S. R., & Dement, W. Effect of REM sleep deprivation on psychological functioning. *Journal of Nervous and Mental Disease*, 1967, *144*, 488-491.

Cohen, D. B. Frequency of dream recall estimated by three methods and related to defense preference and anxiety. *Journal of Consulting and Clinical Psychology*, 1969, *33*, 661-667.

Cohen, D. B. Dream recall and short-term memory. *Perceptual and Motor Skills*, 1971, *33*, 867-871.

Cohen, D. B. Presleep experience and home dream reporting: An exploratory study. *Journal of Consulting and Clinical Psychology*, 1972, *38*, 122-128.

Cohen, D. B. Toward a theory of dream recall. *Psychological Bulletin*, 1974, *81*, 138-154.

Cohen, D. B., & MacNeilage, P. F. Dream salience and postsleep interference factors that differentiate frequent and infrequent dream recallers. *Sleep Research*, 1973, *2*, 111. (Abstract)

Cohen, D. B., & Wolfe, G. Dream recall and repression: Evidence for an alternative hypothesis. *Journal of Consulting and Clinical Psychology*, 1973, *41*, 349-355.

Cohen, G. Hemisphere differences in the affects of cueing in visual recognition tests. *Journal of Experimental Psychology*, 1975, *1*, 366-373.

Cohen, H., & Dement, W. Sleep: Changes in threshold to electroconvulsive shock in rats after deprivation of "paradoxical" phase. *Science*, 1965, *150*, 1318-1319.

Cohen, H., & Dement, W. Sleep: Suppression of rapid eye movement phase in the cat after electroconvulsive shock. *Science*, 1966, *154*, 396-398.

Cohen, H. B., & Dement, W. Electrically induced convulsions in REM deprived mice: Prolongation of the tonic phase. *Psychophysiology*, 1968, *4*, 381. (Abstract)

Cohen, H. B., Duncan, R., & Dement, W. C. The effect of electroconvulsive shock in cats deprived of REM sleep. *Science*, 1967, *156*, 1646-1648.

Cohen, H., Edelman, A., Bowen, R., & Dement, W. Sleep and self-stimulation in the rat. *Sleep Research*, 1972, *1*, 158.

Cohen, H., Mitchell, G., & Dement, W. C. Chlorpromazine and sleep in the cat. *Psychophysiology*, 1968, *5*, 207. (Abstract.)

Cohen, H. D., & Shapiro, A. Vaginal blood flow during sleep. *Psychophysiology*, 1970, *1*, 338. (Abstract)

Cohen, H. D., Shapiro, A., Goodenough, D. R., & Saunders, D. The EEG during stage 4 sleep-talking. Paper presented at the meeting of the Association for the Psychophysiological Study of Sleep, Washington, D. C., March, 1965.

Cohen, H., Thomas, J., & Dement, W. C. Sleep stages, REM deprivation, and electroconvulsive threshold in the cat. *Brain Research*, 1970, *19*, 317-321.

Cohen, J. Some statistical issues in psychological research. In B. B. Wolman, *Handbook of clinical psychology*. New York: McGraw Hill, 1965.

Cohen, J., & Cohen, P. *Applied multiple regression/correlation analysis for the behavioral sciences*. Hillsdale, N. J.: Lawrence Erlbaum Associates, 1975.

Collins, A. M., & Loftus, E. F. A spreading activation theory of semantic processing. *Psychological Review*, 1975, *82*, 4-7-428.

Collins, G., Davison, L., & Breger, L. Dream function in adaptation to threat: A preliminary study. Paper presented at the meeting of the Association for the Psychophysiological Study of Sleep, Santa Monica, 1967.

Cory, T. L., Ormiston, D. W., Simmel, E., & Dainoff, M. Predicting the frequency of dream recall. *Journal of Abnormal Psychology*, 1975, *84*, 261-266.

Critchley, M. The pre-dormitum. *Revue Neurologique*, 1955, *93*, 101-106.

Czaya, J., Kramer, M., & Roth, T. Changes in dream quality as a function of time into REM. Paper presented at the meeting of the Association for the Psychophysiological Study of Sleep, San Diego, 1973.

Dallett, J. Theories of dream function. *Psychological Bulletin*, 1973, *6*, 408-416.

Davis, K. B. *Factors in the sex life of twenty-two hundred women.* New York: Harper & Bros., 1929.

Davison, G. C., Tsujimoto, R. N., & Glaros, A. G. Attribution and the maintenance of behavior change in falling asleep. *Journal of Abnormal Psychology,* 1973, *82,* 124-133.

Delorme, F., Jeannerod, M., & Jouvet, M. Effects remarquables de la reserpine sur l'activite EEG phasique ponto-geniculo-occipitale, *Comptes Rendus des Seances de la Societe de Biologie,* 1965, *159,* 900-903.

De Koninck, J. M., & Koulack, D. Dream content and adaptation to a stressful situation. *Journal of Abnormal Psychology,* 1975, *84,* 250-260.

DeMartino, M R. A review of the literature on children's dreams. *Psychiatric Quarterly Supplement,* 1955, *29,* 90-100.

Dement, W. C. Dream recall and eye movement during sleep in schizophrenics and normals. *Journal of Nervous and Mental Disease,* 1955, *122,* 263-269.

Dement, W. C. The effect of dream deprivation. *Science,* 1960, *131,* 1705-1707. (a)

Dement, W. C. Letter to the editor. *Science,* 1960, *132,* 1420-1422. (b)

Dement, W. C. Experimental dream studies. In J. H. Masserman (Ed.), *Science and psychoanalysis,* Vol. III. New York: Grune & Stratton, 1964. (a)

Dement, W. Eye movements during sleep. In M. Bender (Ed.), *The oculomotor system.* New York: Holber Medical Division, Harper & Row, 1964, (b)

Dement, W. An essay on dreams: The role of physiology in understanding their nature. In F. Barron (Ed.), *New directions in psychology,* Vol. II. New York: Holt, Rinehart & Winston, 1965. (a)

Dement, W. C. Recent studies in the biological role of rapid eye movement sleep. *American Journal of Psychiatry,* 1965, *122,* 404-408. (b)

Dement, W. C. Dreams and dreaming. *International Journal of Neurology,* 1965, *5,* 168-186. (c)

Dement, W. Studies on the function of rapid eye movement (paradoxical) sleep in human subjects. In M. Jouvet (Ed.) *Aspects anatomofonctionnels de la physiologie du sommeil.* Paris: Centre National de la Recherche Scientifique, 1965. (d)

Dement, W. C. Psychophysiology of sleep and dreams. In S. Arieti (Ed.), *American handbook of psychiatry,* Vol. 3. New York: Basic Books, 1966.

Dement, W. C. Possible physiological determinants of a possible dream-intensity cycle. *Experimental Neurology Supplement,* 1967, *4,* 38-55.

Dement, W. C. The biological role of REM sleep (circa 1968). In A. Kales (Ed.), *Sleep: Physiology and pathology.* Philadelphia: Lippincott, 1969.

Dement, W. C. *Some must watch while some must sleep.* San Francisco: W. H. Freeman, 1972.

Dement, W. C. Commentary on "The biological role of REM sleep". In W. B. Webb (Ed.), *Sleep: An active process.* Glenview, Ill.: Scott, Foresman, 1973.

Dement, W. C. Personal communication to Arkin, A. M., 1975.

Dement, W., Cohen, H., Ferguson, J., & Zarcone, V. A sleep researcher's odyssey: The function and clinical significance of REM sleep. In L. Madow, & L. H. Snow, *The psychodynamic implications of the physiological studies on dreams.* Springfield, Ill.: Thomas, 1970.

Dement, W., Ferguson, J., Cohen, H., & Barchas, J. Nonchemical methods and data using a biochemical model: The REM quanta. In A. Mandell & M. Mandell (Eds.), *Psychochemical research in man. Methods, Strategy and theory.* New York: Academic Press, 1969.

Dement, W. C., & Fisher, C. Experimental interference with the sleep cycle. *Canadian Psychiatric Association Journal,* 1963, *8,* 400-405.

Dement, W., & Greenberg, S. Changes in total amount of stage four sleep as a function of partial sleep deprivation. *Electroencephalography and Clinical Neurophysiology,* 1966, *20,* 523-526.

Dement, W., Greenberg, S., & Klein, R. The effect of partial REM sleep deprivation and delayed recovery. *Journal of Psychiatric Research,* 1966, *4,* 141-152.

Dement, W. C., Kahn, E., & Roffwarg, H. P. The influence of the laboratory situation on the dreams of the experimental subject. *Journal of Nervous and Mental Disease,* 1965, *140* 119-131.

Dement, W. C., & Kleitman, N. Cyclic variations in EEG during sleep and their relation to eye movements, bodily motility and dreaming. *Electroencephalography and Clinical Neurophysiology,* 1957, *9,* 673-690. (a)

Dement, W. C., & Kleitman, N. The relation of eye movements during sleep to dream activity: An objective method for the study of dreaming. *Journal of Experimental Psychology,* 1957, *53,* 339-346. (b)

Dement, W. C., & Mitler, M. M. New developments in the basic mechanisms of sleep. In G. Usdin (Ed.), *Sleep research and clinical practice.* New York: Brunner-Mazel, 1973.

Dement, W., & Wolpert, E. Interrelations in the manifest content of dreams occurring on the same night. *Journal of Nervous and Mental Disease,* 1958, *126,* 568-578. (a)

Dement, W., & Wolpert, E. The relation of eye movements, body motility, and external stimuli to dream content. *Journal of Experimental Psychology,* 1958, *55,* 543-553. (b)

Dement, W., Zarcone, V., Ferguson, J., Cohen, H., Pivik, T., & Barchas, J. Some parallel findings in schizophrenic patients and serotonin-depleted cats. In D. V. S. Sankar (Ed.), *Schizophrenia: Current concepts and research.* Hicksville, N.Y.: PJD Publications, 1969.

De Valois, R. L., Abramov, I., & Mead, W. R. Single cell analysis of wavelength discrimination at the lateral geniculate nucleus in the macaque. *Journal of Neurophysiology,* 1967, *30,* 415-433.

Dewan, E. M. The P (programming) hypothesis for REMs. *Psychophysiology,* 1968, *4,* 365-366. (Abstract)

Dewan, E. M. The programming (P) hypothesis for REMs. *Physical Sciences Research Papers,* 1969, No. 388, 1-12. Cambridge: Cambridge Research Laboratories, 1969.

Dewan, E. M. The programming (P) hypothesis for REM sleep. In E. Hartmann (Ed.), *Sleep and Dreaming.* Boston: Little, Brown & Co., 1970.

Dewson, J., Dement, W., & Simmons, F. Middle ear muscle activity in cats during sleep. *Experimental Neurology,* 1965, *12,* 1-8.

Dewson, J. H., Dement, W. C., Wagener, T. E., & Nobel, K. Rapid eye movement sleep deprivation: A central neural change during wakefulness. *Science,* 1967, *156,* 403-406.

Dixon, N. F. Subliminal perception: The nature of a controversy. London: McGraw-Hill, 1971.

Domhoff, B. A quantitative study using an objective indicator of dreaming. Unpublished doctoral dissertation, University of Miami, 1962.

Domhoff, B., & Gerson, A. Replication and critique of three studies on personality correlates of dream recall. *Journal of Consulting Psychology,* 1967, *31,* 431.

Domhoff, B., & Kamiya, J. Problems in dream content study with objective indicators: 1. A. comparison of home and laboratory dream reports. *Archives of General Psychiatry,* 1964, *11,* 519-524.

Dorus, E., Dorus, E., & Rechtschaffen, A. The incidence of novelty in dreams. *Archives of General Psychiatry,* 1971, *25,* 364-368.

Duncan, R., II., Henry, P., Karadzic, V., Mitchell, G., Pivik, T., Cohen, H., & Dement, W. Manipulation of the sleep-wakefulness cycle in the rat: A longitudinal study. *Psychophysiology,* 1968, *4,* 379. (Abstract)

Dunleavy, D. L. F., MacLean, A. W., & Oswald, I. Debrisoquine, guanethidine, propranolol and human sleep. *Psychopharmacologia,* 1971, *21,* 101-110.

Dusan-Peyrethon, D., Peyrethon, J., & Jouvet, M. Etude quantitative des phénoménes phasiques du sommeil paradoxale pendant et après sa déprivation instrumentale. *Comp tes Rendus des Seances de la Société de Biologie,* 1967, *161,* 2530-2537.

Eagle, E. J. An exploratory study of the relationships between cognitive and perceptual styles and drives and defenses in differing states of awareness. An unpublished study cited by H. A. Witkin, R. D. Dyk, H. F. Faterson, D. R. Goodenough, & S. A. Karp *Psychological differentiation.* Potomac, Maryland: Erlbaum, 1974. (Originally published: 1963.)

Eagle, M. Sherwood on the logic of explanation in psychoanalysis. In B. B. Rubenstein (Ed.), *Psychoanalysis and comtemporary science,* Vol 2. New York: Macmillan Publishing Company, 1973.

Ehrlichman, H., & Antrobus, J. S. Sleep mentation and functional hemispheric asymmetry. National Institute of Mental Health Grant Proposal, 1974.

Ekstrand, B. R. Effect of sleep on memory. *Journal of Experimental Psychology,* 1967, *75,* 64-72.

Ekstrand, B., Sullivan, M. J., Parker, D. F., & West, J. Spontaneous recovery and sleep. *Journal of Experimental Psychology,* 1971, *88,* 142-144.

Ellman, S. J. The experimental modification of two aspects of the REM sleep cycle. Unpublished doctoral dissertation, New York University, 1970.

Ellman, S. J. Discussion Presented at Annual Conference of the Center for Research in Cognition and Affect, New York City, May, 1976.

Ellman, S. J., Ackermann, R. F., Farber, J., Mattiace, L., & Steiner, S. S. Relation between dorsal brainstem sleep sites and intracranial self-stimulation. *Physiological Psychology,* 1974, *2,* 31-34.

Ellman, S. J., Antrobus, J. S., Arkin, A. M., Farber, J., Luck, D., Bodnar, R., Sanders, K., & Nelson, W.T. Sleep mentation in relation to phasic and tonic events − REMP and NREM. Paper presented at the meeting of the Association for the Psychophysiological Study of Sleep, Jackson Hole, May, 1974.

Ellman, S. J., & Steiner, S. S. The effect of electrical self-stimulation on REM rebound. Paper presented at the meeting of the Association for the Psychophysiological Study of Sleep, Boston, 1969. (a)

Ellman, S. J., & Steiner, S. S. The effect of REM deprivation on intracranial self-stimulation. Paper presented at the meeting of the Association for the Psychophysiological Study of Sleep, Boston, 1969. (b)

Emerson, R. W. *Lectures and biographical sketches.* Boston: Houghton Mifflin, 1884.

Emmons, W. H., & Simon, C. W. The non-recall of material presented during sleep. *American Journal of Psychology,* 1956, *69,* 79-81.

Empson, J. A., & Clarke, P. R. Rapid eye movements and remembering. *Nature,* 1970, *227,* 287-288.

Ephron, H. S., & Carrington, P. Rapid eye movement sleep and cortical homeostasis. *Psychological Review,* 1966, *73,* 500-526.

Erikson, E. H. The dream specimen of psychoanalysis. In R. Knight, & C. Friedman (Eds.), *Psychoanalytic psychiatry and psychology.* New York: International Universities Press, 1954. (a)

Erikson, E. H. The dream specimen of psychoanalysis. *Journal of the American Psychoanalytic Association,* 1954, *2,* 5-55. (b)

Erikson, E. H. *Childhood and society* (Rev. ed.) New York: W. W. Norton & Company, 1963.

Evans, F. J. Hypnosis and sleep: Techniques for exploring cognitive activity during sleep. In E. Fromm & R. E. Shor (Eds.), *Hypnosis: Research developments and perspectives.* Chicago: Aldine, 1972.

Evans, F. J., Gustafson, L. A., O'Connell, D. N., Orne, M. T., & Shor, R. E. Response during sleep with intervening waking amnesia. *Science,* 1966, *152,* 666-667.

Evans, F. J., Gustafson, L. A., O'Connell, D. N., Orne, M. T., & Shor, R. E. Sleep-induced behavioral response. *Journal of Nervous and Mental Disease,* 1969, *148,* 467-476.

Evans, F. J. Gustafson, L. A., O'Connell, D. N., Orner, M. T., & Shor, R. E. Verbally induced behavior responses during sleep. *Journal of Nervous and Mental Disease,* 1970, *150,* 171-187.

Evans, J. I., Lewis, S. A., Gibb, S. A. M., & Cheetham, M. Sleep and barbiturates: Some experiments and observations. *British Medical Journal,* 1968, *4,* 291-293.

Evans, F. J., & Orchard W. Sleep learning: The successful waking recall of material presented during sleep. *Psychophysiology,* 1969, *6,* 269. (Abstract)

Evans, J. I., & Oswald, I. Some experiments in the chemistry of narcoleptic sleep. *British Journal of Psychiatry,* 1966, *112,* 401-409.

Fahrion, S. L., Davison, L., & Berger, L. The relationship of heart rate and dream content in heart rate responders. Paper presented at the meeting of the Association for the Psychophysiological Study of Sleep, Santa Monica, California, April, 1967.

Farber, J., Arkin, A. M., Ellman, S. J., Antrobus, J. S., & Nelson, W. The effects of sleep interruption, deprivation and elicited verbalizations on sleep speech parameters. Paper presented at the meeting of the Association for the Psychophysiological Study of Sleep, San Diego, California, 1973.

Feinberg, I. Sleep in organic brain conditions. In A. Kales (Ed.), *Sleep: Physiology and pathology.* Philadelphia: Lippincott, 1969.

Feinberg, I., & Evarts, E. V. Some implications of sleep research for psychiatry. In J. Zubin & C. Shagass (Eds.), *Proceedings of the American Psychopathological Association: Neurobiological aspects of psychopathology.* New York: Grune & Stratton, 1969.

Feinberg, I., Hibi, S., Cavness, C., & March, J. Absence of REM rebound after barbiturate withdrawal. *Science,* 1974, *185,* 534-535.

Feldman, R. E. The effect of deprivation of rapid eye movement sleep on learning and retention in humans. *Dissertation Abstracts* (B), 1969, *30,* 4390-4391.

Feldman, R., & Dement, W. Possible relationships between REM sleep and memory consolidation. Paper presented at the meeting of the Association for the Psychophysiological Study of Sleep, Denver, Colorado, 1968, *Psychophysiology,* 1968, *5,* 243. (Abstract)

Feldstein, S. REM deprivation: The effects on ink blot perception and fantasy processes. Doctoral dissertation, City University of New York, 1972.

Feltin, M., & Broughton, R. J. Differential effects of arousal from slow wave sleep versus REM sleep. *Psychophysiology,* 1968, *5,* 231. (Abstract)

Ferguson, J., Cohen, H., Henriksen, S., McGarr, K., Mitchell, G., Hoyt, G., Barchas, J., & Dement, W. The effect of chronic administration of PCPA on sleep in the cat. *Psychophysiology,* 1969, *6,* 220-221. (Abstract)

Ferguson, J., & Dement, W. The effects of variations in total sleep time on the occurrence of rapid eye movement sleep in cats. *Electroencephalography and Clinical Neurophysiology,* 1967, *22,* 2-10.

Ferguson, J., & Dement, W. Changes in intensity of REM sleep with deprivation. *Psychophysiology,* 1968, *4,* 380-381. (Abstract)

Ferguson, J., & Dement, W. The behavioral effects of amphetamine on REM deprived rats. *Journal of Psychiatric Research,* 1969, *7,* 111-118.

Ferguson, J., Henriksen, S., McGarr, K., Belenky, G., Mitchell, G., Gonda, W., Cohen, H., & Dement, W. Phasic event deprivation in the cat. *Psychophysiology,* 1968, *5,* 238-239. (Abstract)

Fingl, E., & Woodbury, A. M. General principles. In L. S. Goodman, & A. Gilman, *The Pharmacological basis of therapeutics* (4th ed.). London: MacMillan, 1970.

Firth, H. Eye movements, dreams and drugs. *Sleep Research,* 1972, *1,* 102.

Firth, H. Habituation during sleep. *Psychophysiology,* 1973, *10,* 43-51.

Firth, H. Sleeping pills and dream content. *British Journal of Psychiatry,* 1974, *124,* 547-553.

Firth, H., & Oswald, I. Eye movements and visually active dreams. *Psychophysiology,* 1975, *12,* 602-605.

Fishbein, W. Paradoxical sleep: A periodic mechanism for securing and maintaining information for long term memory. (Doctoral dissertation, University of Colorado, 1969). *Dissertation Abstracts International,* 1969, *30,* 865B. University Microfilms No. 69-13410.

Fishbein, W. Interference with conversion of memory from short-term to long-term storage by partial sleep deprivation. *Communications in Behavioral Biology* (A), 1970, *5,* 171-175.

Fishbein, W. Disruptive effects of rapid eye movement sleep deprivation on long-term memory. *Physiology and Behavior,* 1971, *6,* 279-282.

Fishbein, W., McGaugh, J. L., & Schwarz, J. R. Retrograde amnesia: Electroconvulsive shock effects after termination of rapid eye movement sleep deprivation. *Science,* 1971, *172,* 80-82.

Fisher, C. A study of the preliminary stages of the construction of dreams and images. *Journal of the American Psychoanalytic Association,* 1957, *5,* 5-60.

Fisher, C. Preconscious stimulation in dreams, associations and images: Classical studies by Otto Pötzl, Rudolf Allers and Jakob Teller. *Psychological Issues,* 1960, *2* (Monograph 7).

Fisher, C. Psychoanalytic implications of recent research on sleep and dreaming. Part I: Empirical findings. Part II: Implications for psychoanalytic theory. *Journal of the American Psychoanalytic Association,* 1965, *13,* 197-303.

Fisher, C. Dreaming and sexuality. In R. Lowenstein, L. Newman, M. Schur, & A. Solnit (Eds.), *Psychoanalysis: A general psychology.* New York: International Universities Press, 1966.

Fisher, C., Byrne, J., Edwards, A., & Kahn, E. A psychophysiological study of nightmares. *Journal of the American Psychoanalytic Association,* 1970, *18,* 747-782.

Fisher, C., & Dement, W. C. Dreaming and psychosis: Observations on the dream cycle during the course of an acute paranoid psychosis. *Bulletin of the Philadelphia Association for Psychoanalysis,* 1961, *11,* 130-132.

Fisher, C., & Dement, W. C. Studies on the psychopathology of sleep and dreams. *American Journal of Psychiatry,* 1963, *119,* 1160-1168.

Fisher, C., Gross, J., & Zuch, J. Cycles of penile erection synchronous with dreaming (REM) sleep. *Archives of General Psychiatry,* 1965, *12,* 29-45.

Fisher, C., Kahn, E., Edwards, A., & Davis, D. Total suppression of REM sleep with Nardil in a patient with intractable narcolepsy. *Sleep Research,* 1972, *1,* 159.

Fisher, C., Kahn, E., Edwards, A., & Davis, D. M. A psychophysiological study of nightmares and night terrors. I: Physiological aspects of the stage 4 night terrors. *Journal of Nervous and Mental Disease,* 1973, *157,* 75-98. (a)

Fisher, C., Kahn, E., Edwards, A., & Davis, D. M. A psychophysiological study of nightmares and night terrors. II: The suppression of stage 4 night terrors with diazepam. *Archives of General Psychiatry,* 1973, *28,* 252-259. (b)

Fisher, C., Kahn, E., Edwards, A., Davis, D. A psychophysiological study of nightmares and night terrors. In L. Goldberger & V. H. Rosen (Eds.), *Psychoanalysis and contemproary science,* Vol. 3. New York: International Universities Press, 1974.

Fisher, C., Kahn, E., Edwards, A., Davis, D. M., & Fine, J. A psychophysiological study of nightmares and night terrors. III: Mental content and recall of stage 4 night terrors. *Journal of Nervous and Mental Disease,* 1974, *158,* 174-188.

Fisher, C., & Paul, I. The effect of subliminal visual stimulation on images and dreams: A validation study. *Journal of the American Psychoanalytic Association,* 1959, *7,* 35-83.

Fisher, J., & Breger, L. (Eds.) *The meaning of dreams: Recent insights from the laboratory.* Research symposium 3 of the State of California Department of Mental Hygiene, 1969.

Fishman, R., & Roffwarg, H. P. REM sleep inhibited by light in the albino rat. *Experimental Neurology,* 1972, *36,* 166-178.

Fiss, H., & Ellman, S. J. REM sleep interruption: Experimental shortening of REM period duration. *Psychophysiology*, 1973, *10*, 510-516.

Fiss, H., Ellman, S. J., & Klein, G. S. Waking fantasies following interrupted and completed REM periods. *Archives of General Psychiatry*, 1969, *21*, 230-239.

Fiss, H., Klein, G. S., & Bokert, E. Waking fantasies following interruption of two types of sleep. *Archives of General Psychiatry*, 1966, *14*, 543-551.

Fiss, H., Klein, G. S., & Shollar, E. "Dream intensification" as a function of prolonged REM-period interruption. In L. Goldberger & V. H. Rosen (Eds.), *Psychoanalysis and contemporary science*, Vol. 3. New York: International Universities Press, 1974.

Fiss, H., Klein, G. S., Shollar, E., & Levine, B. Changes in dream content as a function of prolonged REM sleep interruption. Paper presented at the meeting of the Association for the Psychophysiological Study of Sleep, Denver, 1968. *Psychophysiology*, 1968, *5*, 217, (Abstract.)

Fleiss, J. Estimating the magnitude of experimental effects. *Psychological Bulletin*, 1969, *72*, 273-276.

Foote, S. L. Compensatory changes in REM sleep time of cats during *ad libitum* sleep and following brief REM sleep deprivation. *Brain Research*, 1973, *54*, 261-276.

Foulkes, D. Dream reports from different stages of sleep. Unpublished doctoral dissertation, University of Chicago, 1960.

Foulkes, D. Dream reports from different stages of sleep. *Journal of Abnormal and Social Psychology*, 1962, *65*, 14-25.

Foulkes, D. Theories of dream formation and recent studies of sleep consciousness. *Psychological Bulletin*, 1964, *62*, 236-247.

Foulkes, D. *The psychology of sleep.* New York: Charles Scribners & Sons, 1966.

Foulkes, D. Dreams of the male child: Four case studies. *Journal of Child Psychology and Psychiatry*, 1967, *8*, 81-97. (a)

Foulkes, D. Nonrapid eye movement mentation. *Experimental Neurology*, 1967, *19*, (Supplement 4), 28-38. (b)

Foulkes, D. Review of effects of somatosensory stimulation on dream content. *Sleep Reviews*, Los Angeles: UCLA Brain Information Service, 1970.

Foulkes, D. Longitudinal studies of dreams in children. In J. Masserman (Ed.), *Science and psychoanalysis*, Vol. 19. *Dream dynamics.* New York: Grune & Stratton, 1971.

Foulkes, D. What do we know about dreams and how did we learn it? Paper presented at the meeting of the Association for the Psychophysiological Study of Sleep, San Diego, May, 1973.

Foulkes, D., & Fleisher, S. Mental activity in relaxed wakefulness. *Journal of Abnormal Psychology*, 1975, *84*, 66-75.

Foulkes, D. Larson, J. D., Swanson, E. M., & Rardin, M. Two studies of childhood dreaming. *American Journal of Orthopsychiatry*, 1969, *39*, 627-643.

Foulkes, D., Pivik, T., Ahrens, J., & Swanson, E. M. Effects of "dream deprivation" on dream content: An attempted cross-night replication. *Journal of Abnormal Psychology*, 1968, *73*, 403-415.

Foulkes, D., Pivik, T., Steadman, H. S., Spear, P. S., & Symonds, J. D. Dreams of the male child: An EEG study. *Journal of Abnormal Psychology*, 1967, *72*, 457-467.

Foulkes, D., & Pope, R. PVE and SCE in stage REM: A modest confirmation and an extension. *Sleep Research*, 1972, *1*, 103.

Foulkes, D., & Pope, R. Primary visual experience and secondary cognitive elaboration in stage REM: A modest confirmation and an extension. *Perceptual and Motor Skills*, 1973, *37*, 107-118.

Foulkes, D., & Rechtschaffen, A. Presleep determinants of dream content: Effects of two films. *Perceptual and Motor Skills*, 1964, *19*, 983-1005.

Foulkes, D., & Scott, E. An above-zero waking baseline for the incidence of momentarily hallucinatory mentation. *Sleep Research*, 1973, *2*, 108.

Foulkes, D., & Shepherd, J. Stimulus incorporation in children's dreams. *Sleep Research,* 1972, *1,* 119.

Foulkes, D., Shepherd, J., Larson, J. D., Belvedere, E., & Frost, S. Effects of awakenings in phasic vs. tonic stage REM on children's dream reports. *Sleep Research,* 1972, *1,* 104.

Foulkes, D., Spear, P.S., & Symonds, J. Individual differences in mental activity at sleep onset. *Journal of Abnormal Psychology,* 1966, *71,* 280-286.

Foulkes, D., & Vogel, G. Mental activity at sleep onset. *Journal of Abnormal Psychology,* 1965, *70,* 231-243.

Foulkes, D., & Vogel, G. The current status of laboratory dream research. *Psychiatric Annals,* 1974, *7,* 7-23.

Fowler, M. J., Sullivan, M. J., & Ekstrand, B. R. Sleep and memory. *Science,* 1973, *179,* 302-304.

Fox, R., Kramer, M., Baldridge, B., Whitman, R., & Ornstein, P. The experimenter variable in dream research. *Diseases of the Nervous System,* 1968, *29,* 698-701.

Freedman, A., Luborsky, A., & Harvey, R. Dream time (REM) and psychotherapy correlates of REM time with a patient's behavior in psychotherapy. *Archives of General Psychiatry,* 1970, *22,* 33-39.

Freemon, F. R. *Sleep research: A critical review.* Springfield, Illinois: Charles C. Thomas, 1972.

Friedman, S., & Fisher, C. On the presence of a rhythmic diurnal oral instinctual drive in man: A preliminary report. *Journal of the American Psychoanalytic Association,* 1967, *15,* 317-343.

Friedman, R. C., Kornfeld, D. S., & Bigger, T. J., Jr. Psychological problems associated with sleep deprivation in interns. *Journal of Medical Education,* 1973, *48,* 436-441.

French, T., & Fromm, E. *Dream interpretation: A new approach.* New York; Basic Books, 1964.

Freud, S. *Dreams and telepathy. Standard edition of the complete psychological works of Sigmund Freud.* (J. Strachey, Ed., trans.) Vol. 28. London: Hogarth Press, 1953. (a) (Originally published: 1922)

Freud, S. *Three essays on the theory of sexuality.* London: Hogarth Press, 1953 (b) (originally published: Leipzig & Vienna: Deuticke, 1905).

Freud, S. *The interpretation of dreams. Standard edition of the complete psychological works of Sigmund Freud.* (c) (J. Strachey, Ed., trans.) Vol. 4 London: Hogarth Press, 1953.

Freud, S. *The interpretation of dreams.* New York: Basic Books, 1955. (a) (Originally published: Leipzig & Vienna, Frunze, Deuticke, 1900).

Freud, S. *Introduction to psychoanalysis and the war neurosis. Standard edition of the complete psychological works of Sigmund Freud.* (J. Strachey, Ed., trans.) London: Hogarth Press, 1955 (b) (Originally published Leipzig & Vienna: Internationaler Psychoanalytischer Verlag)

Freud, S. *Mourning and melancholia. Standard edition of the complete psychological works of Sigmund Freud.* (J. Strachey, Ed., trans.) London: Hogarth Press, 1957 (b) (Originally published Leipzig & Vienna: Internationale Zeitschrifte fur Psychoanalyse, 1917, *4,* 288-301)

Freud, S. *Beyond the pleasure principle. Standard edition of the complete psychological works of Sigmund Freud.* (J. Strachey, Ed., trans.) Vol. 18. London: Hogarth Press 1960. (a)

Freud, S. *The interpretation of dreams. Standard edition of the complete psychological works of Sigmund Freud.* (J. Strachey, Ed., trans.) Vol. 4. London: Hogarth Press, 1960. (b)

Freud, S. *An outline of psychoanalysis. Standard edition of the complete psychological works of Sigmund Freud.* (J. Strachey, Ed., trans.) Vol. 23. London: Hogarth Press, 1964.

Fromme, E *The forgotten language.* New York: Holt, 1951.

Gaarder, K. A conceptual model of sleep. *Archives of General Psychiatry,* 1966, *14,* 253-260.

Gahagan, L. Sex differences in recall of stereotyped dreams, sleep-talking and sleep-walking. *Journal of Genetic Psychology,* 1936, *48,* 227-236.

Galin, D. Implications for psychiatry of left and right cerebral specialization. *Archives of General Psychiatry,* 1974, *31,* 572-583.

Gardner, R., Jr., & Grossman, W. I. Normal motor patterns in sleep in man. In E. D. Weitzman (Ed.), *Advances in sleep research,* Vol. 2. New York: Spectrum, 1976.

Gardner, R., Grossman, W., Roffwarg, H., & Weiner, H. The relationship of small limb movements during REM sleep to dreamed limb action. *Psychosomatic Medicine,* 1975, *37,* 147-159.

Gardner, R. A., & Runquist, W. N. Acquisition and extinction of problem-solving set. *Journal of Experimental Psychology,* 1958, *55,* 274-277.

Gardos, G., Cole, J. O., Volicer, J. L., Orzack, M. H., & Oliff, A. C. A dose response study of propranolol in chronic schizophrenia. *Current Therapeutic Research,* 1973, *15,* 314-323.

Garner, W. R., Hake, H. W., & Eriksen, C. W. Operationism and the concept of perception. *Psychological Review,* 1956, *63,* 149-159.

Gassel, M. M., Marchia Fava, P. L., & Pompeiano, O. Phasic changes in muscular activity durduring desynchronized sleep in unrestrained cats. An analysis of the pattern and organization of myoclonic twitches. *Archives Italiennes de Biologie,* 1964, *102,* 449-470. (a)

Gassel, M. M., Marchia Fava, P. L., & Pompeiano, O. Tonic and phasic inhibition of spinal reflexes during deep desynchronized sleep in unrestrained cats. *Archives Italiennes de Biologie,* 1964, *102,* 471-499. (b)

Gastaut, H., & Broughton, R. A clinical polygraphic study of episodic phenomena during sleep – Academic address. In J. Wortis (Ed.), *Recent advances in biological psychiatry,* Vol. 7. New York: Plenum Press, 1965.

German, D. C., & Bowden, D. M. Catecholamine systems as the neutral substrate for intracranial self-stimulation: A hypothesis. *Brain Research,* 1974, *73,* 381-419.

Getter, H., Mulry, R., Holland, C., & Walker, P. Experimenter bias and the WAIS. Unpublished data, University of Connecticut, 1967.

Getzels, J. W., & Jackson, P. W. *Creativity and intelligence.* New York: Wiley, 1962.

Giambra, L. Daydreaming across the life span: Late adolescent to senior citizen. *Developmental Psychology,* 1975 (in press).

Gillam, P. M. S., & Prichard, B. N. C. Use of propranolol in angina pectoris. *British Medical Journal,* 1965, *2,* 337-339.

Gillin, J. C., Buchsbaum, M. S., Jacobs, L. S., Fram, D. H., Williams, R. B. Jr., Vaughn, T. B., Jr., Mellon, E., Snyder, F., & Wyatt, R. J. Partial REM sleep deprivation, schizophrenia and field articulation. *Archives of General Psychiatry,* 1974, *30,* 653-662.

Gillin, J. C., & Wyatt, R. J. Schizophrenia: Perchance a dream? *International Review of Neurobiology,* 1975, *17,* 297-342.

Giora, Z. REM deprivation: An afterthought. *Comprehensive Psychiatry,* 1971, *12,* 321-329.

Globus, G. G. Rapid eye movement cycle in real time. Implications for a theory of the D-State. *Archives of General Psychiatry,* 1966, *15,* 654-659.

Globus, G. G. Rhythmic functions during sleep. In E. Hartmann (Ed.), *Sleep and dreaming.* Boston: Little, Brown & Company, 1970. *International Psychiatry Clinics,* 1970, *7,* (2).

Globus, G. G., Knapp, P. H., Skinner, J. C., & Healy, A. B. An appraisal of telepathic communication in dreams. Paper presented at the meeting of the Association for the Psycholophysiological Study of Sleep, Los Angeles, 1967. *Psychophysiology,* 1968, *4,* 365. (Abstract)

Goblot, E. Sur le souvenir des rêves. *Revue Philosophique,* 1896, *42,* 288. Cited by Giora, Z. Dream recall: Facts and perspectives. *Comprehensive Psychiatry,* 1973, *14,* 159-167.

Goff, W. R., Allison, T., Shapiro, A., & Rosner, B. S. Cerebral somatosensory responses evoked during sleep in man. *Electroencephalography and Clinical Neurophysiology,* 1966, *21,* 1-9.

Goldstein, L., Stolzfus, N. W., & Gardocki, J. F. Changes in interhemispheric amplitude relationships in the EEG during sleep. *Physiology and Behavior,* 1972, *8,* 811-815.

Goodenough, D. R. Some recent studies of dream recall. In H. A. Witkin & H. B. Lewis (Eds.), *Experimental studies of dreaming.* New York: Random House, 1967.

Goodenough, D. R. The phenomena of dream recall. In L. E. Abt & B. F. Riess (Eds.), *Progress in clinical psychology,* Vol. 8. New York: Grune & Stratton, 1968.

Goodenough, D. R., Lewis, H. B., Shapiro, A., Jaret, L., & Sleser, I. Dream reporting following abrupt and gradual awakenings from different types of sleep. *Journal of Personality and Social Psychology,* 1965, *2,* 170-179. (a)

Goodenough, D. R., Lewis, H. B., Shapiro, A., & Sleser, I. Some correlates of dream reporting following laboratory awakenings. *Journal of Nervous and Mental Disease,* 1965, *140,* 365-373. (b)

Goodenough, D. R., Sapan, J., Cohen, H., Portnoff, G., & Shapiro, A. Some experiments concerning the effects of sleep on memory. *Psychophysiology,* 1971, *8,* 749-762.

Goodenough, D. R., Shapiro, A., Holden, M., & Steinschriber, L. A comparison of "dreamers" and "nondreamers": Eye movements, electroencephalograms and the recall of dreams. *Journal of Abnormal Psychology,* 1959, *59,* 295-302.

Goodenough, D. R., Witkin, H. A., Koulack, D., & Cohen, H. The effects of stress films on dream affect and on respiration and eye-movement during rapid-eye movement sleep. *Psychophysiology,* 1975, *15,* 313-320.

Goodenough, D. R., Witkin, H. A., Lewis, H. B., Koulack, D., & Cohen, H. Repression, interference and field dependence as factors in dream forgetting. *Journal of Abnormal Psychology,* 1974, *83,* 32-44.

Gottschalk, L. A. Measuring transient psychological states. In *Research in verbal behavior and some neurophysiological implications.* New York: Academic Press, 1967.

Gottschalk, L. A., Haer, J. L., & Bates, D. E. Effect of sensory overload on psychological state. *Archives of General Psychiatry,* 1972, *27,* 451-457.

Gottschalk, L. A., Stone, W. N., Gleser, G. C., & Iacono, J. M. Anxiety and plasma free fatty acids (FFA). *Life Sciences,* 1969, *8,* 61-68.

Gottschalk, L. A., Winget, C. N., & Gleser, G. C. *Manual of instruction for the Gottschalk-Gleser content analysis scales.* University of California Press, 1969.

Gradess, R. S., Stone, J., Steiner, S. S., & Ellman, S. J. Conditioned motor responding in sleeping human subjects. Paper presented at the meeting of the Association for the Psycholophysiological Study of Sleep, Bruges, Belguim, 1971.

Granda, A. M., & Hammack, J. T. Operant behavior during sleep. *Science,* 1961, *133,* 1485-1486.

Graves, E. A. The effect of sleep upon retention. *Journal of Experimental Psychology,* 1936, *19,* 316-322.

Greenberg, R. Dreaming and memory. *International Psychiatric Clinics,* 1970, *7,* 258-267.

Greenberg, R., & Leiderman, P. H. Perceptions, the dream process and memory: An up-to-date version of notes on a mystic writing pad. *Comprehensive Psychiatry,* 1966, *7,* 517-523.

Greenberg, R., & Pearlman, C. Delirium tremens and dreaming. *American Journal of Psychiatry,* 1967, *124,* 133-142.

Greenberg, R., & Pearlman, C. The source and function of dreams: A study of the psychoanalytic-dream continuum. Paper presented at the Association for the Psychophysiological Study of Sleep, San Diego, May, 1973.

Greenberg, R., & Pearlman, C. Cutting the REM nerve: An approach to the adaptive role of REM sleep. *Perspectives in Biology and Medicine,* 1974, *17,* 513-521.

Greenberg, R., & Pearlman, C. REM sleep and the analytic process: A psychophysiologic bridge. *Psychoanalytic Quarterly,* 1975, *44,* 392-403.

Greenberg, R., Pearlman, C., Brooks, R., Mayer, R., & Hartmann, E. Dreaming and Korsakoff's psychosis. *Archives of General Psychiatry,* 1968, *18,* 203-209.

Greenberg, R., Pearlman, C., Fingar, R., Kantrowitz, J., & Kawliche, S. The effects of dream deprivation: Implications for a theory of the psychological function of dreaming. *British Journal of Medical Psychology,* 1970, *43,* 1-11.

Greenberg, R., Pearlman, C. A., & Gampel, D. War neuroses and the adaptive function of REM sleep. *British Journal of Medical Psychology,* 1972, *45,* 27-33.

Greenberg, R., Pillard, R., & Pearlman, C. The effect of dream (REM) deprivation on stress. *Psychosomatic Medicine,* 1972, *34,* 257-262.

Greenson, R. R. The exceptional position of the dream in psychoanalytic practice. *Psychoanalytic Quarterly,* 1970, *39,* 519-549.

Grieser, C., Greenberg, R., & Harrison, R. H. The adaptive function of sleep: The differential effects of sleep and dreaming on recall. *Journal of Abnormal Psychology,* 1972, *80,* 280-286.

Grob, D., Harvey, A., Langworthy, D., & Lilienthal, J. The administration of di-isopropyl fluorophosphate (DFP) to man. *Bulletin of Johns Hopkins Hospital,* 1947, *81,* 257-266.

Gross, J., Byrne, J., & Fisher, C. Eye movements during emergent stage 1 EEG in subjects with life-long blindness. *Journal of Nervous and Mental Disease,* 1965, *141,* 365-370.

Gross, M. M., Goodenough, D. R., Hastey, J. M., Rosenblatt, S. M., & Lewis, E. Sleep disturbances in alcohol intoxication and withdrawal. In N. K. Mello, & J. H. Mendelson (Eds.), Recent advances in studies of alcoholism. Washington, D. C.: U.S. Government Printing Office (Publication No. (HSM) 71-9045), 1971.

Gross, M. M., Goodenough, D. R., Nagarajan, M., & Hastey, J. M. Sleep changes induced by 4 and 6 days of experimental alcoholization and withdrawal in humans. In M. M. Gross (Ed.), *Alcohol intoxication and withdrawal: Experimental studies.* New York: Plenum Press, 1973.

Grosser, G., & Siegal, A. Emergence of a tonic-phasic model for sleep and dreaming: Behavioral and physiological observations. *Psychological Bulletin,* 1971, *75,* 60-72.

Grossman, W., Gardner, R., Roffwarg, H., Fekete, A., Beers, L., & Weiner, H. Relations of dreamed to actual limb movement. Paper presented at the meeting of the Association for the Psychophysiological Study of Sleep. Bruges, Belgium, June, 1971.

Grossman, W. I., Gardner, R., Roffwarg, A. P., Fekete, A. F., Beers, L., & Weiner, H. Relation of dreamed to actual limb movement, *Psychophysiology,* 1972, *9,* 118-119. (Abstract)

Guilleminault, C., & Brusset, B. Sleep and schizophrenia: Nightmares, insomnia and autonomic discharges. (Study on a young chronic schizophrenic). In U. J. Jovanovic (Ed.), *The nature of sleep.* Stuttgart: Gustav Fischer Verlag, 1973.

Gulevich, G., Dement, W., & Johnson, L. Psychiatric and EEG observations on a case of prolonged (264 hours) wakefulness. *Archives of General Psychiatry,* 1966, *15,* 29-35.

Hacker, F. Systematische Traumbeobachtungen mit besonderer Berucksichtigung der Gedanken. *Archiv für die Gesamte Psycholgie,* 1911, *21,* 1-121.

Hall, C. *The meaning of dreams.* New York: McGraw-Hill, 1966.

Hall, C., & Nordby, V. J. *The individual and his dreams.* New York: New American Library, 1972.

Hall, C., & Van de Castle, R. L. *The content analysis of dreams.* New York: Appleton-Century-Crofts, 1966.

Hall, C. S., Van de Castle, R. L., Hess, R., Dertke, M., Daverso, G., Dupont, G., Nordby, V. J., Scott, J., & Clark, S. *Studies of dreams reported in the laboratory and at home.* Institute of Dream Research Monograph Series, No. 1. Santa Cruz, California, 1966.

Hamilton, M. A rating scale for depression. *Journal of Neurology, Neurosurgery, and Psychiatry,* 1960, *23,* 56-62.

Handwerker, M., & Fishbein, W. Neural excitability after PSD: A replication and further examination. *Physiological Psychology,* 1975, *3,* 137-140.

Hartmann, E. Dauerschlaf: A polygraphic study. *Archives of General Psychiatry,* 1968, *18,* 99-111. (a)

Hartmann, E. The 90-minute sleep dream cycle. *Archives of General Psychiatry,* 1968, *18,* 280-286. (b)

Hartmann, E. A note on the nightmare, In E. Hartmann (Ed.), *Sleep and dreaming.* Boston: Little, Brown & Company, 1970. (a)

Hartmann, E. (Ed.). *Sleep and dreaming.* Boston: Little, Brown & Company, 1970. *International Psychiatry Clinics,* 1970, *7*(2). (b)

Hartmann, E. *The functions of sleep.* New Haven, Conn.: Yale University Press, 1973.

Hartmann, E., Baekeland, F., Zwilling, G., & Hoy, P. Sleep need: How much sleep and what kind? *American Journal of Psychiatry,* 1971, *127,* 1001-1008.

Hartmann, E., Marcus, J., & Leinoff, A. The sleep-dream cycle and convulsive threshold. *Psychonomic Science,* 1968, *13,* 141-142.

Hartmann, E., & Stern, W. C. Desynchronized sleep deprivation: Learning deficit and its reversal by increased catecholamines. *Physiology and Behavior,* 1972, *8,* 585-587.

Hartmann, H. *Ego psychology and the problem of adaptation.* New York: International Universities Press, 1939.

Hauri, P. Evening activity, sleep mentation, and subjective sleep quality. *Journal of Abnormal Psychology,* 1970, *2,* 270-275.

Hauri, P. White noise and dream reporting. Paper presented at the meeting of the Association for the Psychophysiological Study of Sleep, New York, 1972.

Hauri, P. Review of Arkin, A., Antrobus, J., Toth, M., Baker, J., & Jackler, F. A comparison of the content of mentation reports elicited after nonrapid eye movement (NREM) associated sleep utterance and NREM "silent" sleep. *Sleep Research,* 1974, *3,* 324.

Hauri, P. Categorization of sleep mental activity for psychophysiological studies. In G. C. Lairy & P. Salzarulo (Eds.), *The experimental study of human sleep.* Amsterdam: Elsevier, 1975.

Hauri, P. Dreams in patients remitted from reactive depression. *Journal of Abnormal Psychology,* 1976, *85,* 1-10.

Hauri, P., & Hawkins, D. R. Phasic REM, depression, and the relationship between sleeping and waking. *Archives of General Psychiatry,* 1971, *25,* 56-63.

Hauri, P., & Rechtschaffen, A. An unsuccessful attempt to find physiological correlates of NREM recall. Paper presented at the meeting of the Association for the Psychophysiological Study of Sleep. New York, March, 1963.

Hauri, P., Sawyer, J., & Rechtschaffen, A. Dimensions of dreaming. A factored scale for rating dream reports. *Journal of Abnormal Psychology,* 1967, *72,* 16-22.

Hauri, P., & Van de Castle, R. L. Dream content and physiological arousal during REMPs. Paper presented at the meeting of the Association for the Psychophysiological Study of Sleep. Santa Fe, New Mexico, March, 1970. (a)

Hauri, P., & Van de Castle, R. L. Dream content and physiological arousal. *Psychophysiology,* 1970, *7,* 330-331. (b)

Hauri, P., & Van de Castle, R. L. Psychophysiological parallels in dreams. In U. J. Jovanovic (Ed.), *The nature of sleep.* Stuttgart: Fischer, 1973. (a)

Hauri, P., & Van de Castle, R. L. Psychophysiological parallelism in dreams. *Psychosomatic Medicine*, 1973, *35*, 297-308. (b)

Hawkins, D. R. A review of psychoanalytic dream theory in the light of recent psychophysiological studies of sleep and dreaming. *British Journal of Medical Psychology*, 1966, *39*, 85-104.

Hawkins, D. R., Puryear, H. B., Wallace, C. D., Deal, W. B., & Thomas, E. J. Basal skin resistance during sleep and "dreaming". *Science*, 1962, *136*, 321-322.

Hays, W. L. *Statistics for psychologists*. New York: Holt, Rinehart & Winston, 1973.

Head, H. *Aphasia and kindred disorders of speech*. Cambridge, England: Cambridge University Press, 1926.

Hebb, D. O. *The organization of behavior:* A neuropsychological theory. New York: Wiley, 1949.

Heine, R. Über Wiedererkennen und rückwirdende Hemmung. *Zeitschrift für Psychologie und Physiologie der Sinnesorgane*. 1914, *68*, 161-236.

Hicks, R., Paulus, M., & Johnson, J. Effect of REM sleep deprivation on electric shock threshold in rats. *Psychological Reports*, 1973, *32*, 1242.

Hildoff, U., Antrobus, J. S., Farber, J., Ellman, S. J., & Arkin, A. M. Slow eye movements and mental activity at sleep onset. *Sleep Research*, 1974, *3*, 120.

Hilgard, E. R. A neodissociationist interpretation of pain reduction in hypnosis. *Psychological Review*, 1973, *80*, 396-411.

Hinshelwood, R. D. Hallucinations and propranolol. *British Medical Journal*, 1969, *2*, 445.

Hobson, J. A., Goldfrank, F., & Snyder, F. Respiration and mental activity in sleep. *Journal of Psychiatric Research*, 1965, *3*, 79-90.

Hobson, J., & McCarley, R. *Neuronal activity in sleep: An annotated bibliography*. Los Angeles: University of Southern California at Los Angeles Brain Information Service, 1971.

Hockey, G. R. J., Davies, S., & Gray, M. M. Forgetting as a function of sleep at different times of day. *Quarterly Journal of Experimental Psychology*, 1972, *24*, 386-393.

Hodes, R., & Dement, W. C. Depression of electrically induced reflexes ("H"-reflexes) in man during low voltage EEG "sleep". *Electroencephalography and Clinical Neurophysiology*, 1964, *17*, 617-629.

Holdstock, T. L., & Verschoor, G. J. Retention of maze learning following paradoxical sleep deprivation in rats. *Physiological Psychology*, 1973, *1*, 29-32.

Holmes, M. REM sleep patterning and dream recall in covergers and divergers: Evidence for different defensive preferences (Occasional Paper No. 16) Edinburgh: University of Edinburgh, Center for Research in the Educational Sciences, 1973.

Holt, R. R. Motives and thought: Psychoanalytic essays in honor of David Rapaport. *Psychological Issues*, 1967, *5*, (2-3), (Monograph 18-19). New York: *International Universities Press*, 1967.

Holt, R. R. Drive or wish? A reconsideration of the psychoanalytic theory of motivation. *Psychological Issues*, 1976, *9*, (Monograph 36), 158-197. New York: International Universities Press.

Horowitz, M. J. Modes of representation of thought. *Journal of the American Psychoanalytic Association*, 1972, *20*, 793-819.

Horowitz, M. J. Hallucinations: An information processing approach. In R. K. Siegel & L. J. West (Eds.), *Hallucinations: Behavior, experience and theory*. New York: John Wiley and Sons, 1975.

Hospers, J. *An introduction to philosophical analysis* (2nd ed.). Englewood Cliffs, New Jersey: Prentice-Hall, Inc., 1967.

Hudson, L. *Contrary imaginations: A psychological study of the young student*. New York: Shocken, 1966.

Humphrey, M. E., & Zangwill, O. C. Cessation of dreaming after brain injury. *Journal of Neurology, Neurosurgery and Psychiatry*, 1951, *14*, 322-325.

Jackson, H. *Selected writings.* (J. Taylor, G. Holmes, & F. Walshe, Eds.). New York: Basic Books, 1958.

Jackson, H. quoted by Jones, E. The relation between dreams and psychoneurotic symptoms. In E. Jones (Ed.), *Papers in psychoanalysis.* Boston: Beacon Press, 1961.

Jacobs, L., Feldman, M., & Bender, M. Eye movements during sleep. I. The pattern in the normal human. *Archives of Neurology,* 1971, *25,* 151-159.

Jacobs, L., Feldman, M., & Bender, M. Are the eye movements of dreaming sleep related to the visual images of dreams? *Psychophysiology,* 1972, *9,* 393-401.

Jacobson, E., & Kales, A. Somnambulism: All night EEG and related studies. In S. S. Kety, E. V. Evarts, & H. L. Williams (Eds.), *Sleep and altered states of consciousness.* Baltimore: Williams and Wilkins Company, 1967.

Jacobson, A., Kales, A., Lehmann, D., & Hoedemaker, F. S. Muscle tonus in human subjects during sleep and dreaming. *Experimental Neurology,* 1964, *10,* 418-424.

Jacobson, A., Kales, A., Lehmann, D., & Zweizig, J. Somnambulism: All night electroencephalographic studies. *Science,* 1965, *148,* 975-977.

Jacobson, E. Electrophysiology of mental activities. *American Journal of Psychology,* 1932, *44,* 677-694.

Jeannerod, M. Organisation de l'activité électrique phasique de sommeil paradoxal, étude électrophysiologique et neuro-pharmacologique. Thèse de Medicine, Lyon, 1965.

Jenkins, J. G., & Dallenbach, K. M. Obliviscence during sleeping and waking. *American Journal of Psychology,* 1924, *35,* 605-612.

Jenkins, J. J. Remember that old theory of memory? Well, forget it! *American Psychologist,* 1974, *29,* 785-796.

Johnson, L. C. A psychophysiology for all states. *Psychology,* 1970, *6,* 501-516.

Johnson, L. C. Are stages of sleep related to waking behavior? *American Scientist,* 1973, *61,* 326-338.

Johnson, L. C., & Karpan, W. E. Autonomic correlates of the spontaneous K-complex. *Psychophysiology,* 1968, *4,* 444-452.

Johnson, L. C., & Lubin, A. Spontaneous electrodermal activity during waking and sleeping. *Psychophysiology,* 1966, *3,* 8-17.

Johnson, L. C., & Lubin, A. The orienting reflex during waking and sleeping. *Electroencephalography and Clinical Neurophysiology,* 1967, *22,* 11-21.

Johnson, L., Naitoh, P., Lubin, A., & Moses, J. Sleep stages and performance. In P. Colquhoun (Ed.), *Aspects of human efficiency.* London: English Universities Press, 1972.

Johnson, L. C., Naitoh, P., Moses, J. M., & Lubin, A. Interaction of REM deprivation and stage 4 deprivation with total sleep loss: Experiment 2. *Psychophysiology,* 1974, *11,* 147-159.

Jones, E. E., Kanouse, D. E., Kelley, H. H., Nisbett, R. E., Valins, S., & Weiner, B. *Attribution: Perceiving the causes of behavior.* Morristown, New Jersey: General Learning Press, 1971.

Jones, H. S., & Oswald, I. Two cases of healthy insomnia. *Electroencephalography and Clinical Neurophysiology,* 1968, *24,* 378-380.

Jones, R. M. The manifest dream, the latent dream, and the dream work. In E. Hartmann (Ed.), *Sleep and dreaming.* Boston: Little, Brown and Company, 1970. (a)

Jones, R. M. *The new psychology of dreaming.* New York: Grune & Stratton, 1970. (b)

Jones, R. M. The transformation of the stuff dreams are made of. In E. Hartmann (Ed.), *Sleep and dreaming.* Boston: Little, Brown and Company, 1970. (c)

Jouvet, M. Recherches sur les structures nerveuses et les mécanismes responsables des différentes phases du sommeil physiologique. *Archives Italiennes de Biologie,* 1962, *100,* 125-206.

Jouvet, M. Paradoxical sleep. A study of its nature and mechanisms. *Progress in Brain Research*, 1965, *18*, 20-57. (a)

Jouvet, M. Etude de la dualité des états de sommeil at des mécanismes de la phase paradoxale. In: Aspects anatomo-fonctionnels de la physiologie du sommeil. Actes du Colloque Internationale sur les Aspects Anatomo-fonctionnels de la Physiologie de Sommeil. Lyon, 1963, *Colloques Internationaux du Centre Nationale de la Recherche Scientifique*, 1965, *127*, 397-449. (b)

Jouvet, M. Neurophysiology of the status of sleep. *Physiological Reviews*, 1967, *47*, 117-177.

Jouvet, M., Dechaume, J., & Michel, F. Etude des mécanismes du sommeil physiologique. *Lyon Medicale*, 1960, *204*, 479-521.

Jouvet, M., & Delorme, J. Locus coeruleus et sommeil paradoxal. *Comptes Rendus des Séances de la Société de Biologie*, 1965, *159*, 895-899.

Jouvet, M., & Jouvet, D. A study of the neurophysiological mechanisms of dreaming. *Electroencephalography and Clinical Neurophysiology Supplement*, 1965, *24*, 133-157.

Jouvet, M., & Michel, F. Correlations electromyographiques du sommeil chez le chat decortique et mésencephalique chronique. *Comptes Rendus de Séances de la Société de Biologie*, 1959, *153*, 422-425.

Jouvet, D., Vismont, P., & Delorme, F. Etude de la privation séléctive de la phase paradoxale de sommeil chez de chat. *Comptes Rendus de Séances de la Société de Biologie et de Ses Filiales*, 1974, *158*, 576-579.

Joy, R. M., & Prinz, P. N. The effect of sleep altering environments upon the acquisition and retention of a conditioned avoidance response in the rat. *Physiology and Behavior*, 1969, *4*, 809-814.

Jung, C. G. *The integration of the personality* (translated by S. M. Dell). New York: Farrar and Rinehart, 1939.

Jung, C. G. *The psychology of dementia praecox*. New York: Journal of Nervous and Mental Disease Publishing Company, 1944.

Jung, C. On the nature of dreams. In *The structure and dynamics of the Psyche*. New York: Pantheon, 1960. (Originally published: 1945)

Jus, K., & Jus, A. Experimental studies on memory disturbances in humans in pathological and physiological conditions. *International Journal of Psychobiology*, 1972, *2*, 205-218.

Jus, K., Kiljan, A., Losieczko, T., Wilczak, H., & Jus, A. Experimental studies on memory during slow sleep stages and REM stages. *Electroencephalography and Clinical Neurophysiology*, 1969, *27*, 668.

Kahn, E., Dement, W. C., Fisher, C., & Barmack, J. L. The incidence of color in immediately recalled dreams. *Science*, 1962, *137*, 1054.

Kahn, E., Fisher, C., Byrne, J., Edwards, A., & Davis, D. M. The influence of Valium, Thorazine and Dilantin on stage 4 nightmares. *Psychophysiology*, 1970, *7*, 350. (Abstract)

Kahn, E., Fisher, C., Edwards, A., & Davis, D. Mental content of stage 4 night terrors. *Proceedings of the 81st Annual Convention of the American Psychological Association*, 1973, *8(Pt. 1)*, 499-500.

Kahn, E., Fisher, C., & Lieberman, L. Dream recall in the normal aged. *Journal of the American Geriatrics Society*, 1969, *17*, 1121-1126.

Kales, A., Adams, G., Haley, J., Preston, T., & Rickles, W. Sleep patterns during withdrawal from Tuinal: Effects of Dilantin administration. *Psychophysiology*, 1969, *6*, 262. (Abstract) (a)

Kales, A., Bixler, E. O., & Kales, J. D. Role of the sleep research and treatment facility: Diagnosis, treatment and education. In E. D. Weitzman (Ed.), *Advances in sleep research*, Vol. 1. Flushing, New York: Spectrum Publications, 1974.

Kales, A., Hoedemaker, F. S., Jacobson, A., & Lichtenstein, E. L. Dream deprivation: An experimental reappraisal. *Nature*, 1964, *204*, 1337-1338.

Kales, A., Hoedemaker, F., Jacobson, A., Kales, J., Paulson, M., & Wilson, T. Mentation during sleep: REM and NREM recall reports. *Perceptual and Motor Skills*, 1967, *24*, 556-560.

Kales, A., & Jacobson, A. Mental activity during sleep: Recall studies, somnambulism and effects of rapid eye movement deprivation and drugs. *Experimental Neurology*, 1967, *19* (Suppl. 4), 81-91.

Kales, A., Jacobson, A., Paulson, M. J., Kales, J. D., & Walter, R. D. Somnambulsim: Psychophysiological correlates. I. All night EEG studies. *Archives of General Psychiatry*, 1966, *14*, 586-596.

Kales, A., Kales, J., Po, J., & Klein, J. A review of recent sleep and dream studies. *Bulletin of the Los Angeles Neurological Society*, 1966, *31*, 136-151.

Kales, A., Malmstrom, E. J., Rickles, W. H., Hanley, J., Ling Tan, T., Stadel, B., & Hoedemaker, F. S. Sleep patterns of a pentobarbital addict: Before and after withdrawal. *Psychophysiology*, 1968, *5*, 208, (Abstract)

Kales, A., Malmstrom, E. J., Kee, H. K., Kales, J. D., Tan, T. L., Stadel, D., & Hoedemaker, F. S. Effects of hypnotics on sleep patterns dreaming and mood state: Laboratory and home studies. *Biological Psychiatry*, 1969, *1*, 235-241. (b)

Kales, A., Malmstrom, E. J., Scharf, M. B., & Rudin, R. T. Psychophysiological and biochemical changes following use and withdrawal of hypnotics. In A. Kales (Ed.), *Sleep: Physiology and pathology, a symposium.* Philadelphia: Lippincott, 1969. (c)

Kales, A., Preston, T. A., Tan, T., & Allen, C. Hypnotics and altered sleep — dream patterns I and II. *Archives of General Psychiatry*, 1970, *23*, 211-225.

Kamiya, J. Behavioral, subjective and physiological aspects of drowsiness and sleep. In D. W. Fiske, & S. R. Maddi (Eds.), *Functions of varied experience.* Homewood, Illinois: Dorsey Press, 1961.

Kamiya, J., & Fong, S. Dream reporting from NREM sleep as related to respiration rate. Paper presented at the meeting of the Association for the Psychophysiological Study of Sleep, Chicago, March, 1962.

Kanzer, M. The recollection of the forgotten dream. *Journal of the Hillside Hospital*, 1959, *8*, 74-85.

Kanzow, E., Krause, D., & Kuhnel, H. The vasomotor behavior of the cerebral cortex in the phases of desynchronized EEG-activity during natural sleep in the cat. *Pflügers Archiv für die Gesamte Physiologie*, 1962, *274*, 593-607.

Karacan, I., Goodenough, D. R., Shapiro, A., & Starker, S. Erection cycle during sleep in relation to dream anxiety. *Archives of General Psychiatry*, 1966, *15*, 183-189.

Karacan, I., Hursch, C. J., Williams, R. L., & Thornby, J. I. Some characteristics of nocturnal penile tumescence in young adults. *Archives of General Psychiatry*, 1972, *26*, 351-356.

Karacan, I., & Snyder, F. Erection cycle during sleep in Macaca mulatta. Paper presented at the meeting of the Association for the Psychophysiological Study of Sleep. Gainesville, Florida, March, 1966.

Kawamura, H., & Sawyer, C. Differential temperature changes in the rabbit brain during slow wave and paradoxical sleep. Paper presented at the meeting of the Association for the Psychophysiological Study of Sleep, Washington, D.C., March, 1965.

Keenan, R., & Krippner, S. Content analysis and visual scanning in dreams. *Psychophysiology*, 1970, *7*, 302-303.

Keller, H. *The world I live in.* New York: Century Company, 1908.

Kennedy, J., Cook, P., & Crewer, R. An examination of the effects of three selected experimenter variables in verbal conditioning research. Unpublished manuscript, University of Tennessee, 1968.

Kerlinger, F. N., & Pedhazur, E. J. *Multiple regression in behavioral research.* New York: Holt, Rinehart, & Winston, 1973.

Kirtley, D. D. *The psychology of blindness.* Chicago: Nelson-Hall, 1975.

Klein, G. Peremptory ideation: Structure and force. In R. R. Holt (Ed.), Motives and thought. *Psychological Issues*, 1967, 5 (2-3 Monograph), 18-19.

Klein, G. S. Freud's two theories of sexuality. In L. Breger (Ed.), *Clinical-cognitive psychology models and integrations*. Englewood Cliffs, New Jersey: Prentice-Hall, Inc., 1969.

Klein, G. S., Fiss, H., Shollar, E., Dalbeck, R., Warga, C., & Gwozdz, F. Recurrent dream fragments in dreams and fantasies elicited in interrupted and completed REM periods. Paper presented at the meeting of the Association for the Psychophysiological Study of Sleep, Santa Fe, New Mexico, 1970. *Psychophysiology*, 1970, *7*, 331-332. (Abstract)

Kleinsmith, L. J., & Kaplan, S. Paired-associate learning as a function of arousal and interpolated interval. *Journal of Experimental Psychology*, 1963, *65*, 190-193.

Kleitman, N. *Sleep and wakefulness* (2nd ed.). Chicago: University of Chicago Press, 1963.

Kleitman, N. Does dreaming have a function? In E. Hartmann (Ed.) *Sleep and dreaming*. Boston: Little, Brown & Company, 1970, 352-353.   (a)

Kleitman, N. Implications for organization of activities. In E. Hartmann (Ed.), *Sleep and dreaming*. Boston: Little, Brown and Company, 1970, 13-14. (b)

Kling, A., Borowitz, G., & Cartwright, R. Plasma levels of 17-hydroxy-cortico-steroids during sexual arousal in man. *Journal of Psychosomatic Research*, 1972, *16*, 215-221.

Klinger, E. *Structure and functions of fantasy*. New York: Wiley, 1971.

Knapp, P., Greenberg, R., Pearlman, C., Cohen, M., Kantrowitz, J., & Sashin, J. Clinical measurement in psychoanalysis: An approach. *Psychoanalytic Quarterly*, 1975, *44*, 404-430.

Knopf, N. B. The study of heart and respiration rates during dreaming. Unpublished master's thesis, University of Chicago, 1962.

Kohler, W. C., Coddington, R., & Agnew, H. W., Jr. Sleep patterns in 2-year-old children. *Journal of Pediatrics*, 1968, *72*, 228-233.

Kopell, B. S., Zarcone, V., de la Peña, A., & Dement, W. C. Changes in selective attention as measured by the visual averaged evoked potential following REM deprivation in man. *Electroencephalography and Clinical Neurophysiology*, 1972, *32*, 322-325.

Koranyi, E. K., & Lehmann, H. E. Experimental sleep deprivation in schizophrenic patients. *Archives of General Psychiatry*, 1960, *2*, 534-544.

Koukkou, M., & Lehmann, D. EEG and memory storage in sleep experiments with humans. *Electroencephalography and Clinical Neurophysiology*, 1968, *25*, 455-462.

Koulack, D. Repression and forgetting of dreams. In M. Bertini (Ed.), *Psicofisiologia del sonno e del sogno. Proceedings of an international symposium*, Rome, 1967. Milan: Editrice Vita e Pensiero, 1970.

Koulack, D. Dream time and real time. *Psychonomic Science*, 1968, *11*, 202.

Koulack, D. Effects of somatosensory stimulation on dream content. *Archives of General Psychiatry*, 1969, *20*, 718-725.

Koulack, D. Rapid eye movements and visual imagery during sleep. *Psychological Bulletin*, 1972, *78*, 155-158.

Koulack, D., & Goodenough, D. R. Dream recall and dream recall failure: An arousal-retrieval model. *Psychological Bulletin*, 1976, *83*, 975-984.

Kramer, M. Paradoxical sleep. *Postgraduate Medicine*, 1969, *45*, 157-161.

Kramer, M. Manifest dream content in normal and psychopathologic states. *Archives of General Psychiatry*, 1970, *22*, 149-159.

Kramer, M., Baldridge, B. J., Whitman, R. M., Ornstein, P. H., & Smith, P. C. An exploration of the manifest dream in schizophrenic and depressed patients. *Diseases of the Nervous System*, 1969, *30* (Suppl.), 126-130.

Kramer, M., Czaya, J., Arand, D., & Roth, T. The development of psychological content across the REMP. Paper presented at the meeting of the Association for the Psychophysiological Study of Sleep, Jackson Hole, 1974.

Kramer, M., Hlasny, R., Jacobs, G., & Roth, T. Do dreams have meaning? An empirical inquiry. Paper presented at the meeting of the Association for the Psychophysiological Study of Sleep, Edinburgh, 1975.

Kramer, M., & Roth, T. Comparison of dream content in laboratory dream reports of schizophrenic and depressive patient groups. *Comprehensive Psychiatry,* 1973, *14,* 325-329.

Kramer, M., Sandler, C., Whitman, R., & Baldridge, B. J. Hall-Van de Castle scoring of dreams of the depressed. *Psychophysiology,* 1970, *7,* 327. (Abstract)

Kramer, M., Trinder, J., & Roth, T. Dream content analysis of male schizophrenic patients. *Canadian Psychiatric Association Journal,* 1972, *17* (Suppl. 2), 5251-5257.

Kramer, M., Whitman, R. M., Baldridge, B., & Lansky, L. Depression: Dreams and defenses. *American Journal of Psychiatry,* 1965, *122,* 411-417.

Kramer, M., Whitman, R. M., Baldridge, B., & Lansky, L. Dreaming in the depressed. *Canadian Psychiatric Association Journal,* 1966, *11* (Special Suppl.), 178-192.

Kramer, M., Whitman, R. M., Baldridge, B., & Ornstein, P. H. Drugs and dreams III: The effects of imipramine on the dreams of depressed patients. *American Journal of Psychiatry,* 1968, *124,* 1385-1392.

Kramer, M., Whitman, R. M., Baldridge, B. J., & Ornstein, P. H. (Eds.), *Dream psychology and the new biology of dreaming.* Springfield, Illinois: C. C. Thomas, 1969.

Kramer, M., Winget, C., & Whitman, R. M. A city dreams: A survey approach to normative dream content. *American Journal of Psychiatry,* 1971, *127,* 1350-1356.

Kripke, D. An ultradian biologic rhythm associated with perceptual deprivation and REM sleep. *Psychosomatic Medicine,* 1972, *34,* 221-228.

Kripke, D. F., & Sonnenschein, D. A 90 minute daydream cycle. Paper presented at the meeting of the Association for the Psychophysiological Study of Sleep, San Diego, 1973.

Kris, E. *Psychoanalytic explorations in art.* New York: International Universities Press, 1952.

Krippner, S., Calvallo, M., & Keenan, R. Content analysis approach to visual scanning theory in dreams. *Perceptual and Motor Skills,* 1972, *34,* 41-42.

Kubie, L. S. The concept of dream deprivation: A critical analysis. *Psychosomatic Medicine,* 1962, *24,* 62-65.

Lacey, J. I., Bateman, D. E., & Van Lehn, R. Autonomic response specificity: An experimental study. *Psychosomatic Medicine,* 1963, *15,* 8-21.

Lachmann, F. M., Lapkin, B., & Handelman, N. S. The recall of dreams: Its relation to repression and cognitive control. *Journal of Abnormal and Social Psychology,* 1962, *64,* 160-162.

Ladd, G. Contributions to the psychology of visual dreams. *Mind,* 1892, *1,* 299-304.

Langer, S. K. *Philosophy in a new key. A study in the symbolism of reason, rite and act* (3rd ed.). Cambridge, Mass.: Harvard University Press, 1957.

Langs, R. J. Manifest dreams from three clinical groups. *Archives of General Psychiatry,* 1966, *14,* 634-643.

Laplanche, J., & Pontalis, J. B. *The language of psychoanalysis.* New York: W. W. Norton and Company, 1973.

Larson, J. D. Hypnogogic mentation of repressors and sensitizers as influenced by hostile and friendly presleep condtions. *Psychophysiology,* 1971, *7,* 327.

Larson, J. D., & Foulkes, D. Electromyogram suppression during sleep, dream recall and orientation time. *Psychophysiology,* 1969, *5,* 548-555.

Lasaga, J. I., & Lasaga, A. M. Sleep learning and progressive blurring of perception during sleep. *Perceptual and Motor Skills,* 1973, *37,* 51-62.

Laverty, S. G. Sleep disorders and delirium associated with the use of ethanol. In T. J. Boag, & D. Campbell (Eds.), *A triune concept of the brain and behavior*. Toronto: University of Toronto Press, 1969.

Lavie, P., & Kripke, D. F. Ultradian rhythms: The 90- minute clock inside us. *Psychology Today*, 1975, *8*, (11), 54-65.

Lehmann, D., & Koukkou, M. Learning and EEG during sleep in humans. In W. P. Koella & P. Levin (Eds.), *Sleep: Physiology, biochemistry, psychology, pharmacology, clinical implications*. First European Congress on Sleep Research, Basel, 1972. Basel: Karger, 1973.

Lerner, B. Rorschach movement and dreams: A validation study using drug-induced dream deprivation. *Journal of Abnormal Psychology*, 1966, *71*, 75-86.

Lerner, B. Dream function reconsidered. *Journal of Abnormal Psychology*, 1967, *72*, 85-100.

Lester, B. K., Chanes, R. E., & Condit, P. T. A clinical syndrome and EEG-sleep changes associated with amino acid deprivation. *American Journal of Psychiatry*, 1969, *126*, 185-190.

Levine, M., & Spivak, G. *The Rorschach index of repressive style*. Springfield, Illinois: Thomas, 1964.

Levitt, R. A. Paradoxical sleep: Activation by sleep deprivation. *Journal of Comparative and Physiological Psychology*, 1967, *63*, 505-509.

Lewin, B. D. The forgetting of dreams. In R. M. Loewenstein (Ed.), *Drives, affects, behavior*. New York: Intenational Universities Press, 1953.

Lewin, I., & Glaubman, H. The effect of REM deprivation: Is it detrimental, beneficial or neutral? *Psychophysiology*, 1975, *12*, 349-353.

Lewis, H. B. Some clinical implications of recent dream research. In L. E. Abt, & B. F. Riess (Eds.), *Progress in clinical psychology*, Vol. 8. Dreams and dreaming. New York: Grune and Stratton, 1968.

Lewis, H. G. Effects of sleep and dream research on the handling of dreams in psychoanalytic practice. In E. Hartmann (Ed.), *Sleep and dreaming*. Boston: Little, Brown and Company, 1970.

Lewis, H. B., Goodenough, D. R., Shapiro, A., & Sleser, I. Individual differences in dream recall. *Journal of Abnormal Psychology*, 1966, *71*, 52-59.

Lewis, S. A. The quantification of rapid-eye-movement sleep. In A. Herxheimer (Ed.), *A symposium on drugs and sensory functions*. Boston: Little, Brown & Co., 1968.

Linden, E., Bern, D., & Fishbein, W. Retrograde amnesia: Prolonging the fixation phase of memory consolidation by paradoxical sleep deprivation. *Physiology and Behavior*, 1975, *14*, 409-412.

Liddon, S. C. Sleep paralysis and hypnogogic hallucinations. *Arch. Gen. Psychiatry*, 1967, *17*, 88-95.

Lindsay, P. H., & Norman, D. A. *Human information processing: An introduction to psychology*. New York: Academic Press, 1972.

Ling, G. M., & Usher, D. R. Effect of REM and total sleep deprivation on the synthesis and release of ACTH. Paper presented at the meeting of the Association for the Psychophysiological Study of Sleep, Boston, 1969.

Lovatt, D. J., & Warr, P. B. Recall after sleep. *American Journal of Psychology*, 1968, *81*, 253-257.

Loveland, N. T., & Singer, M. T. Projective test assessment of the effects of sleep deprivation. *Journal of Projective Techniques*, 1959, *23*, 323-334.

Luborsky, L. Momentary forgetting during psychotherapy and psychoanalysis: A theory and research method. In R. R. Holt (Ed.), *Motives and thought: Psychoanalytic essays in in honor of David Rapaport. Psychological Issues*, 1967, *5*, (2-3 Monograph 18-19). New York: International Universities Press, Inc.

Luby, E. D., Grisell, J. L., Frohman, C. E., Lees, H., Cohen, B. D., & Gottlieb, J. S. Biochemical, psychological, and behavioral responses to sleep deprivation. *Annals of the New York Academy of Sciences*, 1962, *96*, 71-78.

MacNeilage, L. A. Activity of the speech apparatus during sleep and its relation to dream reports. (Doctoral dissertation, Columbia University) Ann Arbor, Michigan: University Microfilms, 1971. No. 721355.

MacNeilage, P. F., Cohen, D. B., & Macneilage, L. A. Subjects' estimations of sleep-talking propensity and dream recall frequency are positively related. Paper presented at the meeting of the Association for the Psychophysiological Study of Sleep, New York, 1972.

MacNeilage, P. F., & MacNeilage, L. A. Central processes controlling speech production during sleep and waking. In F. J. McGuigan, & R. A. Schoonover (Eds.), *The psychophysiology of thinking*. New York: Academic Press, 1973.

Madow, L., & Snow, L. H. (Eds.), *The psychodymanic implications of the physiological studies on dreams*. Springfield, Illinois: Charles C. Thomas, 1970.

Maggs, R., & Neville, B. Chlordiazepoxide (Librium): A clinical trial of its use in controlling symptoms of anxiety. *British Journal of Psychiatry*, 1964, *120*, 540-543.

Magnussen, G. *Studies on respiration during sleep*. London: H. K. Lewis, 1944.

Malcolm, L. J., Watson, J. A., & Burke, W. PGO waves as unitary events. *Brain Research*, 1970, *24*, 130-133.

Malcolm, N. *Dreaming*. New York: Humanities Press, 1959.

Mandler, G. *Mind and emotion*. New York: John Wiley & Sons, 1975.

Mark, J., Heiner, L., Mandel, P., & Godin, Y. Norepinephrine turnover in brain and stress reactions in rats during paradoxical sleep deprivation. *Life Sciences*, 1969, *8*, 1085-1093.

Masling, J. Differential indoctrination of examiners and Rorschach responses. *Journal of Consulting Psychology*, 1965, *29*, 198-201.

Maury, A. *Le sommeil et les rêves*. Paris: 1861.

Max, L. W. An experimental study of the motor theory of consciousness. III. Action-current responses in deaf-mutes during sleep, sensory stimulation and dreams. *Journal of Comparative Psychology*, 1935, *19*, 469-486.

Max, L. W. An experimental study of the motor theory of consciousness. IV. Action-current responses in the deaf during awakening, kinesthetic imagery and abstract thinking. *Journal of Comparative Psychology*, 1937, *24*, 301-304.

McCarley, R. W., Hobson, J. A., & Pivik, R. T. Cortical PGO spikes: Periodicities. Paper presented at the meeting of the Association for the Psychophysiological Study of Sleep, San Diego, May, 1973.

McDonald, D. G., Johnson, L. C., & Hord, D. J. Habituation of the orienting response in alert and drowsy subjects. *Psychophysiology*, 1964, *1*, 163-173.

McDonald, D. G., Schicht, W. W., Frazier, R. E., Shallenberger, H. D., & Edwards, D. J. Studies of information processing in sleep. *Psychophysiology*, 1975, *12*, 624-629.

McGaugh, J. L. Time-dependent processes in memory storage. *Science*, 1966, *153*, 1351-1358.

McGuigan, F. J., & Tanner, R. G. Covert oral behavior during conversational and visual dreams. *Psychophysiology*, 1970, *7*, 329. (Abstract)

McKellar, P. *Imagination and thinking*. New York: Basic Books, 1957.

Medoff, L., & Foulkes, D. "Microscopic" studies of mentation in stage REM: A preliminary report. *Psychophysiology*, 1972, *9*, 114. (Abstract)

Meier, C., Ruef, H., Ziegler, A., & Hall, C. Forgetting dreams in the laboratory. *Perceptual and Motor Skills*, 1968, *26*, 551-557.

Mendels, J., & Cochrane, C. The nosology of depression: The endogenous-reactive concept. *American Journal of Psychiatry*, 1968, *124* (Suppl.), 1-11.

Mendels, J., & Hawkins, D. R. Sleep and depression: A controlled EEG study. *Archives of General Psychiatry*, 1967, *16*, 344-354.

Mendelson, J. H., Siger, L., & Solomon, P. Psychiatric observations on congenital and acquired deafness: Symbolic and perceptual processes in dreams. *American Journal of Psychiatry*, 1960, *116*, 883-888.

Mendelson, W., Guthrie, R., Frederick, G., & Wyatt, R. Should flower pots be used for flowers, pot, or rats? *Sleep Research*, 1973, *2*, 169.

Mendelson, W., Guthrie, R., Frederick, G., & Wyatt, R. The flower pot technique of rapid eye movement (REM) sleep deprivation. *Pharmacology, Biochemistry and Behavior*, 1974, *2*, 553-556.

Messick, S. The psychology of acquiesence: An interpretation of research evidence. In I. Berg (Ed.), *Response set in personality assessment*. New York: Irvington, 1971.

Michel, F., Jeannerod, M., Mouret, J., Rechtschaffen, A., & Jouvet, M. Sur les mecanismes de l'activité de pointes au niveau du système visuel au cours de la phase paradoxale du sommeil. *Comptes Rendus des Séances de la Société de Biologie*, 1964, *158*, 103-106.

Mikiten, T., Niebyl, P., & Hendley, C. EEG desynchronization during behavioral sleep associated with spike discharges from the thalamus of the cat. *Federation Proceedings*, 1961, *20*, 327. (Abstract)

Miller, J. B. Dreams during varying stages of depression. *Archives of General Psychiatry*, 1969, *20*, 560-565.

Miller, L., Drew, W. G., & Schwartz, I. Effect of REM sleep deprivation on retention of a one-trial passive avoidance response. *Perceptual and Motor Skills*, 1971, *33*, 118.

Minard, J., Loiselle, R., Ingledue, E., & Dautlich, C. Discriminative electro-oculogram deflections (EOGDs) and heart-rate (HR) pauses elicited during maintained sleep by stimulus significance. *Psychophysiology*, 1968, *5*, 232. (Abstract)

Moffat, M. C. Unpublished data, University of British Columbia, 1966.

Molinari, S., & Foulkes, D. Tonic and phasic events during sleep: Psychological correlates and implications. *Perceptual and Motor Skills*, 1969, *29*, 343-368.

Monroe, L. J. Psychological and physiological differences betwen good and poor sleepers. *Journal of Abnormal Psychology*, 1967, *72*, 255.

Monroe, L., Rechtschaffen, A., Foulkes, D., & Jensen, J. Discriminability of REM and NREM reports. *Journal of Personality and Social Psychology*, 1965, *2*, 456-460.

Montgomery, D. D., & Bone, R. N. Dream recall and cognitive style. *Perceptual and Motor Skills*, 1970, *31*, 386.

Moore, S. F. Jr. Therapy of psychosomatic symptoms in gynecology, an evaluation of chlordiazepoxide. *Current Therapeutic Research*, 1962, *4*, 249-257.

Morden, B., Conner, R., Mitchell, G., Dement, W., & Levine, S. Effects of rapid eye movement (REM) sleep deprivation on shock induced fighting. *Physiology and Behavior*, 1968, *3*, 425-432.

Morden, B., Mitchell, G., & Dement, W. Selective REM sleep deprivation and compensation phenomena in the rat. *Brain Research*, 1967, *5*, 339-349.

Morden, B., Mullins, R., Levine, S., Cohen, H., & Dement, W. Effect of REMs deprivation on the mating behavior of male rats. *Psychophysiology*, 1968, *5*, 241-242. (Abstract)

Morrison, A. R., & Pompeiano, O. Vestibular influences during sleep. VI. Vestibular control of autonomic functions during the rapid eye movements of desynchronized sleep. *Archives Italiennes de Biologie*, 1970, *108*, 154-180.

Moruzzi, G. Active processes in the brain stem during sleep. *Harvey Lecture Series*, 1963, *58*, 233-297.

Moruzzi, G. General discussion, In *Aspects anatomo-fonctionnels de la physiologie du sommeil. Actes du Colloque International sur les Aspects Anatomo-fonctionnels de la Physiologie du Sommeil, Lyon, 1963.* Colloques Internationaux du Centre National de la Recherche Scientifique, No. 127, 1965.

Moruzzi, G., & Magoun, H. W. Brain stem reticular formation and activation of the electro-encephalogram. *Electroencephalography and Clinical Neurophysiology,* 1949, *1,* 455-473.

Moskowitz, E., & Berger, R. J. Rapid eye movements and dream imagery: Are they related? *Nature,* 1969, *224,* 613-614.

Mouret, J., Jeannerod, M., & Jouvet, M. L'activité électrique du systèm visuel au cours de la phase paradoxale du sommeil chez le Chat. *Journal de Physiologie,* 1963, *55,* 305-306.

Mouret, J., Pujol, J. F., & Kiyuno, S. Paradoxical sleep rebound in rats: Effects of physical procedures involved in intracranial ingestion. *Brain Research,* 1969, *15,* 501-506.

Muller, G. E., & Pilzecker, A. Experimentelle Beitrage zur Lehre vom Gadächtnis. *Zeitischrift für Psychologie,* 1900, Supplement No. 1.

Muzio, J., Roffwarg, H., Anders, C., & Muzio, L. Retention of rote learned meaningful verbal material and alterations in the normal sleep EEG patterns. Paper presented at the meeting of the Association for the Psychophysiological Study of Sleep, Bruges, Belgium, 1971.

Naiman, J., Poitros, R., & Englesmann, F. The effect of chlorpromazine on REM rebound in normal volunteers. *Canadian Psychiatric Association Journal,* 1972, *17,* 463-469.

Nakazawa, Y., Kotorii, M., Kotorii, T., Tachibana, H., & Nakano, T. Individual differences in compensatory rebound of REM sleep with particular reference to their relationship to personality and behavioral characteristics. *Journal of Nervous and Mental Disease,* 1975, *161,* 18-25.

Nauta, W. J. H. Hippocampal projections and related neural pathways to the midbrain in cats. *Brain,* 1958, *81,* 319-340.

Newman, E. B. Forgetting of meaningful material during sleeping and waking. *American Journal of Psychology,* 1939, *52,* 65-71.

Newton, P. Recalled dream content and the maintenance of body image. *Journal of Abnormal Psychology,* 1970, *76,* 134-139.

Nebes, R. D. Hemispheric specialization in commisurotomized man. *Psychological Bulletin,* 1974, *81,* 1-14.

Nowlis, V., & Nowlis, H. H. The description and analysis of mood. *Annals of the New York Academy of Sciences,* 1956, *65,* 344-355.

Offenkrantz, W., & Rechtschaffen, A. Clinical studies of sequential dreams. I. A patient in psychotherapy, *Archives of General Psychiatry,* 1963, *8,* 497-508.

Offenkrantz, W., & Wolpert, E. The detection of dreaming in a congenitally blind subject. *Journal of Nervous and Mental Disease,* 1963, *136,* 88-90.

Ogden, C. K., & Richards, I. A. *The meaning of meaning.* (7th ed.) London: Kegan Paul, Trench, Trubner and Company, 1945.

Ohlmeyer, P., Brilmayer, H., & Hüllstrung, H. Periodische Vorgänge im Schlaf. *Pflügers Archiv für die Gesamte Physiologie,* 1944, *248,* 559-560.

Okuma, T., Sunami, Y., Fukuma, E., Takeo, S., & Motoike, M. Dream content study in chronic schizophrenics and normals by REMP-awakening technique. *Folia Psychiatrica et Neurologica Japonica,* 1970, *24,* 151-162.

Olds, J. A preliminary mapping of electrical reinforcing effects in the brain. *Journal of Comparative and Physiological Psychology,* 1956, *49,* 281-285.

Olds, J. Hypothalamic substrates of reward. *Physiological Reviews,* 1962, *42,* 554-604.

Oppelt, A. W. & Palmer, R. Cri de coeur: Time out for questions: Therapy. *Emergency Medicine,* 1972, *4,* 56-73.

Orlinsky, D. Psychodynamic and cognitive correlates of dream recall – A study of individual differences. Unpublished doctoral dissertation, University of Chicago, 1962.

Orne, M. T. On the social psychology of the psychological experiment: With particular reference to demand characteristics and their implications. *American Psychologist,* 1962, *17,* 776-783.

Orr, W. J., Dozier, J. E., Green, L., & Cromwell, R. L. Self-induced waking: Changes in dreams and sleep patterns. *Comprehensive Psychiatry*, 1968, *9*, 499-506.

Oswald, I. *Sleeping and waking*. Amsterdam, New York: Elsevier Publishing Company, 1962.

Oswald, I. Sleep, dreams and drugs. *Proceedings of the Royal Society of Medicine*, 1969, *62*, 151-153. (a)

Oswald, I. Human brain protein, drugs and dreams. *Nature*, 1969, *223*, 893-897. (b)

Oswald, I. Drug research and human sleep. In H. W. Elliott, R. Okun, & R. George (Eds.), *Annual review of pharmacology*, Vol. 13. Palo Alto, California: Annual Reviews, Inc., 1973.

Oswald, I., Berger, R. J., Jaramillo, R. A., Keddie, K. M. G., Olley, P. C., & Plunkett, G. B. Melancholia and barbiturates: A controlled EEG, body and eye movement study of sleep. *British Journal of Psychiatry*, 1963, *109*, 66-78.

Oswald, I., Lewis, S. A., Tagney, J., Firth, A., & Haider, I. Benzodiazepines and human sleep. In S. Garratini, E. Mussini, & L. O. Randall (Eds.), *The benzodiazepines*. New York: Raven Press, 1973.

Oswald, I., & Priest, R. Five weeks to escape the sleeping pill habit. *British Medical Journal*, 1965, *2*, 1093.

Oswald, I., Taylor, A. M., & Treisman, M. Discriminative responses to stimulation during human sleep. *Brain*, 1960, *83*, 440-453.

Oswald, I., Thacore, V. R., Adam, K., Brezinova, V., & Burack, R. Alpha-adrenergic receptor blockade increases human REM sleep. *British Journal of Clinical Pharmacology*, 1975, *2*, 107-110.

Othmer, E., Hayden, M. P., & Segelbaum, R. Encephalic cycles during sleep and wakefulness in humans: A 24-hour pattern. *Science*, 1969, *164*, 447-449.

Overton, D. A. State-dependent learning produced by depressant and atropine-like drugs. *Psychopharmacologia*, 1966, *10*, 6-31.

Overton, D. A. State-dependent retention of learned responses produced by drugs. Its relevance to sleep learning and recall. In W. P. Koella, & P. Levin (Eds.), *Sleep – Physiology, biochemistry, psychology, pharmacology, clinical implications*. (Proceedings of the First European Congress on Sleep Research, Basel, 1972). Basel, Switzerland: S. Karger, 1973.

Owen, M., & Bliss, E. L. Sleep loss and cerebral excitability. *American Journal of Physiology*, 1970, *218*, 171-173.

Paivio, A. *Imagery and verbal processes*. New York: Holt, Rinehart & Winston, 1971.

Palmer, J. O. Alterations in Rorschach's experience balance under conditions of food and sleep deprivation: A construct validation study. *Journal of Projective Techniques*, 1963, *27*, 208-213.

Palombo, S. R. The associative memory tree. In B. B. Rubinstein (Ed.), *Psychoanalysis and contemporary science*, Vol. 2. New York: Macmillan Publishing Company, 1973.

Patrick, G. T. W. & Gilberg, J. A. On the effects of sleep loss. *Psychological Review*, 1896, *3*, 469-483.

Pearlman, C. REM sleep deprivation impairs latent extinction in rats. *Physiology and Behavior*, 1973, *11*, 233-237.

Pearlman, C., & Becker, M. REM sleep deprivation impairs barpress acquisition in rats. *Physiology and Behavior*, 1974, *13*, 813-817.

Pearlman, C., & Becker, M. Retroactive impairment of cooperative learning by imipramine and chlordiazepoxide in rats. *Psychopharmacologia*, 1975, *42*, 63-66.

Pearlman, C., & Greenberg, R. Posttrial REM sleep: A critical period for consolidation of shuttlebox avoidance. *Animal Learning Behavior*, 1973, *1*, 49-51.

Perenin, M. T., Maeda, T., & Jeannerod, M. Are vestibular nuclei responsible for rapid eye movements of paradoxical sleep? *Brain Research*, 1972, *43*, 617-621.

Pessah, M., & Roffwarg, H. Middle ear muscle activity during sleep: An important new phasic phenomenon. *Psychophysiology*, 1972, *9*, 127-128. (Abstract) (a)

Pessah, M. A., & Roffwarg, H. P. Spontaneous middle ear muscle activity in man: A rapid eye movement phenomenon. *Science*, 1972, *178*, 773-776. (b)

Peterfreund, E., & Franceschini, E. On information, motivation and meaning. In B. B. Rubinstein (Ed.), *Psychoanalysis and contemporary science*, Vol. 2. New York: Macmillan Publishing Company, 1973.

Peterfreund, E., & Schwartz, J. T. Information, systems and psychoanalysis. An evolutionary biological approach to psychoanalytic theory. *Psychological Issues*, 1971, *7* (Monograph 1-2), 25-26.

Peterson, L. R., & Peterson, M. J. Short-term retention of individual verbal items. *Journal of Experimental Psychology*, 1959, *58*, 193-198.

Piaget, J. *Play, dreams and imitation in childhood*. London: Heinemann, 1951.

Pivik, R. T. Mental activity and phasic events during sleep. (Doctoral dissertation, Stanford University) Ann Arbor, Michigan: University Microfilms, 1971, No. 71-19746.

Pivik, T. Review of Cartwright, R. D., Sleep fantasy in normal and schizophrenic persons. *Sleep Research*, 1974, *3*, 327-328.

Pivik, T., & Dement, W. Amphetamine, REM deprivation and K-complexes. *Psychophysiology*, 1968, *5*, 241. (Abstract)

Pivik, T., & Dement, W. C. Phasic changes in muscular and reflex activity during non-REM sleep. *Experimental Neurology*, 1970, *27*, 115-124.

Pivik, T., & Foulkes, D. "Dream deprivation": Effects on dream content. *Science*, 1966, *153*, 1282-1284.

Pivik, T., & Foulkes, D. NREM mentation: Relation to personality, orientation time, and time of night. *Journal of Consulting and Clinical psychology*, 1968, *37*, 144-151.

Pivik, T., Halper, C., & Dement, W. Phasic events and mentation during sleep. *Psychophysiology*, 1969, *6*, 215. (Abstract) (a)

Pivik, T., Halper, C., & Dement, W. NREM phasic EMG suppression in the human. *Psychophysiology*, 1969, *217*. (Abstract) (b)

Plumer, S., Matthews, L., Tucker, M., & Cook, T. The water tank technique: Avoidance conditioning as a function of water level and pedestal size. *Physiology and Behavior*, 1974, *12*, 285-287.

Pompeiano, O. Muscular afferents and motor control during sleep. In R. Granit (Ed.), *Muscular afferents and motor control*. Stockholm: Almquist and Siksell, 1966.

Pompeiano, O. The neurophysiological mechanism of the postural and motor events during desynchronized sleep. In S. S. Kety, E. V. Evarts, & H. L. Williams (Eds.), *Sleep and altered states of consciousness*. Baltimore: Williams & Wilkins, 1967.

Pompeiano, O. Mechanisms of sensorimotor integration during sleep. In E. Stellar, & J. M. Sprague (Eds.), *Progress in physiological psychology*. Vol. 3. New York: Academic Press, 1970.

Pope, R. A. Psychological correlates of theta burst activity in sleep onset. Unpublished master's thesis, University of Wyoming, 1973.

Portnoff, G., Baekeland, F., Goodenough, D. R., Karacan, I., & Shapiro, A. Retention of verbal materials perceived immediately prior to onset of non-REM sleep. *Perceptual and Motor Skills*, 1966, *22*, 751-758.

Pötzl, O., Allers, R., & Teler, J. Preconscious stimulation in dreams, associations and images. *Psychological Issues*, 1960, *7*, 1-40.

Prichard, B. N. C., & Gillam, P. M. S. Use of propranolol (Inderal) in treatment of hypertension. *British Medical Journal*, 1964, *2*, 725-727.

Prichard, B. N. C., & Gillam, P. M. S. Treatment of hypertension with propranolol. *British Medical Journal*, 1969, *1*, 7-16.

Prigot, A., Barnes, A.L., & Barnard, R. D. Meprobamate therapy. *Harlem Hospital Bulletin*, 1957, *10*, 63-77.

Prince, M. The mechanism and interpretation of dreams. *Journal of Abnormal Psychology,* 1911, *5,* 337-354.

Pujol, J. F., Mouret, J., Jouvet, M., & Glowinski, J. Increased turnover of cerebral norepinephrine during rebound of paradoxical sleep in rats. *Science,* 1968, *159,* 112-114.

Puryear, H. B. Personality characteristics of reporters and non-reporters of dreams. Doctoral dissertation, University of North Carolina at Chapel Hill. Ann Arbor, Michigan: University Microfilms, 1963, No. 64-1884.

Putkonen, P., & Putkonen, A. Suppression of paradoxical sleep (PS) following hypothalamic defense reaction in cats during normal conditions and recovery from PS deprivation. *Brain Research,* 1971, *26,* 333-347.

Quillian, M. R. Semantic memory. Unpublished doctoral dissertation, Carnegie Institute of Technology, 1966. Reprinted in part in M. Minsky (Ed.), *Semantic Information Processing.* Cambridge, Mass.: M. I. T. Press, 1968.

Raffetto, A. Experimenter effects on subjects' reported hallucinatory experience under visual and auditory deprivation. Paper presented at the meeting of the Midwestern Psychological Association, Chicago, May, 1968.

Ramsey, G. V. Studies of dreaming. *Psychological Bulletin,* 1953, *50,* 432-455.

Rao, C. R. *Linear statistical inference and its applications.* New York: Wiley, 1973.

Rapaport, D. The structure of psychoanalytic theory. *Psychological Issues Monograph Series,* Vol. 2. New York: International Universities Press, 1960.

Rapaport, D. The collected papers of David Rapaport, M. M. Gill (Ed.). New York: Basic Books, 1967.

Rapaport, D., & Gill, M. M. The points of view and assumptions of metapsychology. *International Journal of Psychoanalysis,* 1959, *40,* 153-162.

Rechtschaffen, A. Discussion of: Experimental dream studies, by W. C. Dement. In J. H. Masserman (Ed.), *Science and psychoanalysis,* Vol. 1, *Development and research.* New York: Grune and Stratton, 1964.

Rechtschaffen, A. Dream reports and dream experiences. *Experimental Neurology,* 1967, (Suppl. 4), 4-15.

Rechtschaffen, A. The psychophysiology of mental activity during sleep. In F. J. McGuigan, & R. A. Schoonover (Eds.), *The psychophysiology of thinking.* New York: Academic Press, 1973.

Rechtschaffen, A., & Chernik, D. A. The effect of REM deprivation on periorbital spike activity in NREM sleep. *Psychophysiology,* 1972, *9,* 128. (Abstract)

Rechtschaffen, A., Cornwell, P., & Zimmerman, W. Brain temperature variations with paradoxical sleep in the cat. Unpublished manuscript, 1965.

Rechtschaffen, A., & Dement, W. C. Narcolepsy and hypersomnia. In A. Kales (Ed.), *Sleep: Physiology and pathology.* Philadelphia: Lippincott, 1969.

Rechtschaffen, A., & Foulkes, D. Effect of visual stimuli on dream content. *Perceptual and Motor Skills,* 1965, *20,* 1149-1160.

Rechtschaffen, A., Goodenough, D., & Shapiro, A. Patterns of sleep talking. *Archives of General Psychiatry,* 1962, *7,* 418-426.

Rechtschaffen, A., Hauri, P., & Zeitlin, M. Auditory awakening thresholds in REM and NREM sleep stages. *Perceptual and Motor Skills,* 1966, *22,* 927-942.

Rechtschaffen, A., & Kales, A. (Eds.). *A manual of standardized terminology, techniques and scoring system for sleep stages of human subjects.* (National Institute of Health Publication No. 204) Washington, D.C.: United States Government Printing Office, 1968.

Rechtschaffen, A., & Maron, L. The effect of amphetamine on the sleep cycle. *Electroencephalography and Clinical Neurophysiology,* 1964, *16,* 438-445.

Rechtschaffen, A., Michel, F., & Metz, J. T. Relationship between extraocular and PGO activity in the cat. *Psychophysiology,* 1972, *9,* 128. (Abstract)

Rechtschaffen, A., Mollinari, S., Watson, R., & Wincor, M. Extraocular potentials: A possible indicator of PGO activity in the human. Paper presented at the Association for the Psychophysiological Study of Sleep, Santa Fe, New Mexico, 1970, *Psychophysiology*, 1970, *1*, 336. (Abstract)

Rechtschaffen, A., & Verdone, P. Amount of dreaming: Effect of incentive, adaptation to laboratory and individual differences. *Perceptual and Motor Skills*, 1964, *18*, 947-958.

Rechtschaffen, A., Verdone, P., & Wheaton, J. Reports of mental activity during sleep. *Canadian Psychiatric Association Journal*, 1963, *8*, 409-414. (a)

Rechtschaffen, A., Vogel, G., & Shaikun, G. Interrelatedness of mental activity during sleep. *Archives of General Psychiatry*, 1963, *9*, 536-547. (b)

Rechtschaffen, A., Watson, R., Wincor, M., & Molinari, S. Orbital phenomena and mental activity in NREM sleep. Paper presented at the First International Congress of the Association for the Psychophysiological Study of Sleep, Belgium, 1971.

Rechtscaffen, A., Watson, R., Wincor, M. Z., & Molinari, S. Orbital phenomena and mental activity in NREM sleep. *Psychophysiology*, 1972, *9*, 128. (Abstract) (a)

Rechtschaffen, A., Watson, R., Wincor, M. Z., Molinari, S., & Barta, S. G. The relationship of phasic and tonic periorbital EMG activity to NREM mentation. *Sleep Research*, 1972, *1*, 114. (b)

Reed, H. Learning to remember dreams. *Journal of Humanistic Psychology*, 1973, *13(3)*, 33-48.

Reite, M. L., & Pegram, G. U. Cortical temperature during paradoxical sleep in the monkey. *Electroencephalography and Clinical Neurophysiology*, 1968, *25*, 36-41.

Rich, K. D., Antrobus, J. S., Ellman, S. J., & Arkin, A. M. REM rebound following deprivation as a function of changes in dream mentation fantasy. *Sleep Research*, 1975, *4*, 244.

Richardson, A., & Gough, J. E. The long range effect of sleep on retention. *Australian Journal of Psychology*, 1963, *15*, 37-41.

Richardson, G. A., & Moore, R. A. On the manifest dream in schizophrenia. *Journal of the American Psychoanalytic Association*, 1963, *11*, 281-302.

Ricoeur, P. *Freud and philosophy: An essay on interpretation.* New Haven: Yale University Press, 1970.

Roffwarg, H. Inter-model relationships in sleep research. In G. Lairy & P. Salzarulo (Eds.), *The experimental study of human sleep: Methodological problems.* Amsterdam: Elsevier, 1975.

Roffwarg, H., Adrien, J., Herman, J., Lamstein, S., Pessah, M., Spiro, R., & Bowe-Anders, C. The place of the middle ear muscle activity in the neurophysiology and psychophysiology of the REM state. *Sleep Research*, 1973, *2*, 36.

Roffwarg, H., Bowe-Anders, C., Tauber, E., & Herman, J. Dream Imagery: The effect of long term perceptual modification, *Sleep Research*, 164, *4*, 1975. (Abstract)

Roffwarg, H. P., Dement, W., & Fisher, C. Preliminary observations of the sleep-dream pattern in neonates, infants, children and adults. In E. Harms (Ed.), *Problems of sleep and dream in children.* New York: Macmillan Press, 1964.

Roffwarg, H., Dement, W., Muzio, J., & Fisher, C. Dream imagery: Relationship to rapid eye movements of sleep. *Archives of General Psychiatry*, 1962, *7*, 235-258.

Roffwarg, H., Herman, J., & Lamstein, S. The middle ear muscles: Predictability of their phasic activity in REM sleep from dream material. *Sleep Research*, 1975, *4*, 165.

Roffwarg, H. P., & Muzio, J. N. Sleep onset stage I-A re-evaluation. Paper presented at the Association for the Psychophysiological Study of Sleep, Washington, D.C., 1965.

Roffwarg, H. P., Muzio, J. N., & Dement, W. C. Ontogenetic development of the human sleep-dream cycle. *Science*, 1966, *152*, 604-619.

Rommetveit, R. *Words, meanings and messages: Theory and experiments in psycholinguistics.* New York: Academic Press, 1968.

Rorschach, H. *Psychodiagnostics: A diagnostic test based on perception.* Translated by P. Lemkau and B. Kronenburg. Berne: Hans Huber, 1942.

Rosch, E. Reply to Loftus. *Journal of Experimental Psychology: General,* 1975, *104,* 241-243.

Rosen, J. *Direct analysis, selected papers.* New York: Grune and Stratton, 1953.

Rosenthal, R. *Experimenter effects in behavioral research.* New York: Appleton-Century-Crofts, 1966.

Rosenthal, R., & Fode, K. L. The effect of experimenter bias on the performance of the albino rat. *Behavioral Science,* 1963, *8,* 183-189.

Rosenthal, R., Friedman, N., & Kurland, D. Instruction-reading behavior of the experimenter as an unintended determinant of experimental results. *Journal of Experimental Research in Personality,* 1966, *1,* 221-226.

Rosenthal, R., & Rosnow, R. L. (Eds.), *Artifact in behavioral research.* New York: Academic Press, 1969.

Ross, D. *Aristotle* (5th ed.). New York: Barnes and Noble University Paperbacks, 1964.

Roth, T., Kramer, M., & Arand, D. Dreams as a reflection of immediate psychological concern. Paper presented at the meeting of the Association for the Psychophysiological Study of Sleep, Cincinnati, 1976.

Roth, M., Shaw, J., & Green, J. The form, voltage distribution and physiological significance of the K-complex. *Electroencephalography and Clinical Neurophysiology,* 1956, *8,* 385-402.

Routtenberg, A. Neural mechanisms of sleep: Changing views of reticular formation function. *Psychological Review,* 1966, *73,* 481-499.

Routtenberg, A. The two arousal hypothesis: Reticular formation and limbic system. *Psychological Reviews,* 1968, 75, 51-80.

Rubin, F. *Current research in hypnopaedia.* New York: American Elsevier, 1968.

Rubinstein, B. B. Explanation and mere description: A meta scientific examination of certain aspects of the psychoanalytic theory of motivation. In *Psychoanalytic essays in honor of David Rapaport. Psychological Issues,* 1967, *5* (Nos. 2 & 3), Monograph 18-19, 18-77. New York International Universities Press.

Rubinstein, B. B. On the logic of explanation in psychoanalysis, In B. B. Rubinstein (Ed.), *Psychoanalysis and contemporary science,* Vol. 2. New York: Macmillan Company, 1973.

Rubinstein, B. B. On the role of classificatory processes in mental functioning: Aspects of a psychoanalytic theoretical model. In L. Goldberger & V. H. Rosen (Eds.), *Psychoanalysis and contemporary science,* Vol. 3. New York: International Universities Press, 1974.

Rumelhart, D. E., Lindsay, P. H., & Norman, D. A. *A process model of long-term memory.* New York: Academic Press, 1972.

Safer, D. J. The effect of LSD on sleep-deprived men. *Psychopharmacologia,* 1970, *17,* 414-424.

Sagales, T., & Domino, E. Effects of stress and REM sleep deprivation on the patterns of avoidance learning and brain acetylcholine in the mouse. *Psychopharamcologia,* 1973, *29,* 307-315.

Salzinger, K. An hypothesis about schizophrenic behavior. *American Journal of Psychotherapy,* 1971, *25,* 601-614.

Sampson, H. Deprivation of dreaming sleep by two methods: I. Compensatory REM time. *Archives of General Psychiatry,* 1965, *13,* 79-86

Sampson, H. Psychological effects of deprivation of dreaming sleep. *Journal of Nervous and Mental Disease,* 1966, *143,* 305-317.

Satinoff, E., Drucker-Colin, R. R., & Hernandez, P. R. Paleocortical excitability and sensory filtering during REM sleep deprivation. *Physiology and Behavior,* 1971, *7,* 103-106.

Saul, L. J., Sheppard, E., Stelby, D., Lhamon, W., Sachs, D., & Master, R. The quantification of hostility in dreams with reference to essential hypertension. *Science,* 1954, *119,* 382-383.

Schachtel, E. G. *Metamorphosis: On the development of affect, perception, attention, and memory.* New York: Basic Books, 1959.

Schacter, D. L. The hypnogogic state: A critical review of its literature. *Psychological Bulletin,* 1976, *83,* 452-481.

Schimek, J. G. A critical re-examination of Freud's concept of unconscious mental representation. *International Review of Psychoanalysis,* 1975, *2,* 171-188.

Schjelderup, H. K. Time relations in dreams. *Scandinavian Journal of Psychology,* 1960, *1,* 62-64.

Schonbar, R. A. Some manifest characteristics of recallers and nonrecallers of dreams. *Journal of Consulting Psychology,* 1959, *23,* 414-418.

Schonbar, R. A. Differential dream recall frequency as a component of "life style." *Journal of Consulting Psychology,* 1965, *29,* 468-474.

Scott, J. Performance after abrupt arousal from sleep: Comparison of a simple motor, a visual-perceptual, and a cognitive task. *Proceedings of the 77th Annual Convention of the American Psychological Association,* 1969, 225-226. (Summary)

Seligman, M. E. P., On the generality of the laws of learning. *Psychological Review,* 1970, *77,* 406-418.

Selling, L. S. A clinical study of a new tranquilizing drug. *Journal of the American Medical Association,* 1955, *157,* 1594-1596.

Serafetinides, A. A. Speech findings in epilepsy and electrocortical stimulation: An overview. *Cortex,* 1966, *2,* 463-473.

Shapiro, A. Dreaming and the physiology of sleep. *Experimental Neurology,* 1967, *19,* 56-81.

Shapiro, A. Comments on the 90-minute sleep-dream cycle. In E. Hartmann (Ed.), *Sleep and dreaming.* Boston: Little, Brown & Company, 1970.

Shapiro, A., Goodenough, D. R., Biederman, I., & Sleser, I. Dream recall and the physiology of sleep. *Journal of Applied Physiology,* 1964, *19,* 778-783.

Shapiro, A., Goodenough, D. R., & Gryler, R. B. Dream recall as a function of method of awakening. *Psychosomatic Medicine,* 1963, *25,* 174-180.

Shapiro, A., Goodenough, D. R., Lewis, H. B., & Sleser, I. Gradual arousal from sleep: A determinant of thinking reports. *Psychosomatic Medicine,* 1965, *27,* 342-349.

Sharpe, E. F. *Dream analysis. A practical handbook for psychoanalysis.* London: Hogarth Press Ltd., 1949.

Sharpless, S. K. Hypnotics and sedatives. In L. S. Goodman, & A. Gilman (Eds.), *The pharmacological basis of therapeutics* (4th ed.). London: Macmillan, 1970.

Sheffield, R. D., Roby, T. B., & Campbell, B. A. Drive reduction versus consummatory behavior as determinants of reinfocement. *Journal of Comparative and Physiological Psychology,* 1954, *47,* 349-354.

Sherwood, M. *The logic of explanation in psychoanalysis.* New York: Academic Press, 1969.

Sherwood, M. Another look at the logic of explanation in psychoanalysis. In B. B. Rubinstein (Ed.), *Psychoanalysis and contemporary science,* Vol. 2. New York: Macmillan Publishing Company, 1973.

Shevrin, H., & Fisher, C. Changes in the effects of a waking subliminal stimulus as a function of dreaming and non-dreaming sleep. *Journal of Abnormal Psychology,* 1967, *72,* 362-368.

Shope, R. K. Freud's concept of meaning. In B. B. Rubinstein (Ed.), *Psychoanalysis and contemporary science,* Vol. 2. New York: Macmillan Publishing Company, 1973.

Siegel, J., & Gordon, T. P. Paradoxical sleep: Deprivation in the cat. *Science,* 1965, *148,* 978-980.

Simon, C. W., & Emmons, W. H. Responses to material presented during various levels of sleep. *Journal of Experimental Psychology,* 1956, *51,* 89-97.

Singer, J. L. *Daydreaming: An introduction to the experimental study of inner experience.* New York: Random House, 1966.

Singer, J. L. Research applications of the projective methods. In A. Rabin (Ed.), *Projective techniques in personality assessment.* New York: Springer, 1968.

Singer, J. L. Imagery and daydream techniques in psychotherapy. In C. D. Spielberger (Ed.), *Current topics in clinical and community psychology,* Vol. 3. New York: Academic Press, 1971.

Singer, J. L. Daydreaming and the stream of thoughts. *American Scientist,* 1974, *62,* 417-425. (a)

Singer, J. L. *Imagery and daydream methods in psychotherapy and behavior modification.* New York: Academic Press, 1974. (b)

Singer, J. L. *The inner world of daydreaming.* New York: Harper & Row, 1975.

Singer, J. L. Review of Foulkes, D., & Fleisher, S. Mental activity in relaxed wakefulness. *Sleep Bulletin.* Los Angeles: Brain Information Service of the University of California at Los Angeles, 1976.

Singer, J. L., & Antrobus, J. S. A factor analysis of daydreaming and conceptually-related cognitive and personality variables. *Perceptual and Motor Skills,* 1963, *17* (Monograph Supplement), 187-209.

Singer, J. L., & Antrobus, J. S. Eye movements during fantasies. *Archives of General Psychiatry,* 1965, *12,* 71-76.

Singer, J. L., & Antrobus, J. S. Daydreaming, imaginal processes, and personality: A normative study. In P. Sheehan (Ed.), *The function and nature of imagery.* New York: Academic Press, 1972.

Singer, J. L., Greenberg, S., & Antrobus, J. S. Looking with the mind's eye: Experimental studies of ocular motility during daydreaming and mental arithmetic. *Transactions of the New York Academy of Sciences,* 1971, *33,* 694-709.

Singer, J. L., & Schonbar, R. A. Correlates of daydreaming: A dimension of self-awareness. *Journal of Consulting Psychology,* 1961, *25,* 1-6.

Sitaram, N., Wyatt, R. J., Dawson, S., & Gillin, J. C. REM sleep induction by physostigmine infusion during sleep. *Science,* 1976, *191,* 1281-1283.

Skinner, B. F. *Verbal behavior.* New York: Appleton-Century-Crofts, 1957.

Skinner, B. F. The operational analysis of psychological terms. In H. Feigl & M. Brodbeck (Eds.), *Readings in the philosophy of science.* N. Y.: Appleton-Century-Crofts, 1953.

Skinner, J. C. The dream in psychoanalytic practice. In E. Hartmann (Ed.), *Sleep and dreaming.* Boston: Little, Brown and Company, 1970.

Sloan, M. The effects of deprivation of rapid eye movement (REM) sleep on maze learning and aggression in the albino rat. *Journal of Psychiatric Research,* 1972, *9,* 101-111.

Snyder, F. Dream recall, respiratory variability and depth of sleep. Paper presented at the Round Table on Dream Research, Annual Meeting of the American Psychiatric Association, Atlantic City, New Jersey, May, 1960.

Snyder, F. The new biology of dreaming. *Archives of General Psychiatry,* 1963, *8,* 381-391

Snyder, F. Sleep and dreaming: Progress in the new biology of dreaming. *American Journal of Psychiatry,* 1965, *122,* 377-391.

Snyder, F. Toward an evolutionary theory of dreaming. *American Journal of Psychiatry,* 1966, *123,* 121-142.

Snyder, F. In quest of dreaming. In H. A. Witkin & H. B. Lewis (Eds.), *Experimental studies of dreaming.* New York: Random House, 1967.

Snyder, F. Sleep and REM as a biological enigma. In A. Kales (Ed.), *Sleep: Physiology and pathology, a symposium.* London: Lippincott, 1969.

Snyder, F. The phenomenology of dreaming. In H. Madow & L. H. Snow (Eds.), *The psychodynamic implications of the physiological studies on dreams.* Springfield, Illinois: Charles C. Thomas, 1970.

Snyder, F., Hobson, J., & Goldfrank, F. Blood pressure changes during human sleep. *Science,* 1963, *142,* 1313-1314.

Snyder, F., Hobson, J., Morrison, D., & Goldfrank, F. Changes in respiration, heart rate, and systolic blood pressure in human sleep. *Journal of Applied Physiology*, 1964, *19*, 417-422.

Snyder, F., Karacan, I., Thorp, U. R., & Scott, J. Phenomenology of REM dreaming. *Psychophysiology*, 1968, *4*, 375. (Abstract)

Spence, D. P., & Holland, B. The restricting effects of awareness: A paradox and an explanation. *Journal of Abnormal and Social Psychology*, 1962, *64*, 163-174.

Sperry, R. W. A modified concept of consciousness. *Psychological Review*, 1969, *76*, 532-536.

Sperry, R. W. An objective approach to subjective experience: Further explanation of a hypothesis. *Psychological Review*, 1970, *77*, 585-590.

Spevack, A. A., & Suboski, M. D. Retrograde effects of electroconvulsive shock on learned responses. *Psychological Bulletin*, 1969, *72*, 66-76.

Stanfield, C. Clinical experience with chlordiazepoxide (Librium). *Psychosomatics*, 1961, *2*, 179-183.

Starker, S. Aspects of inner experience: Autokinesis, daydreaming, dream recall and cognitive style. *Perceptual and Motor Skills*, 1973, *36*, 663-673.

Starker, S. Daydreaming styles and nocturnal dreaming. *Journal of Abnormal Psychology*, 1974, *83*, 52-55.

Stegie, R. Zur Beziehung Zwischen Traumenhalt und während des Traümens ablaufenden Herz und atmungstätigkeit. Unpublished doctoral dissertation, University of Dusseldorf, 1973.

Steiner, S. S., Bodnar, R. J., Ackerman, R. F., & Ellman, S. J. Escape from rewarding brain stimulation of dorsal brain stem and hypothalamus. *Physiology and Behavior*, 1973, *11*, 589-591.

Steiner, S. S., & Ellman, S. J. Relation between REM sleep and intracranial self-stimulation. *Science*, 1972, *177*, 1122-1124. (a)

Steiner, S. S., & Ellman, S. J. Unpublished data, 1972. (b)

Stekel, W. *The interpretation of dreams – new developments and techniques.* Translated by E. Paul & C. Paul. New York: Liveright, 1943.

Stern, W. C. Stress effects of REM sleep deprivation in rats: Adrenal gland hypertrophy. Paper presented at the meeting of the Association for the Psychophysiological Study of Sleep, Boston, 1969.

Stern, W. Acquisition impairments following rapid eye movement sleep deprivation on rats. *Physiology and Behavior*, 1971, *7*, 345-352. (a)

Stern, W. Effects of desynchronized sleep deprivation upon startle response habituation in the rat. *Psychonomic Science*, 1971, *23*, 31-32. (b)

Stokes, J. P. The effects of rapid eye movement sleep on retention. *The Psychological Record*, 1973, *23*, 521-532.

Storms, M. D., & Nisbett, R. F. Insomnia and the attribution process. *Journal of Personality and Social Psychology*, 1970, *16*, 319-328.

Stoyva, J. The effects of suggested dreams on the length of rapid eye movement periods. Unpublished doctoral dissertation, University of Chicago, 1961.

Stoyva, J. M. Finger electromyographic activity during sleep: Its relation to dreaming in deaf and normal subjects. *Journal of Abnormal Psychology*, 1965, *70*, 343-349. (a)

Stoyva, J. Posthypnotically suggested dreams and the sleep cycle. *Archives of General Psychiatry*, 1965, *12*, 287-294. (b)

Stoyva, J., & Kamiya, J. Electrophysiological studies of dreaming as the prototype of a new strategy in the study of consciousness. *Psychological Review*, 1968, *75*, 192-205.

Strauch, I. Psychological aspects of dream recall. Paper presented at a symposium on sleep and dreaming, 19th International Congress of Psychology, London, July/August, 1969.

Swanson, E. M., & Foulkes, D. Dream content and the menstrual cycle. *Journal of Nervous and Mental Disease*, 1968, *145*, 358-363.

Szabo, L., & Waitsuk, P. Contributions to the problem of nocturnal verbal automatisms. *Electroencephalography and Clinical Neurophysiology*, 1971, *31*, 522. (Summary)

Takeo, S. Relationship among physiological indices during sleep and characteristics of dreams. *Psychiatria et Neurologia Japonica*, 1970, *72*, 1-18.

Tani, K., Yoshii, N., Yoshino, I., & Kobayashi, E. Electroencephalographic study of parasomnia: Sleep-talking enuresis, and bruxism. *Physiology and Behavior*, 1966, *1*, 241-243.

Tart, C. T. Frequency of dream recall and some personality measures. *Journal of Consulting Psychology*, 1962, *26*, 467-470.

Tart, C. T. A comparison of suggested dreams occurring in hypnosis and sleep. *International Journal of Clinical and Experimental Hypnosis*, 1964, *12*, 263-289.

Tart, C. T. Toward the experimental control of dreaming: A review of the literature. *Psychological Bulletin*, 1965, *64*, 81-91.

Tart, C. Personal communication, 1974.

Tart, C., & Dick, L. Conscious control of dreaming: I. The posthypnotic dream. *Journal of Abnormal Psychology*, 1970, *76*, 304-315.

Tatsuoka, M. M. *Multivariate analysis*. New York: Wiley, 1971.

Tauber, E., Roffwarg, H., & Herman, J. The effects of long-standing perceptual alterations on the hallucinatory content of dreams. *Psychophysiology*, *5:*219, 1968. (Abstract)

Tebbs, R. B. Post-awakening visualization performances as a function of anxiety level, REM or NREM sleep, and time of night. NSAF Academy, Colorado. SRL-TR-72-0005. AD-738 630, 1972.

Terman, L. M. *Psychological factors in marital happiness*. New York: McGraw-Hill, 1938.

Thomas, J., & Benoit, O. Individualization of slow wave sleep and phasic activity. *Brain Research*, 1967, *5*, 221-235.

Timm, N. H. *Multivariate analysis*. Monterey, California: Brooks/Cole, 1975.

Tizard, B. Habituation of EEG and skin potential changes in normal and severely subnormal children. *American Journal of Mental Deficiency*, 1968, *73*, 34-40.

Toll, N. Librium as an adjunct to psychotherapy in private practice. *Diseases of the Nervous System*, 1960, *21*, 264-266.

Tomkins, S. *Affect, imagery, consciousness*, Vols. I and II. New York: Springer, 1962.

Torda, C. Dreams of subjects with loss of memory for recent events. *Psychophysiology*, 1969, *6*, 358-365.

Townsend, V. E., Johnson, L. C., Naitoh, P., & Muzet, A. F. Heart rate preceding motility in sleep. *Psychophysiology*, 1975, *12*, 217-219.

Tracy, R. L., & Tracy, L. N. Reports of mental activity from sleep stages 2 and 4. *Perceptual and Motor Skills*, 1974, *38*, 647-648.

Trinder, J., & Kramer, M. Dream recall. *American Journal of Psychiatry*, 1971, *128*, 296-301.

Trosman, H. Dream research and the psychoanalytic theory of dreams. *Archives of General Psychiatry*, 1963, *9*, 9-18.

Trosman, H., Rechtschaffen, A., Offenkrantz, W., & Wolpert, E. Studies in the psychophysiology of dreams. IV. Relations among dreams in sequence. *Archives of General Psychiatry*, 1960, *3*, 602-607.

Tyrer, P. J., & Lader, M. Effects of beta adrenergic blockade with sotalol in chronic anxiety. *Clinical Pharmacology and Therapeutics*, 1973, *14*, 418-426.

Ullman, M. Dreaming, life-style and physiology. A comment on Adler's view of the dream. *Journal of Individual Psychology*, 1962, *18*, 18-25.

Ullman, M., & Krippner, S. *Dream studies and telepathy: Experiments in nocturnal ESP*. New York: Penguin Books, 1974.

Umbarger, C. Problems in the psychology of dreaming: A review of the work of Richard Jones. In L. Goldberger & V. H. Rosen (Eds.), *Psychoanalysis and contemporary science,* Vol. 3. New York: International Universities Press, 1974.

Van de Castle, R. L. Some problems in applying the methodology of content analysis to dreams. Paper presented at the Symposium on Dream Psychology and the New Biology of Dreaming, Cincinnati, 1967.

Van de Castle, R. L. *The psychology of dreaming.* New York: General Learning Corporation, 1971.

Van de Castle, R. L., & Holloway, J. Dreams of depressed patients, non-depressed patients, and normals. *Psychophysiology,* 1970, *7,* 326. (Abstract)

Van Ormer, E. B. Retention after intervals of sleep and waking. *Archives of Psychology,* 1932, No. 137, 49.

Van Ormer, E. B. Sleep and retention. *Psychological Bulletin,* 1933, *30,* 413-439.

Verdone, P. Variables related to the temporal reference of manifest dream content. Unpublished doctoral dissertation, University of Chicago, 1963.

Verdone, P. Temporal reference of manifest dream content. *Perceptual and Motor Skills,* 1965, *20,* 1253-1268.

Verdone, P. Sleep satiation: Extended sleep in normal subjects. *Electroencephalography and Clinical Neurophysiology,* 1968, *24,* 417-423.

Vimont-Vicary, P., Jouvet, D., & Delorme, F. Effets EEG et comportementaux des privations du sommeil paradoxal chez le chat. *Electroencephalography and Clinical Neurophysiology,* 1966, *20,* 439-449.

Viscott, D. S. Chlordiazepoxide and hallucinations. *Archives of General Psychiatry,* 1968, *19,* 370-376.

Vogel, G. W. REM deprivation: III. Dreaming and psychosis. *Archives of General Psychiatry,* 1968, *18,* 312-329.

Vogel, G. Review of Wyatt, R., Termini, B. A., & Davis, J. Biochemical and sleep studies of schizophrenia: A review of the literature, 1960-1970. Part II. Sleep studies. *Sleep Research,* 1973, *2,* 378-379.

Vogel, G. W. Review of REM sleep deprivation. Paper presented at the meeting of the Association for the Psychophysiological Study of Sleep, Jackson Hole, Wyoming, 1974.

Vogel, G. W. Review of REM sleep deprivation. *Archives of General Psychiatry,* 1975, *32,* 749-761.

Vogel, G., Barrowclough, B., & Giesler, D. Limited discriminability of REM and sleep onset reports and its psychiatric implications. *Archives of General Psychiatry,* 1972, *26,* 449-455.

Vogel, G., Foulkes, D., & Trosman, H. Ego functions and dreaming during sleep onset. *Archives of General Psychiatry,* 1966, *14,* 238-248.

Vogel, G. W., Giesler, D. D., & Barrowclough, B. Exercise as a substitute for REM sleep. Paper presented at the meeting of the Association for the Psychophysiological Study of Sleep, Santa Fe, New Mexico, 1970. *Psychophysiology,* 1970, *7,* 300-301. (Abstract)

Vogel, G. W., Thurmond, A., Gibbons, P., Sloan, K., Boyd, M., & Walker, M. REM sleep reduction effects on depression syndromes. *Archives of General Psychiatry,* 1975, *32,* 765-777.

Vogel, G. W., & Traub, A. C. Further studies on REM deprivation of depressed patients. *Psychophysiology,* 1968, *5,* 239. (Abstract) (a)

Vogel, G. W., & Traub, A. C. REM deprivation of depressives. *Psychophysiology,* 1968, *4,* 382. (Abstract) (b)

Vogel, G. W., & Traub, A. C. REM deprivation: I. The effect on schizophrenic patients. *Archives of General Psychiatry,* 1968, *18,* 287-300. (c)

Vogel, G. W., Traub, A. C., Ben-Horin, P., & Meyers, G. REM deprivation: II. The effect on depressed patients. *Archives of General Psychiatry,* 1968, *18,* 301-311.

Volkan, V. Sleep (a bibliographical study). *British Journal of Medical Psychology*, 1962, *35*, 235-244.

Waelder, R. The principle of multiple function. *Psychoanalytic Quarterly*, 1936, *5*, 45-62.

Waldhorn, H. F. The place of the dream in psychoanalysis. In E. D. Joseph (Ed.), *Monograph Series of the Kris Study Group of the New York Psychoanalytic Institute*. Monograph 2. New York: International Universities Press, 1967.

Whitman, R., Pierce, C., Maas, J., & Baldridge, B. The dreams of the experimental subject. *Journal of Nervous and Mental Disease*, 1962, *134*, 431-439.

Williams, H. L. Information processing during sleep. In W. P. Koella & P. Levin (Eds.), *Sleep: Physiology, biochemistry, psychology, pharmacology, clinical implications*. First European Congress on Sleep Research, Basel, 1972. Basel: Karger, 1973.

Walker, P. C., & Johnson, R. F. Q. The influence of pre-sleep suggestions on dream content: Evidence and methodological problems. *Psychological Bulletin*, 1974, *81*, 362-370.

Walker, E. L., & Tarte, R. D. Memory storage as a function of arousal and time with homogeneous and heterogeneous lists. *Journal of Verbal Learning and Verbal Behavior*, 1963, *2*, 113-119.

Wallach, M. A., & Kogan, N. *Modes of thinking in young children*. New York: Holt, Rinehart & Winston, 1965.

Watson, J. B. *Behaviorism*. New York: People's Institute, 1924.

Watson, R. K. Mental correlates of periorbital potentials during REM sleep. Unpublished doctoral dissertation, University of Chicago, 1972.

Waugh, N. C., & Norman, D. A. Primary memory. *Psychological Review*, 1965, *72*, 89-104.

Webb, W. B. Partial and differential sleep deprivation. In A. Kales (Ed.), *Sleep: Physiology and pathology*. Philadelphia: Lippincott, 1969.

Webb, W., & Agnew, H. Sleep: Effects of a restricted regime. *Science*, 1965, *150*, 1745-1747.

Webb, W. B., & Friel, J. Sleep stage and personality characteristics of "natural" long and short sleepers. *Science*, 1971, *171*, 587-588.

Webb, W. B., & Kersey, J. Recall of dreams and the probability of stage 1 – REM sleep. *Perceptual and Motor Skills*, 1967, *24*, 627-630.

Weiss, L. Experimenter bias as a function of stimulus ambiguity. Unpublished manuscript, State University of New York at Buffalo, 1967.

Weisz, R. Phenomenological correlates of discrete events in NREM sleep: The K-complex as a NREM phasic indicator. *Psychophysiology*, 1972, *9*, 127. (Abstract)

Weisz, R. Review of Kramer, M., & Roth, T., A comparison of dream content in laboratory dream reports of schizophrenic and depressive patient groups. *Sleep Research*, 1975, *4*, 371.

Weisz, R., & Foulkes, D. Home and laboratory dreams collected under uniform sampling conditions. *Psychophysiology*, 1970, *6*, 588-597.

Wessler, R. Experimenter expectancy effects in psychomotor performance. *Perceptual and Motor Skills*, 1968, *26*, 911-917.

West, L. T., Janszen, H. H., Lester, B. K., & Cornelisoon, F. S., Jr. The psychosis of sleep deprivation. *Annals of the New York Academy of Sciences*, 1962, *96*, 66-70.

Whitman, R. M. Remembering and forgetting dreams in psychoanalysis. *Journal of the American Psychoanalytic Association*, 1963, *7*, 752-774.

Whitman, R. A decade of dreams: A review. *International Journal of Psychoanalytic Psychotherapy*, 1974, *3*, 217-245.

Whitman, R., Kramer, M., & Baldridge, B. J. Which dream does the patient tell? *Archives of General Psychiatry*, 1963, *8*, 277-282.

Whitman, R., Kramer, M., Ornstein, P., & Baldridge, B. The varying use of the dream in clinical psychiatry. In L. Madow & L. Snow (Eds.), *The psychodynamic implications of physiological studies on dreams*. Springfield, Ill.: Charles Thomas, 1970.

Whitman, R. M., Pierce, C. M., & Maas, J. W. Drugs and dreams. In L. Uhr & J. G. Miller (Eds.), *Drugs and behavior*, New York: John Wiley & Sons, 1960.

Whitman, R. M., Pierce, C. M., Maas, J. W., & Baldridge, B. Drugs and dreams II: Imipramine and prochlorperazine. *Comprehensive Psychiatry*, 1961, *2*, 219-226.

Williams, H. L., Hammack, J. T., Daly, R. L., Dement, W. C., & Lubin, A. Responses to auditory stimulation, sleep loss and the EEG stages of sleep. *Electroencephalography and Clinical Neurophysiology*, 1964, *16*, 269-279.

Williams, H. L., Morlock, H. C., Jr., & Morlock, J. V. Instrumental behavior during sleep. *Psychophysiology*, 1966, *2*, 208-216.

Williams, R. L., Karacan, I., & Hursch, C. J. *Electroencephalography (EEG) of human sleep: Clinical applications*. New York: John Wiley & Sons, 1974.

Wilson, W. P., & Zung, W. W. K. Attention, discrimination, and arousal during sleep. *Archives of General Psychiatry*, 1966, *15*, 523-528.

Winer, B. S. *Statistical principles in experimental design*. New York: McGraw-Hill, 1971.

Winget, C., & Kapp, F. T. The relationship of the manifest content of dreams to duration of childbirth in primiparae. *Psychosomatic Medicine*, 1972, *34*, 313-320.

Winget, C., & Kramer, M. *Dimensions of dreams*. Gainesville: University of Florida Press, 1974.

Winget, C., Kramer, M., & Whitman, R. M. Dreams and demography. *Canadian Psychiatric Association Journal*, 1972, *17* (Special Supplement 2), 203-208.

Winick, C. & Holt, H. Differential recall of the dream and function of audience perception. *Psychoanalysis*, 1962, *49*, 53-62.

Witkin, H. A. Influencing dream content. In M. Kramer, R. M. Whitman, B. J. Baldridge, & P. H. Ornstein (Eds.), *Dream psychology and the new biology of dreaming*. Springfield, Illinois: C. C. Thomas, 1969. (a)

Witkin, H. A. Presleep experiences and dreams. In J. Fisher and L. Berger (Eds.), *The meaning of dreams: Recent insights from the laboratory*. California Mental Health Research, 1969, *3*, 1-37. (b)

Witkin, H. A. Individual differences in dreaming. In E. Hartmann (Ed.), *Sleep and dreaming*. Boston: Little & Brown, 1970.

Witkin, H. A., Dyk, R. B., Faterson, H. F., Goodenough, D. R., & Karp, S. A. *Psychological differentiation*. New York: Wiley, 1962.

Witkin, H. A., & Lewis, H. B. Presleep experiences and dreams. In H. A. Witkin & H. B. Lewis (Eds.), *Experimental studies of dreaming*. New York: Random House, 1967.

Witkin, H. A., & Lewis, H. The relation of experimentally induced presleep experiences to dreams: A report on method and preliminary findings. *Journal of the American Psychoanalytic Association*, 1965, *13*, 819-849.

Witkin, H. A., Lewis, H. B., Hertzman, M., Machover, K., Meisser, P. B., & Wapner, S. *Personality through perception*. New York: Harper & Row, 1954.

Wolin, S. J., & Mello, N. K. The effects of alcohol on dreams and hallucinations in alcohol addicts. *Annals of the New York Academy of Science*, 1973, *215*, 266-302.

Wolpert, E. Studies in psychophysiology of dreams. II. An electromyographic study of dreaming. *Archives of General Psychiatry*, 1960, *2*, 231-241.

Wolpert, E. A. Two classes of factors affecting dream recall. *Journal of the American Psychoanalytic Association*, 1972, *20*, 45-58.

Wolpert, E. A., & Trosman, H. Studies in psychophysiology of dreams. I: Experimental evocation of sequential dream episodes. *American Association Archives of Neurology and Psychiatry*, 1958, *79*, 603-606.

Wood, P. Dreaming and social isolation. Unpublished doctoral dissertation. University of North Carolina, 1962. University Microfilms # 63-3571.

Wyatt, R. J., Fram, D. H., Kupfer, D. J., & Snyder, F. Total prolonged drug-induced REM sleep suppression in anxious depressed patients. *Archives of General Psychiatry*, 1971, *24*, 145-155.

Wyatt, R. J., Gillin, J. C., Green, R., Horowitz, D., & Snyder, F. Measurement of phasic integrated potentials (PIP) during treatment with parachlorophenylalanine (PCPA). *Psychophysiology*, 1972, *9*, 127. (Abstract)

Wyatt, R., Termini, B. A., & Davis, J. Biochemical and sleep studies of schizophrenia: A review of the literature 1960-1970. Part II. Sleep studies. *Schizophrenia Bulletin*, 1971, *4*, 45-66.

Yaroush, R., Sullivan, M. J., & Ekstrand, B. R. Effect of sleep on memory. II: Differential effect of the first and second half of the night. *Journal of Experimental Psychology*, 1971, *88*, 361-366.

Zarcone, V., Azumi, D., de la Peña, A., Cartwright, R., & Dement, W. Individual differences in response to REM deprivation. *Psychophysiology*, 1969, *6*, 239. (Abstract)

Zarcone, V., Azumi, K., Dement, W., Gulevich, G., Kraemer, H., & Pivik, T. REM phase deprivation and schizophrenia II. *Archives of General Psychiatry*, 1975, *32*, 1431-1436.

Zarcone, V., de la Peña, A., Kopell, B., & Dement, W. Visual evoked responses following REM deprivation. Paper presented at the meeting of the Association for the Psychophysiological Study of Sleep, Santa Fe, New Mexico, 1970. *Psychophysiology*, 1970, *7*, 301. (Abstract)

Zarcone, V., Gulevich, G., Pivik, T., Azumi, K., & Dement, W. REM deprivation and schizophrenia. *Biological Psychiatry*, 1969, *1*, 179-184.

Zarcone, V., Gulevich, G., Pivik, T., & Dement, W. Partial REM phase deprivation and schizophrenia. *Archives of General Psychiatry*, 1968, *18*, 194-202.

Zarcone, V., Zukowsky, E., Gulevich, G., Dement, W., & Hodes, E. Rorschach responses subsequent to REM deprivation in schizophrenic and non-schizophrenic patients. *Journal of Clinical Psychology*, 1974, *30*, 248-250.

Zepelin, H. An investigation of age differences in men's dreams. *Sleep Research*, 1972 *1*, 128.

Zetzel, E. R. Is the domain of the psychological still floating? In E. Hartmann (Ed.), *Sleep and Dreaming*. Boston: Little, Brown & Company, 1970.

Zimmerman, W. B. Psychological and physiological differences between "light" and "deep" sleepers. Unpublished doctoral dissertation, University of Chicago, 1967.

Zimmerman, W. B. Sleep mentation and auditory awakening thresholds. *Psychophysiology*, 1970, *6*, 540-549.

Zimmerman, W. B. Psychological and physiological differences between "light" and "deep" sleepers. *Psychophysiology*, 1968, *4*, 387. (Abstract)

Author Index

Numbers in *italics* refer to pages on which the complete references are listed.

Subject Index